The Family Practice

Practice

DESK REFERENCE

THIRD EDITION

The Family Practice

DESK REFERENCE

Charles E. Driscoll, M.D.
Mercy Hospital, Iowa City, Iowa

Edward T. Bope, M.D.
Director, Family Practice Residency Program
Riverside Methodist Hospital, Columbus, Ohio

Charles W. Smith, Jr., M.D.
Executive Associate Dean for Clinical Affairs
Professor of Family and Community Medicine
Medical Director, The University Hospital of Arkansas
University of Arkansas for Medical Sciences
Little Rock, Arkansas

Barry L. Carter, Pharm. D., F.C.C.P.
Professor and Chairman, Department of Pharmacy Practice
School of Pharmacy, University of Colorado, Denver, Colorado

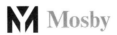 Mosby

St. Louis Baltimore Boston Carlsbad Chicago Naples New York Philadelphia Portland
London Madrid Mexico City Singapore Sydney Tokyo Toronto Wiesbaden

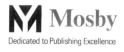 Mosby

Dedicated to Publishing Excellence

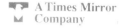 A Times Mirror
Company

Editor: Stephanie Manning
Developmental Editor: Carolyn Malik
Project Manager: Linda McKinley
Production Editor: Cathy Bricker
Designer: Elizabeth Fett
*Cover Photograph: Copyright © The Image Bank
by John R. Ramey*

NOTICE
The authors and publishers have made every effort to ensure that the patient care recommended herein, including choice of drugs and drug dosages, is in accord with the accepted standards and practice at the time of publication. However, since research and regulations constantly change clinical standards, the reader is urged to check the product information sheet included in the package of each drug, which includes recommended dosages, warnings, and contraindications. This is particularly important with new or infrequently used drugs.

THIRD EDITION
Copyright © 1996 by Mosby–Year Book, Inc.

Previous editions copyrighted 1986, 1991

Printed in the United States of America
Composition by Clarinda Company
Printing/binding by R.R. Donnelley & Sons Company

Mosby–Year Book, Inc.
11830 Westline Industrial Drive
St. Louis, Missouri 63146

Library of Congress Cataloging in Publication Data
The family practice desk reference / [edited by] Charles E. Driscoll
  . . . [et al.]. — 3rd ed.
      p.   cm.
   Includes bibliographical references and index.
   ISBN 0-8151-2201-2
   1. Family medicine—Handbooks, manuals, etc.   I. Driscoll,
Charles E.
   [DNLM: 1. Family Practice—handbooks.   WB 39 F198 1995]
RC55.H26   1995
610—dc20
DNLM/DLC
for Library of Congress   95-19477
                                                              CIP

96   97   98   99   00   /   9   8   7   6   5   4   3   2   1

Preface

Like us, you probably remember carrying a small pocket notebook when you were a medical student. We called it the "peripheral brain." All the "pearls" and a few "pellets" of learning were jotted down and kept handy for ready reference. Sometimes, all that was needed to look good on rounds was a nugget of information extracted from that little book at just the right moment. Our fond memories of those medical school notebooks spawned the first edition of this reference 12 years ago, and it is now presented here in this revised third edition. To those of you who would still like to fit it into your pocket, we apologize; with the breadth of family practice, it never will. As a matter of fact, with new developments in medicine reported weekly, we were never quite sure when the book was finished. At least we did not need to issue a set of wheels so you could pull it around with you!

As you browse through the book, notice that we have updated the material that is subject to changing recommendations—for example, STD treatment protocols—while keeping intact much of the standard reference material that was developed in the prior editions. New to this edition are an expanded section on the primary care of HIV-infected patients and the new ACHPR guidelines, for example, treatment of middle ear effusion and prostatic hypertrophy. There are also many new subjects included such as sleep disorders, helping patients to comply with treatment and strategies for smoking cessation. Also new to this edition is the infusion of the drug therapy chapter into every chapter for ease of use.

In the middle of a busy office day, one really never has the time to go to the books for any but the most perplexing of cases. Later, perhaps while reading a book or article, you will find a fact or memory jogger that you wish you would have had to provide better care to your patients. These are the things we have tried to collect and put into one quick reference for your office desk. A few of our readers have also contributed their ideas about what should be in the book, and we thank you all. Undoubtedly we have overlooked something that should be included, and we encourage anyone to submit her or his favorite table or often-used reference to consider for inclusion in the next edition. We would like to thank our secretaries, acknowledge the patience of our wives, and offer a special word of praise for our editor at Mosby–Year Book, Ms. Carolyn Malik, without whose gentle pressure we would still be moving deadlines into the future.

Charles E. Driscoll, M.D., Senior Editor
Edward T. Bope, M.D.
Charles W. Smith, Jr., M.D.
Barry L. Carter, Pharm. D., F.C.C.P.

Contents

1 *Family Practice*

Charles E. Driscoll

CONTENT OF FAMILY PRACTICE

Family practice is the medical specialty that provides continuing and comprehensive health care for the individual and family. It is the specialty in breadth that integrates the biological, clinical, and behavioral sciences. The scope of family practice encompasses all ages, both sexes, each organ system, and every disease entity.

Family practice is the continuing and current expression of the historical medical practitioner and is uniquely defined within the family context (*Academy Policy: 1993-94 Compendium of AAFP Positions on Selected Health Issues*, Kansas City, Mo, American Academy of Family Physicians, p. 24).

Family physicians provide care for patients of all ages, both sexes, and in a variety of settings for up to one third of the ambulatory medical visits in the United States.

TABLE 1-1.—AGE-SEX DISTRIBUTION OF PATIENTS AND 20 MOST COMMON REASONS FOR OFFICE VISITS

		Trend in Past 5 Years
Female (3.1 Visits/Year)		
<15 yr	9%	↓0.2%
15-24 yr	6%	↓1.7%
25-44 yr	18.3%	↓0.3%
45-65 yr	12.4%	↓0.5%
>65 yr	14.1%	↑1.6%
	59.8% of total	↓1.1% overall
Male (2.2 Visits/Year)		
<15 yr	9.7%	↑0.2%
15-24 yr	3.1%	↓0.8%
25-44 yr	9.4%	↑0.4%
45-65 yr	8.8%	↑0.1%
>65 yr	9.2%	↑1.2%
	40.2% of total	↑0.9% overall

Continued.

TABLE 1-1.—Age-Sex Distribution of Patients and 20 Most Common Reasons for Office Visits—cont'd

RANK	REASON FOR VISIT	PERCENT DISTRIBUTION OF VISITS
1	General medical examination	4.4
2	Cough	3.6
3	Routine prenatal examination	2.9
4	Symptoms referable to throat	2.7
5	Postoperative visit	2.4
6	Earache or ear infection	2.0
7	Well baby examination	2.0
8	Back symptoms	1.9
9	Skin rash	1.8
10	Stomach pain, cramps, and spasms	1.7
11	Fever	1.5
12	Headache, pain in head	1.5
13	Vision dysfunctions	1.5
14	Knee symptoms	1.4
15	Nasal congestion	1.3
16	Blood pressure test	1.1
17	Head cold, upper respiratory infection (coryza)	1.1
18	Neck symptoms	1.1
19	Depression	1.1
20	Low back symptoms	1.1
	All other reasons	61.8

Modified from Schappert SM: *NCHS Advance Data* 230:7, 1993.

SCREENING AND HEALTH MAINTENANCE

TABLE 1-2.—THE FOUR *A*'S OF SMOKING CESSATION: A GUIDE FOR PHYSICIANS

Ask about Smoking Status at Every Opportunity
- "Do you smoke? How much? How soon after waking do you have your first cigarette? Are you interested in stopping smoking? Have you ever tried to stop smoking? What happened?"

Advise Every Smoker to Stop Smoking
- State your advice clearly, for example, "As your physician, I must advise you to stop smoking now."
- Personalize the message to quit. Refer to your patient's clinical condition, smoking and family history, personal interests, and/or social role.

Assist Your Patient in Stopping Smoking
- Set a quit date. Help your patient choose a date within the following 4 weeks. Acknowledge that no time is ideal.
- Provide self-help materials. The smoking cessation coordinator or support staff member can review the materials with your patient if desired. (Call 1-800-4-CANCER for the National Cancer Institute's *Quit for Good* materials.)
- Consider prescribing nicotine transdermal patches or gum, especially for the highly nicotine-addicted patient (one who smokes a pack a day or more or who smokes his or her first cigarette within 30 minutes of waking).
- Consider signing a stop-smoking contract with your patient.
- If the patient is not willing to quit now, provide motivating literature. (Call 1-800-4-CANCER for the National Cancer Institute's pamphlet entitled *Why Do You Smoke?*). Ask about smoking status again at the next office visit.

Arrange Follow-up Visits
- Schedule a follow-up visit within 1 to 2 weeks after the quit date.
- Have a member of the office staff call or write to your patient within 7 days after the initial visit to reinforce the decision to stop smoking and remind him of the quit date.
- Ask about your patient's smoking status at the first follow-up visit to provide support and help prevent relapse. Relapse is common; if it happens, encourage your patient to try again immediately.
- Schedule a second follow-up visit in 1 to 2 months. For a patient who has relapsed, discuss the circumstances of the relapse and any special concerns.

From Owens GR: How to help your patients stop smoking, *J Respir Dis* 14(5):644, 1993.

TABLE 1-3.—COMPARISON OF RECOMMENDATIONS FOR PHYSICAL EXAMINATION OF ASYMPTOMATIC ADULTS

CLINICAL TEST OR PROCEDURE	OBOLER AND LAFORCE RECOMMENDATIONS*	U.S. PREVENTIVE SERVICES TASK FORCE RECOMMENDATIONS†	FRANK, STANGE, MOORE, AND SMITH RECOMMENDATIONS‡
Vital Signs			
Temperature	No evidence supporting	Not addressed	In presence of infectious disease symptoms
Pulse	No evidence supporting	Not addressed	In hypertensive patients
Respiration	No evidence supporting	Not addressed	Count respirations often enough to recognize tachypnea without counting
Weight	Every 4 years	Routinely	Baseline, then in patients who look overweight or underweight
Blood Pressure	Every 2 years	Every 2 years if diastolic blood pressure <85 mm Hg; every year if diastolic blood pressure >85 mm Hg	Every visit until normotensive status established, then every 1-2 years
Skin	Screen for moles once; no screening for other lesions	Routinely in high-risk persons (sun exposure, personal or family history of skin cancer)	Observe skin at any opportunity; screen carefully when skin is fair and when observed moles are numerous (>6), large (>0.5 cm), or dysplastic
Hearing	Yearly after age 60 with hand-held audiometer	Routinely after age 65; optimal frequency not determined	With hearing change
Eyes			
Vision	Eye chart annually after age 60	May be appropriate for elderly patients	With vision change
Funduscopy	No evidence supporting	Not recommended	To maintain clinical skills
Tonometry	Not addressed	Not recommended	Not recommended

			Comments
Mouth	Recommend annual dental examination	Recommend regular dental examinations	Reinforce need for dental checkups
Thyroid	No evidence supporting	No evidence supporting	Check for nodules or goiter
Lymph Nodes	No evidence supporting	Not addressed	When examining in the area
Lungs	No evidence supporting	Not addressed	Auscultate while checking for moles; reinforce need for smoking cessation
Breasts	Annual examination for women over age 40	Annual examination for women over age 40; teaching self-examination not recommended	With Pap smear; yearly for women after age 40
Heart	At initial visit, then again at age 60	Not addressed	Patients expect examination; easy to perform, reassuring
Abdomen Abdominal aortic aneurysm	Yearly in men over age 60	Not addressed	While checking for moles
Hepatomegaly	No evidence supporting	Not addressed	"Over-the-liver" test (inquire about alcohol use while palpating liver)
Splenomegaly	No evidence supporting	Not addressed	Low yield
Genitourinary Rectal	No evidence supporting	Insufficient evidence for or against	Only with symptoms
Testicular	No evidence supporting	Insufficient evidence for or against examination by physician or patient	Reinforce need for self-examination during office examination

*Oboler SK, LaForce FM: The periodic physical examination in asymptomatic adults, *Ann Intern Med* 110(3):214, 1989.

†U.S. Preventive Services Task Force: *Guide to clinical preventive services: an assessment of the effectiveness of 169 interventions,* Baltimore, 1989, Williams & Wilkins.

‡Modified from Frank SH, Stange KC, Moore P, Smith CK: The focused physical examination: should checkups be tailor-made? *Postgrad Med* 92(2):182, 1992.

Continued.

TABLE 1-3.—COMPARISON OF RECOMMENDATIONS FOR PHYSICAL EXAMINATION OF ASYMPTOMATIC ADULTS—cont'd

CLINICAL TEST OR PROCEDURE	OBOLER AND LAFORCE RECOMMENDATIONS*	U.S. PREVENTIVE SERVICES TASK FORCE RECOMMENDATIONS†	FRANK, STANGE, MOORE, AND SMITH RECOMMENDATIONS‡
Pelvic			
Speculum	For Pap smear and sexually transmitted diseases twice, then every 3 years	For Pap smear every 1-3 years, depending on risk factors	For Pap smear every 1-3 years, depending on risk factors
Bimanual	No evidence supporting	May be prudent when examining for other reasons	With speculum examination; avoid excessive patient pain or discomfort, recognizing limited value as screening tool
Vascular			
Carotid	No evidence supporting	Auscultation may be prudent in high-risk patients	Palpate on neck examination; auscultate in high-risk patients while examining heart
Peripheral	No evidence supporting	Not recommended for asymptomatic patients	When examination reveals other arteriosclerotic disease
Musculoskeletal			
Back	No evidence supporting	Not recommended	In patients at risk of work- or sport-related injury
Neurological			
Mental status	No evidence supporting	Be alert for changes in functional status and performance	Observation is first screen; test for multiple sclerosis if problems observed
Deep tendon reflexes and sensory	No evidence supporting	Not addressed	Patients expect to see tendons jump

*Oboler SK, LaForce FM: The periodic physical examination in asymptomatic adults, Ann Intern Med 110(3):214, 1989.
†U.S. Preventive Services Task Force: Guide to clinical preventive services: an assessment of the effectiveness of 169 interventions, Baltimore, 1989, Williams & Wilkins.
‡Modified from Frank SH, Stange KC, Moore P, Smith CK: The focused physical examination: should checkups be tailor-made? Postgrad Med 92(2):182, 1992.

TABLE 1-4.—Recommended Schedule for Active Immunization of Infants, Children, and Adults

AGE	IMMUNIZATION		APPROXIMATE COST* (WHOLESALE $)	
Birth	HBV #1		16.00	
2 Months	HBV #2		16.00	
	TOPV #1		12.80	
	DTP #1 ⎱	or Tetramune #1+	5.40	27.50+
	HbCV #1 ⎰		15.70	
4 Months	DTP #2 ⎱	or Tetramune #2+	5.40	27.50+
	HbCV #2 ⎰		15.70	
	TOPV #2		12.80	
6 Months	DTP #3 ⎱	or Tetramune #3+	5.40	27.50+
	HbCV #3 ⎰		15.70	
9 Months	HBV #3		12.80	
12-18 Months	VV		unavailable	
15-18 Months	MMR #1		31.00	
	TOPV #3		12.80	
	DTaP #1		16.00	
	HbCV #4		16.00	
5 Years	MMR #2		31.00	
	DTaP #2		16.00	
	TOPV #4		12.80	
Every 10 years after age 5	Td		7.50 (Pediatric) 6.80 (Adult)	
10 Years and older	HBV series if not given before age 10		120.00/Series	
65 Years	23-Valent polysaccharide pneumococcal vaccine		12.00	
>65 Years and preferred for high-risk adults	Annual inactivated influenza vaccine		1.80	

*1994 prices.
HBV, Hepatitis B vaccine; *TOPV,* trivalent oral polio vaccine (suspension of live attenuated poliovirus types 1, 2, and 3); *DTP,* diphtheria-tetanus-pertussis (inactivated *Corynebacterium diphtheriae, Clostridium tetani,* killed strains of *Bordetella pertussis*); *HbCV,* Haemophilus influenza type-B conjugate vaccine, (conjugate of oligosaccharides of the capsular antigen); *MMR,* measles-mumps-rubella (live attenuated measles, mumps, and rubella viruses); *DTaP,* diphtheria-tetanus-acellular pertussis; *Td,* tetanus (full dose)-diphtheria (reduced dose); *VV,* varivax.

TABLE 1-5.—HEALTH EDUCATION TOPICS FOR ALL PATIENTS

1. Eat foods from each of the basic four food groups; decrease red meat intake; decrease animal fat intake; choose low-fat dairy products; choose polyunsaturated and monosaturated fats.
2. Eat more fish and poultry—remove skins, bake or broil; do not fry.
3. Increase soluble fiber content in diet, such as oat bran, dry beans, and peas; eat high-fiber vegetables.
4. Seek calcium and potassium; avoid sodium and phosphate.
5. Drink 3 or more glasses of water daily.
6. Eat one main meal daily (prior to activity, not sedentary period) and two smaller ones; maintain ideal weight, plus or minus 10%.
7. Be physically active: 30 min, 3-5 times/week at 75% max. pulse.*
8. Avoid excess alcohol (3 drinks or less/week).
9. Do not smoke or use smokeless tobacco.
10. Know your blood pressure (keep it <100 + age/90) and cholesterol (keep <200 mg/dl).
11. Maintain immunity with up-to-date boosters.
12. *Always* wear seatbelts.
13. Do not act irresponsibly in sexual activity; use safe-sex practices.
14. Use protective equipment during dangerous activities (e.g., helmets, eye and ear protection, mask).
15. Read labels on hazardous materials (e.g., household cleaners) and follow directions explicitly.

*Max. pulse = 220 − Patient's age (years).

TABLE 1-6.—Techniques to Improve Patient Adherence

TECHNIQUES	RATIONALE
Tell patients what their "numbers" are at each visit	Encourages ownership, which reinforces reality, particularly in asymptomatic conditions. Leads to an active rather than passive approach
Explain things in simple language and assess for understanding	Patients need to understand what is wrong and what to do before they will act
Set realistic goals for diet, exercise, and use of medication	Success at smaller goals (e.g., 5 lb of weight loss) leads to fulfillment and more effort
Provide written material for patient education	Reinforces the main points and underscores patients' need to know more about themselves. Discourages dependence on the physician
Instruct patient to self-monitor (e.g., blood sugar, blood pressure measurements)	Patients become active participants in their own health care
Ask patients to tell in their own words how they have complied with recommendations/goals	Avoids assumptions about how patients take their medications
At each follow-up, give objective feedback on progress toward goal	Shows patient relationship between behavior and change; shows you care about how they are doing
At each follow-up, be sure to go "heavy" on the praise and "light" on the admonishment	A sense of failure may lead to hopelessness, helplessness, and resistance to change
At the end of a visit, provide a "prescription" on a piece of paper. This can be brief instructions, a diagram, or a copy of their flowsheet	Patients expect some tangible result of their visit. Medication prescriptions are not appropriate for all visits

OCCUPATIONAL HEALTH

The *occupational history* is an integral part of delivering total care to the family. Emotional and physical concerns may arise secondary to the occupation, or preexisting problems may adversely affect the work role. Use all occupational health encounters to screen for risk factors (e.g., tobacco, seatbelts) and health advice (Table 1-7).

TABLE 1-7.—OCCUPATIONAL AND ENVIRONMENTAL ASSESSMENT

1. Describe any health problems or injuries arising from past or present jobs.
2. Has any substance you work with caused a rash on your skin?
3. Has an illness related to work caused you to lose more than 1 day of work?
4. Have you ever worked in a job that caused you to have difficulty breathing?
5. Have you ever had a TB skin test or chest x-ray film as screening for your work?
6. Have you ever had to change jobs because of illness or injury?
7. Do you have frequent low back pain, or have you ever had to see a doctor for back care?
8. Do you come into direct contact with liquid, gaseous, powdered, or other toxic substances?
9. Are you aware of sensory (hearing, visual, smell, taste, touch) disturbances connected to your work?
10. Have you ever had to change homes because of a health problem?
11. Have you in the past or present lived very near an industrial plant? Near high voltage wires or a microwave tower?
12. Which hobbies or crafts do you do at home?
13. Do you use home and garden chemicals?
14. Do you have an air conditioner, humidifier, or fireplace at home?

THE FAMILY LIFE CYCLE AND FAMILY FUNCTION

The patterns of development in most families are relatively consistent and predictable. The family physician can use this knowledge to solve puzzling diagnoses, provide anticipatory guidance, and detect deviations from the norm. The family life cycle is a composite of the individual developmental changes of its members and the marital relationship itself.

A family crisis may occur abruptly or gradually and can have profound effects on the emotional and physical well-being of individuals in the family. Assessment of family function and coping abilities aids in efficient management of these problems. Family function also should be studied whenever (1) a new family enters your practice, (2) family members must render care for chronic illness, (3) psychosomatic illness is suspected, and (4) patient-physician relationships are strained.

TABLE 1-8.—Types of Family Crises

Dismemberment
Hospitalization
Loss of child
Loss of spouse
Prolonged separation (military service, work)

Demoralization
Disgrace (alcoholism, crime, delinquency, drug addiction)
Infidelity
Prolonged unemployment
Sudden impoverishment
Progressive dissension

Accession
Adoption
Relative moves in
Stepmother/stepfather marries in

Demoralization Plus Dismemberment or Accession
Desertion
Divorce
Illegitimacy
Imprisonment
Institutionalization
Runaway
Suicide or homicide

From Rakel RE: *Principles of family medicine*, Philadelphia, 1977, WB Saunders, p. 351.

TABLE 1-9.—DEVELOPMENTAL STAGES OF THE FAMILY

MAJOR STAGES OF THE FAMILY	AVERAGE LENGTH	DEFINITION	TASKS
Newly married	2 Years	Union of couple; no children	Disengage from family of origin; adjust to each other's personality; meet social, economic, and sexual needs; establish effective methods of communication
Birth of first child	2.5 Years	Oldest child age 0-30 months	Assume parental role while maintaining marital role; institute new schedule; deal with fatigue, financial stress, home confinement, and decreased leisure activity
With preschool children	3.5 Years	Oldest child age 30 months to 6 years	Socialization of the children; child learns to relate emotionally to others, undergoes early individuation and sexual identity
With children in school	7 Years	Oldest child age 6-13 years	First official separation from home; parents' social activities widen to include school activities; child develops physically, socially, emotionally, and intellectually
Families with teenagers	7 Years	Oldest child age 13-20 years	Stressful stage; family must maintain closeness and cohesiveness while simultaneously encouraging child's development of independence; child begins disengagement process; adolescent sexual feelings conflict with social restriction
Launching years	8 Years	First child leaves home to last child gone	Parent-child relationship changes to adult-adult type; parents face prospect of time alone and need to reinvest in each other instead of children
Parents alone in middle years	15 Years	Last child leaves; empty nest	Reappraisal of lifetime goals, realignment of priorities; couples who have remained together for sake of children divorce; most difficult time for women, causing emotional crises; adaptation to grandparent role
Retirement and later years	10-15 Years	Retirement; death of both spouses	Coping with aging process; loss of occupation; societal disengagement; depression may arise

Modified from Duvall EM: *Family development*, ed 4, 1971, Philadelphia, JB Lippincott.

TABLE 1-10.—FIVE COMPONENTS OF FAMILY FUNCTION (FAMILY APGAR)

The family Apgar is a five-item family function screening questionnaire in which the patient is asked to describe how family members communicate, eat, sleep, and carry out home, school, and job responsibilities.

1. Adaptation   The utilization of intrafamilial and extrafamilial resources for problem solving in times of crisis

2. Partnership   The sharing of decision making and nurturing responsibilities by family members

3. Growth   The physical and emotional maturation and self-fulfillment that are achieved by family members through mutual support and guidance

4. Affection   The caring or loving relationship that exists among family members

5. Resolve   The commitment to devote time to other members of the family for physical and emotional nurturing, involving a decision to share wealth and space

From Rosen GM, Geyman JP, Layton RH: *Behavioral science in family practice,* New York, 1980, Appleton-Century-Crofts, p. 145; Smilkstein G: The family APGAR: a proposal for a family function test and its use by physicians, *J Fam Pract* 6:1231, 1978.

TABLE 1-11.—FAMILY APGAR QUESTIONNAIRE

	ALMOST ALWAYS	SOME OF THE TIME	HARDLY EVER
I am satisfied that I can turn to my family when something is troubling me.	_____	_____	_____
I am satisfied with the way my family talks things over with me and shares problems with me.	_____	_____	_____
I am satisfied that my family accepts and supports my wishes to take on new activities or directions.	_____	_____	_____
I am satisfied with the way my family expresses affection and responds to my emotions, such as anger, sorrow, and love.	_____	_____	_____
I am satisfied with the way my family and I share time together.	_____	_____	_____

From Rosen GM, Geyman JP, Layton RH: *Behavioral science in family practice,* New York, 1980, Appleton-Century-Crofts, p. 147; Smilkstein G: The family APGAR: a proposal for a family function test and its use by physicians, *J Fam Prac* 6:1231, 1978.

Scoring: The patient checks one of the three choices, which are scored as follows: "Almost always" (2 points), "Some of the time" (1 point), or "Hardly ever" (0). The scores for each of the five questions are then totaled. A score of 7-10 suggests a highly functional family. A score of 4-6 suggests a moderately dysfunctional family. A score of 0-3 suggests a severely dysfunctional family.

TABLE 1-12.—Family CAGE* Screening for Family Alcohol Problems

---

The following questions help us understand the way you and your family use alcohol, including beer, wine, and wine coolers. Please check the answer that best describes you and your family.

Have you ever felt that *you* or *anyone in your family* should *cut down* on your/ their drinking?

You?	_____ 0 Never	_____ 1 Occasionally	_____ 2 Often
Family?	_____ 0 Never	_____ 1 Occasionally	_____ 2 Often

Have *you* or *anyone in your family* ever felt *annoyed by complaints* about drinking?

You?	_____ 0 Never	_____ 1 Occasionally	_____ 2 Often
Family?	_____ 0 Never	_____ 1 Occasionally	_____ 2 Often

Have *you* or *anyone in your family* ever felt bad or *guilty* about your/their drinking?

You?	_____ 0 Never	_____ 1 Occasionally	_____ 2 Often
Family?	_____ 0 Never	_____ 1 Occasionally	_____ 2 Often

Have *you* or *anyone in your family* ever had a *drink first thing in the morning* to steady your/their nerves or get rid of a hangover?

You?	_____ 0 Never	_____ 1 Occasionally	_____ 2 Often
Family?	_____ 0 Never	_____ 1 Occasionally	_____ 2 Often

Modified from Frank SH, Graham AV, Zyzanski SJ, White S: Use of the Family CAGE in screening for alcohol problems in primary care, *Arch Fam Med* 1:209, 1992.

*CAGE is an acronym indicating *Cut* down on drinking; *Annoyed* by complaints about drinking; *Guilty* about drinking; had an *Eye-opener* first thing in the morning.

The Family CAGE Screening is appropriate for patients presenting with emotional or family problems; for high utilizers of care; for patients with multiple, vague symptoms; or for use during prenatal or pediatric visits when family dysfunction is suspected. Be aware of appropriate community resources for referral (Table 1-15).

Scoring: Add up the numbers next to the checked responses. A score of ≥ 2 is a positive screen.

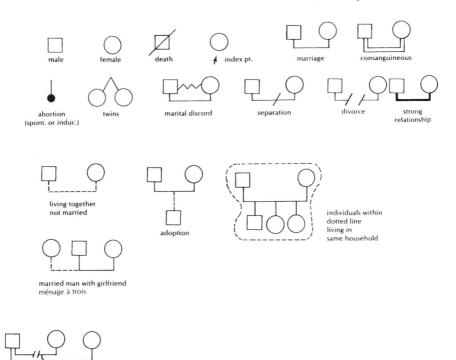

FIG 1-1.
Using a family genogram to understand family structure. Standard symbols are illustrated here. Genograms help to (1) record data on repetitive conditions (e.g., bipolar illness, Down syndrome), (2) understand family interactions and relationships (e.g., conflict, enmeshment, roles), and (3) establish a plan for follow-up and screening (e.g., familial poliposis, cancer family syndrome). Completion of the genogram often supplies the "missing link" to diagnosing illness or family dysfunction. (From McGoldrick M, Gerson R: *Genograms in family assessment,* New York, 1985, WW Norton.)

FAMILY-CENTERED CARE

TABLE 1-13.—GUIDELINES FOR INVOLVING THE FAMILY IN A PATIENT'S CARE

See patient only	Minor acute problems (URI, laceration) Routine self-limiting problems (back strain, influenza, fracture)
Family conference desirable	Treatment failure or regular recurrence of symptoms Routine preventive/educational visits (premarital exam, prenatal care, well child care)
Family involvement essential	Chronic illness (diabetes, obesity, cancer, hypertension) Serious acute illness (major trauma, acute myocardial infarction) Psychosocial problems (anxiety and depression, trouble with the law, substance abuse) Diagnostic or treatment errors, undiagnosed cases Death

TABLE 1-14.—BASIC STRATEGIES FOR FAMILIES COPING WITH CHRONIC ILLNESS

1. Provide regular physician contact for empathetic guidance; explain the diagnosis and management (carefully, clearly, slowly, and repeatedly).
2. Have a family meeting and involve all members in decisions and care.
3. Involve competent assistants in the family's care (social worker, visiting nurse, clergy member).
4. Assist family in recognizing financial and legal issues.
5. Suggest resources that can provide respite for the caregivers (hospice, church groups) and places available for placement if it should eventually be needed.
6. Focus on the needs of the entire family, not just the patient. Have family develop a "coping notebook" with names and phone numbers of doctor, friends, agencies, self-help support groups, and emergency care services.
7. Strive to maintain patient's general health, mental status, and skills for independent activities.
8. Ensure patient safety. Reduce objects that may cause falls; install tub/toilet rail; reduce bathwater temperature; wear ID bracelet; install intercom or call bell system; use lifeline system (automatic dialing of emergency number by single button push).
9. Provide names of other families who have successfully dealt with a similar medical problem.
10. Provide periodic written summary of patient's course and your assessment and plans to family caregivers and any other physicians or professionals involved in patient's care.

COMMUNITY RESOURCES

To provide comprehensive health care, the family physician must use community resources to serve physical, emotional, sociological, and rehabilitative needs. Use appropriate referral and consultation request letters to provide information, ask questions, and give notice that the family physician will remain involved in the patient's care. Written documentation of services or care provided should be requested.

TABLE 1-15.—COMMUNITY RESOURCES USED BY FAMILY PHYSICIAN'S PATIENTS

Physical Health Care
Child Development Clinics—diagnoses of various handicaps
County health department—TB and STD case follow-up
Community dental services
National Black Women's Health Project (1-800-275-2947)
Public health nurses—immunization program
Planned Parenthood and family planning clinics—contraception and venereal
  disease treatment (1-800-230-7526)
Veterinarian—zoonoses control
WIC (women-infants-children) programs providing food supplements

Home Care
Hospice—terminal illness care
Homemakers, Inc.—housekeeping assistance
Home Intravenous Therapy Team
La Leche League—breastfeeding (1-800-525-3243)
Medical equipment and supply companies—home oxygen and sick care items
Manpower Health Care Services
Occupational therapist
Visiting Nurses Association—home nursing assistance
Others listed in Yellow Pages under "nurses" or "health"

Social Services
ADC (Aid to Dependent Children)
Child Welfare Services—foster care, child abuse intervention
Department of Public Assistance
Eldercare Locator (1-800-677-1116)
Food Stamp Program—food assistance
GAU (General Assistance to Unemployed)
Health Foundation National Clearinghouse on Postsecondary Education for
  People with Disabilities (1-800-544-3284)
Hill-Burton Funds—free or reduced hospital services provided by some hospi-
  tals

Continued.

TABLE 1-15.—Community Resources Used by Family Physician's Patients—cont'd

Lutheran Social Services—social and psychological services
Medicaid—financial aid for medical services
Medicare Hotline (1-800-638-6833)
National Council for Adoption
National Information Center for Children/Youth with Disabilities
National Information Clearinghouse for Infants with Disabilities and Life-
    Threatening Conditions (1-800-922-9234)
National Rehabilitation Information Center (1-800-346-2742)
United Cerebral Palsy Association (1-800-872-5827)

Psychological Services
Al-Anon (1-800-443-4525)
Al-Anon Family Groups (1-800-356-9996)
Alcohol and Drug Information Referral Line (1-800-252-6465)
Association for Retarded Citizens
Cocaine Hotline (1-800-262-2463)
Community mental health services
Crisis center—all types of emotional problems
Marriage and family service
National Clearinghouse on Family Support/Children's Mental Health (1-800-628-
    1696)
National Council on Alcoholism and Drug Dependence Hopeline (1-800-622-
    2255)
National Down Syndrome Congress (1-800-232-6372)
National Down Syndrome Society (1-800-221-4602)
National Institute on Drug Abuse Hotline (1-800-662-4357)
National Runaway Switchboard (1-800-621-4000)
Parents Anonymous, Inc.
Pastoral care through local churches
Phoenix Society for Burn Survivors (1-800-888-2876)
Rape crisis center—sexual assault

Disease-Related Associations and General Information Services
Alzheimer's Association (1-800-272-3900)
American Cancer Society (1-800-227-2345)
American Diabetes Association (1-800-232-3472)
American Heart Association (1-800-242-8721)
American Liver Foundation (1-800-223-0179)
American Lung Association (1-800-362-1643-Iowa only)
American Parkinson Disease Association (1-800-223-2732)
American Society for Deaf Children (1-800-942-2732)

TABLE 1-15.—Community Resources Used by Family Physician's Patients—cont'd

Birthright (1-800-848-5683)
Cancer Information and Counseling Line (1-800-525-3777)
Cancer Information Service of the National Cancer Institute (1-800-422-6237)
Candlelighters Childhood Cancer Foundation (1-800-366-2223)
CDC National AIDS Clearinghouse (1-800-458-5231)
CDC National AIDS Hotline (1-800-342-2437)
    Deaf Consumers (1-800-243-7889)
    Spanish Speaking Consumers (1-800-344-7432)
CDC National Sexually Transmitted Diseases Hotline (1-800-227-8922)
Cystic Fibrosis Foundation (1-800-344-4823)
Easter Seals
Epilepsy Foundation of America (1-800-332-1000)
Hearing AID Help Line (1-800-521-5247)
International Shriners Hospital (1-800-237-5055)
Leukemia Society of America (1-800-955-4572)
Lupus Foundation of America, Inc. (1-800-558-0121)
Multiple Sclerosis Association (1-800-798-6677, Iowa only)
Muscular Dystrophy Association
National Abortion Federation Hotline (1-800-772-9100)
National Center for the Blind (1-800-638-7518)
National Marrow Donor Program for Cancer Patients (1-800-654-1247)
National Organization for Rare Disorders (1-800-999-6673)
National Parkinson Foundation (1-800-327-4545)
National Spinal Cord Injury Hotline (1-800-962-9629)
Senior Citizens Center
Simon Foundation for Continence/Help for Incontinent People (1-800-237-4666)
Social Security Office
Spina Bifida Association of America (1-800-621-3141)
United Ostomy Association (1-800-826-0826)
United Way (1-703-836-7100)
University of Iowa Cancer Information Service (1-800-237-1225)
Volunteer Groups
Y-ME for Breast Cancer (1-800-221-2141)

Short-Term Emergency Assistance
American Red Cross (1-202-737-8300)
Community churches
Community food pantry
REACT and Civil Defense
Salvation Army (1-703-684-5500)

HOME VISITS

The proportion of elderly and home-bound patients is increasing. Rising medical costs have led to earlier discharge from hospitals and pressure on the family to give home care. Reasonable guidelines for home care are included in Table 1-16.

TABLE 1-16.—INDICATIONS FOR HOME VISITS

Initial assessment/management of an acute illness when:
  Patient is too elderly to come to office (no transportation capabilities).
  Patient is too ill (acute back injury, severe influenza).
  Pain is exacerbated by movement (febrile hospice patient with malignancy).
  Ambulation is impaired (elderly person with casted leg).
  Patient would be infectious to other patients (chicken pox).
  Patient's problem needs treatment before transport to hospital can be effected (acute asthma in elderly single patient, CPR, relief of pain).
  Need to assess indications for admission to the hospital.
When patient needs follow-up after release from the hospital:
  Assess rehabilitation progress and adaptation to illness.
  Assess coping abilities of family members to deal with chronic disease.
  To help patients who need more time to recover from disfiguring trauma or surgery.
Patients with chronic diseases:
  Patients confined to the home (severe arthritis, multiple sclerosis, COPD, CHF).
  Patients with a dementing illness or problems with toileting control.
  Patients with terminal illness.
When disturbed home situation or family dysfunction is suspected:
  Assess financial capabilities, hygiene, family's ability to care for patient.
  Recommend family counseling to include members who won't come to office.

TABLE 1-17.—ON A HOME VISIT, A PHYSICIAN *OBSERVES*

O—*Outside*
   Type of neighborhood
   Type of house
   Play area for children
   Condition of patient's home and other homes in area
   Environmental hazards
B—*Behavior of family members*
   How do they relate to one another? (Degree of love and intimacy; strength;
      nature of nurturing process; character of communication; exchange of
      looks; verbal exchange; nature of physical contact [warm and supportive;
      quarrelsome and rejecting]; if different ethnic group, don't misinterpret
      signs.)
   How do they relate to the children?
   How do they relate to the physician? Is the TV on?
   Is there a caretaker (hidden patient)? How is caretaker coping?
   Cultural or ethnic activities?
S—*Safety*
   High rate of accidents in home?
   Is there much clutter around?
   Are there exposed wires, fans, hot water vaporizers, poor lighting, flaking
      paint, smoke detectors?
   Is it poison proof? Presence of ipecac?
   Medicines?
E—*Eating area: Habits and patterns*
   Where does the family eat? (Kitchen, dining room; in front of TV; at round
      table or long, narrow one?)
   Sanitation of the kitchen?
   Is garbage disposed of properly?
   What about cooking and storage facilities?
   What food is available?
R—*Relationships and support groups in wider community*
   Is there extended family nearby?
   Do they know neighbors? Are they supportive? Hostile? Indifferent?
   Do they have friends they can contact in an emergency?
   Do they belong to a church or civic organization?
   Do family members work nearby? Who works? Economic background?
   When do they shop?
V—*Variations*
   Had you expected the home to be different? More adequately furnished?
      Less? Does the inside look different from the outside?
   Family member or friend present who was not previously mentioned?
   Evidence of children's toys, etc.?

Courtesy Antonnette V. Graham, RN, LISW, Assistant Professor of Family Medicine, Case
Western Reserve University, Cleveland, Ohio.

Continued.

TABLE 1-17.—On a Home Visit, A Physician *Observes*—cont'd

E—*Environment within the home setting*
   Furnishings, pets?
   Housekeeping?
   Bathroom sanitation?
   Homey? (Family pictures, mementos, religious artifacts, hobbies, etc.)
   Study area? Play area for children?
   Family space? Private space? Where does the family congregate? (What
      people do in a physical setting turns a space into a place. For example,
      the bathroom may be the library, a think tank, an escape from the family,
      or a haven for suicides.)
   Sleeping arrangements? (The stage of the family in its life cycle; use of
      space; communal versus private space within the home.)
S—*Sickness*
   Medications?
   Provisions for ill persons (bed-bound patient locations; dust-proofing for
      asthmatics; handrails for cardiac patients)? How does the family perceive
      the illness?

CARE OF OLDER PERSONS

There is an increasing percentage (11%) of elderly in our population, which is projected to reach 12.5% by the year 2000. Family and social support for the elderly may be lacking, so direct your careful attention toward early discovery of their common, major problems: (1) impaired intellectual functioning, (2) instability and immobility, and (3) incontinence.

TABLE 1-18.—THE MINI-MENTAL STATUS EXAM

	MAXIMUM SCORE
Orientation	
1. What is the year, season, day, month, date?	5
2. Where are we (state, county, town, hospital, floor)?	5
Registration	
3. Name three objects, then have the patient name them. Give one point per each correct answer; repeat until all three are named (record number of tries).	3
Attention/Calculation	
4. Begin with 100 and serially subtract seven until stopped. Stop patient after five correct responses, or ask patient to spell "world" backwards.	5
Recall	
5. Ask patient to name the three objects named earlier. Give one point per correct answer.	3
Language	
6. Have patient identify a pencil (pen) and watch.	2
7. Ask patient to repeat "no ifs, ands, or buts."	1
8. Have patient follow a three-step command, for example, "Take the paper in your right hand, fold it in half, and put it on the floor."	3
9. Have the patient read this statement and obey it: "Close your eyes."	1
10. Ask patient to write a sentence.	1
11. Have patient copy a design.	1
	TOTAL* 30

Modified from Folstein MF, Folstein SE, McHugh PR: *J Psychiatr Res* 12:189, 1975.
*Significant cognitive impairment ≤23.

TABLE 1-19.—Assessment of Functional Status (Activities of Daily Living)

Pulses Profile*

Rate each area on a scale of 1 to 4 (no, mild, moderate, or severe impairment).
   P—Physical condition, health/illness problems
   U—Upper limb function in self-care activities
   L—Lower limb function in mobility
   S—Sensory (vision, hearing, communication) function
   E—Excretory (bowel/bladder) control
   S—Support by others for psychological, emotional, and financial functions

Activities of Daily Living†

Rate each area on a scale of 1 to 3 (no, minimal, or moderate assistance required).
   Bathing—either sponge, tub bath, or shower
   Dressing—gets clothes from closet/drawers, including underwear; does fasteners
   Toileting—goes to the "bathroom" and cleans self afterward; rearranges clothes
   Transfer—movement in and out of bed/chair
   Continence—bladder and bowel control
   Feeding—act of feeding self, not cooking

Instrumental Activities of Daily Living Scale‡

Shopping
Transportation
Use telephone
Prepare meals
Take medications
Manage money
Keep house
Do laundry

*Modified from Granger CV, Albrecht GL, Hamilton BB: *Arch Phys Med Rehabil* 60:145, 1979.
†Modified from Katz S et al: *JAMA* 185:94, 1963.
‡Modified from Lawton MP, Brody EM: Assessment of older people: self-maintaining and instrumental activities of daily living, *Gerontologist* 9:179, 1969.

OFFICE MANAGEMENT

TABLE 1-20.—Time Management for the Family Physician

1. Do not interrupt patient care for phone calls except for emergencies or long-distance calls that would be expensive to return. No phones in exam rooms.
2. Have clearly stated, written protocols for handling telephone calls. Instruct receptionist and nurse which patients to bring into office and which ones to instruct by phone. When doubt exists regarding management, have a period of the day set aside for returning phone calls.
3. When you are running late or called to the hospital for an emergency, have the receptionist notify patients with appointments.
4. Use the first or last hour of the day for extended visit scheduling (e.g., counseling, minor office operations, complete exams).
5. Use preprinted or computerized questionnaires for database collection prior to your visit with the patient.
6. Delegate tasks to professional staff (nurses, clinical pharmacist, social worker) and formulate a complete set of written patient instructions for routine care.
7. Schedule weekly time regularly for house visits and nursing home rounds. Make hospital rounds at same time each day.
8. Use three exam rooms per physician for maximum efficiency.
9. Dictate office records and clearly delegate to nurse in "Plans" section what to carry out prior to your next visit with the patient (e.g., "patient should be weighed and pulse/BP checked prior to each visit"). Instruct the nurse to read "Plans" section of prior office note when placing patient in exam room.
10. Write notes to yourself about patient data that is not medical. Place photos and newspaper clippings about your patients in their record.
11. Delay dealing with noncrisis, nonthreatening "second" problems until another visit. Document what needs to be addressed at that next visit.
12. Use flowsheets and preprinted forms to shorten documentation time for routine care (e.g., hypertension, prenatal visits, well child care).
13. Regularly reserve time in your schedule for self and family, personal fitness, and continuing education.
14. Develop system to ensure all laboratory, x-ray reports, and written communications get your attention and then are properly filed.
15. Have routine period set aside to see pharmaceutical representatives; if none visit, use the time for office administration.

TABLE 1-21.—Occupational Safety and Health Administration Regulations for the Family Physician's Office

1. General employee communication and reporting
   - Employees are obligated to follow office rules, wear protective equipment, and report hazardous conditions.
   - Employers are required to become familiar with all OSHA standards and communicate them to employees. Employers must enforce the rules.
2. Employees must have access to a Material Safety Data Sheet (MSDS) for each hazardous product in the workplace.
3. Blood borne pathogens protection
   - Employers must enforce the concept of universal precautions and workers must have access to needed safety equipment.
   - There must be an employee training program.
   - Each office must create an exposure control plan.
   - Occupationally exposed workers must be offered vaccination against hepatitis B.
   - Engineering controls should reduce pathogen hazards by confining potentially infectious material.
   - In event of exposure, follow-up for 1 year is required.
4. State consultation project directory
   - Consultation programs funded by OSHA must be available and staffed by professionals from each state's government.

Educational Resources: Occupational Safety and Health Administration, Washington, DC, U.S. Department of Labor, U.S. Government Printing Office.

2 The Skin

Edward T. Bope

COMMON DERMATOLOGICAL DISEASES

In the following pages you will find dermatological diseases organized according to the type of skin lesion they produce. To conserve space, treatments are listed below in broad groups and identified by number where they are indicated.

1. Topical steroids (see Table 2-9)
2. PO steroids (see Table 2-8)
3. Topical antibiotics
4. PO or IM antibiotics
5. Antihistamines
6. Selenium sulfide shampoo
7. Pain medication
8. Treatment of underlying disorder
9. Topical scabicide
10. Excision (see Figs. 2-1 and 2-2)
11. Observation
12. Curettage
13. Topical or PO antifungal agents
14. PO or topical acyclovir
15. Drying agent (e.g., calamine lotion)

MACULES

TABLE 2-1.—ANNULAR LESIONS

DISEASE	SITES	LESION	ETIOLOGY	TREATMENT*	DIAGNOSTIC AIDS
Erythema annulare centrifugum	Extremities, trunk	Annular lesions with slight peripheral scale	Allergy, sarcoid, TB, fungus	Organism specific	Biopsy
Erythema multiforme	Palms, soles, generalized	Target lesions	Drug allergy, viral infection	2	Biopsy, immunofluorescence
Lyme disease	Generalized	Target lesions	Tick-borne spirochete	4	Fever, headache, myalgia, arthritis
Pityriasis rosea	Trunk, extremities, rarely on face	Herald patch, flame-shaped lesions in lines of cleavage	Unknown	5	None
Purpura annularis telangiectodes	Legs	Purpuric with brown pigmentation after involution	Unknown		Biopsy
Seborrheic dermatitis	Scalp, face, chest, midback, genitalia	Oily, yellow scale	Unknown	6, 1, 13	Biopsy

Tinea circinata and other tinea	Generalized	Concentric circles, may have raised border	Fungus	13	Examination of scrapings, culture
Erythema infectiosum (fifth disease)	Arms and face, then to trunk	Erythematous "slapped cheeks"	Virus	11	Clinical appearance
Enterovirus, Coxsackievirus Echovirus	Generalized	Red macules; vesicles may also be seen	Virus	11	Clinical appearance, history of viral syndrome
Adenovirus	Generalized	Red macules	Virus	11	Clinical appearance, history of viral syndrome
Rubella	Face, then trunk	Enlarged post-auricular nodes; rash less intense than rubeola	Virus	11	Clinical appearance
Rubeola	Ears, forehead, then trunk	Morbilliform rash, Koplik spots	Virus	11	Clinical appearance
Roseola	Trunk	Faint red, appears after fever subsides	Virus	11	Clinical appearance, history of high fever

*Numbers refer to treatments listed on p.27.

PAPULES

TABLE 2-2.—ANNULAR LESIONS

DISEASE	SITES	LESION	ETIOLOGY	TREATMENT	DIAGNOSTIC AIDS
Erythema multiforme	Palms, soles, generalized	Target lesions; macules and vesicles may also be present	Drug allergy, viral infection	2, 5	Biopsy, immunofluorescence
Granuloma annulare	Over bony prominences	Palpable, deep, faintly erythematous papules with elevated borders	Unknown	1	Biopsy
Lichen planus	Flexor surfaces of forearms; genitalia; mouth	Linear groups of violaceous polygonal flat lesions; on mucous membrane—white reticulated	Unknown; anxiety	5, 2, 1	Biopsy
Pityriasis rosea	Trunk, extremities, rarely on face	Herald patch, flame-shaped lesions in lines of cleavage	Unknown	5	Clinical appearance

	Location	Description	Cause	Treatment	Diagnosis
Psoriasis	Scalp, elbows, knees, trunk; rarely on face	Profuse scale; bleeding points follow removal of scale	Unknown	1, Tar, PUVA	Biopsy
Sarcoid	Nose, mouth, hands	Plaques, papules, or nodules	Unknown	Intralesional steroids	Biopsy, Kveim test
Secondary syphilis	Face, palms, soles	Brownish red with scale at margin	*Treponema pallidum*	4	Darkfield microscopic examination, STS
Urticaria	Generalized	Transitory, branched	Allergy or psychogenic	5	History, clinical appearance
Scarlet fever	Begins on neck and spreads	Scarlet eruption with pinpoint papules	Streptococcal infection	4	History, throat culture, ASO titer
Molluscum contagiosum	Trunk, face, arms, genitalia	Umbilicated, firm waxy papule	Virus	12	Clinical appearance

VESICLES

TABLE 2-3.—Vesicles

DISEASE	SITES	LESION	ETIOLOGY	TREATMENT	DIAGNOSTIC AIDS
Bullous pemphigoid	Trunk, extremities	Pruritic, annular vesicles which are flaccid and break easily	Unknown	5	Biopsy, immunofluorescence
Dermatitis herpetiformis	Trunk, palms, extremities	Pruritic; vesicles and papules	Unknown	5	Biopsy, potassium iodide test, patch test, add IgA before immunofluorescence, small bowel biopsy
Dermatitis venenata	Where exposed to sensitizer	Vesicles on edematous base; pruritic	Contact sensitivity	5	Patch test
Erythema multiforme	Mouth, genitalia, trunk	Occurs with macules and papules	Drug allergy, viral infection	2	Biopsy, immunofluorescence
Herpes simplex	Lips or genitalia	Pruritic groups	Virus	14	Tissue culture, serology, Tzanck test, biopsy
Impetigo contagiosa	Face and other areas	Blood or pus-filled, yellow crust	*Staphylococcus, Streptococcus*	3, 4	Culture, Gram stain, serology
Lymphangioma circumscriptum	Generalized	Round or irregular groups of lymph vesicles with hyperkeratotic top	Congenital		Biopsy

Pemphigus vulgaris	Mucous membranes, any part	Unknown	Annular vesicles, which break easily	2	Biopsy, immunofluorescence
Varicella	Starts on trunk and then involves extremities	Virus	Lesions in various stages of age	5	Tzanck test, tissue culture, serology, biopsy
Zoster	Unilateral, follows nerve	Virus	Tense vesicles on edematous base; painful	5, 7	Tissue culture, serology, Tzanck test, biopsy
Acute eczema	Cheeks, diaper area, flexor surfaces	Many; atopy	Pruritic, vesicles, excoriation, crusting	1, 2, 5	Skin test to confirm sensitivity
Burns	Exposed surfaces	Thermal agent	Bullae	1, 2	History of burn
Enteroviruses, Coxsackievirus, Echovirus	Generalized; hand; foot and mouth possible	Virus	Vesicle	11, 5	Tissue culture
Staphylococcal, scalded skin	Face first, then neck, chest, groin	Staphylococci	Thin fragile bullae	4	Culture
Vasculitis*	Dependent parts	Mostly idiopathic	Often urticarial, necrotic and ulcerated	2	Biopsy if needed
Poison ivy	Exposed skin	Rhus allergy	Pruritic vesicles, linear streaking	1, 15, 2	History of outdoor exposure

*May also be purpuric.

EXCORIATED LESIONS

TABLE 2-4.—Excoriated Lesions

DISEASE	SITES	LESION	ETIOLOGY	TREATMENT	DIAGNOSTIC AIDS
Atopic eczema	Face, trunk, flexor surfaces	Macules, papules, and vesicles progressing to crusting and scaling	Atopy	1, 2, 5	None
Dermatitis herpetiformis	Trunk	Vesicles and papules becoming blood encrusted	Unknown	6	Biopsy, potassium iodide test, patch test, IgA immunofluorescence
Dermatitis venenata	Exposed parts of body	Linear vesicles progressing to blood and serous crusts	Often secondary infection		Patch test
Hodgkin's disease	Generalized	Macular lesions becoming blood encrusted, excoriations	Hodgkin's disease	8	Biopsy of skin lymph nodes or involved tissue
Jaundice	Generalized	Pruritic icterus leading to linear bloody excoriations	Hepatic dysfunction	8	Liver function studies, serum bilirubin

Leukemic cutis	Generalized; may be in only one area	Plaques, nodules, or tumors with blood-encrusted excoriations	Leukemia	8	Biopsy of skin, sternal marrow studies, blood count
Neurotic excoriations	Within reach of hands	Deep bloody excoriations	Psychiatric	8	Psychiatric examination
Papular urticaria	Face, trunk, extremities	Papules and vesicles with blood crusts	Bites—usually fleas	6	Clinical appearance
Pediculosis capitis	Scalp and forehead and back of neck	Blood-encrusted excoriations with pus	Louse	9	Microscopic examination of ova attached to hair
Pediculosis corporis	Trunk	Bloody excoriations, furuncles	Louse	9	Microscopic examination of parasites
Pediculosis pubis	Pubic area	Blood- and pus-encrusted excoriations	Louse	9	Microscopic examination of ova attached to hair
Scabies	Between fingers, palms, wrists, buttock, genitalia; not on face	Linear papule with blood, serous, and pus crusting	Mite	9	Microscopic study of vesicle contents for *Acarus scabiei* or ova and feces

ULCERS

TABLE 2-5.—Ulcers

DISEASE	SITES	LESION	ETIOLOGY	TREATMENT	DIAGNOSTIC AIDS
Blastomycosis	Face, hands, feet	Granulomatous ulcer, which spreads peripherally with pustules in margin	*Blastomyces dermatitidis*	Amphotericin B	Biopsy, culture, direct microscopic examination of exudate
Bromoderma	Legs	Granulomatous ulcer	Bromide ingestion	Withdraw offender	Biopsy, blood bromide; rule out blastomycosis by direct examination and culture
Chancroid	Genitalia	Papule or vesicle, which becomes a superficial, irregular, soft ulcer with granular base, covered with pus; inguinal adenopathy	*Haemophilus ducreyi*	4	Culture, Gram stain of ulcer
Ecthyma	Legs, buttock, vulva	One or more well-defined ulcers, covered with pus crusts and surrounded by zones of erythema; heals by scar formation	Streptococci, staphylococci	4	Culture, Gram stain, serology
Epithelioma (basal cell)	Face, ears	Papule or nodule that spreads peripherally; ulcer is shallow and surrounded by pearly rolled margin	Carcinoma	10	Biopsy

Condition	Location	Characteristics	Cause	Treatment	Diagnostic Tests
Epithelioma (squamous cell)	Face, lips, hands	More rapidly growing than basal cell; superficial or deep ulcer with granulomatous, irregular central portion that bleeds freely	Carcinoma	10	Biopsy
Erythema induratum	Legs, calves	Deep-seated nodules that grow and ulcerate; little discharge	TB	Anti-TB agents	Biopsy
Factitious ulcer	Areas accessible to hands	Single or multiple well-demarcated ulcers; new ones appearing	Self-inflicted; psychiatric	8	History of scratching, psychiatric examination
Frostbite	Ears, fingers, toes, nose	Erythema, edema, blebs, leading to ulcers	Freezing	Rewarming	History of exposure
Granuloma inguinale	Perineum, genital area	Papule that ulcerates and spreads peripherally; granulomatous-based raised, rolled margin	*Donovania granulomatis*	4	Microscopic examination of Wright's-stain or Giemsa-stain smear of marginal tissue for Donovan bodies
Perforating ulcer of the foot	Plantar surface of foot	Begins as callus, which eventually covers a deep ulcer	Multiple pressure		VDRL, spinal fluid examination, neurological examination, blood sugar
Radiation dermatitis	Irradiated area	Superficial ulcer surrounded by zones of atrophy and telangiectasia	Radiation	None	Biopsy

Continued.

TABLE 2-5.—ULCERS—cont'd

DISEASE	SITES	LESION	ETIOLOGY	TREATMENT	DIAGNOSTIC AIDS
Sickle cell anemia ulcer	Lateral aspects of lower third of legs	Round or oval punched-out ulcer, with indurated edge; purulent drainage	Sickle cell	8	Hemoglobin electrophoresis
Stasis ulcer	Lower third of legs	Superficial or deep with profuse seropurulent discharge; surrounded by stasis eczema	Multiple venous insufficiency	8	Clinical appearance
Syphilis (ecthymatous)	Trunk, scalp, extremities	Large round, flat pustules with red-brown areola; thick crust over ulcer	*Treponema pallidum*	4	Darkfield microscopic examination, VDRL
Syphilis, chancre	Genitalia, lips, nipples	Single, hard, indurated ulcer with scant discharge, lymph nodes enlarged, hard and painless	*Treponema pallidum*	4	Darkfield microscopic examination, STS

Syphilis, gumma	Legs, forehead, scalp	Subcutaneous nodule with necrosis to form a deep ulcer	*Treponema pallidum*	4	RPR
Thermal burns	Exposed areas	Well-circumscribed that sheds cover to form ulcer with granulomatous base	Burn	Dependent on degree	History of burn
Tuberculosis	Face, neck	Round, oval, ulcer that bleeds easily; nodules in margins	TB	Anti-TB drugs	Biopsy, culture
Unusual cutaneous infections: Amebic Diphtheria Chromobacteria *Salmonella* *Listeria* Anaerobes	Anywhere	Abscess that ulcerates	Infectious	8	Biopsy, culture on various media

*Numbers refer to treatments listed on p.27.

COMMON PROBLEMS AND TREATMENTS

TABLE 2-6.—Common Problems and Treatments

Diaper Rash

A good history and examination may reveal whether the rash is due to an irritant or a yeast infection. Yeast generally affects the skin creases more than irritants do.

Irritant

Remove irritant. If urine, leave the baby undiapered several times per day. Use very mild topical steroid such as 1% hydrocortisone cream.

Yeast (*Candida albicans* or other species)
Use a nystatin or nystatin-steroid compound such as Mycolog or clotrimazole.

Corns and Calluses

These are areas of thickened skin over areas where repeated, prolonged friction or pressure occur. These areas are very painful, but pain is eradicated on the removal of thickened skin.

Surgical Debridement

Use a no. 15 blade and 1% xylocaine for anesthesia, if needed.

Intermittent Debridement

Use 40% salicylic acid plaster, applied with tape, for 1-7 days and then remove. Soak foot and debride dead tissue. Repeat as needed to keep the lesion flat.

Warts (nongenital)

There will be spontaneous regression in two thirds of children within 2 years. Warts that are treated by one or more of the treatments below should have a 60%-70% cure rate but may require repeated treatments from several weeks to months. Some of the modalities also can be used for genital warts.

Chemical Agents

Acids: trichloroacetic, bichloroacetic, salicylic

Chemotherapeutics: podophyllum, 5-fluorouracil, interferons

Immunotherapy

Physical Agents

Cryotherapy

Electrodesiccation

CO_2 laser

Surgical excision

Topical Preparations for Home Therapy
10% salicylic acid, 10% lactic acid in flexible collodion
40% salicylic acid plaster

TABLE 2-7.—Disorders of the Hair and Scalp

DISEASE	DESCRIPTION	ETIOLOGY	TREATMENT
Alopecia areata	Well-defined single or multiple patches of balding	Probably autoimmune	Reassurance, intralesional steroids
Dandruff	Noninflammatory scaling occurring on scalp	Physiological desquamation	Selenium sulfide 2.5%
Seborrheic dermatitis	Inflammatory scaling in sebaceous areas: scalp, face, trunk	*Pityrosporum ovale*	Selenium sulfide 2.5%, corticosteroid cream, ketoconazole shampoo
Psoriasis	Chronic proliferative epidermal disease	Unclear	Tar shampoo, intralesional steroids
Fungal infection	Superficial epidermis infections	Dermatophytes	Antifungal agents topically and rarely orally
Hair loss	Loss of hair in front or crown	Male pattern baldness	Minoxidil topically for crown balding
Folliculitis	Infection around hair follicles	*Staphylococcus*	Antibiotics

STEROID USAGE

TABLE 2-8.—Steroids

Oral

For a burst of steroids with a taper lasting a total of 20 days, prescribe prednisone, 5 mg #100.

Prescription: Days 1-3, take 12 in AM (total, 60 mg)
Days 4-6, take 8 in AM (total, 40 mg)
Days 7-9, take 4 in AM (total, 20 mg)
Then 2 in AM until finished

Indications: Severe poison ivy, sunburn, acne

Steroid Preparation	Equivalent Dosage (mg)
Prednisone	5
Prednisolone	5
Methylprednisolone	4
Triamcinolone	4
Cortisone	25
Hydrocortisone	20
Betamethasone	0.6
Dexamethasone	0.75

Intralesional

Provides high local concentration with minimal systemic side effects and a prolonged depot effect.

Use a 1:4 dilution of one of the following with saline or lidocaine:
Betamethasone acetate suspension
Triamcinolone acetonide
Triamcinolone diacetate
Triamcinolone hexacetonide
Methylprednisolone

Indications: acne cysts, psoriatic plaques, circumscribed neurodermatitis, keloids

Topical Steroids

The most potent topical steroids are fluorinated and should be used only for a short time. In general, ointment and gel vehicles are superior to cream or lotion vehicles.

TABLE 2-9.—Prescribing Guidelines for Creams and Ointments

Amount needed for one application	2 g	3 g	4 g	30-60 g
	Hands Head Face Anogenital area	One arm Anterior trunk Posterior trunk	One leg	Entire body

TABLE 2-10.—TOPICAL STEROID POTENCY

DRUG	BRAND NAME	DOSAGE FORM	STRENGTH
Very High Potency			
Augmented Betamethasone Dipropionate	Diprolene	Ointment	0.05%
Clobetasol propionate	Temovate	Cream, ointment	0.05%
Diflorasone diacetate	Florone, Maxiflor, Psorcon	Ointment	0.05%
Halobetasol propionate	Ultravate	Cream, ointment	0.05%
High Potency			
Amcinonide	Cyclocort	Cream, lotion, ointment	0.1%
Augmented betamethasone dipropionate	Diprolene AF	Cream	0.05%
Betamethasone dipropionate	Generic, Diprosone, Maxivate, others	Cream, ointment	0.05%
Betamethasone valerate	Generic, Betatrex, Beta-Val, Valisone	Ointment	0.1%
Desoximetasone	Generic, Topicort	Cream, ointment	0.25%
		Gel	0.05%
Diflorasone diacetate	Florone, Maxiflor, Psorcon	Cream, ointment (emollient)	0.05%
Fluocinolone acetonide	Synalar-HP	Cream	0.2%
Fluocinonide	Generic, Fluonex, Lidex, Lidex-E	Cream, ointment, gel	0.05%
Halcinonide	Halog, Halog-E	Cream, ointment	0.1%
Triamcinolone acetonide	Generic, Kenalog	Ointment	0.1%
Medium Potency			
Betamethasone benzoate	Uticort	Cream, gel, lotion	0.025%
Betamethasone dipropionate	Generic, Diprosone, Maxivate	Lotion	0.05%
Betamethasone valerate	Generic, Betatrex, Beta-Val, Valisone	Cream	0.1%
Clocortolone pivalate	Cloderm	Cream	0.1%
Desoximetasone	Generic, Topicort LP	Cream	0.05%
Fluocinolone acetonide	Generic, Flurosyn, Synalar, Synemol	Cream, ointment	0.025%

Continued.

TABLE 2-10.—TOPICAL STEROID POTENCY—cont'd

DRUG	BRAND NAME	DOSAGE FORM	STRENGTH
Flurandrenolide	Generic, Cordran	Cream, ointment	0.025%
	Cordran SP	Cream, ointment, lotion	0.05%
	Cordran	Tape	4 µg/cm^2
Fluticasone propionate	Cutivate	Cream	0.05%
		Ointment	0.005%
Hydrocortisone valerate	Westcort	Cream, ointment	0.2%
Mometasone furoate	Elocon	Cream, ointment, lotion	0.1%
Triamcinolone acetonide	Generic, Kenalog	Cream, ointment, lotion	0.025%
	Aristocort	Cream, ointment, lotion	0.1%
		Cream, ointment	0.5%
Low Potency			
Aclometasone dipropionate	Aclovate	Cream, ointment	0.05%
Desonide	Desonide, DesOwen, Tridesilon	Cream	0.05%
Dexamethasone	Aeroseb-Dex	Aerosol	0.01%
	Decaspray	Aerosol	0.04%
Dexamethasone sodium phosphate	Decadron Phosphate	Cream	0.1%
Fluocinolone acetonide	Generic, Flurosyn, Synalar, Synemol, Fluonid	Cream, solution	0.01%
Hydrocortisone	Cetacort	Lotion	0.25%
	Generic	Cream, ointment, lotion, aerosol	0.5%
	Generic	Cream, ointment, lotion, solution	1%
	Generic	Cream, ointment, lotion	2.5%
Hydrocortisone acetate	Cortaid,	Cream, ointment	0.5%
	Lanacort, others	Cream, ointment	1%

TABLE 2-11.—Mucocutaneous Manifestations of HIV

Often skin and oral changes are presenting signs of HIV. Careful inspection may lead to early detection of infection.

Herpes simplex	Bacterial skin infections
Herpes zoster	Seborrhea
Warts, common and venereal	Psoriasis
Molluscum contagiosum	Telangiectasis and angiomas
Fungal infections	Aphthous stomatitis
Periodontal disease and gingivitis	Kaposi's sarcoma

TABLE 2-12.—Characteristics of Malignant and Benign Pigmented Skin Lesions

FEATURE	MELANOMA	BENIGN SKIN LESION
Size	Over 1 cm, increasing in size	Less than 1 cm, stable size
Color	Varied, resembling an autumn maple leaf, "flag sign"*	Brown, often becomes pale with increasing age
Surface (palpable)	Hard, elevated area; scaling; oozing; bleeding	Macule progresses to soft papule with increasing age
Surrounding skin	Fingers of pigment penetrate, erythematous	Unremarkable or white, halo
Patient-reported sensations	Itchiness, tenderness	None
Location	Back most common	Over entire body but more common on sun-exposed surfaces
Precursors	Family history, dysplastic nevi, congenital nevi, giant hairy nevus, excess sun exposure, type I/II (easily burned) skin	Excess sun exposure in youth; family history of similar lesions at same or mirror image site
Skin marking†	Absent	Often present

From Love RR: *Principles of oncology.* Monogr ed 125, *Home study self-assessment program.* Kansas City, Mo, American Academy of Family Physicians, October 1989.
*The "flag sign" is the appearance of red, white, and blue colors in a pigmented lesion.
†With a magnifying glass, normal skin has crisscrosses of grooves. These normal lines are obliterated by the disordered malignant growth of melanomas.

TABLE 2-13.—Drugs Causing Photosensitity

TOPICAL

ANTIBACTERIAL AGENTS	FRAGRANCES	SUNSCREEN PRODUCTS	ANTIPSORIATIC AGENTS
Bithionol	Musk ambrette	Oxybenzone	Products containing coal tar
Dichlorophen	6-Methylcoumarin	Paraaminobenzoic acid (PABA)	Psoralens
Fenticlor	Oil of bergamot	Paraminobenzoic acid esters	
Halogenated salicylanilides	Sandalwood oil		

PO OR IV

ANTIBIOTICS	CHEMOTHERAPEUTIC DRUGS	DIURETICS	PHENOTHIAZINES	HYPOGLYCEMIC AGENTS	FUROCOUMARINS
Griseofulvin	Dacarbazine	Furosemide	Chlorpromazine	Sulfonylurea	8-Methoxypsoralen
Nalidixic acid	5-Fluorouracil	Thiazides	Promethazine		Trimethylpsoralen
Sulfonamides	Vinblastine				
Tetracyclines					

TABLE 2-14.—TOPICAL ACNE PRODUCTS

DRUG	CONCENTRATIONS AND STRENGTHS	ACNE SEVERITY	COMMENTS
Benzoyl peroxide liquid, lotion, gel, soap (generic)	2.5%, 5%, 10%	Mild to moderate	Wash face before applying. Begin with 2.5% once daily for several days, then bid. Slowly increase strength if needed. Most are nonprescription.
Sulfur, salicylic acid, resorcinol combinations	Various strengths and combinations	Mild to moderate	Some products have alcohol, phenol, or zinc oxide. Most are nonprescription.
Erythromycin solution (generic, ETS-2%)	1.5%, 2%	Moderate	Wash face and apply bid. All products require a prescription.
Clindamycin gel, solution (Cleocin T)	10 mg/ml	Moderate	Apply bid. Diarrhea and pseudomembranous colitis have occurred with topical and systemic clindamycin. Prescription only.
Metronidazole gel (MetroGel)	0.75%	Moderate	Apply bid. Prescription only.
Tetracycline solution (Topicycline)	2.2 mg/ml	Moderate	Apply bid. Safety in pregnancy not established. Prescription only.
Tretinoin (Retin-A)	*Cream:* 0.025%, 0.05%, 0.1% *Gel:* 0.025%, 0.01% *Liquid:* 0.05%	Moderate to severe	Apply at bedtime. Not contraindicated in pregnancy, but it should be avoided. Prescription only.

TABLE 2-15.—ORAL THERAPY FOR ACNE

DRUG	CONCENTRATIONS AND STRENGTHS	ACNE SEVERITY	COMMENTS
Erythromycin capsules and tablets (generic)	250 mg, 500 mg	Moderate to severe	Dose of 250 mg bid up to 500 mg tid.
Tetracycline capsules (generic)	250 mg, 500 mg	Severe	Contraindicated in pregnancy. Initial dose is 250 mg qid followed by 125-500 mg daily. Do not take with diary products, iron, or antacids.
Isotretinoin capsules (Accutane)	10 mg, 20 mg, 40 mg	Severe recalcitrant cystic acne	Absolutely contraindicated in pregnancy. Dose is 0.5-2.0 mg/kg/day divided into two doses over 15-20 weeks. Numerous adverse reactions may occur.

TABLE 2-16.—Drugs Which Commonly Cause Dermatological Reactions

DRUG	MOST COMMON REACTIONS
Ampicillin	Urticaria, maculopapular
Allopurinol	Epidermal necrolysis, maculopapular
Antimetabolites	Alopecia, maculopapular
Barbiturates	Epidermal necrolysis; exfoliative dermatitis; Stevens-Johnson syndrome, bullous, erythema multiforme
Cephalosporins	Maculopapular, urticaria, eczematous
Chlordiazepoxide	Maculopapular
Codeine	Urticaria, erythema nodosum
Corticosteroids	Acneiform
Griseofulvin	Photosensitive, erythema multiforme, maculopapular, urticaria
Gold	Purpura, maculopapular, exfoliative dermatitis, urticaria, photosensitive, bullous, erythema multiforme
Iodides	Acneiform, bullous, erythema nodosum, urticaria
Isoniazid	Acneiform, maculopapular, exfoliative dermatitis
Lithium	Acneiform, maculopapular, urticaria, alopecia
Nitrofurantoin	Urticaria, maculopapular, exfoliative dermatitis
Nonsteroidal antiinflammatory drugs	Urticaria, maculopapular, bullous
Oral contraceptives	Photosensitive, acneiform, erythema nodosum, urticaria, alopecia
Penicillins	Urticaria, maculopapular, epidermal necrolysis, erythema nodosum, erythema multiforme, exfoliative dermatitis, Stevens-Johnson syndrome
Phenothiazines	Photosensitive, erythema multiforme, urticaria, epidermal necrolysis, exfoliative dermatitis
Phenytoin	Epidermal necrolysis, exfoliative dermatitis, Stevens-Johnson syndrome, erythema multiforme, urticaria, acneiform
Quinidine	Purpura, maculopapular, photosensitive
Salicylates	Maculopapular, erythema nodosum, urticaria, purpura
Sulfonamides	Epidermal necrolysis, urticaria, photosensitive, maculopapular, bullous, erythema nodosum, erythema multiforme, Stevens-Johnson syndrome, purpura
Sulfonylureas	Epidermal necrolysis, Stevens-Johnson syndrome, photosensitive, exfoliative dermatitis, urticaria, maculopapular
Tetracycline	Epidermal necrolysis, urticaria, photosensitive, maculopapular, erythema multiforme
Thiazides	Photosensitive, erythema multiforme, urticaria, purpura, maculopapular

Modified from: Young LY et al: *Handbook of applied therapeutics,* Vancouver, 1989, Applied Therapeutics, Inc., p. 56.8.

PROCEDURES

Wood's Light Examination

A Wood's light produces an invisible longwave ultraviolet radiation that will induce visible fluorescence that can aid in differential diagnosis. It is very safe.

Technique

1. A Wood's lamp must be on for several minutes to get to optimum intensity.
2. Seat the patient securely so that she or he does not fall in the dark.
3. Turn off room lights and allow the patient's eyes to adjust.
4. Hold Wood's lamp 4 to 5 inches from area being inspected.

TABLE 2-17.—Wood's Light Examination Diagnostic Table

	FINDINGS
CONDITION	FLUORESCENT COLOR
Tinea Capitis	
Microsporum audouinii	Brilliant green
Microsporum canis	Brilliant green
Trichophyton schoenleinii	Pale green
Erythrasma	Coral-red or pink*
Pigmentary Alterations	
Depigmentation	Cold bright white
Hypopigmentation	Blue-white
Hyperpigmentation	Purple-brown
Vitiligo	Cold bright white and blue-white
Albinism	Cold bright white
Leprosy	Blue-white
Ash-leaf spot of tuberous sclerosis	Blue-white
Pseudomonas aeruginosa infections	Aqua-green or white-green (rarely yellow-green)
Porphyria cutanea tarda (urine)	Pink to pink-orange
Tinea versicolor	Yellow

Modified from Eaglstein WH, Pariser DM: *Office techniques for diagnosing skin disease,* Chicago, 1978, Mosby.
*Patients who bathe shortly before Wood's light examination may show little or no fluorescence.

SKIN BIOPSY TECHNIQUE

Punch Biopsy

Punch biopsy for diagnosis of most inflammatory diseases and tumors.

1. Clean the lesion with 70% alcohol.
2. Use infiltration with 0.5% to 1.0% lidocaine for anesthesia.
3. Use a 3 to 4 mm punch. Simultaneously twist and press the cutting edge into the tissue (Fig. 2-1, *A*).
4. Incise as deeply as possible.
5. Elevate the specimen, handling the edges only, and cut the base with scissors or a scalpel (Fig. 2-1, *B*). Put the specimen in a specimen container.

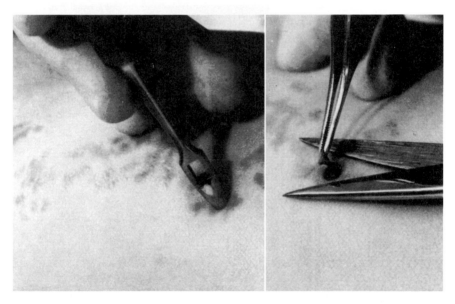

FIG 2-1.
A and **B,** Punch biopsy technique.

Shave Biopsy

Parallel incisional (shave) biopsy for removing superficial benign lesions and biopsy of basal cell and squamous cell carcinomas. This procedure is contraindicated in patients with melanoma.

1. Clean the biopsy site with 70% alcohol.
2. Inject 0.5% to 1.0% lidocaine beneath or directly into the lesions.
3. With scalpel parallel to the skin, shave the lesion from the skin. Pinching the skin may facilitate this step (Fig. 2-2, *A* and *B*).
4. Complete the incision, and place the thin disk of tissue in a specimen bottle.
5. Achieve hemostasis with either pressure, silver nitrate, or ferric subsulfate solution.

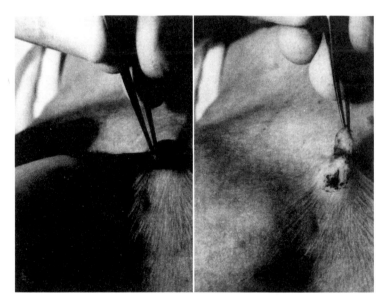

FIG 2-2.
A and **B,** Shave biopsy technique.

SCABIES DETECTION

Preparing a Scabies Slide

1. Select an unexcoriated papule or tract.
2. Place a drop of immersion oil over the lesion. Scrape off the epidermis over the tract or tease the tract open with a scalpel blade. The mite (Fig. 2-3, *B*[5]) will grasp the scalpel blade and can be transferred to a slide.

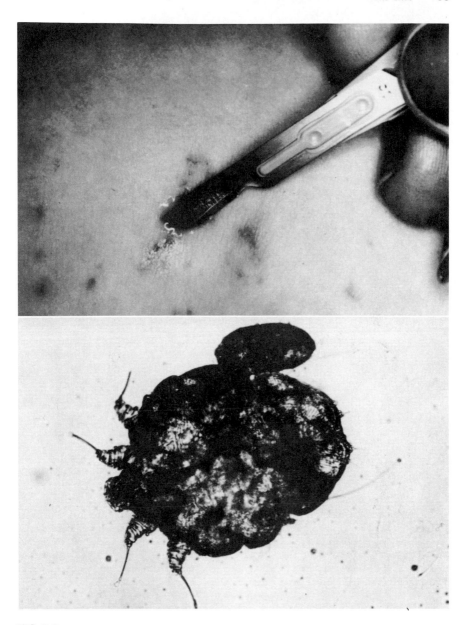

FIG 2-3.
A, With immersion oil over the lesion, use scalpel blade to scrape off epidermis. **B,** Female mite with four of eight legs in focus. An egg is adjacent to the mite at the top of the picture. (From Eaglstein WH, Pariser DM: *Office techniques for diagnosing skin disease,* Chicago, 1978, Mosby.)

KOH PREP

Potassium Hydroxide (KOH) Examination

KOH causes a destruction of the stratum corneum cells and thus a cleaning of debris so that exogenous materials like hyphae, spores, and fiberglass fibers can be seen (Fig. 2-4, *A* and *B*).

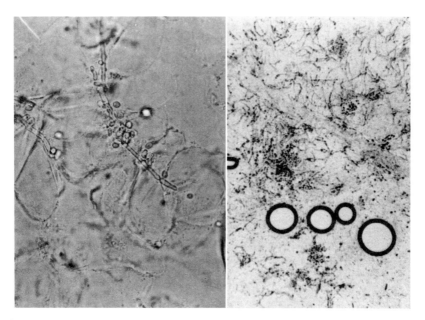

FIG 2-4.
A, Spores, budding spores, and hyphae of *Candida.* (×400.) *Candida* hyphae cross the epidermal cell walls, as do dermatophyte hyphae. **B,** Hyphae and spores of tinea versicolor. (×100.) The findings are often called "spaghetti and meatballs." Short and long hyphae and clusters of spores are seen. In this field, long hyphae predominate. Large circles are oil droplets. (From Eaglstein WH, Pariser DM: *Office techniques for diagnosing skin disease,* Chicago, 1978, Mosby.)

Indications

1. Scaling disorders.
2. Blisters of the hands and feet.
3. Patches of missing or broken hair.
4. Disorders of the nails.
5. Excoriated papules in skin creases.
6. Warty nodules containing tiny black dots (chromomycosis).

Technique

1. Remove all powders or creams with acetone or alcohol.
2. Collect scale on a clean slide by scraping the advancing edge of the lesion with a round-bellied blade.
3. Place a drop of 10% KOH solution on the material and apply the coverslip.
4. Gently warm but do not boil the slide over an alcohol burner.
5. Examine microscopically.

3 *The Eye*

Edward T. Bope

VISION EVALUATIONS

TABLE 3-1.—Percentage of Visual Loss (AMA Method)*

Use best correcting glasses and measure both distance vision by the Snellen chart and near vision by the Jaeger test. In this method, near and distant vision are weighted equally.

Snellen Chart for Distance Visual Acuity	% Loss
20/20	0
20/25	5
20/40	15
20/50	25
20/80	40
20/100	50
20/160	70
20/200	80
20/400	90

Jaeger Test for Near Visual Acuity (Fig. 3-1)	% Loss
1	0
2	0
3	10
6	50
7	60
11	85
14	95

*% Vision acuity $= 100 - \dfrac{\text{% Near loss } + \text{ % Distant loss}}{2}$.

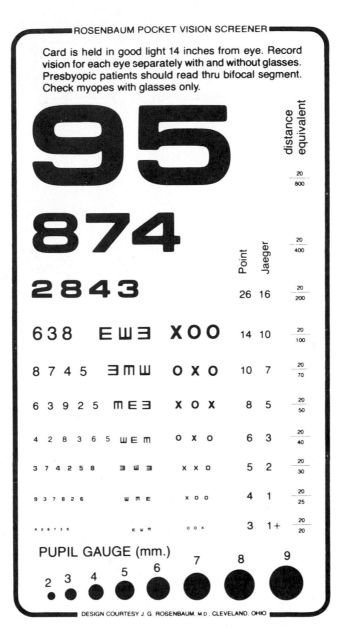

FIG 3-1.
Jaeger test for near visual acuity. (Courtesy J.G. Rosenbaum, M.D., Cleveland, Ohio.)

TABLE 3-2.—PEDIATRIC EYE AND VISION SCREENING GUIDELINES

TEST	0-3 MONTHS	6-12 MONTHS	3½ YEARS	5 YEARS
Red reflex	X	X	X	X
Symmetric corneal reflex	X	X	X	X
Inspection	X	X	X	X
Differential occlusion (resisting one eye being covered more than the other)		X		
Ability to fix and follow		X		
Cover/uncover (See Table 3-9)		X	X	X
Visual acuity			X	X

From Gerald R. Page O.D., Columbus, Ohio.

EXTRAOCULAR MUSCLES

TABLE 3-3.—Extraocular Muscle Innervation

NERVE	CRANIAL NO.	MUSCLE	FUNCTION	RESULTS OF DEFICIT
Oculomotor	III	Medial rectus	Moves eye toward nose	Eye looks downward because of unopposed action of lateral rectus and superior oblique
		Superior rectus	Upward gaze	Weakness of upward gaze
		Inferior rectus	Downward gaze	Weakness of downward gaze
		Inferior oblique	Moves eye up when looking nasally	Vertical diplopia; head remains tilted to compensate
			Rotates eye when looking temporally	
			Moves eye up and out when in forward gaze	
		Levator of upper eyelid (levator palpebrae superioris)	Elevates upper lid	Severe ptosis
Trochlear	IV	Superior oblique	Moves eye down when looking nasally	Vertical diplopia; head remains tilted to compensate
			Rotates eye when looking temporally	
			Moves eye down and out when in forward gaze	
Abducens	VI	Lateral rectus	Moves eye temporally	Inability to look temporally
Cervical sympathetics		Müller's	Elevates upper lid	Mild ptosis

RETINAL EXAMINATION

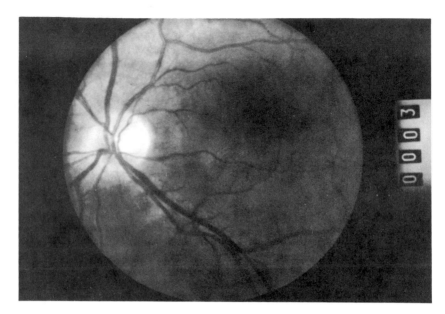

FIG 3-2.
Normal retina.

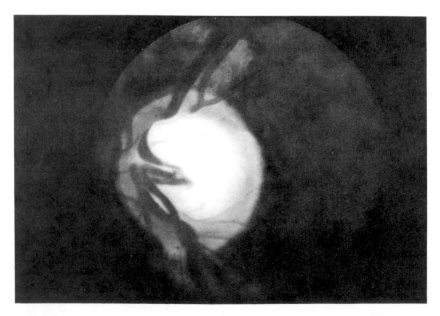

FIG 3-3.
Glaucoma. Cupping due to glaucoma extends to edge of the optic disc.

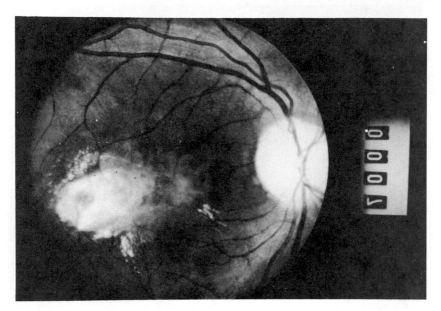

FIG 3-4.
Senile macular degeneration. Note scattered exudates in the macular area and absent foveal light reflex. There may be scattered hemorrhages.

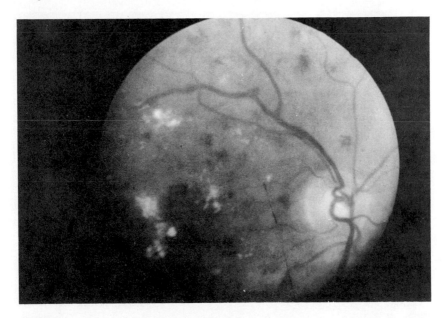

FIG 3-5.
Diabetic retinopathy. Note small hemorrhages and scattered exudates.

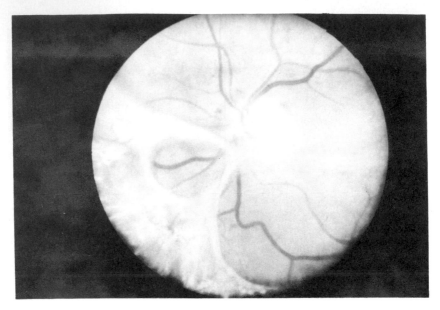

FIG 3-6.
Diabetic retinitis proliferans. Note sheets of connective tissue and new blood vessels near the optic disc.

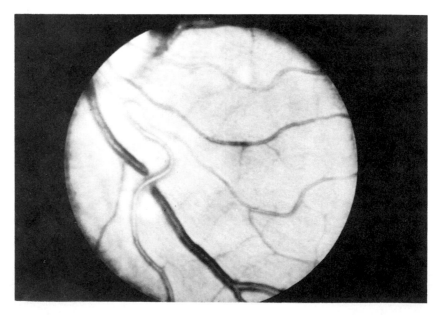

FIG 3-7.
Hypertensive retinopathy. Note AV nicking and hard exudates.

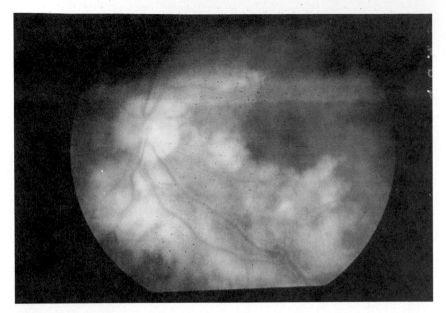

FIG 3-8.
CMV retinitis. Chorioretinitis characterized by hemorrhages and exudates described as "cotton wool" patches.

COMMON EYE SYMPTOMS

TABLE 3-4.—Common Eye Symptoms

EYE SYMPTOMS	MOST COMMON DIAGNOSES
Acute spontaneous loss of vision in one eye, transient	Transient ischemic attack involving blood circulation to retina; lasting deficit may indicate central retinal artery occlusion or arteriolar or venous hemorrhage Migraine
Acute spontaneous loss of vision in both eyes, transient	Transient ischemic attack involving blood circulation to visual areas of the brain Migraine
Floaters (particles of dust, spots, cobwebs); no other visual difficulties	Vitreous opacities, usually insignificant
Lightning flashes	Migraine (often also manifest as "wavy" appearance of environment) May accompany traction on retina or retinal detachment
Curtain drawn over an eye	Retinal detachment or hemorrhage
Blurred vision—far only	Myopia
Blurred vision—near only	Hyperopia; use of cycloplegic drops; presbyopia
Double vision	Nerve or muscle damage; if monocular, may reflect lens dislocation or cataract
Vertigo (sensation of spinning, either the patient or the environment)	Dysfunction of vestibular apparatus or its connection in the brainstem
Loss of central vision in one eye	Macular or optic nerve disease

COMMON EYE SIGNS

TABLE 3-5.—Common Eye Signs

SIGN	DIAGNOSIS	TREATMENT
Tender pimple on lid margin	Hordeolum (stye)	Warm compresses qid Topical antibiotic Referral for I&D if persistent
Tender nodule in lid away from margin	Chalazion	Warm compresses Antibiotics of little value Referral for excision if persistent
Ulcerated lesion with pearly border (lower lid)	Basal cell carcinoma	Excision or referral for excision
Soft, yellow, raised lid lesions	Xanthelasma	Can be cosmetically removed Check for diabetes and hyperlipidemia
Lower conjunctiva exposed and red	Ectropion	Plastic repair
Foreign body sensation; lid margin not seen	Entropion	Plastic repair
Ecchymosis of lid	Black eye	Examine eye for diplopia Ice for 24 hours
Red hemorrhagic sclera	Subconjunctival hemorrhage	No treatment
Warm, tender swelling in superolateral aspect of upper lid	Lacrimal gland inflammation	Treat infection Rule out tumor
Warm, tender swelling of nasal aspect of lower lid	Lacrimal sac inflammation	Antistaph topical antibiotics Warm compresses Massage lacrimal sac
Crusty, sore eyelids with scaling	Blepharitis	Topical antibiotics Dandruff control
Ocular pain—eye injected temporally	Episcleritis	Consultation Steroids
Ocular pain—halos around lights	Glaucoma	Schiøtz tonometry Consultation
Soft yellow patches on sclera at 3 o'clock and 9 o'clock	Pinguecula	No treatment
Scleral vascularization extending to nasal cornea	Pterygium	Can be cosmetically removed
Mild ptosis, small pupil and same-sided decreased facial sweating	Horner's syndrome	Consultation, chest x-ray film A large differential, including tumor

DIFFERENTIAL DIAGNOSIS OF RED EYE

TABLE 3-6.—DIFFERENTIAL DIAGNOSIS OF RED EYE

ASPECT	DIAGNOSIS			
	ACUTE CONJUNCTIVITIS	ACUTE IRITIS	ACUTE GLAUCOMA	CORNEAL ULCER OR TRAUMA
Redness	Diffuse	Circumcorneal	Diffuse	Diffuse
Vision	Normal	Slightly blurred	Markedly blurred	Blurred
Discharge	Large	None	None	Watery or purulent
Pain	None	Moderate	Severe	Moderate to severe
Cornea	Clear	Anterior chamber may be cloudy	Cloudy	Opacity, fluorescein positive
Pupil—size	Normal	Small	Dilated	Normal or small if secondary iritis
Pupil—light response	Normal	Poor	Poor	Normal
Intraocular pressure	Normal	Normal	Increased	Normal
Therapy	Antibiotics	Atropine, Cortisone	Pilocarpine, Diamox, surgery	Antibiotics
Prognosis	3-5 Days	Definitive treatment needed to avoid serious complications		

OCULAR MANIFESTATIONS OF SYSTEMIC DISEASE

TABLE 3-7.—OCULAR MANIFESTATIONS OF SYSTEMIC DISEASE

AIDS: Retinopathy with "cotton wool" spots on retina; Kaposi's sarcoma of eyelids and conjunctiva; keratitis; herpes zoster; uveitis; candida chorioretinitis

Albinism: Light fundus background (choroidal vessels seen easily with the ophthalmoscope as pigment epithelium is unpigmented; nystagmus; poor vision (high refractive errors and poor macular development); pink-blue iris (iris transilluminates).

Alkaptonuria: Melanin deposits in sclera (at 9 o'clock and 3 o'clock positions around the cornea).

Amyloidosis: Weakness of extraocular muscles; vitreous opacities; pupillary abnormalities; amyloid nodules in lids and conjunctiva.

Anemia: Conjunctiva appears pale; retinal hemorrhages and exudates present.

Ankylosing spondylitis: Uveitis; scleritis; scleromalacia perforans (thinning of the sclera with exposure of the uveal tissue).

Atopic dermatitis: Cataracts; keratoconus.

Behçet's syndrome: Uveitis.

Cystic fibrosis: Papilledema; retinal hemorrhages.

Cystinosis: Deposits of cystine crystals in cornea and conjunctiva.

Cytomegalic inclusion disease (congenital): Chorioretinitis cataracts.

Dermatomyositis: Extraocular muscle palsies; lid edema, scleritis; uveitis; retinal exudates.

Diabetes mellitus: Extraocular muscle palsies; xanthelasmas; retinal microaneurysms; hemorrhages, exudates, and neovascularization of the retina; cataracts; rubeosis iridis (neovascularization of the iris); glaucoma.

Down syndrome: Up-and-out obliquity to the lids; Brushfield's spots (white speckling of iris); cataracts; myopia; strabismus.

Ehlers-Danlos syndrome: Blue sclera; strabismus; epicanthal folds.

Friedreich's ataxia: Nystagmus; strabismus; retinitis pigmentosa.

Galactosemia: Cataracts.

Glomerulonephritis: Periorbital edema; hypertensive retinopathy.

Gout: Episcleritis, uveitis; deposition of uric acid crystals in cornea.

Hereditary hemorrhagic telangiectasia (Osler-Weber-Rendu disease): Telangiectasis of conjunctiva and retina.

Herpes zoster: Dermatitis along ophthalmic branch of cranial nerve V; uveitis; keratitis.

Histoplasmosis: Chorioretinal scars, retinal hemorrhage.

Homocystinuria: Dislocated lens.

Hyperlipidemia: Xanthelasma, arcus juvenilis, lipemia retinalis (milky retinal vessels secondary to excessive lipids in the blood).

Hyperparathyroidism: Band keratopathy (gray-white band containing calcium deposits, extending horizontally across the cornea); optic atrophy.

Hyperthyroidism: Proptosis, lid retraction; infrequent blinking (staring): lid lag on downward gaze, weakness of upward gaze; poor convergence; diplopia, corneal erosion (from poor lid closure); papilledema; papillitis.

From Goldberg S: *Ophthalmology made ridiculously simple,* Miami, 1991, MedMaster.

TABLE 3-7.—Ocular Manifestations of Systemic Disease—cont'd

Hypoparathyroidism: Cataracts; papilledema; optic neuritis.

Hypothyroidism (congenital cretinism): Strabismus; farsightedness; cataracts; swollen lids with narrow slits between lids; wide-set eyes; retrobulbar neuritis; optic atrophy; loss of outer half of eyebrows.

Impending stroke: Amaurosis fugax (transient blindness from intermittent vascular compromise in arteriosclerotic disease); Hollenhorst plaques (glistening emboli seen at branch points of retinal arterioles).

Kernicterus (erythroblastosis fetalis): Strabismus; nystagmus; retinal hemorrhage.

Lead poisoning: Papilledema; optic atrophy.

Lupus erythematosus: Retinal hemorrhages; cotton wool exudates; papilledema; lid lesions similar to lesions elsewhere; episcleritis; keratitis; uveitis; nystagmus; extraocular muscle palsies; cataracts.

Macroglobulinemia: Venous occlusion (engorged retinal veins with hemorrhages and exudates); papilledema.

Marchesani's syndrome: Dislocated lens.

Marfan syndrome: Dislocated lens.

Migraine: Throbbing eye pain; transient visual compromise (e.g., flashing lights, waves, hemianopia); miotic (small) pupil (sympathetic axon compromise with carotid artery wall edema).

Mucopolysaccharidoses: Corneal clouding.

Multiple sclerosis: Retrobulbar neuritis; optic atrophy; internuclear ophthalmoplegia; strabismus.

Myasthenia gravis: Ptosis; extraocular muscle paresis.

Myotonia: Cataracts.

Neurofibromatosis: Lid and orbital tumors; optic gliomas.

Osteogenesis imperfecta: Blue sclera (choroid shows through thin sclera).

Polyarteritis nodosa: Episcleritis; corneal ulcers, uveitis; retinal hemorrhages and exudates; papilledema; hypertensive retinopathy; arteriolar occlusion.

Polycythemia: Markedly dilated retinal veins; papilledema.

Pseudoxanthoma elasticum: Angioid streaks (reddish bands radiating from disc region, resembling blood vessels), probably representing defects in the choroidal membrane (Bruch's membrane) just outside the pigment epithelium. Also found in Paget's disease of the bone and sickle cell disease.

Radiation exposure: Cataracts; retinopathy.

Reiter's syndrome: Uveitis; retinal vasculitis.

Rheumatoid arthritis: Uveitis; band keratopathy; scleromalacia perforans (degeneration and thinning of anterior sclera with bulging out of underlying bluish choroid).

Riley-Day syndrome (familial dysautonomia): Decreased tear production; decreased corneal sensation with subsequent exposure keratitis.

Rosacea: Blepharitis; conjunctivitis; keratitis; episcleritis.

Rubella (congenital): Cataracts; microphthalmia; cloudy corneas; uveitis; pigmentary retinopathy.

Sarcoid: Uveitis; whitish perivenous infiltrates in retina band keratopathy.

Continued.

TABLE 3-7.—Ocular Manifestations of Systemic Disease—cont'd

Sickle cell anemia: Retinal hemorrhages, exudates, microaneurysms, neovascularization (vascular and hemorrhagic changes are worse in sickle cell-hemoglobin C disease than in sickle cell-hemoglobin S disease); papilledema; angioid streaks.

Sjögren's syndrome: Dry eyes; corneal erosions.

Stevens-Johnson syndrome: Purulent conjunctivitis with scarring of conjunctiva and cornea.

Subacute bacterial endocarditis: Congenital and retinal hemorrhages; Roth spots (retinal hemorrhages with white centers).

Sturge-Weber syndrome: Congenital glaucoma on side of facial nevus.

Syphilis: Interstitial keratitis (inflammation, edema, and vascular infiltration of the cornea, particularly the corneal periphery); uveitis; optic neuritis; cataracts; chorioretinitis; lens dislocation; Argyll Robertson pupil.

Tay-Sachs disease: Cherry red spot (cloudiness of retina, except in fovea region).

Temporal arteritis: Transient or permanent loss of vision from vasculitis affecting the optic nerve.

Toxemia: Hypertensive retinopathy.

Toxoplasmosis: Chorioretinitis.

Trichinosis: Inflammation of extraocular muscles.

Tuberculosis: Uveitis; chorioretinitis.

Tuberous sclerosis: Retinal tumor.

Ulcerative colitis: Uveitis.

Vitamin deficiencies:
  Vitamin A deficiency. Night blindness; xerophthalmia (drying of cornea and conjunctiva).
  Thiamine deficiency (beriberi). Optic neuritis; extraocular muscle weakness.
  Niacin deficiency (pellagra). Optic neuritis.
  Riboflavin deficiency. Photophobia; inflammation of conjunctiva and cornea.
  Vitamin C deficiency (scurvy). Hemorrhages within the outside of the eye.
  Vitamin D deficiency. Cataracts; papilledema (as in hypoparathyroidism).

Von Hippel-Landau disease: Retinal hemangiomas.

Wilms' tumor: Aniridia (absence of iris).

Wilson's disease: Copper deposits in Descemet's membrane in the peripheral cornea (Kayser-Fleischer ring) and in the lens (copper cataracts).

TABLE 3-8.—Herpes Infections of the Eye

Simplex: Ulcers on the eyelid may be inoculated into the eye, and this forms a dendritic corneal ulcer (a zigzag surface lesion). These are difficult to treat and may cause corneal scarring. Note: Topical corticosteroids should not be used because they will encourage corneal spread of this virus.

Zoster: When involving the eye, it is in the typical unilateral trigeminal distribution. The conjunctiva is red, and the cornea shows discrete white subepithelial opacities. Fine dendritic ulcers may occur. Mydriatics, antibiotics, and topical corticosteroids should be used.

STRABISMUS, PSEUDOSTRABISMUS, AND AMBLYOPIA

TABLE 3-9.—Strabismus, Pseudostrabismus, and Amblyopia

Amblyopia
Loss of vision in one eye caused by (1) physical occlusion (e.g., cataract, ptosis), (2) refractive error (unilateral), or (3) strabismus
Mechanism
The brain receives a confusing image from the affected eye and selectively suppresses the image.

Strabismus
Deviation of the eye in an inward direction (esotropia, cross-eyed), outward direction (exotropia, walleyed), or vertical direction (hypertropia).
Classification
Paralytic: Caused by damage to cranial nerves III, IV, or VI or by a lesion in the extraocular muscle itself. May be caused by brain tumor, encephalitis, intracranial aneurysm, vascular accident, thyrotropic exophthalmos, myasthenia gravis, or orbital cellulitis.
Nonparalytic: The most common form, resulting in suppression amblyopia.
Detection
Normal eye position will show a penlight reflected in the exact center of each pupil.
Alternate cover test: (1) Have patient fixate eyes on a penlight. (2) Cover one eye. (3) Remove cover and observe movement of uncovered eye. (4) Alternate eyes in 1-second intervals. (5) Interpret movement according to the chart below.
Cover/uncover test: To diagnose strabismus, cover the disconjugate eye and then remove the cover. The eye remains deviated.

Continued.

TABLE 3-9.—Strabismus, Pseudostrabismus, and Amblyopia—cont'd

Interpretation of alternate cover and cover/uncover tests:

Test	Movement	Meaning
Alternate cover	Inward	Eye rests in outward position (exophoria)
	None	Normal
	Outward	Eye rests in inward position (esophoria)
Cover/uncover	Deviated	Strabismus

Treatment

If not corrected, seek consultation soon after age 6 months. The ophthalmologist will probably follow this outline:

Nonparalytic

Refractive error: Correct it. Remember that if the eye is farsighted, it will converge to accommodate, producing esotropia.

No refractive error: Alternately patch the eyes to exercise the extraocular muscles and stimulate vision in both eyes. Consider surgical intervention if this fails.

Paralytic: Specific to neurological disease.

Pseudostrabismus

An optical illusion, usually secondary to broad epicanthal folds.

EYE TRAUMA

TABLE 3-10.—Treatment for Chemical Burn

Irrigate eye with water or saline for 15-20 minutes.

Clear cornea: Stain with fluorescein to estimate damage.

Mild to moderate epithelial damage:
Topical antibiotic
Patch
Examine daily until healed (2-3 days)

Marked epithelial damage:
Consult ophthalmologist

Pupillary constriction (indicates intraocular irritation):
Consult ophthalmologist
Consider emergency use of cycloplegic drops on recommendation of ophthalmologist

Cloudy cornea: Irreversible damage; consult ophthalmologist

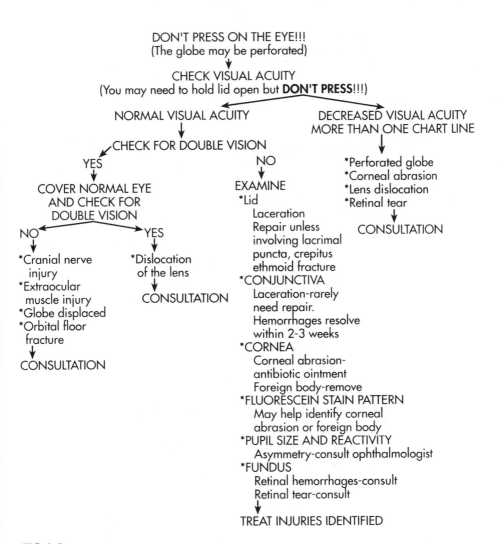

DON'T PRESS ON THE EYE!!!
(The globe may be perforated)
↓
CHECK VISUAL ACUITY
(You may need to hold lid open but **DON'T PRESS**!!!)

NORMAL VISUAL ACUITY

DECREASED VISUAL ACUITY
MORE THAN ONE CHART LINE
↓
*Perforated globe
*Corneal abrasion
*Lens dislocation
*Retinal tear
↓
CONSULTATION

CHECK FOR DOUBLE VISION

YES
↓
COVER NORMAL EYE
AND CHECK FOR
DOUBLE VISION

NO
↓
*Cranial nerve
injury
*Extraocular
muscle injury
*Globe displaced
*Orbital floor
fracture
↓
CONSULTATION

YES
↓
*Dislocation
of the lens
↓
CONSULTATION

NO
↓
EXAMINE
*Lid
Laceration
Repair unless
involving lacrimal
puncta, crepitus
ethmoid fracture
*CONJUNCTIVA
Laceration-rarely
need repair.
Hemorrhages resolve
within 2-3 weeks
*CORNEA
Corneal abrasion-
antibiotic ointment
Foreign body-remove
*FLUORESCEIN STAIN PATTERN
May help identify corneal
abrasion or foreign body
*PUPIL SIZE AND REACTIVITY
Asymmetry-consult ophthalmologist
*FUNDUS
Retinal hemorrhages-consult
Retinal tear-consult
↓
TREAT INJURIES IDENTIFIED

FIG 3-9.
Blunt injury to the eye.

REMOVAL OF A FOREIGN BODY

Persistent pain in the eye suggests the presence of a foreign body or corneal abrasion.

TABLE 3-11.—REMOVAL OF A FOREIGN BODY

Technique
1. Use proparacaine (Ophthaine) or tetracaine (Pontocaine) drops to achieve anesthesia. It will last 10-25 minutes.
2. Inspect globe in all gazes.
3. Inspect conjunctiva by pulling down the lower lid during upward gaze.
4. Evert the upper lid by grasping the upper lid margin and applying pressure over the tarsal plate with a cotton-tipped applicator or tongue blade (Figs. 3-10 and 3-11).
5. Magnifying glasses may be very helpful.

Continued.

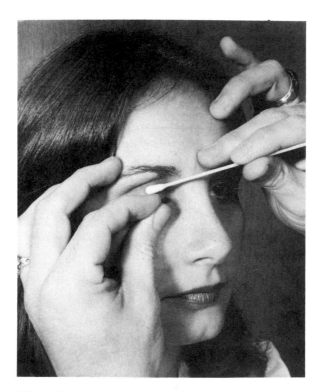

FIG 3-10.
Proper positioning of cotton-tip applicator to eyelid for eversion of lid.

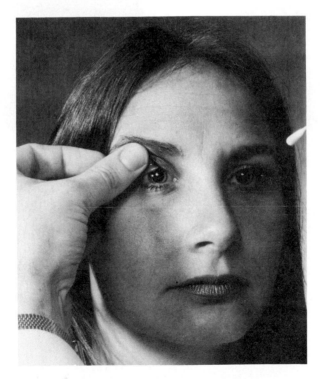

FIG 3-11.
Eyelid everted for visual inspection for a foreign body.

TABLE 3-11.—REMOVAL OF A FOREIGN BODY—cont'd

Removal of Foreign Body
1. Prior practice on a porcine or bovine globe is essential.
2. Make sure anesthetic is still effective.
3. Attempt irrigation with saline under pressure.
4. Attempt removal by *light* touch of sterile cotton-tipped applicator.
5. Attempt removal with 26-gauge needle on a sterile cotton tip (Fig. 3-12) or an eye spud.
6. If unsuccessful, consult an ophthalmologist for slit lamp removal.
7. Prophylactic topical antibiotics should be prescribed for 24-48 hours.
8. Eye patch is optional, depending on patient comfort.

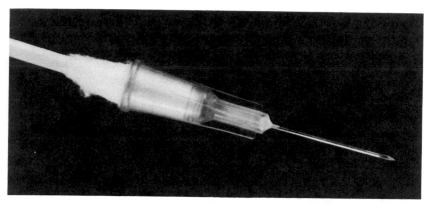

FIG 3-12.
26-gauge needle on cotton-tip applicator for use as eye spud.

TABLE 3-12.—Ocular Manifestations of Common Drugs

Allopurinol: Cataracts.
Amantadine: Visual hallucination more common in the elderly (reversible).
Amiodarone: Corneal deposits.
Antianxiety agents: Diplopia.
Antihistamines: Blurred vision, mydriasis, decreased lacrimal secretions.
Antimalarials: Corneal deposits and edema, ptosis, decreased accommodation.
Antituberculosis drugs: Optic neuritis and optic atrophy.
Contraceptives: Corneal edema (may interfere with contact lens wearing), papill-
   edema, migraine.
Corticosteroids: Cataracts, increased intraocular pressure, retinal edema, papill-
   edema.
Digitalis: Yellow hue to vision (xanthopsia), conjunctivitis, decreased vision.
Diuretics: Retinal edema, retinal hemorrhages, myopia.
Gold: Corneal, Conjunctival and lens gold deposits, ptosis.
Haloperidol: Oculogyric crisis.
Ibuprofen: Reduced vision and change in color vision.
Indomethacin: Reduced vision and change in color vision.
Metoclopramide: Oculogyric crisis.
Pentazocine (Talwin): Constriction of pupils and visual hallucinations.
Phenothiazines: Posterior corneal deposits, Horner's syndrome, oculogyric
   crisis.
Phenytoin: Frequent nystagmus, ophthalmoplegia and resulting diplopia,
   cataracts.
Tamoxifen: Corneal opacities, reduced vision, retinopathy.
Tetracycline: Blurring of vision, diplopia, papilledema (reversible).
Thioridazine (Mellaril): Pigment deposits on retina.
Tricyclic antidepressants: Mydriasis, angle-closure glaucoma, cycloplegia.
Vitamin A: Papilledema, nystagmus, diplopia, color vision disturbance.
Vitamin D: Band keratopathy.

TABLE 3-13.—Ophthalmic Antimicrobials

DRUG	DOSAGE FORM/STRENGTH
Bacitracin	Ointment (500 U/g)
Chloramphenicol	Ointment (1%); solution (0.05%, 0.16%, 0.5%, 1.0%)
Ciprofloxacin	Solution (0.3%)
Erythromycin	Ointment (0.5%)
Gentamicin	Ointment or solution (0.3%)
Norfloxacin	Solution (0.3%)
Sulfacetamide	Solution (10%, 15%, 30%); ointment (10%)
Sulfisoxazole	Solution (4%); ointment (4%)
Tetracycline	Ointment (1%)
Chlortetracycline	Ointment (1%)
Tobramycin	Solution (0.3%); ointment (0.3%)

Combination Products
Neomycin 0.35%; polymyxin B 10,000 U/g, bacitracin 500 U/g in ointment
Polymyxin B 10,000 U/g; bacitracin 500 U/g in ointment
Polymyxin B 10,000 U/g or ml; neomycin 0.35% in ointment or solution
Oxytetracycline 0.5% and polymyxin B 10,000 U/g in ointment
Tetramethoprim 0.1% and polymyxin B 10,000 U/g in ointment

From Herfindal ET, Gourley DR, Hart LL: *Clinical pharmacy and therapeutics,* ed 5, Baltimore, Md, 1992, Williams & Wilkins.

TABLE 3-14.—AGENTS FOR ALLERGIC CONJUNCTIVITIS

DRUG	DOSAGE	COMMENTS
Oral Therapy		
Chlorpheniramine (generic)	4-12 mg once (hs) or twice daily	Reserve for patients with systemic allergic symptoms. Other oral antihistamines are acceptable but much more expensive.
Topic Antiallergic Drops		
Levocabastine (Livostin)	One drop in affected eye(s) four times daily for up to 14 days	Potent antihistamine actions.
Lodoxamide (Alomide)	One or two drops in affected eye(s) four times daily for up to 3 months	Mast cell stabilizer indicated for vernal keratoconjunctivitis, vernal conjunctivitis, and vernal keratitis.
Topical Decongestant/Antihistamine Combinations		
Antazoline 0.5% with naphazoline 0.05% (generic, Vasocon-A)	One or two drops in affected eye(s) every 3-4 hours or less to relieve symptoms	
Pheniramine 0.3% with naphazoline 0.025% (generic, Naphcon-A)	One of two drops in affected eye(s) every 3-4 hours or less to relieve symptoms	

TABLE 3-15.—Ophthalmic Decongestant Product Table

PRODUCT (MANUFACTURER)	VISCOSITY AGENT	VASOCONSTRICTOR	PRESERVATIVE
Allerest Eye Drops (Pharmacraft)		Naphazoline HCl 0.012%	Benzalkonium Cl, EDTA
Clear Eyes (Ross)		Naphazoline HCl 0.012%	Benzalkonium Cl 0.01%; EDTA 0.1%
Collyrium Fresh Eye Drops (with tetrahydrozoline) (Wyeth-Ayerst)		Tetrahydrozoline HCl 0.05%	Benzalkonium Cl 0.005%; EDTA 0.02%
Comfort Eye Drops (Sola/Barnes-Hind)	Hydroxyethylcellulose; polyvinyl alcohol	Naphazoline HCl 0.03%	Benzalkonium Cl 0.01%; EDTA
OcuClear (Schering)		Oxymetazoline HCl 0.025%	
Relief (Allergan)	Polyvinyl alcohol 1.4%	Phenylephrine HCl 0.12%	Benzalkonium Cl 0.004%; EDTA
Soothe Eye Drops (Alcon)	Povidone	Tetrahydrozoline HCl 0.05%	0.1%
Vasoclear A (Iolab)	Polyvinyl alcohol 0.25%	Naphazoline HCl 0.02%	Benzalkonium Cl 0.005%; EDTA
Visine Eye Drops (Leeming)		Tetrahydrozoline HCl 0.05%	Benzalkonium Cl 0.01%; EDTA 0.1%
Visine Extra* (Leeming)		Tetrahydrozoline HCl 0.05%	Benzalkonium Cl 0.013%; EDTA 0.1%

Modified from Herfindal ET, Gourley DR, Hart LL: *Clinical pharmacy and therapeutics*, ed 5, Baltimore, Md, 1992, Williams & Wilkins.
*Includes PEG-400 1%.

TABLE 3-16.—Artificial Tear Products

PRODUCT	VISCOSITY AGENT	PRESERVATIVE
Artificial Tears Solution	Polyvinyl alcohol 1.4%	Edetate disodium, chlorobutanol
Comfort Tears	Hydroxyethylcellulose; polyvinyl alcohol	Edetate disodium 0.005%; benzalkonium Cl 0.02%
Hypotears	Polyvinyl alcohol 1%	Benzalkonium Cl 0.01%
Isopto Plain	Hydroxypropyl methylcellulose 0.05%	Benzalkonium Cl 0.01%
Just Tears	Hydroxypropyl methylcellulose	Benzalkonium Cl 0.01%; edetate disodium 0.025%
Liquifilm Tears	Polyvinyl alcohol 1.4%	Chlorobutanol 0.5%
Murine	Polyvinyl alcohol 1.4%; povidone 0.6%	Benzalkonium Cl; edetate disodium
Tears Naturale	Hydroxypropyl methylcellulose; dextran 70	Benzalkonium Cl 0.01%; edetate disodium 0.05%
Tears Naturale II	Hydroxypropyl methylcellulose 0.3%; dextran 70, 0.1%	Edetate disodium

Modified from Herfindal ET, Gourley DR, Hart LL: *Clinical pharmacy and therapeutics*, ed 5, Baltimore, Md, 1992, Williams & Wilkins.

SCHIØTZ TONOMETRY AND GLAUCOMA

TABLE 3-17.—Schiøtz Tonometry and Glaucoma

Tonometry

Indication Routine exam after age 40 since elevated intraocular pressure (glaucoma) is responsible for 12% of cases of blindness in the United States.

Contraindications Superficial eye infections, corneal edema or damage, uncooperative patients.

Technique (using Schiøtz tonometer)

1. Place patient in a comfortable position, supine, with the face straight upward.
2. Instill one drop of 0.5% proparacaine.
3. While waiting 1 minute for anesthesia, check to see that the 7.5-g weight is in place. Use 5.5-g weight for very soft eyes and 10-g weight for hard eyes (Fig. 3-13).
4. Test tonometer accuracy on metal test block. It should read "0."
5. With patient staring at point on ceiling, gently separate lids with thumb and forefinger applied to orbital rims (Fig. 3-14).
6. Gently place tonometer perpendicularly on center of cornea.
7. Read scale and interpret from Table 3-18. Pressures of 24 mm Hg or higher suggest glaucoma.

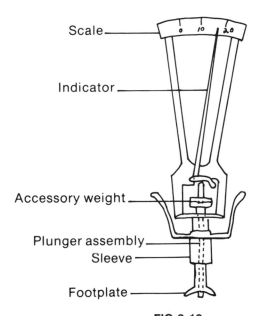

Scale

Indicator

Accessory weight

Plunger assembly

Sleeve

Footplate

FIG 3-13.
Schiøtz tonometer.

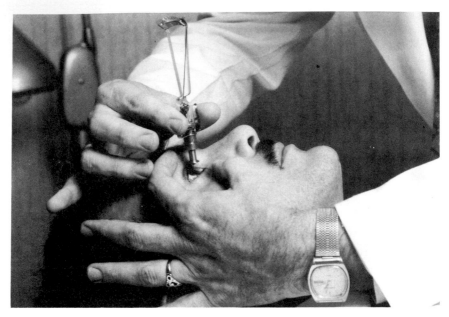

FIG 3-14.
Correct positioning and use of Schiøtz tonometer.

TABLE 3-18.—Calibration Scale for Schiøtz Tonometer

SCALE READING	PLUNGER LOAD (g)			
	5.5	7.5	10.0	15.0
0	41	59	82	127
.5	38	54	75	118
1.0	35	50	70	109
1.5	32	46	64	101
2.0	29	42	59	94
2.5	27	39	55	88
3.0	24	36	51	82
3.5	22	33	47	76
4.0	21	30	43	71
4.5	19	28	40	66
5.0	17	26	37	62
5.5	16	24	34	58
6.0	15	22	32	54
6.5	13	20	29	50
7.0	12	19	27	46
7.5	11	17	25	43
8.0	10	16	23	40
8.5	9	14	21	38
9.0	9	13	20	35
9.5	8	12	18	32
10.0	7	11	16	30
10.5	6	10	15	27
11.0	6	9	14	25
11.5	5	8	13	23
12.0		8	11	21
12.5		7	10	20
13.0		6	10	18
13.5		6	9	17
14.0		5	8	15
14.5			7	14
15.0			6	13
15.5			6	11
16.0			5	10
16.5				9
17.0				8
17.5				8
18.0				7

4 The Ears, Nose, and Throat

Charles W. Smith, Jr.

EXAMINATION TECHNIQUES

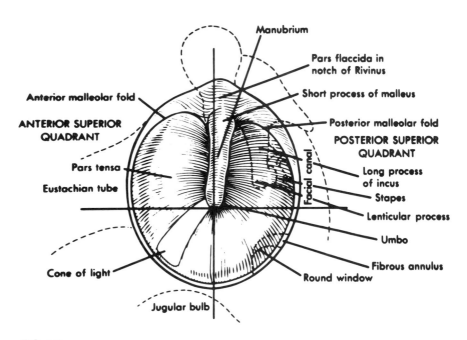

FIG 4-1.
Important middle ear landmarks. (From Miglets A, Saunders WH, Paparella MM: *Atlas of ear surgery,* ed 4, St. Louis, 1986, Mosby.)

Office Hearing Tests

TABLE 4-1.—OFFICE HEARING TESTS

TEST	METHOD	INTERPRETATION
Weber's test	512-Hz tuning fork placed on top of the head; patient is asked which ear tone is heard	*Normal:* sound heard in midline *Conductive loss:* sound heard on affected side *Neurosensory loss:* sound heard on unaffected side
Rinne's test	512-Hz tuning fork held against mastoid; when sound is no longer heard, duration of bone conduction is noted; fork transferred to ½ inch from ear; air conduction should be twice as long as bone and louder	*Air > bone:* normal (+) test *Bone > air:* conductive hearing loss (−) test
Whispered voice	Occlude opposite ear; whisper softly, from 2 feet away. Do not use a question that is answered by "yes" or "no"	Usually indicates 20-dB hearing loss if not perceived.
Watch tick	Hold watch 2 inches from ear	Indicates high frequency loss if not perceived. If heard, there is a 98% chance of hearing all lower frequencies normally.
Schwabach's test	512-Hz tuning fork is pressed alternately to examiner's mastoid then to patient's mastoid	When hearing is normal, both patient and examiner cease to hear the tuning fork at the same time. If patient hears the tuning longer than an examiner with normal hearing, this indicates middle ear (conductive) loss. If examiner with normal hearing hears the tuning longer, the patient has sensorineural loss.

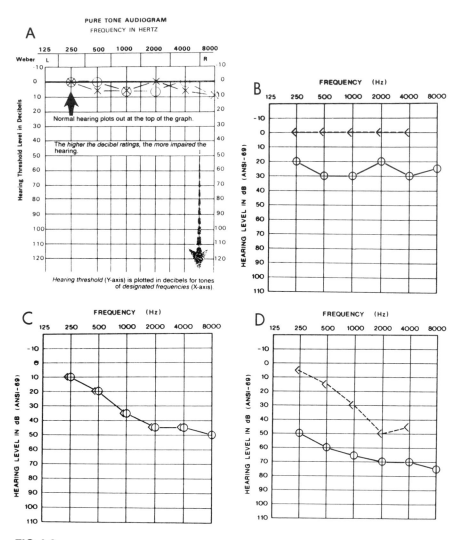

FIG 4-2.
Audiograms. **A,** Normal hearing. **B,** Conductive hearing loss. **C,** Sensorineural hearing loss. **D,** Combined sensorineural and conductive hearing loss. *Air conduction:* O, right; *X,* left. *Bone conduction:* < right; > left. (**A** from Hoffman SR: *Hosp Med;* 20:204, 1984; **B** to **D** from Adams GL, Boies LR, Paparella MM: Audiology. In Boies LR, ed: *Fundamentals of otolaryngology,* ed 5, Philadelphia, 1978, WB Saunders.)

Tympanometry

Tympanometry records the same movements of the tympanic membrane (TM) elicited during pneumatic otoscopy. It records compliance of the TM with pressures varying from -200 to 200 mm Hg.

TABLE 4-2.—TYMPANOMETRY

TYMPANOGRAM PATTERN	INTERPRETATION
Type A	Normal
Type A$_S$	Stiff ossicles (tympanosclerosis)
Type A$_D$	High TM compliance (monomeric TM)
Type B	Middle ear fluid, thickened drum, impacted cerumen
Type C	Retracted TM, eustachian tube dysfunction

From Jerger JJ, Jerger SJ: Measurements of hearing in adults. In Paparella MM, Shumrick DA, eds: *Otolaryngology,* ed 2, vol 2, p 1232, Philadelphia, 1980, WB Saunders Co. Reproduced by permission.

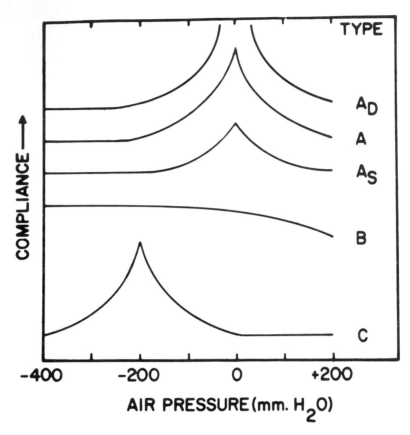

FIG 4-3.
Patterns of tympanograms (see also Table 4-2). (From Jerger JJ, Jerger JS: Measurements of hearing in adults. In Paparella MM, Shumrick DA, eds: *Otolaryngology,* ed 2, Philadelphia, 1980, WB Saunders.)

TABLE 4-3.—Audiometric Testing

TEST	INDICATION	INTERPRETATION
Pure tone audiometry	Persistent abnormality on office hearing screening tests	Conductive, sensorineural, or combined deficit identified
Speech audiometry	Learning disability; poor school performance; evaluation of need for speech therapy	Shows altered speech reception threshold or diminished speech discrimination
Békésy audiogram	Sensorineural hearing loss	Helps differentiate between cochlear and eighth nerve hearing loss
Short Increment Sensitivity Index	Sensorineural hearing loss	Positive in early cochlear disease
Threshold tone decay	Sensorineural hearing loss	Positive in cochlear disease

TABLE 4-4.—Technique of Indirect Mirror Laryngoscopy

Approach should be calm but firm.

Topical anesthetic spray, 5% cocaine or 4% lidocaine, best delivered with a bulb-type atomizer.

May use IV Valium, 5-10 mg, over a 2-minute period if patient gags excessively.

Patient should sit erect with chin forward and feet on floor.

Tongue is held with gauze.

Warm mirror over alcohol lamp to prevent fogging. Test on hand for being too hot.

Hold mirror midway on shaft like a pen.

Place mirror with back side against the uvula.

Ask patient to breathe regularly; if patient gags, ask her or him to "pant like a dog."

Ask patient to say "EEE" so that approximation of the cords can be seen.

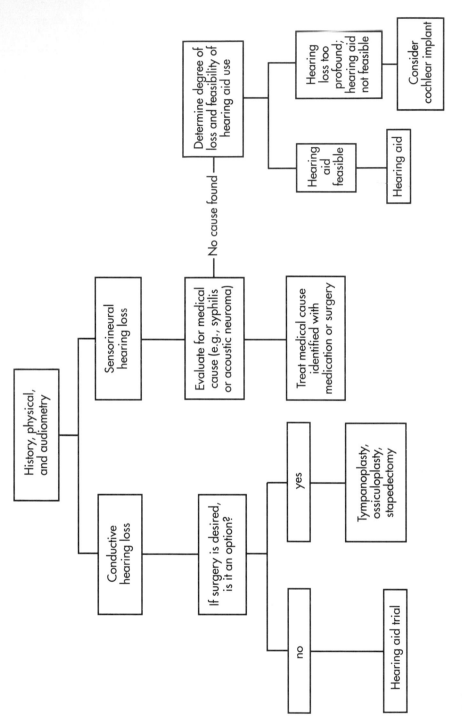

FIG 4-4.
Diagnosis and treatment of hearing loss.

COMMON EAR PROBLEMS

TABLE 4-5.—Usual Bacterial Organisms in Otitis Media

ORGANISM	PERCENT OF CASES
Streptococcus pneumoniae	35
Haemophilus influenzae	25
Moraxella catarrhalis	15
Streptococcus pyogenes	5
Other organisms	5
Sterile aspirates	15

From *Medical Letter* 36(917):19-21, 1994. Drugs for treatment of acute otitis media in children.

TABLE 4-6.—Tympanocentesis Technique

1. Restrain child well.
2. Remove cerumen with irrigation or cerumen spoon.
3. Anesthetize tympanic membrane with 1-2 gtt of 2% Xylocaine.
4. Use 1-ml syringe with 0.2 ml of nonbacteriostatic saline and an 18-gauge, 3½-inch spinal needle. Make a double bend in the needle so that the TM can be visualized.
5. Visualize posteroinferior portion of the TM with the otoscope.
6. Perforate the TM with the needle and apply brief negative pressure.
7. Send one drop for culture and one drop for Gram stain. Place one drop each on blood and chocolate agar plates. Place remainder in thioglycolate broth.

Modified from Johnson KB: *The Harriet Lane handbook,* ed 13, St. Louis, 1993, Mosby.

Outcomes of Treating Otitis Media with Effusion*

Table 4-7 summarizes the benefits and harms identified for management interventions in the target child with otitis media with effusion.

*The target patient is an otherwise healthy child age 1 through 3 years with no craniofacial or neurological abnormalities or sensory deficits.

TABLE 4-7.—Benefits and Harms Associated with Treatment
of Otitis Media with Effusion in Children

INTERVENTION	BENEFITS*	HARMS*
Observation	Base case	Base case
Antibiotics	Improved clearance of effusion at 1 month or less, 14.0% (95% CI [3.6%, 24.2%]) Possible reduction in future infections	Nausea, vomiting, diarrhea (2%-32% depending on dose and antibiotic) Cutaneous reactions ($\leq$5%) Numerous rare organ system effects, including very rare fatalities Cost Possible development of resistant strains of bacteria
Antibiotics plus steroids	Possible improved clearance at 1 month, 25.1% (95% CI [-1.3%, 49.9%])† Possible reduction in future infections	See antibiotics and steroids separately

From *Otitis media with effusion: clinical practice guideline,* Pub #94-0623, Washington, D.C., July 1994, U.S. Dept of Health & Human Services.

*Outcomes are reported as differences from observation, which is treated as the base case. When possible, metaanalysis was performed to provide a mean and associated confidence interval (CI).

†Difference from base case not statistically significant.

TABLE 4-7.—Benefits and Harms Associated with Treatment
of Otitis Media with Effusion in Children—cont'd

INTERVENTION	BENEFITS*	HARMS*
Steroids alone	Possible improved clearance at 1 month, 4.5% (95% CI [−11.7%, 20.6%])†	Possible exacerbation of varicella Long-term complications not established for low doses Cost
Antihistamine/ decongestant	Same as base case	Drowsiness and/or excitability‡ Cost
Myringotomy with tubes	Immediate clearance of effusion in all children Improved hearing	Invasive procedure Anesthesia risk Cost Tympanosclerosis Otorrhea Possible restrictions on swimming
Adenoidectomy	Benefits for young children have not been established	Invasive procedure‡ Anesthesia risk Cost
Tonsillectomy	Same as base case	Invasive procedure‡ Anesthesia risk Cost

‡Risks were not examined in detail because no benefits were identified.

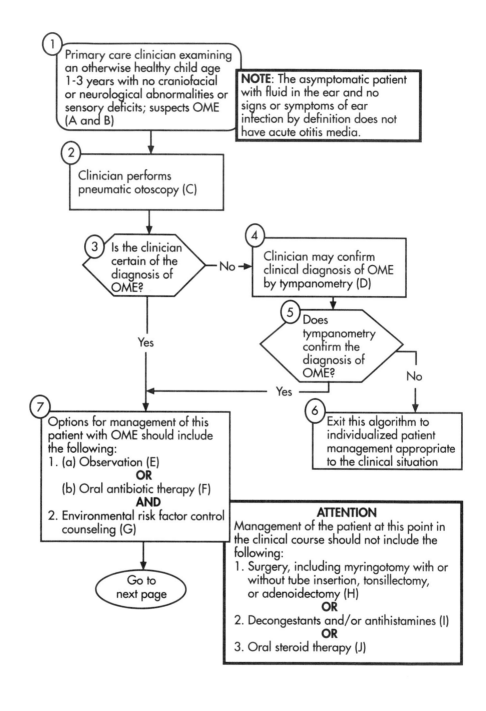

FIG 4-5.

Algorithm for managing otitis media with effusion in an otherwise healthy child age 1 to 3 years. **A,** Otitis media with effusion (OME) is defined as *fluid in the middle ear without signs or symptoms of infection.* OME is not to be confused with acute otitis media (inflammation of the middle ear with signs of infection). The Guideline (see Table 4-7 footnote) and this algorithm apply only to the child with otitis media with effusion. This algorithm assumes follow-up intervals of 6 weeks. **B,** The algorithm applies only to a child age 1 to 3 years with no craniofacial or neurological abnormalities or sensory deficits (except as noted) who is healthy except for otitis media with effusion. The Guideline recommendations and algorithm do not apply if the child has any craniofacial or neurological abnormality (e.g., cleft palate or mental retardation) or sensory deficit (e.g., decreased visual acuity or preexisting hearing deficit). **C,** There is found some evidence that pneumatic otoscopy is more accurate than otoscopy performed without the pneumatic test of eardrum mobility. **D,** Tympanometry may be used as confirmation of pneumatic otoscopy in the diagnosis of OME. Hearing evaluation is recommended for the otherwise healthy child who has had bilateral OME for 3 months; before 3 months, hearing evaluation is a clinical option. **E,** In most cases, OME resolves spontaneously within 3 months. **F,** The antibiotic drugs studied for treatment of OME were amoxicillin, amoxicillin-clavulanate potassium, cefaclor, erythromycin, erythromycin-sulfisoxazole, sulfisoxazole, and trimethoprim-sulfamethoxazole. **G,** Exposure to cigarette smoke (passive smoking) has been shown to increase the risk of OME. For bottle-feeding versus breast-feeding and for child-care facility placement, associations were found with OME, but evidence did not show decreased incidence of OME with breast-feeding or with removal from child-care facilities. **H,** The recommendation against tonsillectomy is based on the lack of added benefit from tonsillectomy when combined with adenoidectomy to treat OME in older children. Tonsillectomy and adenoidectomy may be appropriate for reasons other than OME. **I,** The Panel found evidence that decongestants and/or antihistamines are ineffective treatments for OME. **J,** Metaanalysis failed to show a significant benefit for steroid medications without antibiotic medications in treating OME in children.   *Continued.*

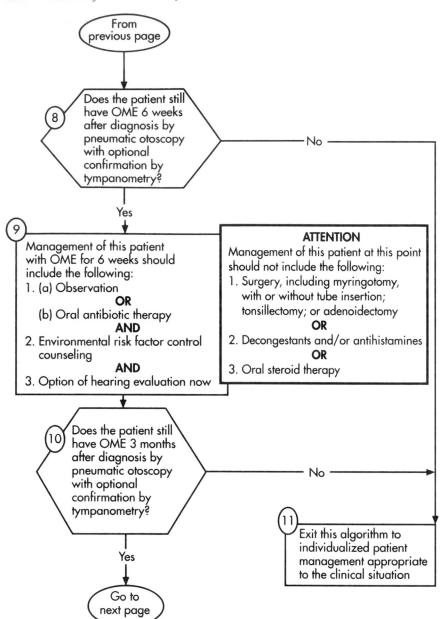

FIG 4-5, *cont'd.*

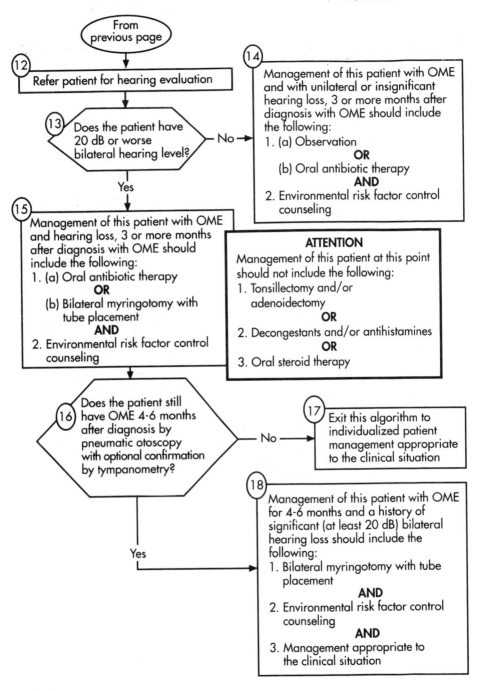

FIG 4-5, *cont'd.*

TABLE 4-8.—Antibiotic Dosing and Cost for Upper Respiratory Tract Infections in Pediatric Patients

ANTIBIOTIC	TOTAL DAILY DOSE	DOSING FREQUENCY (HOURS)	COST*
Amoxicillin	30-50 mg/kg	8	$ 6.03
Amoxicillin-clavulanate (Augmentin)	30-40 mg/kg	8	$46.40
Penicillin V	50 mg/kg	6-8 (On empty stomach)	$ 4.20
Cefaclor (Ceclor)	40 mg/kg	8	$49.69
Cefixime (Suprax)	8 mg/kg	8-12	$54.74
Cefpodoxime (Vantin)	10 mg/kg	12 (With food)	$54.00
Loracarbef (Lorabid)	15-30 mg/kg†	12 (On empty stomach)	$48.68
Erythromycin-sulfixoxazole (Pediazole)‡	40-50 mg/kg of erythromycin	8	$23.24
Erythromycin Ethylsuc-cinate (EES)	50-80 mg/kg§	6-8	$15.42
TMP-SMX (Bactrim‡)	8 mg/kg (TMP) 40 mg/kg (SMX)	12	$ 4.49

*Cost is based on a 10-day course in a 20-kg child, calculated by the average wholesale price (Redbook, 1993). Costs are approximate and based on generic prices where available.

†Dosage not established for children less than 6 months of age.

‡Contraindicated in children less than 2 months of age.

§400 mg of the ethylsuccinate is equivalent to 250 mg of erythromycin base and higher doses must be used.

SINUSITIS AND LARYNGITIS

TABLE 4-9.—CLINICAL EVALUATION AND TREATMENT OF SINUSITIS

I. Best Predictors of the Presence of Sinusitis include:
1. Maxillary toothache
2. Poor response to nasal decongestants
3. Abnormal transillumination
4. Colored nasal discharge by history
5. Colored nasal discharge by exam
All five present, likelihood ratio = 6.4
None present = Sinusitis virtually ruled out

II. Most Common Organisms Causing Acute Sinusitis†

Organism	Frequency (%)
Streptococcus pneumoniae	36
Haemophilus influenzae	27
Moraxella catarrhalis	2-23 (more common in children)
Streptococcus pyogenes	5
α-Hemolytic streptococcus	5
Staphylococcus aureus	4

III. Differential Diagnosis of Nasal Congestion/Rhinorrhea*
Allergic rhinitis
Vasomotor rhinitis
Rhinitis medicamentosa
Mechanical obstruction of nasal airway
Chronic inflammatory condition (e.g. sarcoid)
Acute viral infection
Acute or chronic bacterial sinusitis

IV. Treatment of Sinusitis
1. Antibiotic treatment with ampicillin or amoxicillin for 14 days.
2. If the response to number 1 is inadequate, try amoxicillin/clavulanate, erythromycin/sulfisoxazole, cefaclor, cefixime, or cefuroxime axetil.
3. If chronic, and choices 1 and 2 are not working well, give patient a course of clindamycin, directed at anaerobic bacteria.
4. Use topical decongestants (e.g. xylometazoline HCl 0.1%, every 3-4 hours for no more than 4 or 5 days.
5. Use systemic decongestants (e.g. pseudoephedrinc HCl 60 mg qid).
6. Elevate head of bed 20 degrees to promote drainage.
7. Consider use of nasal corticosteroid spray such as beclomethasone or flunisolide.

*From Williams JW, Simel DL: Does this patient have sinusitis? Diagnosing acute sinusitis by history and physical examination, *JAMA* 270(10):1242, 1993.
†From Stafford CH: Successful medical management of sinusitis. Clinical Focus, A Medical Education Supplement to *Patient Care,* p. 19, Dec., 1994.

TABLE 4-10.—Epiglottitis Versus Croup: Comparative Clinical Features

VARIABLE	EPIGLOTTITIS	CROUP
Age	Usually 3 to 7 years	Less than 3 years
Seasonal occurrence	Anytime	Spring or fall
Organism	*H. influenzae,* type B	Parainfluenza virus
Clinical course	Rapidly progressive	Slow
Presentation	Toxic appearance, sits up to breathe easier	Lies supine, not acutely ill, barking cough
Dysphagia	Usually marked, drools	None present
Fever	>103° F	<103° F
Stridor	Rare	Frequent
White blood count	>18,000	Usually normal
Treatment	IV antibiotics, intubate	Cool mist, racemic epinephrine
Recurrence	Rare	Common

Adapted from DiPiro, JT et al: *Pharmacotherapy: a physiologic approach,* ed 2, Appleton and Lange, 1993, Norwalk, Conn., p. 1574.

DIZZINESS AND VERTIGO

Dizziness must be differentiated from true vertigo. *Dizziness* is a disturbed sense of relationship to space. *Vertigo* is a sensation of whirling or turning in space.

TABLE 4-11.—Dizziness and Vertigo

Causes of Dizziness
Ocular muscle imbalance
Refractive error
Glaucoma
Proprioceptive defect (e.g., tabes dorsalis)
Mild CNS anoxia (e.g., atherosclerosis, anemia)
CNS infection
Trauma
CNS tumor
Migraine
Petit mal epilepsy
Endocrine lesion (e.g., hypoglycemia)
Functional

Causes of Vertigo
  Central (brain, spinal tract, or nuclear lesion)
CNS infection
Trauma
CNS hemorrhage
Posterior/inferior cerebellar artery thrombus
CNS tumor
Multiple sclerosis
  Peripheral (lesion in external, middle, or inner ear, or along eighth nerve)
Wax or foreign body in canal
Otitis media or serous otitis media
Labyrinthitis
Cholesteatoma
Trauma with middle ear hemorrhage
Lesion in vestibular vessels
Ménière's disease
Motion sickness
Postural vertigo
Eighth nerve infection
Meningitic involvement of eighth nerve
Acoustic neuroma

Evaluation of Vertigo
Perform positional test by observing for nystagmus after placing the patient in
  the following positions:
1. Upright position
2. Recumbent position with left ear down
3. Recumbent with right ear down
4. Head hanging, pointing at the floor
Observe for latency of onset of nystagmus, fatigability (sustained or brief), any
  directional change with positional change, and any unexpected types, considering the position of the patient.
Perform caloric tests (see below for technique).
Refer for audiography, electronystagmography (ENG), and intraauditory canal
  tomography and/or CT scanning, if indicated.
Refer for otolaryngological evaluation if cause is still undetermined.

Caloric Testing
Inject 5 ml of ice water over 5 seconds at posteroinferior quadrant of TM.
Observe for nystagmus, nausea, and vertigo.
If no response, increase to 10 ml and then to 20 ml.
If no response, vestibular apparatus is not functioning.

TABLE 4-12.—Comparative Characteristics of Central and Peripheral Vestibular Disease

CENTRAL VESTIBULAR DISEASE	PERIPHERAL VESTIBULAR DISEASE
Insidious onset	Sudden onset
Continuous episode	Intermittent episodes
Duration—months	Duration—seconds, minutes, or, at most, a few days
Mild disequilibrium	True vertigo and intense disequilibrium during episodes
Little aggravation with head motion	Marked aggravation with head motion
Absence of associated unilateral auditory phenomena	Auditory phenomena (fullness, unilateral hearing loss, and tinnitus)
Presence of other neurological or vascular signs and symptoms	Absence of other neurological signs and symptoms
Positional nystagmus: immediate onset, no fatigue, does not adapt, direction changing with different head positions	*Positional nystagmus:* latent period, fatigue, adapts, direction fixed or changing
Spontaneous nystagmus: horizontal, rotary, or vertical	*Spontaneous nystagmus:* horizontal, rotary, not vertical
Caloric reaction: normal, perverted, or dissociated, rarely hypoactive	*Caloric reaction:* normal or hypoactive, not perverted or dissociated

From DeWeese DD, Saunders WH: *Textbook of otolaryngology,* ed 6, St Louis, 1982, Mosby.

TABLE 4-13.—Comparative Characteristics of Central and Peripheral Spontaneous Nystagmus

FEATURE	PERIPHERAL	CENTRAL
Form	Horizontal/rotary	Horizontal, vertical, diagonal rotatory, multiple, pendular, alternating
Frequency	0.05 to 6 times/second	Any frequency, usually low or variable, of long intervals (weeks to months)
Intensity	Decreasing intensity	Constant
Direction of fast component	Toward "stimulated" labyrinth or away from "destroyed" labyrinth	Toward side of CNS lesion
Duration	Minutes to weeks	Weeks to months
Dissociation between eyes	None	Possible
Unidirectional	Present	Seldom present
Multidirectional	Seldom present	Present
Past pointing and falling	Direction of slow phase	Direction of fast phase

From DeWeese DD, Saunders WH: *Textbook of otolaryngology,* ed 6, St Louis, 1982, Mosby.

TEMPOROMANDIBULAR JOINT SYNDROME

Temporomandibular joint (TMJ) syndrome is a condition of dysfunction and pain related to the TMJ and its articulating tissues.

TABLE 4-14.—TEMPOROMANDIBULAR JOINT SYNDROME

TMJ is characterized by the following:
Unilateral dull aching pain
Gradual onset
Worsened by chewing
Crepitation and clicks in the TMJ
Facial muscle tenderness/spasm
Bruxism
Deviation of jaw
Pain on wide opening and on closure
Women affected 4:1

Treatment Approaches
Eliminate muscle tenderness and pain with physical therapy (heat, ultrasound, cryotherapy, local anesthetic, topical anesthetic)
Eliminate occlusal problems with orthopedic repositioning device (bite block); may require dental referral
Attempt to eliminate bruxism
Exercises designed to stretch and strengthen oral muscles
Attention to associated tension and stress
Systemic therapy if indicated for pain or arthritis

CHRONIC RHINITIS

TABLE 4-15.—ANTIHISTAMINES FOR ALLERGIC RHINITIS

DRUG	DOSAGE	SEDATIVE EFFECTS	COST PER MONTH	COMMENTS
Chlorpheniramine (generic)	4-8 mg hs then slowly titrate to 16-28 mg daily (low doses can be given hs, higher doses twice daily)	++	$2.46 (based on 20 mg daily)	Start the titration several weeks before the anticipated season to minimize drowsiness and maximize efficacy
Diphenhydramine	25-50 mg every 8 hours	+++	$4.00 (50 mg tid)	
Clemastine (Tavist)	1.34-2.68 mg every 12 hours	++	$54.40 (2.68 mg bid)	
Astemizole (Hismanal)	10 mg once daily on an empty stomach (safety and dosing not established in children <12 years)	±	$47.76	Ventricular arrythmias and torsades de pointes have occurred when the recommended dose is exceeded, with hepatic impairment or drug interactions (erythromycin, ketoconazole, or itraconazole), and these are contraindicated with astemizole

| Loratidine (Claritin) | 10 mg once daily on an empty stomach (safety and dosing not established in children <12 years) | ± | $53.17 | |
| Terfenadine (Seldane) | Adults: 60 mg every 12 hours; 6-12 years: 30-60 mg every 12 hours; 3-6 years: 15 mg every 12 hours | ± | $51.37 | Ventricular arrythmias and torsades de pointes have occurred when the recommended dose is exceeded, with hepatic impairment or drug interactions (erythromycin, ketoconazole, or itraconazole) and these are contraindicated with terfenadine |

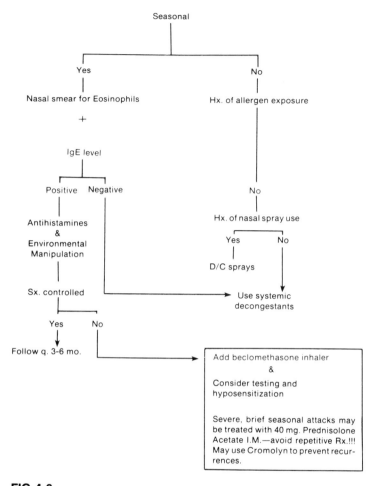

FIG 4-6.
Evaluation and treatment of chronic rhinitis.

EPISTAXIS

TABLE 4-16.—TECHNIQUE OF POSTERIOR PACKING

1. Insert a small rubber catheter through the nose. Clasp, and pull from nasopharynx through oropharynx with Kelly clamp.
2. Roll a 4 × 4 and tie two 8-inch and one 3-inch lengths of 3—0 silk suture to the middle of the roll. Apply vaseline to gauze pad.
3. Attach two of the ties to the catheter.
4. Pull the catheter and the pad back through the nose, placing the pad, if necessary, with the index finger.
5. Fix by tying two sutures around another 4 × 4 placed across the nares.
6. The third, shorter string hangs from the nasopharynx for removal of the pack in 48 hours.
7. Anterior pack may then be placed if bleeding continues.

Materials for Epistaxis Management and Nasal Packing (Fig. 4-7)
Head mirror
Nasal speculum
Suction equipment
Tongue blades
Cotton balls
Lidocaine with epinephrine (1 : 1000)
Bayonet forceps
Silver nitrate sticks
Scissors
Vaseline gauze (½ inch)
Cotton-tipped applicators
Kelly clamp
Posterior packs or Epistat catheter (Xomed, Inc.)
Gauze pads (4 × 4 inches)
Long, 25-gauge needle
5-ml syringe
Cetacaine spray

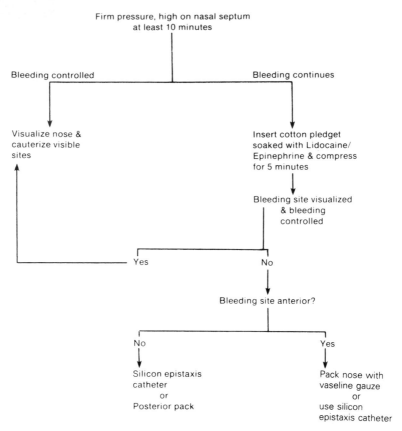

FIG 4-7.
Management of epistaxis.

EMERGENCY AIRWAY

TABLE 4-17.—CRICOTHYROTOMY

1. Place patient supine with support under shoulders and neck hyperextended.
2. Palpate space between thyroid and cricoid cartilage.
3. Make horizontal incision about 1 inch wide over this space (cricothyroid membrane).
4. Bluntly dissect tissues down to membrane.
5. Make 1-cm incision through CT membrane.
6. Insert flat instrument (e.g., scalpel handle) through incision and rotate 90 degrees to hold incision open.
7. If available, insert small tube through incision.
8. As soon as possible, convert cricothyrotomy to standard tracheostomy.

TONSILLITIS

TABLE 4-18.—Using Clinical Findings to Estimate the Probability of Group A Streptococcal Isolation in Adult Patients

CLINICAL FINDINGS	PROBABILITY OF POSITIVE CULTURE (%)	PROBABILITY OF POSITIVE CULTURE AND ANTIBODY RISE (%)	RECOMMENDED ACTION
Temperature <37.8° C (100° F) *and* no tonsillar exudate *and* no anterior cervical adenitis	3.4	0.4	No culture, no treatment. A false-positive culture could lead to unnecessary and potentially risky treatment.
Temperature >37.8° C (100° F) *or* tonsillar exudate *or* anterior cervical adenitis	13.5	5.6	Culture, and treat patients with positive cultures.
Temperature >37.8° C (100° F) *and* tonsillar exudate *and* anterior cervical adenitis	42.1	16.5	Treat immediately. A false-negative culture could prevent necessary treatment.
Special "Risk Factors" Past history of acute rheumatic fever, *or* Documented strep exposure in past week, *or* Known strep epidemic in community, *or* Patient is diabetic or otherwise immunocompromised, *or* Patient has scarlatiniform rash			Treat immediately. Patient is at special risk from strep throat.

From Komaroff AL et al: *J Gen Intern Med* 1:1, 1986.

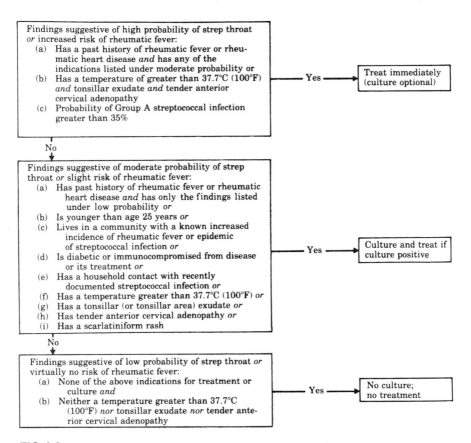

FIG 4-8.
Algorithm describing an evaluation of the probability of group A streptococcal pharyngitis and the risk of developing acute rheumatic fever. NOTE: Rapid (10-minute) strep test may be substituted for culture. Immediate treatment is preferred for those individuals whose throat culture results will not be complete for 9 days into the illness (since treatment after that time has not been shown to be protective against rheumatic fever). (From Komaroff AL: Coryza, pharyngitis, and related infections in adults. In Branch WT, ed: *Office practice of medicine,* ed 2, Philadelphia, 1987, WB Saunders.)

TABLE 4-19.—INDICATIONS FOR TONSILLECTOMY

ABSOLUTE	RELATIVE	NOT INDICATED OR CONTRAINDICATED
Cor pulmonale secondary to tonsillar airway obstruction Pharyngeal or peritonsillar abscess Hypertrophy causing dysphagia and weight loss Suspected malignancy	Recurrent tonsillitis documented more than 3 times/year Tonsillar hyperplasia causing some obstruction to swallowing Residual hyperplasia following mononucleosis History of rheumatic fever with heart damage associated with recurrent tonsillitis	Colds Focal infection Fever of unknown origin Cervical adenopathy Enlarged tonsils (unless there are obstructive symptoms) Allergic rhinitis Asthma

Normal lymphatics and glandular cervical structures

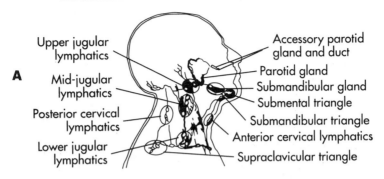

A

Upper jugular lymphatics
Mid-jugular lymphatics
Posterior cervical lymphatics
Lower jugular lymphatics

Accessory parotid gland and duct
Parotid gland
Submandibular gland
Submental triangle
Submandibular triangle
Anterior cervical lymphatics
Supraclavicular triangle

Sites of origin of cervical nodal metastases

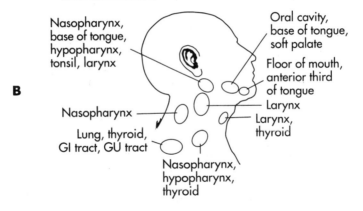

B

Nasopharynx, base of tongue, hypopharynx, tonsil, larynx

Nasopharynx

Lung, thyroid, GI tract, GU tract

Oral cavity, base of tongue, soft palate
Floor of mouth, anterior third of tongue
Larynx
Larynx, thyroid

Nasopharynx, hypopharynx, thyroid

FIG 4-9.
A, Head and neck lymphatics. (From Fried MP: Evaluation of the adult neck mass, *Med Times* 110(1):101, 1982.) **B,** Site of origin of cervical nodal metastases. (From Fried MP: Evaluation of the adult neck mass, *Med Times* 110(1):101, 1982.)

5 *Gynecological Care*

Charles E. Driscoll

PEDIATRIC AND ADOLESCENT GYNECOLOGY

TABLE 5-1.—FETAL DEVELOPMENT

Intrauterine sexual development of the fetus is responsible for most early gynecological disorders in children. Genital structures arise as follows:

Gonad	Derived from	Differentiation
Internal	Genital ridge	6-7 weeks
External	Genital tubercle	10-12 weeks

The genital system is susceptible to teratogens from 26 to 46 days after conception. Careful examination of the neonate is necessary before the parents are informed of the child's sex. If ambiguity exists, tell the parents: "Like a cleft lip, the external sex organ is unfinished. The child will need further laboratory testing to decide what is needed to finish the development." Assign sex only after genetic studies and surgical planning have been completed.

TABLE 5-2.—GYNECOLOGICAL EXAMINATION OF THE NEWBORN AND INFANT

Inspect external genitalia and palpate inguinal areas of abdomen.
Pass soft, neonate feeding catheter through introitus to check patency.
Rectal examination for adnexal mass and palpation of uterus (4 cm length of newborn is larger than at 9 years old secondary to estrogen stimulation in utero).
To visualize vagina and cervix, a veterinarian's otoscope speculum may be used (vagina 4 cm at birth).

TABLE 5-3.—GYNECOLOGICAL CONDITIONS OF THE INFANT

CONDITION	ETIOLOGY	DIAGNOSIS	TREATMENT	PROGNOSIS
Labial agglutination	Congenital or inflammatory process with adhesions	Visible adhesion of labia, thin livid line; vaginal orifice, usually partially patent	Topical estrogen cream bid for 7-14 days	Normal, may recur
Vaginal bleeding age 3-5 days	Withdrawal of placental estrogens	Normal examination; bleeding stops spontaneously	None; reassurance	Normal
Urethral prolapse	?	Painful, friable mass at vaginal orifice; catheter inserted in center of mass enters bladder	Topically applied estrogen and antibiotic creams; surgical excision if medical therapy fails	Fertile
Adrenal virilization (pseudohermaphroditism)	Inborn error of cortisol metabolism (1/15,000 births)	Labial fusion, clitoral enlargement, uterus palpable; buccal chromatin-positive; elevated urinary 17-ketosteroids and pregnanetriol; check electrolytes	Cortisone; surgical excision of large clitoris, reconstruct vagina; estrogens at puberty	Sterile
Nonadrenal virilization	Maternal progestins taken before 12 weeks and up to 16 weeks	Labial fusion, clitoral enlargement, uterus palpable; buccal chromatin-positive; normal urinary 17-ketosteroids and pregnanetriol, history of progestins to mother	Reassurance, surgical correction of fused labia and clitoral enlargement before age 3; no hormone therapy	Fertile

Continued.

TABLE 5-3.—Gynecological Conditions of the Infant—cont'd

CONDITION	ETIOLOGY	DIAGNOSIS	TREATMENT	PROGNOSIS
Vaginal atresia	Dysplasia or aplasia of müllerian ducts	Absent uterus on palpation, no vaginal orifice, may have associated urinary tract anomaly	Emergency urinary drainage, surgical vaginal construction	Sterile
Gonadal agenesis	21 Different abnormal chromosome complements associated (1/2500 births)	Edema of hands and feet of newborn; somatic anomalies (low hairline, low-set ears cubitus valgus, growth failure, high palate); abnormal karyotype	Surgical removal of ovarian streaks if Y chromosome is present to prevent malignancy; estrogens to develop secondary sex characteristics	Sterile
Testicular feminization	Congenital insensitivity to androgens, familial tendency	Girl with inguinal "hernias," blind vaginal pouch, absent uterus; buccal chromatin-negative; 46 XY; primary amenorrhea	Surgical removal of testes, hormone therapy with estrogens, female sex assigned	Sterile
True hermaphroditism	Ovotestis develops often in absence of Y chromosome (rare)	Hypospadic, small phallus; small vagina; gonads may be palpable in labial or scrotal folds; buccal chromatin-positive	Gonads excised to prevent dysgerminoma, surgical sex assignment carried out, hormones for secondary sex characteristics	Sterile

Pediatric Vulvovaginitis

Perhaps the most common gynecological problem in childhood (85%-90%) is vulvovaginitis. Treatment without an examination is a dangerous practice because the symptoms are similar to those of urinary tract infections (itching, burning, dysuria, discharge).

The presence of *Trichomonas*, gonorrhea, or *Chlamydia* may imply sexual abuse.

TABLE 5-4.—PEDIATRIC VULVOVAGINITIS

General Rules:
Perform examination, cultures, vaginal smears, and urinalysis.
Vaginal pH should be 7.0-8.0 in children and 5-5.5 in adolescents.
Foreign bodies cause about 5% of cases.
Teach perineal hygiene, wiping front to back.
About 20% of cases will resolve with sitz baths and good hygiene.
When pus or *Trichomonas* is present, think of gonorrhea and *Chlamydia.*
If a bloody vaginal discharge is present *without* a foreign body, think of
    β-streptococcal infection (indications may include recent respiratory or skin
    infection).
Topical estrogen cream for 5-6 days speeds resolution.
Look for pinworms.

TABLE 5-5.—TREATMENT FOR SPECIFIC CAUSES OF PEDIATRIC VAGINITIS

Candida	Miconazole nitrate vaginal cream* nightly for 7-14 nights
Gardnerella vaginalis or *Trichomonas*	Metronidazole, 35-50 mg/kg/day, in 3 doses, for 7 days
Gonorrhea	If less than 45 kg, ceftriaxone 125 mg IM 1×. Children ≥8 years of age should also receive doxycycline, 100 mg PO bid × 7 days. Children ≥45 kg: use adult regimen.
Pinworms	One mebendazole 100-mg tablet PO
β-Streptococcus	Penicillin G, 200,000 units orally qid for 10 days

*When vaginal infections of children require placement of intravaginal medication (miconazole, estrogen, etc.), use a 10-ml syringe with butterfly IV tubing (needle removed) attached.

TABLE 5-6.—Chickenpox Vulvitis

Pain and itching: Cold compresses, Burow's solution soaks, baking soda, or oatmeal baths. Hydroxyzine HCl 15 mg PO tid may be given.
Urinary retention: Sit in tub of warm water to urinate or apply small amounts of Xylocaine jelly topically.
Infection: Topical Betadine solution diluted 1:4 with water.

TABLE 5-7.—Acute Adolescent Menorrhagia

Bleeding moderate, hemoglobin > 10 g/dl	Observe, evaluate for cause, and follow-up Oral iron supplements Rule out chronic illness, coagulation disorder, pregnancy, and clear cell adenocarcinoma Oral contraceptive 30-50 μg of estrogen one qid × 2 d then low dose oral contraceptives may be prescribed for 3 or 4 months

Bleeding severe, hemoglobin ≤10 g/dl	*Admit to hospital:*
	1. Initial hemostasis
	   Conjugated estrogens, 25-40 mg IV every 4 hours (maximum 6 doses)
	   Progestin (norethindrone acetate), 5 mg every 6 hours orally
	   If still bleeding heavily after 24 hours, examine under anesthesia and perform D & C
	2. Cyclic regulation of menses
	   Concurrent oral administration of estrogen-progestin (norethindrone/mestranol 0.05 mg), 2 tablets stat and 1 every 6 hours, tapered over 3 weeks to usual dose of 1 tablet daily
	   Follow with 3 months of cyclic therapy with conventional low-dose combination oral contraceptive (35-50 μg of estrogen)
	3. Long-term observation, reevaluate at regular intervals
	   5% of patients will never ovulate

Modified from Altchek A: Dysfunctional uterine bleeding in the adolescent, *The Female Patient* 18:45, 1993.

Tanner

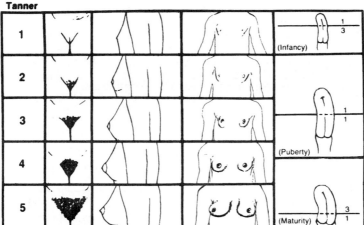

	Pubic Hair		Breast

Pubic Hair

1 Infantile pattern. No true pubic hair present, although there may be a fine downy hair distribution.
2 Sparse growth of lightly pigmented hair, longer than the fine down of the previous stage, appearing on the mons or the labia.
3 The pubic hair becomes darker, coarser, and curlier. Distribution is still minimal.
4 The pubic hair is adult in character, but not yet as widely distributed as in most adults.
5 The pubic hair is distributed in the typical adult female pattern, forming an inverse triangle.

Breast

1 Infantile or childhood pattern.
2 Early pubertal breast development, sometimes referred to as a "breast bud." A small mound of breast tissue causes a visible elevation.
3 The areola and the breast undergo more definite pronouncement in size, with a continuous rounded contour.
4 The areola and nipple enlarge further and form a secondary mound projecting above the contour of the remainder of the breast.
5 The adult breast stage. The secondary mound visible in the preceding stage has now blended into a smooth contour of the breast.

FIG 5-1.

Sexual maturation of girl may be assessed using the normal appearance of the external genitalia as described by Tanner and the usual expected sequence and tempo.

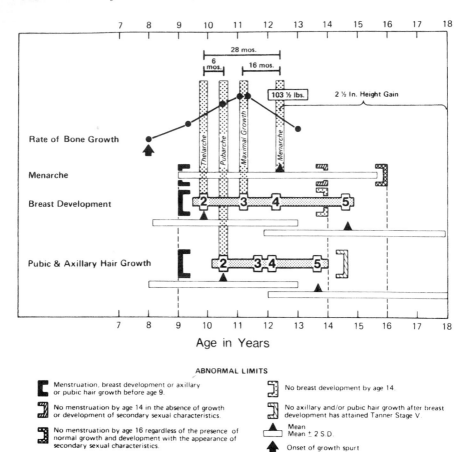

FIG 5-2.
Expected sequence and tempo of sexual development. Numbers in boxes represent Tanner's stages. (From Robie GF Jr: Pediatric gynecology. In Duenholter JH, ed: *Greenhill's office gynecology,* ed 10, Chicago, 1983, Mosby.)

TABLE 5-8.—SIGNS OF SEXUAL ABUSE IN THE PREPUBERTAL GIRL

FINDINGS IN ACUTE SEXUAL ABUSE	FINDINGS IN CHRONIC SEXUAL ABUSE
Perineal contusions	Multiple healed hymenal transections
Perihymenal erythema, swelling, petechiae	Rounded hymenal remnants, synechiae
Abrasions, avulsions, lacerations	Spacious introitus ≥ 4 mm (≥ age 5 years)
Spasm of pubococcygeus muscle	
Seminal products	Fourchette-hymenal lacerations, scarring, neovascularization
Tense rectal sphincter	
Anal fissures	Capacity to relax pubococcygeus muscle
Rectal-perianal contusions or ecchymoses	Leukorrhea, vaginitis, cervicitis
Perianal edema	Anal fissures, scarring, skin tags, pigmentation
	Reflex relaxation of the anal sphincter
	Laxity of vaginal-pubococcygeal muscles

From Abrams ME, Shah RZ, Keenan-Allyn S: *The Female Patient* 13:17, 1988.

CONTRACEPTION

TABLE 5-9.—RELATIVE EFFECTIVENESS OF VARIOUS METHODS OF CONTRACEPTION

METHOD	EFFECTIVENESS*
Hysterectomy	0.0001
Abortion	0.01
Vasectomy	0.02
Tubal ligation	0.13
Oral contraceptives†	0.25
Progestin injection	0.35
Progestin implants	0.5
Progestin alone, oral	1.2
Intrauterine device (copper or progestin)	1.4
Foam and condom	1.5
Diaphragm and jelly	1.9
Female condom (sheath)	2.6
Cervical cap	3-5
Condom	3.6
Foam or jelly alone	11.9
Symptothermal method	22
Coitus interruptus	15-23
Calendar rhythm method	25-40
Chance	80

Modified from Romney SL, Gray MJ, Little AB, et al: *Gynecology and obstetrics: the health care of women,* ed 2, New York, 1981, McGraw-Hill, p. 820, and Mishell DR: *N Engl J Med* 320:777, 1989 (Revised 1994).

*Expressed as pregnancy rate per 100 woman-years.

†Medications may interfere with oral contraceptive effectiveness. Patients taking anticonvulsants, antibiotics, and tranquilizers should consider using additional contraceptive protection (e.g., condoms or spermicide).

TABLE 5-10.—CONTRAINDICATIONS TO ORAL CONTRACEPTIVE USE

Absolute Contraindications
Pregnancy
Breast cancer
Undiagnosed vaginal bleeding
Estrogen-dependent neoplasia
History of or active thromboembolic disorder
History of or active cardiovascular or cerebrovascular disease
Acute or chronic liver disease

Relative Contraindications
Hypertension
Hyperlipidemia
Diabetes mellitus
Lactation
Epilepsy
Pituitary dysfunction
Smoking > 15 cigarettes/day
Age > 35 years
Sickle cell disease
Migraine headaches
Raynaud's disease
Collagen vascular disease
Porphyria
Bleeding diatheses
Retinal disease
Active inflammatory bowel disease
Dermatological disorders (erythema nodosum, melasma)
Cholelithiasis

TABLE 5-11.—LABORATORY TESTS AFFECTED BY ORAL CONTRACEPTIVES

A. Values that are increased (serum values, unless otherwise stated)
1. Erythrocyte sedimentation rate (sometimes the hematocrit, white blood count, and platelets)
2. Serum iron and iron-binding capacity
3. Sulfobromophthalein and sometimes bilirubin
4. Serum glutamic oxaloacetic transaminase, serum glutamic pyruvic transaminase, and serum γ-glutamyl transpeptidase
5. Alkaline phosphatase
6. Clotting factors I, II, VII, VIII, IX, X, and XII; also increased antiplasmins and antiactivators of fibrinolysis
7. Triglycerides, phospholipids, and high-density lipoproteins (sometimes serum cholesterol)

From Greydanus DE: *Semin Perinatol* 5:53, 1981.

Continued.

TABLE 5-11.—LABORATORY TESTS AFFECTED BY ORAL CONTRACEPTIVES—cont'd

8. Serum copper and ceruloplasmin
9. Increase in various binding proteins (transferrin, transcortin, thyroxine-binding globulin)
10. Renin, angiotensin, angiotensinogin, and aldosterone
11. Insulin, growth hormone, and blood glucose
12. C-reactive protein
13. Globulins (α_1 and α_2)
14. α_1-Antitrypsin
15. Total estrogens (urine)
16. Coproporphyrin (feces and urine) and porphobilinogen (urine)
17. Vitamin A
18. Xanthurenic acid (urine)
19. Positive antinuclear antibody test and LE preparation
20. Total T_4

B. Values that are decreased
1. Antithrombin II
2. LH and FSH
3. Pregnanediol and 17-ketosteroids
4. Folate and vitamin B_{12}
5. Glucose tolerance
6. Ascorbic acid
7. Zinc and magnesium
8. T_3 resin uptake
9. Fibrinolytic activity
10. Haptoglobin
11. Cholinesterase
12. T_3 resin uptake

TABLE 5-12.—INTERACTION BETWEEN ORAL CONTRACEPTIVES AND OTHER DRUGS

CONTRACEPTIVE, UNCHANGED; DRUG DECREASED	CONTRACEPTIVE, UNCHANGED; DRUG INCREASED	CONTRACEPTIVE, INCREASED; DRUG UNCHANGED	CONTRACEPTIVE, DECREASED; DRUG UNCHANGED
Acetaminophen*	Chlordiazepoxide	Ascorbic acid	Antibiotics‡
Aspirin*	Corticosteroids†	Co-trimoxazole	Anticonvulsant‡
Clofibrate	Diazepam†		Griseofulvin§
Lorazepam	Imipramine HCl†		Purgatives
Morphine*	Meperidine†		Rifampin§
Oxazepam*	Metoprolol tartrate†		
Temazepam*	Theophylline†		
	Triazolam†		
	Vitamin A		

Modified from Williams RS: Benefits and risks of oral contraceptive use, *Postgrad Med* 92:155, 1992.
*Increase dose of drug.
†Decrease dose of drug needed; decrease by about one third.
‡With spotting increase oral contraceptive dose, otherwise no management change needed.
§Increase oral contraceptive dose or change contraceptive method to avert contraceptive failure.

TABLE 5-13.—RELATION OF SIDE EFFECTS TO HORMONE CONTENT

ESTROGEN EXCESS	PROGESTIN EXCESS	
	PROGESTATIONAL	ANDROGENIC

General Symptoms
Chloasma
Chronic nasal pharyngitis
Gastric influenza and varicella
Hay fever and allergic rhinitis
Urinary tract infections
 	
Premenstrual Syndrome
Bloating
Dizziness—syncope
Edema
Headaches (cyclic)
Irritability
Leg cramps
Nausea and vomiting
Visual changes (cyclic)
Weight gain (cyclic)
 	
Reproductive System
Breast cystic changes
Cervical extrophy
Dysmenorrhea, menstrual
  cramps
Hypermenorrhea, menorrhagia,
  heavy flow and clots
Increase in breast size
Mucorrhea
Uterine enlargement
Uterine fibroid growth
 	
Cardiovascular System
Capillary fragility
Cerebrovascular accident
Deep vein thrombosis hemipa-
  resis (unilateral weakness
  and numbness)
Telangiectasis
Thromboembolic disease
Vascular headaches (migraine)
	General Symptoms
	Appetite increased
	Depression
	Fatigability
	Hypoglycemia symptoms
	Libido decreased
	Neurodermatitis
	Tiredness
	Weight gain (noncyclic)
	
	Cardiovascular System
	Hypertension
	Leg veins dilated
	Hyperlipidemia
	
	Reproductive System
	Cervicitis
	Flow length decreased
	Moniliasis
		Androgenic Symptoms
		Acne
		Cholestatic jaundice
		Hirsutism
		Libido increased
		Oily skin and scalp
		Rash and pruritus

Modified from Dickey R: *Managing contraceptive pill patients*, ed 7, Durant, Oklahoma, 1993, Essential Medical Information Systems, Inc, pp. 146-147.

Continued.

TABLE 5-13.—RELATION OF SIDE EFFECTS TO HORMONE CONTENT—cont'd

ESTROGEN DEFICIENCY	PROGESTIN DEFICIENCY
Bleeding and spotting continuous Bleeding and spotting early (pill day 1 to 9) Flow decreased, hypomenorrhea Nervousness Pelvic relaxation symptoms Vaginitis atrophic Vasomotor symptoms Withdrawal bleeding none	Breakthrough bleeding and spotting late (pill day 10 to 21) Dysmenorrhea (also estrogen excess) Heavy flow and clots (also estrogen excess), hyper- menorrhea, menorrhagia Withdrawal bleeding delayed (also see symptoms listed under Estrogen Excess, Premenstrual Syndrome)

Modified from Dickey R: *Managing contraceptive pill patients*, ed 7, Durant, Oklahoma, 1993, Essential Medical Information Systems, Inc, pp. 146-147.

TABLE 5-14.—SUBDERMAL CONTRACEPTIVE IMPLANTS

Six capsules of levonorgestrel (36 mg each) are implanted subdermally and can be left in place for 5 years. Initial plasma levels of levonorgestrel are 1600 pg/ml, falling to 300-400 pg/ml after 3 months.
Protection begins within 24 hours after insertion.

Contraindications
Active thrombophlebitis
Undiagnosed abnormal genital bleeding
Acute liver disease
Known or suspected carcinoma of the breast
Known or suspected pregnancy

Indications
Do not desire children for 3-5 years and without contraindications
Considering but not yet ready for permanent sterilization
Women for whom other methods are contraindicated
Women who cannot comply with other methods
Women who believe they can tolerate menstrual irregularities for 1 year

Insertion/Removal
Make certain that the woman is not pregnant
Can insert immediately after abortion or during lactation
Use inner aspect of nondominant arm, 8-10 cm above elbow crease
Use template and insert close to skin surface using 5 ml of anesthetic
Trocar is introduced through a 2-mm incision
Direct capsules about 15 degrees apart without removing trocar between placements
Apply firm pressure, and close incision with steristrips
Removal generally takes twice as long as insertion
Fibrous capsule forms around the implant and must be opened
If a new set of implants is desired, they can be inserted in the same incision

TABLE 5-15.—Postcoital Contraception

Indications
Prevent pregnancy after unprotected intercourse
Victims of rape or incest
Patient's physical or emotional well-being is in jeopardy from potential pregnancy

Regimen
Diethylstilbestrol (DES) 25 mg PO bid for 5 days given within 24 to 72 hours
NOTE: Pregnancies that continue despite treatment may be complicated by reproductive tract anomalies in female fetuses; risk < 0.1%

Or   Norgestrel 0.5 mg plus ethinyl estradiol 0.05 mg, 2 tabs within 72 hours after unprotected intercourse and a second dose of 2 tabs 12 hours later; failure rate is 2%

Or   Conjugated estrogens 30 mg PO every day for 5 days, given within 24 hours

Modified from DeMarco JJ: Postcoital contraception underrecognized and underutilized, *The Female Patient* 17:29, 1992.

MENSTRUATION AND ABNORMAL UTERINE BLEEDING

TABLE 5-16.—Definitions of Abnormal Vaginal Bleeding

CONDITION	SYMPTOMS
Menorrhagia	Menstrual blood loss > 80 ml/cycle, anemia
Polymenorrhea	Menstrual interval < 21 days
Oligomenorrhea	Menstrual interval > 36 days
Metrorrhagia	Irregular menstrual bleeding
Menometrorrhagia	Irregular, heavy menstrual bleeding

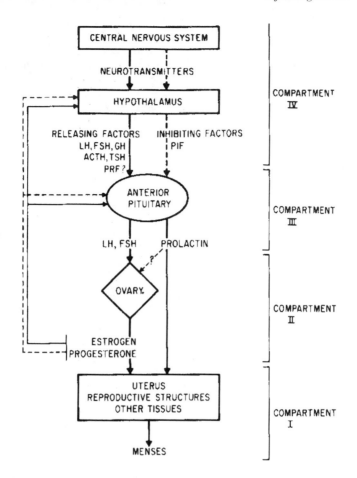

EXCITATORY STIMULUS
INHIBITORY STIMULUS
LH   LUTEINIZING HORMONE
FSH   FOLLICLE STIMULATING HORMONE
GH   GROWTH HORMONE
ACTH ADRENOCORTICOTROPIC HORMONE
TSH   THYROID STIMULATING HORMONE
PRF   PROLACTIN RELEASING FACTOR
PIF   PROLACTIN INHIBITING FACTOR

FIG 5-3.
A, Coordinated interactions among the CNS, hypothalamus, pituitary, and ovaries required for normal menstruation. *Continued.*

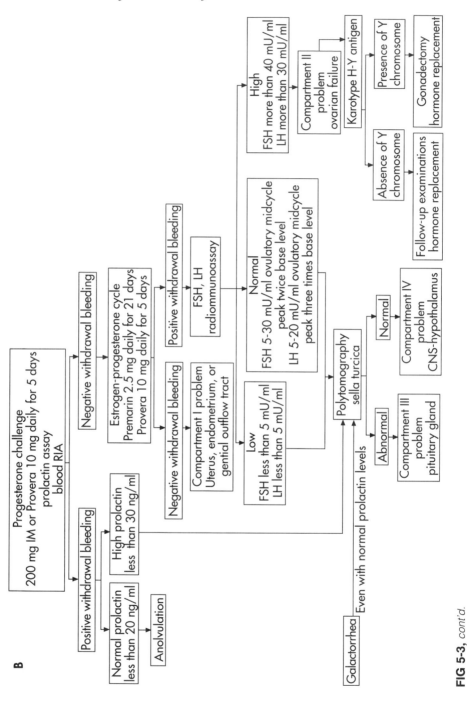

FIG 5-3, *cont'd.*
B, Office workup for amenorrhea. Compartments I to IV are defined in **A.** (From Pelosi MA: *J Med Soc NJ* 78:195, 1981.)

TABLE 5-17.—PREMENSTRUAL SYNDROME

Symptoms (occur cyclically beginning 7-14 days before menses)
Anxiety, depression, emotional lability, weight gain, edema, abdominal bloating, breast tenderness, headache, food craving, painful cramping, backache, fatigue, thirst, muscle pain

Differential Diagnosis
Dysmenorrhea, PID, endometriosis, chronic mental disorders, lupus, thyroid disease

Therapy
Aerobic exercise; reduce salt, sugar, fat, and caffeine intake; pyridoxine (B$_6$), 100 mg/day; spironolactone, 25 mg tid; calcium supplement, 1 g/day; oral contraceptives; prostaglandin synthetase inhibitors (ibuprofen, 600 mg PO qid), natural progesterones, 600 mg/day, vaginal suppositories; teach stress reduction techniques; supportive counseling; family education

TABLE 5-18.—MAJOR CAUSES OF HIRSUTISM IN WOMEN

Idiopathic Hirsutism
Increased sensitivity and/or utilization of androgens

Ovarian Causes
Polycystic ovarian disease
Neoplasms

Adrenal Causes
Congenital adrenal hyperplasia
Cushing's syndrome
Neoplasms

Medications
Danazol, phenytoin, minoxidil, phenothiazines, androgenic steroids

Miscellaneous
Hyperprolactinemia
Y-bearing mosaics in Turner's syndrome
Partial androgen insensitivity

Modified from Hatasaka HH, Wentz AC: Hirsutism: facts and folklore, *The Female Patient* 16:29, 1991.

TABLE 5-19.—Causes of Abnormal Uterine Bleeding

DISORDER	DIAGNOSTIC STRATEGY
Pregnancy disorders	Serum or urine hCG, U.S.
Thyroid disorder	Thyroid function tests
Synthetic sex steroids	Hx of estrogen/progestin use
Intrauterine device	Look for string, x-ray, infection
Carcinoma of cervix or endometrium	Inspection, PAP, Hx of DES, endometrial aspiration, D & C
Coagulation disorder	Platelets, PT, PTT, bleeding time
Dysfunctional uterine bleeding	
Polycystic ovary syndrome	Hirsutism, acne, testosterone, and androstenedione
Liver disease and obesity	Excessive estrone production
Ovarian neoplasm	Androgen excess
Theca cell tumor of the ovary	Increased Estradiol-17β
Transient disruption of hypothalamic-pituitary-ovarian axis	Environmental stresses
Organic lesions of the uterus	Polyps, leiomyomas
Endometritis	Plasma cell infiltrates in endometrial tissue and GC culture positive
Atrophic vaginitis	Inspect vagina, estrogen index of vaginal smear

INFERTILITY

Infertility is the inability to conceive after 1 year of unprotected intercourse. In the United States, 15% to 17% of couples are affected. Factors accounting for infertility are 40% male, 20% ovulatory, 20% tubal, 10% other (e.g., endometrial, cervical), and 10% unexplained.

EVALUATING THE INFERTILE COUPLE

TABLE 5-20.—Common Causes of Hyperprolactinemia

Drugs
Amoxapine, phenothiazines, butyrophenones, thioxanthenes, methyldopa, reserpine, metoclopramide

Hypothyroidism
Prolactinoma
Neural Stimulation
Chest wall and intrathoracic disease (e.g., herpes zoster, chest wall burns, thoracoplasty)
Nipple stimulation

Hypothalamic Disease
Craniopharyngioma
Hypothalamic and/or pineal tumors
Pseudotumor cerebri
Inflammation (e.g., sarcoidosis, encephalitis)

From Veldhuis JD: *Hosp Pract* Nov. 30, 1988, pp 40-56.

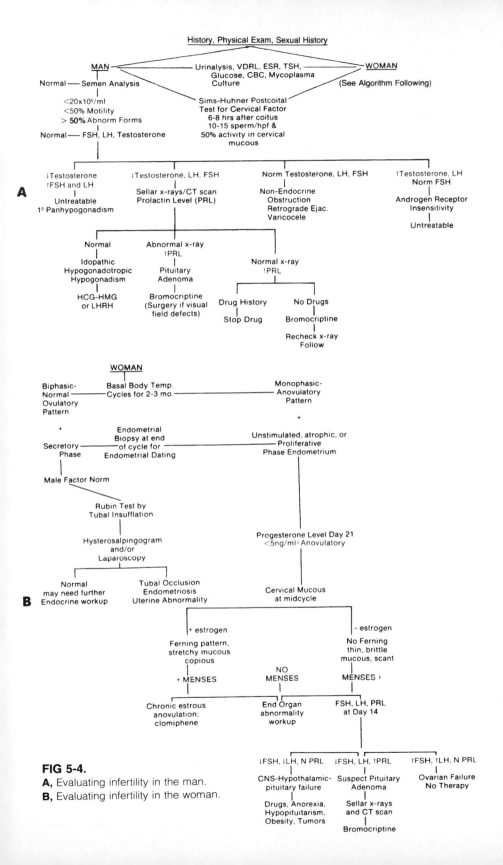

FIG 5-4.
A, Evaluating infertility in the man.
B, Evaluating infertility in the woman.

GYNECOLOGICAL INFECTIONS

TABLE 5-21.—Case Definition of Toxic Shock Syndrome

Major Symptoms and Signs
Fever: Temperature ≥38.9° C (102° F)
Rash: Diffuse macular erythroderma. Desquamation usually occurs 1-2 weeks
after onset of illness, most prominently on the palms and soles
Hypotension: Systolic blood pressure ≤ 90 mm Hg for adults or below 5th per-
centile by age for children less than 16 years of age, or orthostatic syncope

Multisystem Involvement—Three or More of the Following:
Gastrointestinal: Vomiting or diarrhea at onset of illness
Muscular: Severe myalgia or creatine phosphokinase (CPK) level ≥ 2 × ULN*
Mucous membrane: Vaginal, oropharyngeal, or conjunctival hyperemia
Hepatic: Total bilirubin, SGOT, or SGPT ≥ 2 × ULN
Renal: BUN or creatinine ≥ 2 × ULN or pyuria (≥5 white blood cells per high
power field) in the absence of a urinary tract infection
Hematological: Platelets ≤ 100,000/mm^3
CNS: Disorientation or alterations in consciousness without focal neurological
signs when fever and hypotension are absent

Reasonable Evidence for Absence of Other Causes
Negative results on the following tests, if performed:
Blood, throat (group A, β-hemolytic streptococci), or cerebrospinal fluid cultures.
Rise in serological titers to Rocky Mountain spotted fever, leptospirosis, or
measles

From Dan BB, Shands KN: *Pediatr Ann* 10:29, 1981.
*Two times upper limit of normal for laboratory.

TABLE 5-22.—Management of Toxic Shock Syndrome

Primary Treatment
Remove inciting focus, obtain culture and sensitivity
Fluid resuscitation
    Crystaloids and colloids to support blood pressure (may take ≥ 10 L/24
    hour)
    Swan-Ganz catheterization indicated

Ancillary Treatment
Corticosteroids controversial, probably useful
Discontinue future tampon use
β-Lactamase-resistant antistaphylococcal antibiotics (lowers recurrence rate
with subsequent menses from 40% to 10%)

TABLE 5-23.—VAGINITIS AND SEXUALLY TRANSMITTED INFECTIONS

TYPE	SYMPTOMS	CLINICAL FEATURES	LABORATORY	TREATMENT	COMMENTS
Trichomonas vaginalis	Itching, swollen vagina; odor; discharge	Petechiae; "strawberry vagina"; malodorous, frothy yellow-green discharge	Motile trichomonads on saline prep; pH 5.5-5.8*	Metronidazole, 2-g single dose or 500 mg PO bid for 7 days	Transmitted in postmenstrual phase; avoid alcohol while taking metronidazole; treat male sexual partner
Candida albicans	Discharge; itching; dyspareunia	Red, edematous vulva and vagina; scant to thick creamy discharge adherent to vagina	10% KOH prep reveals spores and hyphae; pH 4.0-4.5 (Fig. 5-6)	Butoconazole, clotrimazole, miconazole, terconazole or Tioconazole vaginal cream hs for 7 days (fluconazole 150 mg PO once)	Nickerson's culture may confirm; exacerbated by pregnancy and diabetes
Gardnerella vaginalis	Mild pruritis or burning; odor	Grayish, homogeneous thin discharge gives "fishy" amine odor when mixed with a drop of 10% KOH	Dark, stippled epithelial cells (clue cells) on saline prep (see Fig. 5-5); pH 5.0-5.5	Metronidazole, 500 mg bid for 7 days (or clindamycin, 300 mg PO bid for 7 days)	Probably sexually transmitted
Chlamydia trachomatis	Discharge, spotting after coitus	Cervicitis; acute PID; mucopurulent discharge	Many WBCs, no organisms on saline prep; pH of mucus 7+	Doxycycline, 100 mg PO bid for 7 days or Azithromycin, 1 g PO once (erythromycin in pregnancy)	Associated with gonorrhea in 30%-60% of cases; may cause LGV

Revised according to Centers for Disease Control guidelines, Jan. 1993; Drugs for sexually transmitted diseases. *Med Let* 36:1, 1994.
*Normal vaginal pH, 3.8-4.2.

Continued.

TABLE 5-23.—VAGINITIS AND SEXUALLY TRANSMITTED INFECTIONS—cont'd

TYPE	SYMPTOMS	CLINICAL FEATURES	LABORATORY	TREATMENT	COMMENTS
Neisseria gonorrhoeae	Discharge, abdominal pain, urethritis	Profuse yellow discharge; cervicitis; PID	Intracellular gram-negative diplococci; Thayer-Martin culture	Ceftriaxone 125 mg IM once *plus* doxycycline 100 mg PO bid for 7 days	Usually effective for incubating syphilis, repeat VDRL in 6 weeks; *C. trachomatis, M. hominis, U. urealyticum* may coexist
Herpes genitalis	Painful ulcers, dysuria, pelvic pain	Shallow ulcers; clear or serous discharge without odor	Positive Tzanck smear; multinucleated giant cells	Acyclovir 400 mg PO tid for 7-10 days and tub soaks	Primary infection most symptomatic (prevention of recurrence, Acyclovir 400 mg PO bid)
Syphilis—T. pallidum	Painless sores, swollen glands	Chancre with lymphadenopathy	Positive VDRL; FTABS	Benzothine penicillin G, 2.4 million U IM (early); BPG 2.4 million U weekly for 3 weeks (late)	21-day incubation period; tetracycline 500 mg PO qid, for 15 days in penicillin allergy
Chancroid	Pain on voiding, dyspareunia, vaginal discharge	Ragged ulcer at vaginal introitus, tender inguinal lymph nodes in 50% of patients	Calcium alginate swab of ulcer for *Haemophilus ducreyi* culture	Ceftriaxone 250 mg IM once or Azithromycin 1 g PO once	Relapse rate is 5%; 3-10 day incubation period
Condyloma acuminatum—HPV	Warts, mild irritation	Vulvar/perineal and anal location	Acetowhite change with 4% acetic acid	10% podophyllin on for 6-8 hours, then wash off, or trichloroacetic acid	Sexually transmitted virus, long-term follow-up for types 6/11 and 16/18
Atrophic vaginitis	Vaginal bleeding, pruritus, dyspareunia	Postmenopausal; thin epithelium; scant serous discharge	No abnormal organisms; pH 6.7-7.0	Topical estrogen cream once daily for 14 days, then qod for 14 days	Usually only 4 weeks of therapy needed

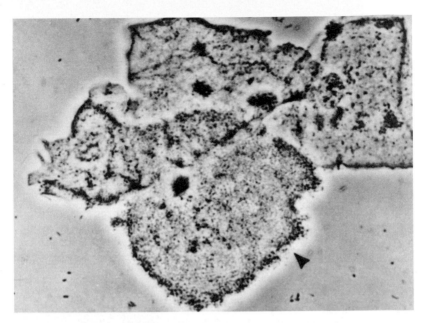

FIG 5-5.
Clue cell *(arrowhead).* Vaginal epithelial cell with organisms stippling the surface and border. (From Eschenbach D: Vaginal discharge. In Duenhoelter JH, ed: *Greenhill's office gynecology,* ed 10, Chicago, 1983, Mosby, p. 91.)

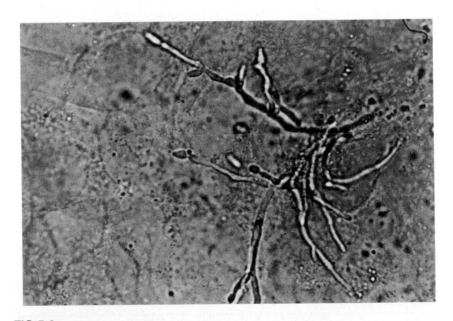

FIG 5-6.
Candida. Branching mycelia and spores are seen with 10% KOH smear. (From Eschenbach D: Vaginal discharge. In Duenhoelter JH, ed: *Greenhill's office gynecology,* ed 10, Chicago, 1983, Mosby, p. 92.)

TABLE 5-24.—Pelvic Inflammatory Disease (PID)

Minimum Criteria for Clinical Diagnosis (All Three Needed)
Lower abdominal, bilateral adnexal, and cervical motion tenderness

Additional Useful Criteria
Oral temperature $\geq$ 101° F
Abnormal cervical/vaginal discharge
Elevated ESR or CRP
WBC > 10,500/μl
Evidence for cervical infection with GC or chlamydia

Deciding Factors that Favor Hospitalization
Pregnancy
Surgical abdomen
Noncompliant patient
Adolescent patient
Concurrent HIV infection
Failed prior outpatient treatment
Severe illness, nausea, and vomiting

Outpatient Therapy
Regimen A: Cefoxitin sodium 2 g IM plus probenecid 1 g PO
                               Or
                  Ceftriaxone sodium 250 mg IM

                  PLUS: Doxycycline hyclate 100 mg PO bid for 14 days

Regimen B: Ofloxacin 400 mg PO bid for 14 days
                  PLUS: Metronidazole 500 mg PO bid for 14 days

Inpatient Therapy
Regimen A: Cefoxitin sodium 2 g IV every 6 hours
                               Or
                  Cefotetan disodium 2 g IV every 12 hours

                  PLUS: Doxycycline hyclate 100 mg IV or PO every 12 hours

                  (Continue this regimen for at least 48 hours after clinical im-
                     provement. After discharge, patient continues doxycycline 100
                     mg PO bid for 14 days.)

Regimen B: Clindamycin phosphate 900 mg IV every 8 hours
                  PLUS: Gentamicin sulfate 2 mg/kg IV loading dose followed by 1.5
                     mg/kg every 8 hours

                  (Continue for 48 hours after clinical improvement and discharge
                     on doxycycline 100 mg PO bid for 14 days or clindamycin HCl
                     450 mg PO qid for 14 days.)

Modified from Howes DS, Marrazzo JM, Scott C: Recognizing and treating PID, *Patient Care Clinical Focus,* March 1994.

TABLE 5-25.—HIV Infection in Women

Women with HIV/AIDS account for 20% of cases; majority are black or Hispanic
Transmission is by IV drug use (51%), heterosexual contact (29%), blood trans-
fusion (11%), unknown (9%)
Maternal-fetal transmission rate during pregnancy is 65%
Opportunistic infections seen in women
   Pneumocystis carinii, cryptococcal meningitis, toxoplasmosis, nonpulmonary
      tuberculosis, atypical tuberculosis *(Mycobacterium avium-intracellulare),*
      esophageal candidiasis, enteric pathogens, herpes viral infections
AIDS symptoms
   Diarrheal syndromes, weight loss, anorexia, dementia, amenorrhea and dys-
      functional uterine bleeding (30%)
High-risk women who should be screened
   Women who received a blood transfusion before 1985; prostitutes; IV drug
      users; sexual partner is HIV+ or high risk
Patient counseling
   Sexual monogamy with seronegative partner, limit number of partners
      Use condoms during *all* sexual contacts, use nonoxynol-9 spermicide
      avoid IUD use; if HIV+ obtain regular PAP smears
   Oral-genital sex and anal intercourse increase risk
   There are no physical or behavioral characteristics of HIV+ persons
   Never share needles

Telephone Numbers for Information:

AIDS Hotline	1-800-342-AIDS
Retrovir (AZT) Hotline	1-800-843-9388
CDC	
Printed information	1-404-329-3534
Recorded information	1-404-329-1290

Modified from Holmes VF, Fernandez F: *The Female Patient* 13:47, 1988; Kapila R,
Kloser P: *Med Aspects Hum Sexuality* pp. 92-94, July 1988.

SEXUAL DYSFUNCTION

TABLE 5-26.—Assessment for Sexual Dysfunction

Routine Sexual History Taking Should Include the Following Questions:
"How satisfactory is your sexual functioning?"
"At sometime in their lives most people experience a sexual problem.
   What type of sexual problems have you experienced?"
"Many people have unanswered questions or need information about sexual
   functioning. What questions do you have?"

A Modified Sexological Examination Includes the Following:
Sensitivity of vulva to touch
Clitoris is free from adhesions to prepuce
Bulbocavernosus contractions are normal
Urethra and vagina have normal sensitivity
Absence of infection, masses, mucosal lesions
Valsalva negative for pelvic relaxation
Uterus palpation is normal
Breast and nipple examination is normal

TABLE 5-27.—Phase-Specific Sexual Disorders in Women

PHASE OF SEXUAL CYCLE	COMMENT/MANAGEMENT
Desire	Most common clinical problem
	Primary (upbringing) versus secondary (depression, disappointment, pain, fear, anger, drugs)
	Unless secondary treatable form, refer for sex therapy
Excitement/plateau	Sexual anesthesia from drugs or disease
	General dysfunction with lack of lubrication
	Lack pleasure in sexual experiences
	Try ban on intercourse and sensate focus therapy
	Referral
Orgasm	Primary, secondary, or situational
	Directed masturbation exercises, guided caress, fantasy
	Assume responsibility for own orgasm
	Deal with negative body image and provide education
	Increase awareness of foreplay and clitoral stimulation
Resolution	Delay causes pelvic congestion; more common during pregnancy
	Enhance stimulation to shorten excitement/plateau phases by teaching Kegel's pubococcygeus muscle exercises (see Table 5-38)
Vaginismus	Not easily classified, involuntary vaginal muscle spasms
	Primary (upbringing) versus secondary (after rape, trauma, vaginitis)
	"No sex life" most common complaint
	Increase stimulation to increase lubrication
	Kegel's exercises and progressive vaginal dilators
	Have sexual activity to orgasm other than intercourse

TABLE 5-28.—MANAGEMENT OF THE RAPE VICTIM*

Introduce self and assure patient of safety; never leave patient alone
Empathetic listening about her ordeal; encourage reporting of crime
Give patient total control; involve her in decision making
    Patient determines rate of questioning and examination
    Inform patient of each procedure and obtain permission
    Patient decides when to contact family
Perform methodical history, physical examination, and collection of well-
    documented evidence according to written protocol
    History of assault, violence, use of weapon, number of attackers
    Type of assault (vaginal, oral, anal, instrument, other)
    Penetration, ejaculation
    Bathed, douched, defecated, brushed teeth, or used mouthwash?
    OB/gyn and general medical history, LMP, contraception
Place collected evidence in sealed, documentation envelopes
    Wood's light examination of pelvic area—semen has bright bluish white fluo-
        rescence
    Vaginal pool aspirate (acid phosphatase, ABH group antigens, motile sper-
        matozoa, wet mount, dry smear slide, DNA typing)
    Urine for pregnancy test
    Rectal, oral specimens if indicated
    Vulva (pubic hair combing for foreign material, patient's pubic hair clipped for
        sample)
    Fingernail scrapings
    Clothing she wore at the time of attack
    Blood typing, VDRL, serum or urine hCG, HIV, HB_SAg
    Cultures for *N. gonorrhoeae, C. trachomatis*
    Pap smear with water-moistened speculum, bimanual examination
Examination of vulva may be done with colposcope, toluidine blue staining
A vaginal washing may be done by irrigating the vaginal vault (avoid the cervix)
    with 10 ml of NaCl. Aspirate the fluid and place in a test tube, which is then
    sealed and labeled. Aspirate can be examined for motile sperm, acid phos-
    phatase, blood group antigens, and sperm precipitins.
Nongynecological examination for bruises, abrasions, contusions, penetrating
    injuries, fractures (photography of wounds)
Discuss the usual psychological sequelae of rape; alleviate guilt and self-
    reproach
Provide patient advocate skilled in rape crisis intervention
Arrange for supportive follow-up care of patient's choice
If patient chooses, VD prophylaxis (probenecid, 1 g, with ampicillin, 3.5 g orally)
    and pregnancy prophylaxis (DES, 25 mg PO bid for 5 days)
Tetanus toxoid if indicated

*USEFUL REFERENCE: Hicks DJ: The patient who's been raped, *Emerg Med* 20:106, 1988.

PAP SMEARS AND COLPOSCOPY

Conducting Pap Smears

Conduct Pap testing on two specimens, one from the ectocervix obtained by spatula scraping and the second from the endocervix by means of a cytobrush. Cytobrush usage yields endocervical cells in nearly 100% of samples. Smear both specimens together on the same slide and fix immediately. If no endocervical cells are present, the smear is inadequate and must be repeated. If atypical endometrial cells are reported, endometrial aspiration or D & C is needed.

TABLE 5-29.—CLASSIFICATION AND MANAGEMENT OF CERVICAL PAP SMEARS

BETHESDA CLASSIFICATION	FINDINGS	COURSE OF ACTION
Within normal limits	Adequate smear endocervical cells present, no abnormal cells	Repeat smear in 1 year
Atypical squamous cells of undetermined significance	Atypical cells present, inflammatory	Treat infection and cervical trauma Repeat smear in 3-4 months If repeat is atypical, do colposcopy
Low-grade squamous intraepithelial lesion	Smear contains abnormal cells consistent with mild dysplasia (CIN1) or cellular changes of HPV	Colposcopy, endocervical curettage, directed biopsies, HPV/DNA Pap Microinvasion or CIN1 = excisional cone biopsy of cervix, LEEP/LETZ, cryotherapy, laser, or hysterectomy
High-grade squamous intraepithelial lesion	Smear contains abnormal cells consistent with moderate dysplasia (CIN2) or severe dysplasia (CIN3) or carcinoma in situ	Colposcopy with directed biopsy CIN2 treat as above for CIN1 CIN3 = excisional cone biopsy
Squamous cell carcinoma	Smear contains abnormal cells suggestive of invasive squamous cell carcinoma	Metastatic survey, radical surgery or radiation

Colposcopy

Nonresolving atypia and all dysplastic Pap smears require colposcopy to confirm the abnormal cytology. There are no contraindications to the procedure.

TABLE 5-30.—Colposcopy: Technique and Findings

Materials Needed

Colposcope, 3%-5% acetic acid, Kervokian-Younge biopsy forceps, vaginal speculum, endocervical curette, endocervical speculum, ferric subsulfate solution, cotton-tipped swabs (large and small), specimen jars with 10% formalin

Procedure

1. Explain procedure to patient
2. Patient in lithotomy position, vaginal speculum in place
3. Remove excess mucus with saline soaked swabs
4. Green filter examination to enhance vascular pattern identification
5. White light examination of vulva, vagina, and cervix
6. Visualize entire squamocolumnar junction under magnification
7. Enhance visualization of abnormalities with 3%-5% acetic acid (clears away mucus and causes transient vasoconstriction). Schiller's or Lugol's solution may be used as alternatives (see Table 5-31 for findings)
8. Perform endocervical curettage and submit as separate specimen
9. Biopsy abnormal patterns (anesthetic seldom needed), achieve hemostasis with ferric subsulfate
10. No special aftercare

TABLE 5-31.—LOCALIZATION OF CERVICAL ABNORMALITIES*

Schiller's iodine test is a simple method of detecting abnormal cervical cells by revealing the absence of glycogen. Schiller's (0.3%) or Lugol's (5%) iodine solution is painted onto the cervix. (Toluidine blue 1% aqueous solution is also effective.) Scars, eversion, endocervical glandular epithelium, erosions, reepithelialization, nonmalignant leukoplakia, and CIN appear pale.

Acetic acid 3% to 5% cause dysplastic and neoplastic areas to briefly appear white in the aceto-white reaction. Green-filtered light enhances the vascular pattern identification.

Iodine-Stained Appearance	Interpretation	Action
Mahogany brown	Normal	None
All surface iodine pale (glycogen-negative) from os to squamocolumnar junction	Erosion	Limit trauma, treat infection, follow-up
Flame-shaped areas contiguous with but outside squamocolumnar junction	Dysplasia	Punch biopsy
Very pale (white) within or contiguous with iodine-pale areas	Leukoplakia	Punch biopsy
Punctate areas	*Trichomonas*	Treat infection
Acetic Acid Appearance		
Well-demarcated areas of:		
Epithelium that appears white "chicken wire" pattern	White dysplasia with mosaic pattern, CIN 1-3	Biopsy
Arboreal, fungating, exophytic white lesion	Hyperkeratinized cervical condylomata	Biopsy, cryotherapy, laser, or trichloracetic acid (TCA)
Green-Filtered Light		
Abnormal vessels with nonarboreal branching, "commas," "squiggles"	Atypical blood vessels, possible invasive carcinoma	Biopsy
Segments of avascular pathological epithelium outlined by capillaries	Mosaic mucosal pattern, CIN 1-3	Biopsy
Dilated, elongated hairpin capillaries, often irregular and slightly twisted	Punctate lesions, CIN 1-3	Biopsy
Punctation (fine red stippling)	Possible HPV or CIN 1-3	Biopsy

*Useful reference: Felmar E, et al: Colposcopy: a necessary adjunct to Pap smears, *Fam Pract Recertification* 10(11):21, 1988.

TUMORS AND MALIGNANT DISEASE

TABLE 5-32.—Clinical Findings Suggestive of Benign or Malignant Adnexal Masses

BENIGN	MALIGNANT
<5 cm	>5 cm
Unilateral	Bilateral
Cystic	Solid
Mobile	Fixed
Smooth	Irregular, lobulated
No ascites	Ascites
Slow growth	Rapid growth
Young patient	Older patient
Tender	Nontender

Modified from Meyers P, Mann WJ: A pelvic mass: malignant or not? *Prim Care and Cancer,* June 1993, pp. 11-13.

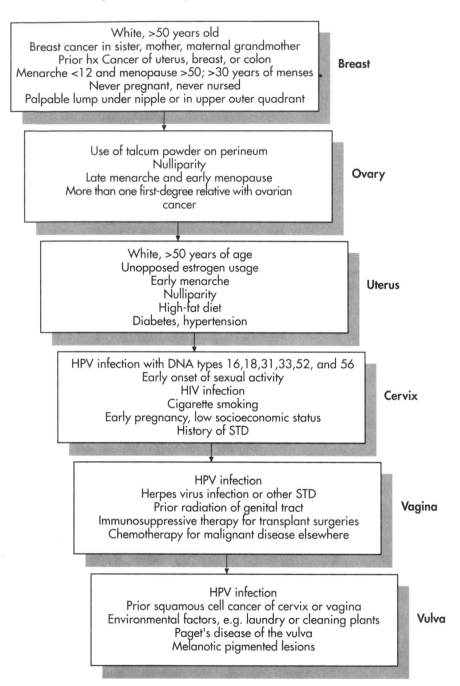

FIG 5-7.
Cancer risk factor screening for women.

TABLE 5-33.—SCREENING FOR OVARIAN CANCER

Ovarian cancer occurs in 1 out of 70 women in the general population (1.4% lifetime risk)

Women at High Risk Should Be Identified for Screening
Family history is the best predictive risk factor
   One second-degree relative with ovarian cancer; lifetime risk becomes 2.9%
   One first-degree relative with ovarian cancer; lifetime risk becomes 4% to 5%
   Two or more first degree relatives affected; lifetime risk is 30% to 50%
Additive risk factors include the following:
   Nulliparity, perineal talc exposure, infertility, high-fat diet, or previous breast cancer; each increases lifetime risk by 2.0%

Screening Methods

Review history	Look for symptoms of bloating, distention, nausea, pelvic discomfort, weight loss, urinary frequency, or shortness of breath
Pelvic examination	Least sensitive but most cost-effective, look for adnexal mass
CA-125 serum antigen	A value above 35 U/ml is abnormal but nonspecific. Elevations may result from cancer of the cervix, endometrium, or fallopian tube. Also, pregnancy, PID, endometriosis, and leiomyoma
Transabdominal ultrasound	May be limited by obesity, prior history of pelvic surgery, bowel gas pattern, or inadequately filled bladder
Transvaginal ultrasound	Can be combined with pulsed, color-flow Doppler to show neovascularity and vascular flow to enhance diagnostic accuracy

Modified from Piver SM, Fernando OR: Ovarian cancer: who needs screening? *Patient Care,* December 15, 1993; Anderson PS, Goldberg GL, Runowicz CD: Ovarian carcinoma: on whom should you carry out screening? *Consultant,* February 1994.

OTHER GYNECOLOGICAL CONDITIONS

Endometriosis

Endometriosis is usually slowly progressive over a number of years. It is invasive but nonmalignant and regresses at menopause.

TABLE 5-34.—Endometriosis

Symptoms
1. Progressive, acquired severe pelvic pain with or just prior to menses
2. Dyspareunia
3. Lower abdominal pain, backache, sciatica
4. Painful defecation
5. Suprapubic pain, dysuria, hematuria
6. Infertility

Signs
1. Tender uterosacral ligaments
2. Thickened, nodular uterosacral ligaments
3. Thickened, rectovaginal septum; fullness in cul-de-sac with tenderness
4. Fixed ovarian or adnexal masses
5. Cutaneous nodules in surgical scars or in vaginal or perineal areas

Diagnosis
Laparotomy, laparoscopy, pelvic ultrasound (for ovarian lesions), MRI (for adnexal masses)

Treatment

Mild	Observe, analgesics, nonsteroidals (e.g., ibuprofen 600 mg PO qid)
Moderate/severe	Low-estrogen/high-androgen hormone therapy; danazol 200-400 mg PO/day when patient desires later fertility. High-dose medroxyprogesterone or Gn-RH agonist may also be used
	A total abdominal hysterectomy with bilateral oophorectomy (TAH-BSO) for patient finished with childbearing
	Wait 3-6 months before estrogen replacement therapy

Recurrence Rate
20% per year recurrence after hormone therapy
50% failure rate if one ovary left behind at time of hysterectomy
<10% recurrence if TAH-BSO is done and FSH is allowed to rise to menopausal level before estrogen replacement

Modified from Barbieri RL (ed): *Curr Probl Obstet Gynecol Fert* 12:1, 1989; Olive DL, Schwartz LB: Endometriosis, *N Engl J Med* 328:1759, 1993.

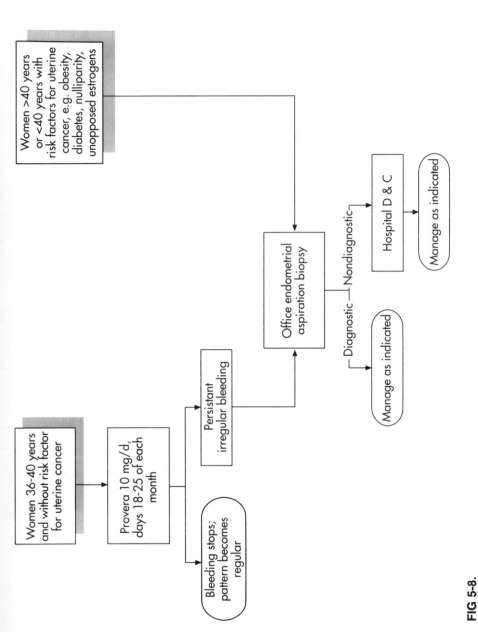

FIG 5-8.
Dysfunctional uterine bleeding in the "transitional" woman.

Menopause

TABLE 5-35.—DIAGNOSIS AND MANAGEMENT OF MENOPAUSE

Definition
Perimenopausal (climacteric)—ovarian function waxes and wanes
Menopause—last menses occurred ≥12 months ago

Diagnosis
Cyclical menstrual function ceases
Estrogen index obtained from upper third of lateral vaginal wall
  Estratrophy = 0/100/0* with slight variability
  Teleatrophy = 100/0/0* with moderate variability
  NOTE: Digitalis therapy shifts maturation index to right

Asymptomatic Patient
Progesterone in oil 100 mg IM or Provera 10 mg PO bid for 5 days produces no
  withdrawal bleeding. (If withdrawal occurs, give cyclical progesterone chal-
  lenge.)
Serum FSH values are >30 mU/ml
Elective estrogen replacement therapy (ERT)

Symptomatic Patient
Conjugated estrogens 0.625 mg PO daily plus Provera 5-10 mg PO the first
  12-14 days of each month
Withdrawal should occur after day 14 or not at all. Withdrawal bleeding usually
  stops after age 65
Continue estrogen-progestin cyclic therapy
  Or
Conjugated estrogens 0.625 mg PO daily plus Provera 2.5 mg PO daily
Irregular spotting may occur for the first 4-5 months of use, then the patient
  should become amenorrheic

Variations in ERT
If triglycerides are >300 mg/dl, consider a transdermal estradiol patch in lieu of
  an oral estrogen
If persistent urogenital symptoms, consider adding a vaginal estrogen
If headache or breast pain, reduce estrogen to 0.3 mg per day
If insufficient relief of vasomotor symptoms, increase estrogen to 1.25 mg per
  day then taper back to 0.625 mg per day after 3-6 months
After hysterectomy, estrogen alone may be used
Androgens may be added to increase libido, relieve breast tenderness, and help
  with control of vasomotor symptoms

Indications for ERT
1. Vasomotor symptoms
2. Genitourinary atrophy
3. Osteoporosis prophylaxis
4. Cardioprotection

[*% parabasal cells/% intermediate cells/% superficial cells.]

TABLE 5-35.—Diagnosis and Management of Menopause—cont'd

Contraindications to ERT
1. Breast or endometrial cancer
2. Impaired liver function, acute liver disease
3. Gallbladder disease
4. Thromboembolism or thrombophlebitis
5. Unexplained vaginal bleeding

Aftercare and Counseling
Supplement calcium intake to achieve 1200 mg daily
Regular exercise is beneficial
Serum lipids and blood pressure should be rechecked periodically
Report unexplained vaginal bleeding at once
Endometrial cytology is recommended every 1-2 years

TABLE 5-36.—Technique for In-Office Endometrial Sampling

Indications:
  Age >35 with dysfunctional uterine bleeding
  Absence of pregnancy or PID
  Women with additional risk factors for endometrial hyperplasia or cancer
    (e.g. diabetes, obesity, hypertension, chronic anovulation, polycystic ovary
    disease)
Pretreat 1 hour before sampling with ibuprofen 600 mg PO
Patient in lithotomy position cervix cleansed with povidone-iodine solution
Anesthetic usually unnecessary
Tenaculum or anterior lip or cervix with gentle traction
Uterus sounded and depth recorded in centimeters
Sampling device passed into endometrial cavity
  Cell sampling may be cytological via Endocyte, EndoPap, Isaacs, or Mi-Mark
    samplers or histological via biopsy with vacuum curettage cannula, Novak
    or Randall curette, or Pipelle
Sample in all quadrants; aspirate tissue and place in formalin. If cytology, smear
  on glass slide and fix immediately
With cervical stenosis and office procedure not possible, do D & C

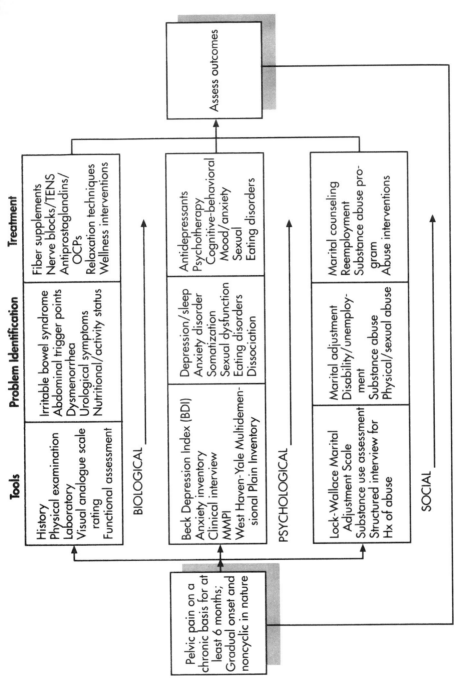

FIG 5-9.
Multidisciplinary approach to chronic pelvic pain.

PELVIC RELAXATION AND INCONTINENCE

TABLE 5-37.—PELVIC RELAXATION AND INCONTINENCE: TREATMENT
OF URINARY INCONTINENCE

TREATMENT	COMMENT
Kegel's exercises	See Table 5-38
Diapers	Up to 500-ml capacity
Diet	Weight reduction, control obesity
Estrogens	Topical or systemic
Drugs	
Bethanechol	Increase tone in hypotonic bladder
Propantheline	Decrease tone in hypertonic bladder (urge incontinence)
Phenylpropanolamine, imipramine	Stimulates urethral sphincter tone (stress incontinence)
Phenoxybenzamine	Reduce urethral sphincter tone (overflow incontinence)
Propranolol	Increase outlet resistance (stress incontinence)
Electric devices	Implantable, intravaginal, external
Occlusive devices	Inflatable Bonnar balloon, pessary, implantable Scott artificial sphincter
Surgery	Marshall-Marchetti; Krantz

TABLE 5-38.—KEGEL'S PUBOCOCCYGEAL MUSCLE EXERCISES

The patient locates the correct muscle by sitting on the toilet with knees as far apart as possible and begins urination, contracting perineum only (not bringing legs together) to stop urine flow. Exercises are to be practiced three times daily and do not require urination after muscle control has been learned. Begin with 10 and work up to 30.
1. Contract the muscle and hold for a count of 3, then relax muscle.
2. Contract and release rapidly in a flicking motion.
3. Breathe deeply imagining that air is being drawn into the vagina, tightening the muscle as you inhale. Begin with 5 and work up to 15.
Practice over a period of months may be necessary before results are noted.

TABLE 5-39.—UTERINE PROLAPSE/PESSARY USE

Symptoms	"Bearing down" perineal sensation, pelvic pressure, and the feeling of "sitting on something"
Physical examination	Descent of uterus, cervix, and vagina visualized on speculum or perineal examination after patient is asked to Valsalva
Indications for pessary	Symptomatic prolapse relieved by the pessary
	Symptomatic prolapse during or after pregnancy
	Where patient wishes to delay attempt at surgical repair
	After unsuccessful prolapse surgery
	Patient has increased risk of surgery and must be managed medically
	As a preoperative diagnostic aid prior to reconstructive surgery
Fitting the pessary	Adequate estrogenization should be achieved first (oral or topical) to prevent vaginal erosions with bleeding
	Start with either Ring pessary or Ring with Support (Milex Products, Inc.). Sizes, like diaphragms, range 0-13 (5, 6, 7 most common)
	Determine distance between pubic symphysis and vaginal apex with bimanual examination as in fitting a diaphragm
	Try ring that most closely approximates this distance. If Valsalva causes pessary ring to pop out, choose next larger size
	If patient senses discomfort with pessary in place, remove it immediately. Walking, sitting, or lying should be tried to ensure patient remains asymptomatic
	Caution patient that she may need to remove pessary to defecate and that urinary incontinence may occur when the pessary replaces the prolapse
	Recheck patient after 72 hours
	Pessary may be removed for intercourse. Remove and wash pessary at least every 1-2 weeks
	Recheck patient in 6-8 weeks for vaginal erosions or granulation tissue
Discontinue pessary if	Recurrent vaginal erosions
	Unacceptable urinary incontinence
	Desire for surgery
	Progression of symptoms and prolapse despite pessary use

DISEASES OF THE BREAST

TABLE 5-40.—BENIGN BREAST DISEASES

DISORDER	CLINICAL FINDINGS	TREATMENT
Fibrocystic disease	Often multiple lesions, generally mobile, commonly tender and cycle with menses; most common between ages 30 and 55 years; commonly associated with multiple cysts	Symptomatic; rarely diuretics, rarely multiple aspirations
Sclerosing adenosis	Lump that is commonly irregular nodularity	Excisional biopsy
Fibroadenoma	Firm, mobile mass; may change with menses; *unreliably* distinguishable from cancer	Excisional biopsy
Solitary large cyst ("blue-domed cyst")	Firm, mobile mass, not necessarily fluctuant or cystlike	Aspiration and follow-up; excisional biopsy if recurrent or bloody fluid
Intraductal papilloma	Serous or serosanguineous nipple discharge; mass-variable pruritus or nipple pain	Nipple fluid cytology, ductography and possible excision; exclude Paget's disease
Galactocele	Milky or opalescent nipple discharge in the postpartum period; possible mass	Symptomatic and breast pumping; biopsy if resolution does not occur
Duct ectasia	Nipple discharge of any description; possible mass; nipple erythema or pruritus	Nipple fluid cytology, ductography and possible excision; exclude Paget's disease
Fat necrosis	Poorly defined mass; possibly symptomatic; variably associated with trauma	Excisional biopsy

From Lippman ME: Approach to the management of breast cancer. In Kelley WN, et al, eds; *Textbook of internal medicine,* Philadelphia, 1988, JB Lippincott, p. 1236.

Continued.

TABLE 5-40.—Benign Breast Diseases—cont'd

DISORDER	CLINICAL FINDINGS	TREATMENT
Acute mastitis with or without evidence of acute abscess	Hot red, swollen breast or any part thereof; more common during lactation	A trial of antibiotics and heat; if *rapid* resolution does not occur, rule out inflammatory breast cancer; I & D if mass present
Mondor's disease (localized thrombophlebitis)	Superficial warm tender cord; most commonly postpartum	Heat, analgesic; biopsy if prompt resolution does not occur
Cystosarcoma phylloides	One or multiple rapidly growing masses	Wide excision if 10%-15% are malignant

6 *Pregnancy*

Charles E. Driscoll

PRECONCEPTION CARE

Women entering their childbearing years should receive evaluation and counseling to optimize health before conception. It is estimated that 50% of pregnancies in the United States are unplanned, therefore all sexually active women are candidates for preconception care. This care can be delivered routinely during visits for other reasons. Patient management is dictated by the findings from the evaluation (Table 6-1).

TABLE 6-1.—CHECKLIST FOR PRECONCEPTION CARE

AREA OF CONCERN	COMMENT
Health Promotion	
Nutrition	Decrease fat, caffeine, salt; ensure adequate nutrients (especially iron and folic acid 0.4 mg per day)
Exercise	Maintain fitness and desired weight
Alcohol, tobacco, and drugs	Identify and treat addictions
Safer sex	Reduce risk of STDs
Family/social	Identify risks for violence, abuse, and supports
Risk Assessments	
Medical status	Infection, reproductive history of patient and spouse, prescribed and OTC medications for chronic conditions, rubella/hepatitis immunities
Genetic risks	Sickle cell, Tay-Sachs disease, cystic fibrosis, neural tube defects, mental retardation, or other birth defects
Psychosocial	Readiness for pregnancy, stress, anxiety, or chronic emotional illness
Financial	Family planning, suggest social services

Modified from Scherger JE: Preconception care: a neglected element of prenatal services, *The Female Patient* 18:78, 1993.

Continued.

TABLE 6-1.—CHECKLIST FOR PRECONCEPTION CARE—cont'd

AREA OF CONCERN	COMMENT
Environmental Conditions	
Workplace hazards	High-risk jobs (e.g. day care and nursing)
Toxic chemicals	Agriculture and home or job use
Radiation	Dental or x-ray technician
Physical Examination	
Breast and pelvic	Infection or structural abnormalities
Cardiovascular	Heart murmurs, hypertension
Respiratory	Exercise-induced asthma
Laboratory Studies	
CBC and urine	Anemia, nutritional status, infection, sugar
Rubella titer	Immunity
Hepatitis B	Environmentally-exposed and high-risk patients
PAP, cultures	HPV, GC, and chlamydia
HIV screen	High-risk patients
Genetic screen	Sickle cell trait, Tay-Sachs disease, thalassemia

DIAGNOSIS OF PREGNANCY

TABLE 6-2.—DIAGNOSIS OF PREGNANCY

The "pregnancy test" is a measurement of human chorionic gonadotropin (hCG) (6% is cleared in the urine) secreted by trophoblastic tissue. Clinical applications include the following:
  Confirmation of a clinical diagnosis of pregnancy in the first trimester
  To exclude pregnancy before surgery, drug treatment, radiation, or rubella vaccination
  To detect ectopic pregnancy in women with abdominal pain (see Table 6-23)
  To evaluate pregnancy threatened by abortion
  To diagnose and guide treatment of trophoblastic tumors
The following three methods are in general use:

Immunoassay
Hemagglutination inhibition (HAI)
Latex particle agglutination inhibition (LAI)
Direct latex particle agglutination (DAP)

Radioimmunoassay (RIA)
Whole molecule or β-subunit

Modified from Krieg A: Pregnancy tests and evaluation of placental function. In Todd, et al, eds: *Clinical diagnosis and management by laboratory methods,* Philadelphia, 1979, WB Saunders.

TABLE 6-2.—Diagnosis of Pregnancy—cont'd

Radioreceptor Assay (RRA)
Serum hCG is detectable 24 hours after implantation (0.005 IU/ml). In the case of inevitable abortion, urine hCG levels of <3000 IU/24 hr will be seen 50-90 days after the LMP.

False Negatives: 50% Rate (HAI, LAI, DAP)
Caused by low-level hCG in early pregnancy, ectopic pregnancies, or threatened abortion (hCG levels in ectopic pregnancy are in the range of 0.14-0.77 IU/ml).
In second and third trimesters, when hCG normal values are 5-10 IU/ml.

False Positives (HAI, LAI, DAP)
Caused by increased LH levels; exogenous hCG; phenothiazines; promethazine; methadone; proteinuria of ≥1 g/24 hr; trophoblastic tumor; carcinomas of ovary, lung, tuboovarian abscess; deteriorated reagents; occasionally RRA may be false positive because of cross-reactivity of LH.

TABLE 6-3.—Gestational Age Assessment

Prolonged pregnancy may have as many adverse effects on the fetus as prematurity. Careful clinical assessment of gestational age should include the following:
Dating by LMP and LNMP
Estimation of dates by size of uterus at first prenatal exam
Appearance of FHTs on Doppler (~10-12 weeks)
Quickening (16-20 weeks)
Appearance of FHTs with unamplified fetoscope (~20 weeks)
Uterine size at 20 weeks (at the navel)
When all these parameters coincide, the EDC may be established with reasonable confidence. If discrepancy exists, order ultrasonographic measurement of the biparietal diameter (BPD) at 12-18 weeks. Ultrasonographic measurements are inaccurate predictors of fetal age in the third trimester. Additional accuracy of estimation of EDC can be obtained from a repeat sonogram 4 weeks after the first. Correlate BPDs with clinical assessment.

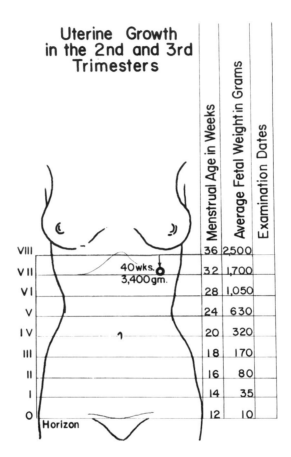

FIG 6-1.
Assessing gestational age by uterine growth. (From Iffy L: *1982-1983 Modern medicine ob-gyn pocket guide.* New York, 1982, Harcourt Brace Jovanovich, p. 66.

Pregnancy Table for Expected Date of Delivery

Find the date of the last menstrual period in the top line (light-face type) of the pair of lines. The dark number (bold-face type) in the line below will be the expected day of delivery.

Month	1	2	3	4	5	6	7	8	9	10	11	12	13	14	15	16	17	18	19	20	21	22	23	24	25	26	27	28	29	30	31	→
Jan.	1	2	3	4	5	6	7	8	9	10	11	12	13	14	15	16	17	18	19	20	21	22	23	24	25	26	27	28	29	30	31	
Oct.	**8**	**9**	**10**	**11**	**12**	**13**	**14**	**15**	**16**	**17**	**18**	**19**	**20**	**21**	**22**	**23**	**24**	**25**	**26**	**27**	**28**	**29**	**30**	**31**	**(1**	**2**	**3**	**4**	**5**	**6**	**7**	**Nov.**
Feb.	1	2	3	4	5	6	7	8	9	10	11	12	13	14	15	16	17	18	19	20	21	22	23	24	25	26	27	28				
Nov.	**8**	**9**	**10**	**11**	**12**	**13**	**14**	**15**	**16**	**17**	**18**	**19**	**20**	**21**	**22**	**23**	**24**	**25**	**26**	**27**	**28**	**29**	**30**	**(1**	**2**	**3**	**4**	**5**				**Dec.**
Mar.	1	2	3	4	5	6	7	8	9	10	11	12	13	14	15	16	17	18	19	20	21	22	23	24	25	26	27	28	29	30	31	
Dec.	**6**	**7**	**8**	**9**	**10**	**11**	**12**	**13**	**14**	**15**	**16**	**17**	**18**	**19**	**20**	**21**	**22**	**23**	**24**	**25**	**26**	**27**	**28**	**29**	**30**	**31**	**(1**	**2**	**3**	**4**	**5**	**Jan.**
April	1	2	3	4	5	6	7	8	9	10	11	12	13	14	15	16	17	18	19	20	21	22	23	24	25	26	27	28	29	30		
Jan.	**6**	**7**	**8**	**9**	**10**	**11**	**12**	**13**	**14**	**15**	**16**	**17**	**18**	**19**	**20**	**21**	**22**	**23**	**24**	**25**	**26**	**27**	**28**	**29**	**30**	**31**	**(1**	**2**	**3**	**4**		**Feb.**
May	1	2	3	4	5	6	7	8	9	10	11	12	13	14	15	16	17	18	19	20	21	22	23	24	25	26	27	28	29	30	31	
Feb.	**5**	**6**	**7**	**8**	**9**	**10**	**11**	**12**	**13**	**14**	**15**	**16**	**17**	**18**	**19**	**20**	**21**	**22**	**23**	**24**	**25**	**26**	**27**	**28**	**(1**	**2**	**3**	**4**	**5**	**6**	**7**	**Mar.**
June	1	2	3	4	5	6	7	8	9	10	11	12	13	14	15	16	17	18	19	20	21	22	23	24	25	26	27	28	29	30		
Mar.	**8**	**9**	**10**	**11**	**12**	**13**	**14**	**15**	**16**	**17**	**18**	**19**	**20**	**21**	**22**	**23**	**24**	**25**	**26**	**27**	**28**	**29**	**30**	**31**	**(1**	**2**	**3**	**4**	**5**	**6**		**April**
July	1	2	3	4	5	6	7	8	9	10	11	12	13	14	15	16	17	18	19	20	21	22	23	24	25	26	27	28	29	30	31	
April	**7**	**8**	**9**	**10**	**11**	**12**	**13**	**14**	**15**	**16**	**17**	**18**	**19**	**20**	**21**	**22**	**23**	**24**	**25**	**26**	**27**	**28**	**29**	**30**	**(1**	**2**	**3**	**4**	**5**	**6**	**7**	**May**
Aug.	1	2	3	4	5	6	7	8	9	10	11	12	13	14	15	16	17	18	19	20	21	22	23	24	25	26	27	28	29	30	31	
May	**8**	**9**	**10**	**11**	**12**	**13**	**14**	**15**	**16**	**17**	**18**	**19**	**20**	**21**	**22**	**23**	**24**	**25**	**26**	**27**	**28**	**29**	**30**	**31**	**(1**	**2**	**3**	**4**	**5**	**6**	**7**	**June**
Sept.	1	2	3	4	5	6	7	8	9	10	11	12	13	14	15	16	17	18	19	20	21	22	23	24	25	26	27	28	29	30		
June	**8**	**9**	**10**	**11**	**12**	**13**	**14**	**15**	**16**	**17**	**18**	**19**	**20**	**21**	**22**	**23**	**24**	**25**	**26**	**27**	**28**	**29**	**30**	**(1**	**2**	**3**	**4**	**5**	**6**	**7**		**July**
Oct.	1	2	3	4	5	6	7	8	9	10	11	12	13	14	15	16	17	18	19	20	21	22	23	24	25	26	27	28	29	30	31	
July	**8**	**9**	**10**	**11**	**12**	**13**	**14**	**15**	**16**	**17**	**18**	**19**	**20**	**21**	**22**	**23**	**24**	**25**	**26**	**27**	**28**	**29**	**30**	**31**	**(1**	**2**	**3**	**4**	**5**	**6**	**7**	**Aug.**
Nov.	1	2	3	4	5	6	7	8	9	10	11	12	13	14	15	16	17	18	19	20	21	22	23	24	25	26	27	28	29	30		
Aug.	**8**	**9**	**10**	**11**	**12**	**13**	**14**	**15**	**16**	**17**	**18**	**19**	**20**	**21**	**22**	**23**	**24**	**25**	**26**	**27**	**28**	**29**	**30**	**31**	**(1**	**2**	**3**	**4**	**5**	**6**		**Sept.**
Dec.	1	2	3	4	5	6	7	8	9	10	11	12	13	14	15	16	17	18	19	20	21	22	23	24	25	26	27	28	29	30	31	
Sept.	**7**	**8**	**9**	**10**	**11**	**12**	**13**	**14**	**15**	**16**	**17**	**18**	**19**	**20**	**21**	**22**	**23**	**24**	**25**	**26**	**27**	**28**	**29**	**30**	**(1**	**2**	**3**	**4**	**5**	**6**	**7**	**Oct.**

FIG 6-2.
Pregnancy table for expected date of delivery. (From Thomas CL, ed: *Taber's cyclopedic medical dictionary*, ed 16, Philadelphia, 1983, FA Davis, p. 1470.)

PRENATAL MATERNAL CARE

TABLE 6-4.—PRENATAL MATERNAL CARE

Complete History
Risk assessment, genetic history (Tay-Sachs disease, Down syndrome, muscular dystrophy, mental retardation, CNS anomaly), tobacco and drug use, hepatitis and HIV risk, diet, activity, general medical history, occupational (industrial, chemical, day care, health care)

Physical Examination
Height, weight, BP, general examination, especially of thyroid, dentition, heart and vascular system, reflexes, breasts, genitalia, and rectum

Laboratory Screening
First Visit
VDRL, Pap smear, GC culture, CBC, rubella titer, type and RH, irregular antibodies, urinalysis, $HB_S Ag$, (sickle cell anemia, Tay-Sachs disease, HIV test, herpes simplex culture, and *Chlamydia* test when indicated)
16-18 Weeks
Serum α-fetoprotein; consider need for ultrasound
18-22 Weeks
Glucose screen 1 hour after 50 g PO glucose load; recheck hematocrit
28 Weeks
Administer RhoGAM to Rh-negative women
36 Weeks
Reassess hemoglobin/hematocrit if previously low, repeat GC and *Chlamydia* cultures if previously positive

Clinical Assessment of Pelvis
Pelvic angle >90 degrees, diagonal conjugate >11.5 cm, intertuberous >8 cm

Patient Education
Drugs, diet, activity, costs, plan for care, travel, smoking, alcohol, analysis of risk assessment, weight gain, intercourse, fetal development, danger signals, father's role, childbirth classes, symptoms of labor, breast care, electronic fetal monitoring, delivery, cesarean delivery indications, analgesia/anesthesia, baby care, newborn circumcision, postpartum depression, contraception, effects on siblings, postpartum care and follow-up

For further information see *Caring for our future: the content of prenatal care,* A Report of the Public Health Service Expert Panel on the Content of Prenatal Care, Washington, D.C., 1989, U.S. Public Health Service, Department of Health and Human Services.

TABLE 6-5.—IDENTIFICATION OF HIGH-RISK PREGNANCY

Risk Assessment
About 70%-80% of perinatal mortality and morbidity is seen in 20%-30% of the obstetrical population. Early identification of risk is aided by combined antenatal and intrapartum risk assessment scoring. Carefully applied, these scoring scales will identify better than 80% of pregnancies with problem newborns. Only 20%-30% of problem newborns originate from the low-risk population.

Maternal-Child Health Care Index*
The scoring system below is an attempt to categorize the degree of maternal and fetal risk based on the information available at the initial history and physical on registration in our obstetrical clinics. Please circle the numbers under each of the 8 categories that you feel apply, and at the bottom of this sheet, add up these numbers and subtract from a perfect score of 100.

I. Maternal Age (years)		II. Race and Marital Status		III. Parity	
<15	20	White	0	0	10
15-19	10	Nonwhite	5	1-3	0
20-29	0	Single	5	4-7	5
30-34	5	Married	0	8+	10
35-39	10				
>40	20				

IV. Past Obstetrical History

Abortions		Premature Births		Fetal Death		Neonatal Death		Congenital Anomaly		Damaged Infants	
1	5	1	10	1	10	1	10	1	10	Physical	10
2	15	2+	20	2+	30	2+	30	2+	20	Neurological	20

V. Medical-Obstetrical Disorders and Nutrition

Systemic Illness	Specific Infections	Diabetes	Chronic Hypertension
Acute, mild 5	*Urinary:*	Pre 20	Mild 15
Acute, serious 15	Acute 5	Overt 30	Severe 30
Chronic nondebilitating 5	Chronic 25		Nephritis 30
Chronic debilitating 20	*Syphilis:*	Heart Disease	
	Treated 0	Class I or II 10	
	Untreated 20	Class III or IV 30	
	At term 30	History of prior failure 30	

*From Aubry RH, Pennington JC: *Clin Obstet Gynecol* 16:6, 1973.

Continued.

TABLE 6-5.—IDENTIFICATION OF HIGH-RISK PREGNANCY—cont'd

Endocrine Disorders		Anemia	
Definite adrenal, pituitary, or thyroid problem	30	Hb, 10-11 g	5
Recurrent menstrual dysfunction	10	Hb, 9-10 g	10
Involuntary sterility: <2 years	10	Hb, <9 g	20
>2 years	20		

Rh Problem		Nutrition	
Sensitized	30	Malnourished	20
Prior infant affected	30	Very obese	30
Prior ABO incompatibility	20	Inadequate diet but not malnourished	10

VI. Generative Tract Disorders

Prior fetal malpresentations	20
Prior cesarean section	30
Known anomaly or incompetent cervix	20
Myomas:	
>5 cm	20
Submucous	30
Contracted pelvis:	
Borderline	10
Any contracted plane	30
Ovarian masses:	
>6 cm	20
Endometriosis	5

VII. Emotional Survey (grade 0-20, based on):

Fears, attitudes, biases, hostilities, motivations, and behavioral patterns; prior pregnancies without supervision at time of registration; standard of child care and responsibilities; family unit, marital relationship; history of psychiatric illness in family

VIII. Social and Economic Survey (grade 0-10, based on):

Employment—husband, patient; annual income adequacy, public assistance; education—husband, patient; housing—location, quality, facilities, neighborhood environment

IX. Score

Total score of all 8 categories   -------------------
100 minus above score equals MCH Care Index   -------------------
High risk: score of 70, moderate risk: score of 71-84, low risk: 85
Perform antenatal risk assessment at initial visit and again at 36 weeks

TABLE 6-6.—Labor Index (LI)

FACTORS	PENALTY POINTS
Maternal Factors	
Prenatal Care	
<3 Prenatal visits	−10
No prenatal visits	−20
Toxemia	
Mild	−20
Severe	−20
Undetected diabetes	−20
Anemia: Hb < 10 g	−10
Fever	−20
Placental Factors	
Bleeding before 20 weeks	−10
Bleeding 20 weeks to term	−20
Bleeding with pain and/or hypotension	−30
Ruptured membranes > 24 hours	−20
Fetal Factors	
Gestational age	
<34 weeks	−30
34-37 weeks	−20
>42 weeks	−20
Multiple pregnancy	−20
Previously undetected Rh sensitization	−20
Meconium staining	−30
Fetal heart rate abnormality (<115, >165)	−30

Scoring
Labor index score = 100 − above penalties
Total index = 200 − (penalties from MCHI + LI)
High-risk group: Total index (MCHI + LI) ≤150

From Aubry RH, Pennington JC: *Clin Obstet Gynecol* 16:6, 1973.

TABLE 6-7.—Estimates for Dietary Need for Pregnancy and Lactation (U.S. RDA)

	NONPREGNANT BY AGES				FOR PREGNANCY ADD	FOR LACTATION ADD
	11-14 YR	15-18 YR	19-22 YR	23-50 YR		
kcal	2200	2100	2100	2000	+300	+500
Protein, g	46	46	44	44	+30	+20
Vitamin A, RE	800	800	800	800	+200	+400
Vitamin D, IU	400	400	300	200	+200	+200
Vitamin E, α-TE	8	8	8	8	+2	+3
Vitamin C, mg	50	60	60	60	+20	+40
Folacin, mg	0.4	0.4	0.4	0.4	0.4	0.1
Niacin, mg NE	15	14	14	13	+2	+5
Riboflavin, mg	1.3	1.3	1.3	1.2	+0.3	+0.5
Thiamin, mg	1.1	1.1	1.1	1.0	+0.4	+0.5
Vitamin B_6, mg	1.8	2.0	2.0	2.0	+0.6	+0.5
Vitamin B_{12}, μg	3.0	3.0	3.0	3.0	+1.0	+1.0
Calcium, mg	1200	1200	800	800	+400	+400
Phosphorus, mg	1200	1200	800	800	+400	+400
Iodine, μg	150	150	150	150	+25	+50
Iron, mg	18	18	18	18	+20*	+20*
Magnesium	300	300	300	300	+150	+150
Zinc	15	15	15	15	+5	+10

Modified from Food and Nutrition Board, National Academy of Sciences–National Research Council: *Recommended Dietary Allowances,* ed 9, revised 1989. Prenatal vitamin supplements usually contribute more than what is needed to satisfy U.S. RDAs. Iron and folacin are probably necessary even if an ordinary diet is taken. Vegetarians require more careful evaluation.

*The increased requirement for iron cannot be met by ordinary diets and supplementation is needed.

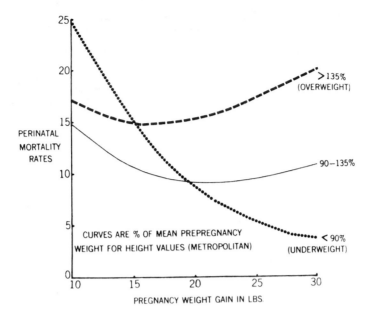

FIG 6-3.
Pregnancy weight gain and perinatal mortality. Overweight mothers had the fewest fetal and neonatal deaths with a 15- to 16-lb weight gain in term pregnancies. The optimal gain for normally proportioned mothers was 20 lb, and 30 lb for underweight mothers. With weight gains of more than 20 lb, underweight mothers had significantly lower perinatal mortalities than did mothers who were not underweight ($P < 0.005$). The underweight mothers in question had fewer losses to amniotic fluid infections, premature rupture of fetal membranes, and major congenital anomalies. (From Naeye RL: *Am J Obstet Gynecol* 135:3, 1979.)

TABLE 6-8.—Physiological Norms of Pregnancy (32-36 Weeks)

PARAMETER	NONPREGNANT	PREGNANT
Thyroid		
T_4 (μg/dl)	3.4-6.4	5.5-10.0
T_3 (%)	25-38	12-25
FTI (μg/dl)	1.2-1.6	0.9-1.4
Blood Count		
Hb (g/dl)	12-16	10-14
HCT (%)	37-47	32-42
WBC (total/mm^3)	4500-10,000	5000-15,000
ESR (mm/hr)	20	30-90
Iron Studies		
Serum Fe (μg)	75-150	65-120
TIBC	240-450	300-500
Blood Pressure	120/80	114/65
Pulse	70	80
Cardiac Output (L/min)	4.5	6.0
ECG	Normal	15-degree left axis deviation
V_1 and V_2	Normal	Inverted T wave
V_4	Normal	Low T
III	Normal	Q and inverted T
aV_R	Normal	Small Q
Respiratory		
Respirations (rate/min)	15	16
Tidal volume (ml)	475	675
Vital capacity (ml)	3150	3300-3400
Residual volume (ml)	950	750
Pao_2 (mm Hg)	95-100	95-100
$Paco_2$ (mm Hg)	35-40	25-35
Renal		
GFR (creatinine clearance, ml/min)	80-120	110-180
BUN (mg/dl)	10-18	4-12
Creatinine (mg/dl)	0.6-1.2	0.4-0.9
Uric acid (mg/dl)	2.0-6.4	2.0-5.5

Modified from Henry JB: *Postgrad Med* 52:110, 1972; 53:221, 1973.

TABLE 6-9.—Zɪᴅᴏᴠᴜᴅɪɴᴇ (ZDV) ғᴏʀ ᴛʜᴇ Pʀᴇᴠᴇɴᴛɪᴏɴ ᴏғ HIV Tʀᴀɴsᴍɪssɪᴏɴ ғʀᴏᴍ Mᴏᴛʜᴇʀ ᴛᴏ Iɴғᴀɴᴛ

Patient Selection
Known HIV-positive mother
No other indications for antiviral therapy exist
Has not received antiretroviral treatment during current pregnancy
CD4+ T-lymphocyte count is >200/μl at initial assessment

ZDV Regimen
100 mg ZDV PO 5 times per day, started at 14-34 weeks of pregnancy and
  continued until delivery
During labor, 2 mg/kg ZDV IV over 1 hour, followed by continuous infusion of 1
  mg/kg/hr until delivery
2 mg/kg ZDV syrup PO every 6 hours to the infant for the first six weeks of life
  beginning 8-12 hours after birth
Culture infant's blood for HIV at birth and at 12, 24, and 78 weeks. A positive
  culture indicates infection with HIV
Test infant for HIV antibody at 15 and 18 months

Modified from *MMWR* 43:285, 1994.

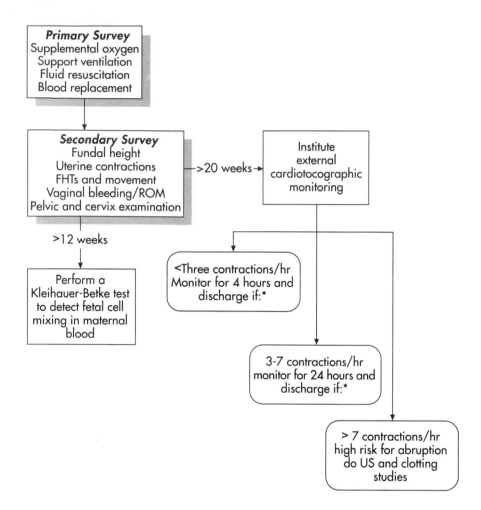

Primary Survey
Supplemental oxygen
Support ventilation
Fluid resuscitation
Blood replacement

Secondary Survey
Fundal height
Uterine contractions
FHTs and movement
Vaginal bleeding/ROM
Pelvic and cervix examination

→>20 weeks→

Institute
external
cardiotocographic
monitoring

>12 weeks

Perform a
Kleihauer-Betke test
to detect fetal cell
mixing in maternal
blood

<Three contractions/hr
Monitor for 4 hours and
discharge if:*

3-7 contractions/hr
monitor for 24 hours and
discharge if:*

> 7 contractions/hr
high risk for abruption
do US and clotting
studies

Discharge Criteria:
Resolution of contractions
Reassuring fetal heart tracing
Intact membranes
No uterine tenderness
No vaginal bleeding
All Rh-negative mothers receive 300µg of RhoGAM
(more if indicated by Kleihauer-Betke testing)

FIG 6-4.
Management of trauma in the pregnant patient. (Modified from Agnoli FL, Deutchman ME: Trauma in Pregnancy, *J Fam Pract* 37:588, 1993.)

GENETIC COUNSELING

TABLE 6-10.—MATERNAL AGE-SPECIFIC RISK ESTIMATES FOR SIGNIFICANT
CHROMOSOMAL DISORDER*

MATERNAL AGE (YEARS)	DOWN SYNDROME PER 1000 LIVEBORN	OTHER CHROMOSOMAL DISORDERS PER 1000 LIVEBORN	TOTAL SIGNIFICANT CHROMOSOMAL DISORDERS PER 1000 LIVEBORN	AS FRACTION†
15	1.0	1.3	2.3	1/450
16	0.9	1.3	2.2	1/450
17	0.8	1.3	2.1	1/500
18	0.7	1.3	2.0	1/500
19	0.6	1.3	1.9	1/500
20	0.6	1.3	1.9	1/500
21	0.6	1.3	1.9	1/500
22	0.6	1.3	1.9	1/500
23	0.7	1.3	2.0	1/500
24	0.8	1.3	2.1	1/500
25	0.8	1.3	2.1	1/500
26	0.9	1.3	2.2	1/450
27	1.0	1.3	2.3	1/450
28	1.0	1.3	2.3	1/450
29	1.1	1.4	2.5	1/400
30	1.1	1.4	2.5	1/400
31	1.2	1.5	2.7	1/350
32	1.4	1.6	3.0	1/333
33	1.7	1.7	3.4	1/300
34	2.2	1.8	4.0	1/250
35	2.7	2.2	4.9	1/200
36	3.5	2.4	5.9	1/170
37	4.5	2.8	7.3	1/140
38	5.7	3.2	8.9	1/110
39	7.2	3.7	10.9	1/90
40	9.2	4.5	13.7	1/70
41	11.7	5.4	17.1	1/60
42	14.9	6.6	21.5	1/50
43	19.0	8.1	27.1	1/37
44	24.2	10.1	34.3	1/30
45	30.8	12.6	43.4	1/25
46	39.3	16.0	55.3	1/20
47	50.0	20.3	70.3	1/14
48	63.8	26.1	89.9	1/10
49	81.2	33.7	114.9	1/9

From Iffy L, Kaminetzky H: *Principles and practice of obstetrics and perinatology,* New York, 1981, John Wiley & Sons, vol 1, p. 398.
*Numbers are based on various estimates, especially those of Hook and Cross. Clinically significant conditions include Down syndrome, trisomies 18 and 13, XXY, and XYY, but not XXX.
†This column provides useful approximations for genetic counseling.

TABLE 6-11.—Maternal Serum α-Fetoprotein Screening (MSAFP)

Elevations Occur in 4% of Those Tested and are Caused by:
Fetus
Anencephaly, spina bifida, encephalocele, omphalocele, gastroschisis, cystic hygroma
Maternal
Hepatitis, persistent AFP production, hepatocellular carcinoma, herpes infection, black race
Pregnancy
Incorrect estimate of gestation, preeclampsia, twins, fetal to maternal bleed, abruption, Rh isoimmunization, ataxia-telangiectasia, congenital nephrosis, epidermolysis bullosa simplex, severe oligohydramnios, spontaneous abortion, stillbirth, prematurity, acardiac twin, cyst or chorioangiomata of the placenta

Depressed Levels Caused by:
Fetus
Trisomies 21 and 18, sex-chromosomal aneuploidy
Maternal
Insulin-dependent diabetes mellitus, obesity

If screening test is abnormal, order a level II (high-resolution) sonogram. Consider amniocentesis for amniotic fluid α-fetoprotein (AF-AFP), chromosome analysis, and amniotic fluid acetylcholinesterase assay.

TABLE 6-12.—Indications for Midtrimester Amniocentesis for Genetic Diagnosis

Clear-cut Indications; High-Risk Situations
Parent is heterozygote for a serious autosomal dominant trait that can be diagnosed in fetus (e.g., achondroplasia; recurrence risk 1 in 2)
Both parents are carriers of a recessively inherited severe metabolic disorder that can be diagnosed in utero (e.g., Tay-Sachs disease; recurrence risk 1 in 4)
Mother is carrier of severe X-linked recessive disorder that can be diagnosed in utero (recurrence risk 1 in 4). If not diagnosable, determinations of fetal sex with a view to termination of male conceptus can be considered
Parents are carriers of a recessive or X-linked recessive malformation syndrome that may be diagnosable (e.g., Meckel' syndrome; recurrence risk 1 in 4)
One parent is a carrier of a translocation chromosome likely to cause serious chromosomal imbalance in the fetus (e.g., D/G translocation; risk is 1 in 10 when the mother is the carrier)
Maternal age over 40 (risk of Down syndrome more than 1 in 100)
Parent or sibling has neural tube defect (recurrence risk 1 in 20)
Previous trisomy, Down syndrome, or other major chromosome anomaly (risk approximately 1 in 100)
Elevated MSAFP, abnormal level II sonogram

Indications Less Clear-cut; Moderate or Uncertain Risk
Maternal age 35-39 (risk of Down syndrome approximately 1 in 200)
Severe maternal anxiety

Indication Controversial or Not Accepted
Amniocentesis only to determine sex, with a view to termination of pregnancy of undesired sex

Modified from Iffy L, Kaminetzky H: *Principles and practice of obstetrics and perinatology,* New York, 1981, John Wiley & Sons, vol 1, p. 397.

TABLE 6-13.—Possible Effects on the Fetus and Newborn of Maternal Drug Ingestion

DRUG	EFFECT
Alcohol	Fetal alcohol syndrome; intrauterine growth retardation (IUGR)
Amphetamines	Cardiac defects; irritability and poor feeding
Androgens	Masculinization
Antineoplastics	Congenital anomalies; growth delay
Barbiturates	Neonatal withdrawal
Cephalothin	Positive direct Coombs' test
Chloramphenicol	"Gray baby" syndrome
Diethylstilbestrol	Vaginal or adenosis adenocarcinoma
Heroin, other narcotics, and propoxyphene	Narcotic withdrawal, convulsions, neonatal death; growth retardation
Ibuprofen	Prolonged pregnancy and labor
Isotretinoin	Many major fetal abnormalities; wastage
Lithium	Congenital heart disease; facial clefts
Novobiocin	Hyperbilirubinemia
Phenylpropanolamine HCl	Eye and ear problems; hypospadias
Phenytoin	Cleft lip and palate; congenital height disorder; hydantoin syndrome; skeleton anomalies, IUGR
Potassium iodide	Goiter; mental retardation
Progestins	Masculinization; septal defects; limb reduction anomalies; hypospadias; VACTERL syndrome
Propylthiouracil	Congenital goiter, cretinism
Quinine	Thrombocytopenia
Radioactive iodine	Thyroid ablation
Reserpine	Nasal congestion; drowsiness
Salicylates	Neonatal bleeding; postmaturity; maternal bleeding
Sodium warfarin (Coumadin)	Fetal death; hemorrhage; blindness; mental retardation; and stippled epiphyses; nasal hypoplasia
Streptomycin	Acoustic nerve damage
Sulfonamides	Hyperbilirubinemia; kernicterus
Tetracyclines	Discoloration of teeth; inhibition of bone growth
Thiazides	Thrombocytopenia, hyperbilirubinemia, hypokalemia
Thiocarbamides	Goiter, hyperthyroidism
Trimethadione	Cleft lip and palate; congenital heart disorder; hydantoin syndrome; skeletal anomalies, IUGR
Trimethoprim	Hyperbilirubinemia at term
Valproic acid	Neural tube defects

Data from Iffy L, Kaminetzky H: *Principles and practice of obstetrics and perinatology,* New York, 1981, John Wiley & Sons, vol 2, p. 724; Rayburn WF, Zuspan FP: *Drug therapy in obstetrics and gynecology,* ed 3. Norwalk, Conn, 1992, Mosby.

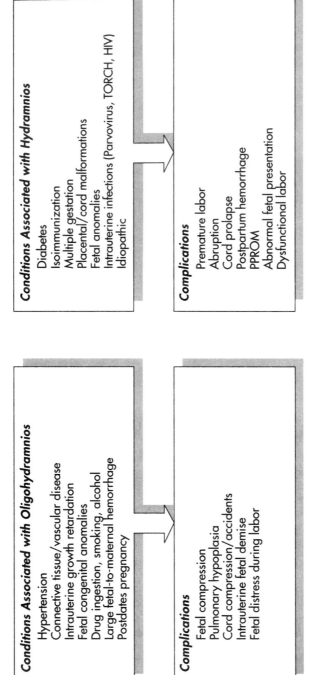

FIG 6-5.
Abnormalities of amniotic fluid volume: causes and complications. (Modified from Smith CS, Weiner S, Bolognese RJ: Amniotic fluid volume: importance and assessment. *The Female Patient* 15:87, 1990.)

Conditions Associated with Hydramnios

Diabetes
Isoimmunization
Multiple gestation
Placental/cord malformations
Fetal anomalies
Intrauterine infections (Parvovirus, TORCH, HIV)
Idiopathic

Complications

Premature labor
Abruption
Cord prolapse
Postpartum hemorrhage
PPROM
Abnormal fetal presentation
Dysfunctional labor

Conditions Associated with Oligohydramnios

Hypertension
Connective tissue/vascular disease
Intrauterine growth retardation
Fetal congenital anomalies
Drug ingestion, smoking, alcohol
Large fetal-to-maternal hemorrhage
Postdates pregnancy

Complications

Fetal compression
Pulmonary hypoplasia
Cord compression/accidents
Intrauterine fetal demise
Fetal distress during labor

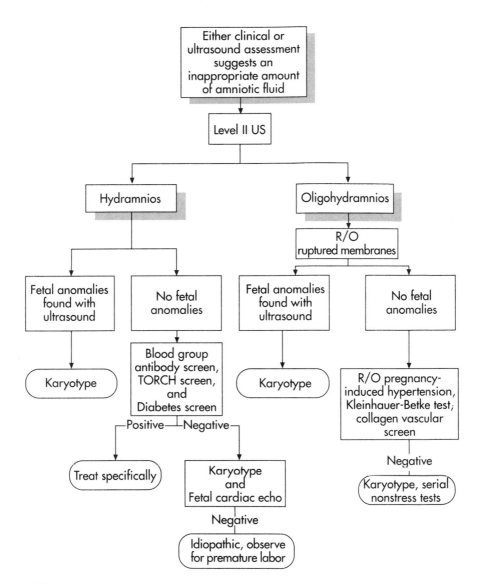

FIG 6-6.
Managing abnormalities of amniotic fluid volume. (Modified from Smith CS, Weiner S, Bolognese RJ: Amniotic fluid volume: importance and assessment, *The Female Patient* 15:85, 1990.)

MEDICAL COMPLICATIONS OF PREGNANCY

Diabetes

The perinatal mortality rate in insulin-dependent diabetics is 6.5%. Fluctuating maternal glucose levels and hyperglycemia are largely responsible for morbidity and mortality of the fetus. The classic triad of infant morbidity consists of hyperbilirubinemia, hypoglycemia, and hypocalcemia. The congenital major malformation rate in insulin-dependent diabetics is 9.0%. These rates may approach near normal with tight control.

TABLE 6-14.—DIABETES IN PREGNANCY

Diagnosis
Suspect if woman has prior history of elevated blood sugar, urine glycosuria, strong family history of diabetes, prior delivery of very large infant (>10 lb), anomalous or stillborn infant, hydramnios, habitual abortion, excessive maternal obesity, or fails glucose screen (see Table 6-4).

Diagnosis of Diabetes by Oral Glucose
Tolerance Test (OGTT) (after 100-g glucose load)

FBS	125 mg/dl
1 hour	185 mg/dl
2 hour	165 mg/dl
3 hour	145 mg/dl

Care during pregnancy should include home glucose monitoring and use of the hemoglobin A_{1C} test.

TABLE 6-15.—WHITE CLASSIFICATION OF DIABETES IN PREGNANCY

CLASS	AGE AT ONSET (YEAR)	DURATION (YEAR)	VASCULAR DISEASE	INSULIN
A	Any	Pregnancy	0	0
B	>20	<10	0	+
C	10-19	10-19	0	+
D	<10	20	Benign retinopathy	+
F	Any	Any	Nephropathy	+
R	Any	Any	Proliferative retinopathy	+
H	Any	Any	Heart disease	+

Modified from White P: *Am J Med* 7:609, 1949.

Cardiovascular Disease

Cardiac disease during pregnancy has a 2% incidence in all pregnant women; 90% is due to rheumatic heart disease (usually mitral stenosis); 1%-3% is due to congenital heart disease. Management is aimed at the prevention of CHF (Table 6-16).

TABLE 6-16.—CARDIOVASCULAR DISEASE DURING PREGNANCY

Prevention Factors	
Infection	Nutritional deficiencies
Anemia	Physical stress
Venous congestion	Fluid retention

Peak cardiac output occurs at 25-32 weeks (30%-50% above nonpregnant levels).

Steps in Management
Diagnose early and classify heart condition according to the New York Heart Association criteria
Auscultate heart frequently; check for anemia often
Class 1 and 2: Frequent rest, housekeeping aid, avoid stairs
Class 3: Greatly reduced activity, bed rest for mild failure
Class 4: Consider therapeutic abortion
Diet low in salt, lower water intake to 800-1000 ml/day for failure
Diuretics for moderate or advanced disease plus edema or venous congestion
Digitalis for failure apparent by signs and symptoms
Hospitalize patient before EDC to evaluate cardiac status
Careful monitoring during labor. Avoid hypotension
Shorten second stage with forceps. Regional block (caudal) recommended
SBE prophylaxis

Dermatoses

TABLE 6-17.—DIFFERENTIAL DIAGNOSIS OF THE MAJOR DERMATOSES ASSOCIATED WITH PREGNANCY*

DISEASE PROCESS	ONSET	TYPE AND LOCATION OF LESIONS	SYMPTOMS	ASSOCIATED LABORATORY ABNORMALITIES	THERAPY	MATERNAL-FETAL MORBIDITY/ MORTALITY
Herpes gestationis	Second half of pregnancy and postpartum, rare	Erythematous papules, vesicules, bullae on extremities, abdomen, buttocks, mucous membranes (20%) (tendency to symmetry)	Pruritus, few mild systemic manifestations (fever, chills)	Eosinophilia positive immunofluorescence, elevated chorionic gonadotropin level	Systemic corticosteroids	*Maternal:* None *Fetal:* Reports variable
Papular dermatitis of pregnancy	Anytime during gestation, rare	Erythematous papules (3-5 mm), generalized eruption	Pruritus, no associated systemic symptoms	Elevated urinary chorionic gonadotropin levels, decreased estrogen and cortisol level	Systemic corticosteroids	*Maternal:* None *Fetal:* Increased mortality
Prurigo gestationis of Besnier	Second half of gestation, 2% of all pregnancies	Small papules (1-2 mm) extensor surface	Pruritus, no associated systemic symptoms	None	Antipruritics	*Maternal:* None *Fetal:* None

Pruritus gravidarum (idiopathic jaundice of pregnancy)	Last trimester common, 17% of all pregnancies	*Extremities:* trunk (tendency to symmetry) No primary lesion, localized to abdomen or generalized	Pruritus, no associated systemic symptoms	Elevated bilirubin (in idiopathic jaundice of pregnancy)	Antipruritics	*Maternal:* None *Fetal:* Increased
Impetigo herpetiformis	Second half of gestation (usually), rare	Small pustules (may coalesce) Groin, inner thighs, extremities, mucous membranes (occasionally)	Pain, severe systemic symptoms common (high fever, chills, vomiting, diarrhea, arthritis, splenomegaly, lymphadenopathy, septicemia)	Hypercalcemia, hyperphosphatemia	Systemic corticosteroids	*Maternal:* Increased mortality *Fetal:* Increased stillbirths

Modified from Wade TR, et al: *Obstet Gynecol*, 52:233, 1978.

*These rashes will be progressive throughout pregnancy and will resolve with delivery; all but impetigo herpetiformis are prone to recurrence with subsequent pregnancies.

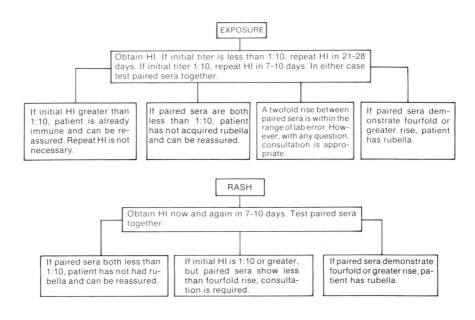

There are special indications for complement fixation antibody, fluorescent antibody, rubella-specific IgM and other determinations. Consult a specialist in Infectious Disease or the Center for Disease Control if:

1. Exposure has occurred more than two weeks prior to initial consultation.

2. Rash has occurred more than one week prior to initial consultation.

3. Paired sera demonstrate some rise but the rise is less than fourfold.

FIG 6-7.
How to diagnose rubella during pregnancy. (From McCubbin JH, Smith JS: *Am Fam Physician* 23:205, 1981.)

Back Pain

There are 3 common back pain syndromes associated with pregnancy:

1. High-back pain (above lumbar area) related to muscle fatigue
2. Low-back (lumbar) pain related to lifting and forward bending
3. Sacroiliac pain (buttock/thigh) related to subluxation of SI joint (Table 6-18).

The first two usually *decrease* in frequency as patients near term. The third syndrome, with or without radicular pattern, usually *increases* as pregnancy progresses toward term, and it is readily treatable.

TABLE 6-18.—BACK PAIN DURING PREGNANCY

Criteria for Diagnosis of Sacroiliac Subluxation

Sacral pain—usually unilateral, radiates like sciatica

Positive Piedallu's sign—forward flexion results in asymmetrical movement of posteriosuperior iliac spines; one becomes higher than the other

Positive pelvic compression—pain provoked by direct, downward pressure on anteriosuperior iliac spines

Asymmetry of anteriosuperior iliac spines—examine in the supine position; one appears higher than the other

Confirmatory Signs of Sacroiliac Subluxation

Straight leg raise—causes pain at highest elevation

Flexion block—with patient supine, flex knee at 90 degrees, then passively flex knee toward chest; flexion of thigh is blocked to one half the expected range on painful side

Positive Patrick's test—pain is provoked by placing one heel on the opposite knee in the supine position and simultaneously rotating the leg outward

Pain at Baer's point—tenderness just to the side and 2-3 inches below the umbilicus on the painful side, one-third of the distance between the umbilicus and the anteriosuperior iliac spine

Management of Sacroiliac Subluxation

One to two rotational manipulations of the SI joint and lumbar spine is usually sufficient to resolve the SI pain. Patient is placed supine, and the ipsilateral shoulder is held to the table. The patient's painful side is manipulated by flexing the thigh toward the abdomen with the knee in full flexion, then internally rotating the knee toward the contralateral side.

Modified from Ostgaard HC, Anderson GBJ, Karlsson K: Prevalence of back pain in pregnancy, *Spine* 16:549, 1991; Daly JM, Frame PS, Rapoza PA: Sacroiliac subluxation: a common, treatable cause of low-back pain in pregnancy, *Fam Pract Res J* 11:149, 1991.

OBSTETRICAL COMPLICATIONS OF PREGNANCY

Abortion

TABLE 6-19.—OBSTETRICAL COMPLICATIONS OF ABORTION

Loss of the products of conception before twentieth week of pregnancy
At least 10% of all pregnancies end in spontaneous abortion
Most spontaneous abortions occur in first 8 weeks; few occur after 13 weeks
Abnormalities of ovum in 60% of cases
Most common causes are polyploidy, trisomy, and sex chromosome aberrations

Six Types of Abortion
Threatened: 70% will go to term; decrease activity and restrict intercourse
Inevitable: Cervix dilated, conceptus at os; may complete with Pitocin
Incomplete: More common after 10 weeks; remaining material removed by
    D & C or suction curettage
Missed: Prolonged retention of nonviable conceptus, uterus does not grow and
    weight decreases 3-4 lb; check coagulation factors and empty uterus
Septic: Usually caused by induced abortion contaminated by *Streptococcus,*
    Staphylococcus, or *E. coli*
Habitual: Three or more consecutive spontaneous abortions; do CBC, blood
    sugar, liver and renal function studies, thyroid studies, rubella test, Coombs'
    test, and TORCH titers; culture for *T. mycoplasma*

TABLE 6-20.—POSSIBLE CAUSES OF ABORTION

Chromosomal abnormality of ovum	Age of gametes
Radiation	Viruses
Chemical exposure	Hypothyroidism
Hyperthyroidism	Diabetes
Chronic infection (*Mycoplasma,* toxoplas-mosis, parvovirus)	Chronic renal vascular disease
	Septate uterus
Chronic glomerular nephritis	Endometrial polyp
Bicornuate uterus	Incompetent cervix
Uterine myomas	Acute illness
Cervical laceration	Parental chromosomal abnormality
Severe mental shock	

From AAFP Home Study Self-Assessment, Monograph 33: *Complications of pregnancy,*
Kansas City, Mo, 1982, American Academy of Family Physicians, p. 12.

Ectopic Pregnancy

TABLE 6-21.—SITES AND INCIDENCE OF ECTOPIC PREGNANCY

SITE	PERCENT OF CASES	INCIDENCE
Ampular	47.0	The incidence of ectopic pregnancy is increasing and is between 1 in 100 and 1 in 200 pregnancies. The typical high-risk patient is older, has a higher parity, has had prior infertility, and has had a prior ectopic pregnancy or PID. Also current IUD use and prior tubal surgery.
Isthmic	21.6	
Fimbrial	5.8	
Interstitial	3.7	
Infundibular	2.5	
Other	19.4	

TABLE 6-22.—PHYSICAL FINDINGS IN ECTOPIC PREGNANCY

ABDOMINAL	PERCENT OF CASES	PELVIC	PERCENT OF CASES
Tenderness/pain	100	Adnexal tenderness	72
Amenorrhea	80	Cervix tenderness	43
Rebound	41	Adnexal fullness	35
Guarding	24	Adnexal mass (infrequent)	30
Distention	29	Cul-de-sac fullness	29
Diminished bowel sounds	18	Uterine enlargement	26
Absent bowel sounds	6	Cervix discoloration	25
Mass	3.5	Cervix softness	21

From AAFP Home Study Self-Assessment, Monograph 33: *Complications of pregnancy,* Kansas City, Mo, 1982, American Academy of Family Physicians, p. 18.

TABLE 6-23.—ULTRASOUND, SERUM hCG, AND PROGESTERONE IN THE DIAGNOSIS
OF NORMAL AND ABNORMAL PREGNANCIES

In a normal gestation, the hCG doubling time is 1.98 days.
Abnormal pregnancies are associated with <66% increase in hCG in a 2-day
  interval.

Ultrasound Findings	Days From LMP	hCG mIU*
Sac	32-38	914 ± 106
Fetal pole	37-44	3783 ± 683
Fetal heart motion	41-53	13,178 ±2898

Above 6000-6500 mIU of hCG, a normal intrauterine gestation can be visualized with transabdominal ultrasound 94% of the time.
The absence of an intrauterine gestational sac when hCG is >6000-6500 mIU
  is diagnostic of ectopic pregnancy in 86% of cases.
Adnexal masses can be found in ≥83% of ectopic pregnancies by ultrasound.
  (Transvaginal ultrasound is proving to be more accurate earlier in the pregnancy than transabdominal ultrasound.)
Serum progesterone (P$_4$) may be helpful in that most ectopics are associated
  with <15 ng/mL; intrauterine pregnancies show >20 ng/mL.

Modified from Leach RE, Ory SJ: *J Reprod Med* 34:324, 1989.
*Second International Standard.

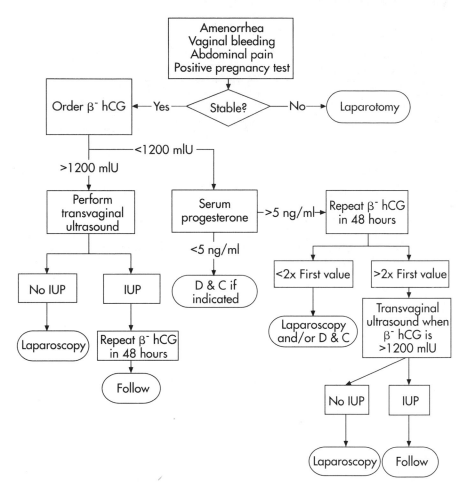

FIG 6-8.
Diagnosis of suspected ectopic pregnancy.

TABLE 6-24.—Culdocentesis Technique

Obtain informed consent; risks are hemorrhage and organ puncture.
Swab vagina and cervix with povidine-iodine.
Grasp posterior lip of cervix with tenaculum, and apply gentle traction.
Subcutaneous lidocaine anesthetic may be used in posterior fornix.
Insert spinal needle on a 10-ml Luer-lock syringe in posterior fornix into transitional fold.
Keep parallel to uterus and apply continuous, gentle negative pressure while inserting into cul-de-sac.
More than 5 ml of nonclotting blood is 99% diagnostic of ectopic pregnancy.
If bowel is inadvertently punctured, no harm should result; withdraw needle and observe.

TABLE 6-25.—Therapy for Ectopic Pregnancy*

Untreated, mortality is 69%

Surgical Therapy
Salpingostomy is used for unruptured ampullary gestations
Segmental resection preferred for gestations within isthmus (ruptured or unruptured so long as patient is stable)
Fimbrial expression for distal ectopic pregnancies already in process of extrusion
Salpingectomy for ruptured tubes with overt hemorrhage
    Subsequent intrauterine pregnancy rates range from 23% to 72%; ectopic risk is about 1 in 4

Nonsurgical Therapy
Indications for methotrexate dissolution therapy†
    Serum hCG < 1500 mIU/ml
    Sac measures ≤4 cm on transvaginal ultrasound
    Loss of blood into abdomen <100 ml
Methotrexate, 1 mg/kg of body weight IM every odd day (e.g., days 1, 3, 5, 7)
Leucovorin, 0.1 mg/kg IM every even day (e.g., 2, 4, 6, 8)
Continue until β-hCG levels drop ≥15% in 48 hours or 4 doses of each drug given
Monitor β-hCG level until undetectable; CBC, platelets, and LFTs
Monitor posttreatment hCG levels to identify persistent trophoblastic tissue

*Modified from Leach RE, Ory SJ: *J Reprod Med* 34:324, 1989.
†Modified from Ory S, et al: *Am J Obstet Gynecol* 154:1229, 1986; Carson SA, Buster JE: Ectopic pregnancy, *N Engl J Med* 329:1174, 1993.

TABLE 6-26.—MANAGEMENT OF THE INCOMPETENT CERVIX

The incidence of this disorder is about 1% and accounts for 20% of second-trimester abortions. Etiological factors include congenital, cervical laceration of prior delivery, prior surgery on cervix, overzealous D & C or therapeutic abortion, and exposure to DES in utero. Fetal survival rate ranges from 90% (if detected early) to 50% (with advanced cervical dilation).

Diagnosis
History of recurrent second trimester loss
Painless dilation and effacement of the cervix
Bulging membranes
Feeling of vaginal pressure with associated discharge
Premature rupture of membranes
Gray scale ultrasound reveals:
    Cervical length <3 cm
    Internal os >2 cm wide
    Bulging of membranes into endocervical canal

Treatment
Referral to obstetrician for either:
    Medical therapy—cervical cultures for GC, *Chlamydia,* and β-hemolytic strep-tocci; bed rest; possibly short-term use of NSAIDs
    Surgical therapy—cerclage placement (McDonald—purse-string with Mer-silene band; or Shirodkar—submucosal suture)

Third-Trimester Bleeding

Any third-trimester bleeding should be presumed to be caused by the placenta, and the fetus should be considered endangered until proven otherwise. As a general rule, any third-trimester bleeding should be investigated in the hospital where surgical care is immediately available. The bleeding may be painful or painless (Table 6-27).

TABLE 6-27.—THIRD-TRIMESTER BLEEDING

Common Causes of Third-Trimester Bleeding

Placenta previa: 1 in 125 pregnancies; maternal mortality is 1%; fetal mortality is up to 30%

Abruptio placentae: 1 in 100 pregnancies; maternal mortality is less than 1%; fetal mortality is up to 35%

Marginal sinus rupture: One third to one half of all cases of third-trimester bleeding; maternal mortality is 0; fetal mortality is 4%

Velamentous insertion of cord/vasa previa: Very rare; maternal mortality is 0, condition may be rapidly fatal for fetus

Ruptured uterus: Rare

Lesions: Cervical, vaginal, or vulvar

General Rules

Do not do a vaginal exam in an unprepared setting; do not insert a finger in the cervix.

Have blood for transfusion available.

Surgical team should be alerted and standing by before double setup examination is attempted.

Try to distinguish maternal from fetal bleeding using Apt test.

Apt Test

Mix equal parts of blood from vagina and 0.25% sodium hydroxide

If bleeding is fetal in origin, no color change (fetal hemoglobin resists alkali)

If maternal in origin, turns light brown (maternal hemoglobin is nonresistant)

Also may look for nucleated RBCs (fetal) by Wright's stain

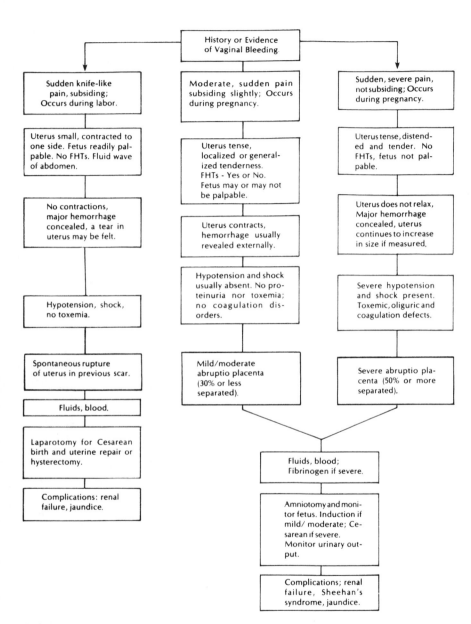

FIG 6-9.
Third-trimester bleeding with pain.

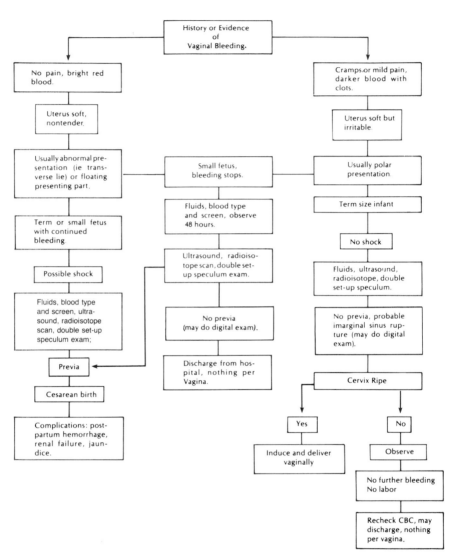

FIG 6-10.
Painless third-trimester bleeding.

TABLE 6-28.—Preterm Premature Rupture of Membranes

Spontaneous premature rupture of the membranes (SPROM) usually occurs at or near term, and 80% of patients may proceed with labor over the next 24 hours. In some patients SPROM occurs before 37 weeks and may be associated with the following:
Amniotic bands leading to fetal malformation if <18 weeks
Chorioamnionitis with maternal and fetal risk for morbidity and mortality
Premature birth with attendant complications in the infant

Diagnosis
History of sudden gush of fluid or a continuous leakage
Palpate uterus for estimation of fetal size and presence of contractions
Auscultate for FHTs
Sterile speculum examination to visualize cervix for draining of fluid through os
Examination of vaginal fluid:
    Swab for C&S for group B streptococcus, *N. Gonorrhoeae,* and chlamydia
    Swab fluid onto glass slide and air dry for fern test—amniotic fluid arborizes and ferns
    Microscopic examination for fetal squamous cells or fat cells, which will stain blue with Nile blue sulfate
    Presence of alkaline pH (touching upper one third of vaginal wall in sampling fluid will give false positive)
    Meconium staining
    Heat a sample of fluid from external os on a glass slide for 1 minute. Amniotic fluid turns white; endocervical mucus of pregnant patients turns brown

TABLE 6-29.—Observed Malformations Useful in Dating of Amniotic Rupture

EVENT IN NORMAL MORPHOGENESIS	DATE BY WHICH STRUCTURE IS DETERMINED	MALFORMATION THAT RESULTS WHEN PROCESS IS INTERRUPTED
Formation of frontonasal process	28 days	Proboscis
Limb budding	28 days	Absent extremity
Flexion of embryo	28 days	Omphalocele with deficiency of abdominal wall
Fusion of maxillary and medial nasal processes	35 days	Cleft lip
Perforation of nasal passages	45 days	Choanal atresia
Closure of palatal shelves	9 weeks	Cleft palate
Return of intestines to abdominal cavity	10 weeks	Omphalocele
Eruption of scalp hair	16 weeks	Lack of normal hair whorl
Formation of dermal ridges	18 weeks	Altered dermal pattern

From Higginbottom MC: *J Pediatr* 95:544, 1979.

TABLE 6-30.—RECOMMENDED MANAGEMENT OF PRETERM PREMATURE RUPTURE OF MEMBRANES (PPROM) IN PATIENTS WITHOUT EVIDENCE OF AMNIONITIS

FETUS	MANAGEMENT
<20 weeks gestation	Termination of pregnancy
500-749 g (20-27 weeks)	Bed rest; await onset of spontaneous labor; monitor temperature and WBC count
750-1749 g (28-33 weeks)	Consider corticosteroid induction of pulmonary maturation. Nothing per vagina and monitor temperature and WBC count; deliver after 24 hours
1740-2249 g (34-35 weeks)	Induction after 16 hours of PPROM; do not stop if in labor; consider β-Lactam antibiotic prophylaxis for GBS
2250 g (>35 weeks)	Induce within 8-12 hours

TABLE 6-31.—DIAGNOSIS OF AMNIONITIS

CLINICAL	LABORATORY
Fetal tachycardia	Leukocytosis
Maternal tachycardia	Amniotic fluid leukocytes
Maternal fever	Amniotic fluid bacteria (smear)
Uterine tenderness	Amniotic fluid culture (quantitative)
Foul cervical discharge	
Uterine contractions	

From Iffy L, Kaminetzky H: *Principles and practice of obstetrics and perinatology,* New York, 1981, John Wiley & Sons, vol 2, p. 1038.

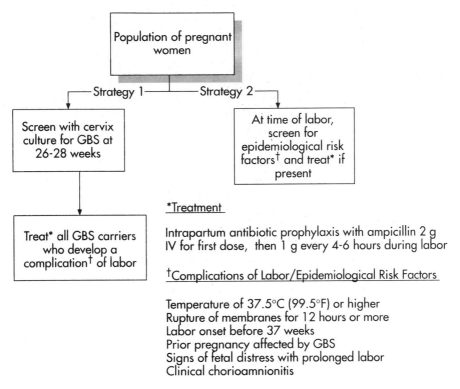

FIG 6-11.
Strategies for prevention of group B streptococcal (GBS) infection.

Premature Labor

Premature labor (<36 weeks) resulting in low birth weight is the major cause of neonatal morbidity and mortality (Table 6-32). Inhibiting premature labor is possible in 50% of patients with bed rest alone since the supine position increases uterine blood flow, thereby decreasing laborlike activity. When unwanted uterine activity persists, ritodrine may be expected to arrest labor in approximately 60% of patients (Table 6-33).

TABLE 6-32.—RECOMMENDED CRITERIA FOR SELECTING PATIENTS FOR TREATMENT OF PRETERM LABOR WITH TOCOLYSIS

Qualifying (all)
Gestation of 20-36 weeks
Fetal weight <2500 g
Regular contractions
Labor progressing, cervix dilating and/or effacing

Disqualifying
Active vaginal bleeding
Eclampsia or severe preeclampsia
Dead fetus or major fetal malformation incompatible with survival
Intrauterine infection
Maternal cardiac disease
Maternal hyperthyroidism
Any obstetrical or medical condition that contraindicates prolongation of pregnancy

Conditions Limiting Chances of Success
Incompetent cervix
Ruptured fetal membranes
Advanced labor, cervical dilation of more than 4 cm
Untreated urinary tract infection

Modified from Barden TP, et al: *Obstet Gynecol* 56:1, 1980.

TABLE 6-33.—Management of Preterm Labor with Tocolysis

Review record for accuracy of gestational dating
Monitor fetal heart tones and contractions with external monitor
If PPROM, culture cervix for GC, chlamydia, and group B streptococci
Follow success of tocolysis with sterile cervical exams every 1-2 hours until
  contractions stop
Monitor maternal respirations, blood pressure, and heart rate
Recheck maternal cardiovascular examination frequently

Alternative Treatment Regimens
1. *Terbutaline:* 0.25 mg subcutaneously every 1-4 hours or 2.5-10 mg PO every
   4-6 hours
   Hold dose if FHTs >180 or maternal vital signs show BP <90 mm Hg sys-
     tolic, respirations >28/min or pulse >120/min
   Can also be given IV at 0.01 mg/min, increasing by 0.005 mg/min every 10
     minutes to maximum of 0.025 mg/min; titrate down to minimum effective
     rate
2. *Ritodrine:* Initial dose, 50-100 μg/min (150 mg diluted in 500 ml of solution
   gives 300 μg/ml); then increase dose by 50 μg/min every 10 minutes until
   contractions stop or unacceptable side effects develop
   Reduce dose if side effects are poorly tolerated. *Side effects:* Maternal
     tachycardia and hypotension, reduced serum potassium, maternal palpita-
     tions, nervousness, nausea, headache
   Maximum dose: 350 μg/minute
   Discontinue ritodrine if labor persists at the maximum dose
   If labor is successfully arrested, continue the infusion for at least 12 hours
     before beginning oral therapy
   Oral Therapy
   Initial dose, 10 mg administered 30 minutes before stopping infusion; then 10
     mg every 2 hours, or 20 mg every 4 hours, for 24 hours; then, if the uterus
     remains quiescent, 10-20 mg every 4-6 hours until further inhibition of la-
     bor is not indicated
   Maximum dose: 120 mg/day.
   If labor recurs during oral administration, infusion may be repeated if the pa-
     tient is qualified
3. *Magnesium sulfate:* 4 g of a 10% solution IV over 20 minutes then 1 g/hr IV
   for maintenance
   Obtain serum magnesium 1 hour after start of therapy, then every 4 hours;
     therapeutic levels are 4-8 mg/dl
   Decrease dose if absent DTRs or respirations <10-12/min
4. *Nifedipine:* 20 mg PO every 8 hours

TABLE 6-34.—Diagnosis of Hypertension in Pregnancy

PARAMETER	PREECLAMPSIA		ECLAMPSIA
	MILD	SEVERE	
Blood pressure (on 2 or more consecutive readings)	≥140/90 mm Hg, or systolic rise of 30 mm Hg or diastolic rise of 15 mm Hg; Mean Arterial Pressure > 95 during the second trimester (MAP = diastolic pressure + [systolic − diastolic pressure]/3)	≥160/110 mm Hg	Usually elevated
Proteinuria	1-2+ (>300 mg/24 hr)	3-4+ (>5 g/24 hr)	3-4+
Edema	1-2+ (1 kg or more weight gain)	3-4+	3-4+
Reflexes	Hyperreactive	Markedly hyperreactive with clonus	Convulsions
Other	Headache	Oliguria (<500 ml/24 hr); visual blurring; right upper quadrant or epigastric pain; elevated serum creatinine, ALT, AST levels; uric acid, and thrombocytopenia <10 × 10^9 per liter	Coma

When these signs appear before the twentieth week, consider hydatidiform mole or nonimmune fetal hydrops.

From 7% to 10% of all pregnancies are complicated by hypertension. Of these, half are due to preeclampsia, and half are the result of chronic hypertension.

Many of those who will later develop preeclampsia may be predicted by observing blood pressures between 28 and 32 weeks. After 10 to 15 minutes of stabilization in the lateral recumbent position, check blood pressure, then roll patient to the supine position and recheck. This is the Gant rollover test. A rise of 20 mm Hg or more in diastolic pressure has approximately 90% predictive accuracy. Adequate dietary protein intake during pregnancy, calcium supplementation and aspirin (60 mg/day in high-risk patients) is the only preventive measure that can be taken. If aspirin therapy is to be tried, start at 12 weeks.

Modified from Carroll J, et al: *Complications of pregnancy,* AAFP Home Study Self-Assessment, Monograph 120, Kansas City, Mo, 1989, American Academy of Family Physicians.

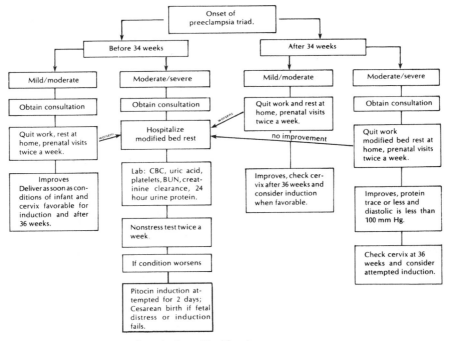

During Labor and Delivery of Pre-Eclampsia

* Artificial rupture of membranes as soon as safe and possible (unless malpresentation or CPD)
* IV oxytocin induction (see oxytocin induction protocol)
* IV Magnesium Sulfate if hyperreflexic (see magnesium sulfate protocol)
* IV Apresoline if diastolic BP greater than 110 (see apresoline protocol)
* Monitor I & O—output should average 100 cc/3 hrs

FIG 6-12.
Preeclampsia management strategies.

TABLE 6-35.—Bishop Scoring of Labor Inducibility

	SCORE†			
FACTOR	0	1	2	3
Dilation (cm)	Closed	1-2	3-4	≥5
Effacement (%)	0-30	40-50	60-70	≥80
or length (cm)*	4	2-4	1-2	<1
Station of head from spines (cm)	−3	−2	−1.0	+1, +2
Consistency	Firm	Medium	Soft	
Position of os	Posterior	Mild	Anterior	

Modified from Romney, et al: *The health care of women,* New York, 1981, McGraw-Hill.
*Use either effacement or length but not both.
†A score from 0 to 13 indicates increasing ease of inducibility.

TABLE 6-36.—HELLP Syndrome

Definition
Intravascular *H*emolysis
*E*levated *L*iver enzymes
*L*ow *P*latelet count

Syndrome
Occurs early (~34 weeks) in third trimester
Occurs in patients with preeclampsia or eclampsia
More frequent in whites and when diagnosis of preeclampsia is delayed or
when delivery is postponed
Screen for this condition in all women with preeclampsia

Clinical Features
High blood pressure, edema, ≥2+ proteinuria and right upper quadrant tenderness

Complications
Disseminated intravascular coagulation is most common
Placental abruption ~20%
Acute renal failure ~8%

Management
Assess cardiovascular status
Monitor liver enzymes and platelet count
Institute seizure prophylaxis
Treat disseminated intravascular coagulation disorder
Deliver as soon as possible

TABLE 6-37.—Drug Management Protocols for Preeclampsia and Eclampsia

Magnesium Sulfate Protocol (for Anticonvulsant and Sedation)
Begin IV infusion of 5% dextrose.
Give 2-4 g of $MgSO_4$ (10% solution) IV, not to exceed 1.5 ml (150 mg) per min.
Maintain $MgSO_4$ by infusion pump, using 20 g in 1000 ml of IV fluid (2% solution).
Usual maintenance dose is 1 g/hr, maximum dose 7.5 ml (150 mg) per min, depending on 30-min assessments of reflexes and respirations. Watch urinary output, and if <30 ml/hr, decrease infusion rate.
Have 10% calcium gluconate for IV use at hand to counteract $MgSO_4$ if respiratory depression (rate <10-12/min) occurs.
Continue $MgSO_4$ for 24-48 hours after delivery.
Therapeutic serum magnesium 4-8 mg/dl. Higher doses are toxic. Patellar reflexes are lost at ~10 mg/dl, respiratory depression at ~12-15 mg/dl, cardiac arrest at ~ 25 mg/dl.

Hydralazine (Apresoline) Protocol (for Diastolic BP >110 mm Hg)
Mix 20 mg of hydralazine in 20 ml of 5% dextrose (1 mg/ml).
Give 5-ml IV bolus over 2-4 minutes and observe BP for 30 minutes.
If no decline of BP in 30 minutes, give 5-10 ml IV slowly every 20-30 minutes.
Repeat 20-ml dose every 1-2 hours as needed.
Keep diastolic BP between 90 and 110 mm Hg.
Watch for tachycardia or hypotension
Diazoxide or labetalol are second line agents if BP refractory to hydralazine.

TABLE 6-38.—Cervical Ripening and Oxytocin Induction Protocol to Stimulate Onset of Labor

Labor induction may be aided by the prior use of prostaglandin E_2 gel, 0.5 mg applied intracervically every 6 hours × 2 or 3 doses.

Begin IV infusion with 5% dextrose.

Monitor externally if cervix is unfavorable for internal monitoring.

Perform amniotomy and attach fetal scalp monitor electrode as soon as presentation is safe or favorable.

A second IV of 1000 ml of 5% dextrose with 1 ml (10 IU) of oxytocin is connected through an infusion pump and attached piggyback to the first IV tubing.

Each 1 ml contains 10 mU of oxytocin.

Start infusion at 0.5 mU/min and increase by 1 mU every 20 minutes until labor is satisfactory (contractions every 2-3 minutes lasting 60-90 seconds). With an intrauterine pressure monitor in place, the desired contraction amplitude is 50-80 mm Hg.

If infusion pump is unavailable, add 2.5 units to 1000 ml, giving 2.5 mU/ml; if the apparatus delivers 1 ml every 15 drops, 3 drops/min will equal 0.5 mU/min.

Antidiuretic effect (increase renal tubular absorption of water) may begin around 15 mU/min and reach maximum at 45 mU/min. This may produce water intoxication and convulsions.

The half-life of IV oxytocin is less than 4 minutes, so if overstimulation (uterine contractions with less than 1 minute between) occurs, stop infusion.

Contraindications to induction: Abnormal fetal presentation, absolute fetopelvic disproportion, uterine scar from prior surgery, women of high parity.

TABLE 6-39.—CT Pelvimetry

Radiation dose is reduced over conventional plain film pelvimetry

Computer enhancement precludes repeat films because of underexposure or overexposure

Efficient and highly accurate measurements

Measurements taken during suspended respiration:

>11.0 cm = True conjugate/pelvic inlet (from horizontal pilot scan). Measure from prominence of S_1 to upper region of pubic symphysis

>12.0 cm = Transverse diameter/widest point of true pelvis (from vertical pilot scan). Measure below ischial spines at widest diameter

>10.0 cm = Interspinous distance/midpelvic diameter (from axial image) Measure between points of ischial spines

TABLE 6-40.—VAGINAL BIRTH AFTER CESAREAN (VBAC) SECTION

Advantages
Lower maternal morbidity and mortality; shorter hospital stay
Increased maternal satisfaction
Better immediate bonding with the newborn
Less blood loss
Less costly

Disadvantages
Sense of failure if repeat cesarean section required after labor
Potential for uterine rupture (7% with classical incision/0.5% with low transverse)
Less safe if 3 or more prior cesarean sections

Management Guidelines for Lowering the Risk
1. Accurate documentation of number (<3) and type of prior cesarean sections
2. Prior incision was low transverse or low vertical not extending into active myometrium
3. No recurrent indications (e.g., fetal-pelvic disproportion, maternal herpes, hemorrhage, fetal distress, maternal systemic disease, hypertension, uncorrectable uterine inertia, malpresentation)
4. No new indication in current pregnancy (e.g., IUGR, previa, abruption, nonvertex presentation)
5. Patient counseled carefully for informed consent and patient motivation high
6. Admit patient as soon as signs of active labor appear
7. Type and screen for 2 units of packed cells
8. Intravenous line in place during labor
9. Electronic fetal monitoring during labor's progress
10. Patient must follow normal course of labor; failure to progress requires repeat cesarean section
11. Emergency cesarean section can be done within 30 minutes of decision and primary physician in constant attendance during labor. Alert surgeon when patient admitted

Modified from Beguin EA: *The female patient* 14:119, 1989; ACOG Committee on Obstetrics: *Maternal and fetal medicine: guidelines for vaginal delivery after cesarean birth,* Washington, DC, 1985.

ANTEPARTUM FETAL SURVEILLANCE

A number of serial antepartum assessments may be used to ensure that the fetus is not adversely affected by the pregnancy (Table 6-41).

TABLE 6-41.—Monitoring Fetal Well-Being

Indications for Assessment
High-risk pregnancy; SGA; LGA; postdatism; trauma; decrease in fetal movements; prior poor obstetrical performance; diabetes, hypertension, or other chronic maternal condition; antepartum bleeding; suspected fetal abnormality.

Biochemical Assessments
Estriols; minimum urinary value at term is 12 mg/24 hr. Obtain weekly (30-33 weeks), then biweekly (34-35 weeks), then every 2 days beginning at 36 weeks.
Norm may be approximated:
$$\text{Minimum} = \left(\frac{\text{Weeks of gestation}}{10}\right)^2 - 4$$

Amniocentesis
Fluid analyses for meconium or fetal blood and to assess fetal maturity
    Alkaline pH; 98% water + 2% solids
    L/S ratio: 2:1 or more indicates fetal lung maturity (use 2.5:1 for diabetic patients)
    Creatinine: 2 mg/100 ml indicates maturity
    Cells: ≥25% anuclear cells or ≥20% fat cells; fetus should weigh >2500 g.
    Foam test: 0.5 ml of normal saline + 1 ml of amniotic fluid + 1 ml 95% ethanol; shake vigorously for 15 seconds. Complete bubble ring is positive and indicates maturity; L/S ratio unnecessary
    Genetic screening may be performed
    Bilirubin concentration (Rh sensitization)
        Zone I: None-to-mild fetal effects
        Zone II: Moderate fetal effects
        Zone III: Severe fetal effects

Fetoscopy
Most accurate for direct examination of fetus and genetic studies. Cannula and trocar placed under ultrasound guidance and sampling of fetal skin and fetal blood taken under direct fiberoptic visualization. Risk of fetal mortality is 7.5%-9.0%. Can lead to premature labor.

Continued.

TABLE 6-41.—Monitoring Fetal Well-Being—cont'd

CONDITION	PARAMETER	SCORE 2	SCORE 0

Biophysical Profile
Combines five parameters to give score of 0-10 (0 being the worst). A score of
8 or 10 indicates fetal well-being. Requires ultrasound. If <8, suspect chronic
asphyxia and deliver if favorable cervix and ≥36 weeks.

CONDITION	PARAMETER	SCORE 2	SCORE 0
Hypoxia/acute stress	Conventional NST*	Reactive	Nonreactive†
	Fetal breathing	Sustained for 30 seconds	Not sustained for 30 seconds
	Fetal movement	≥3 gross body movements (axial rotation) in 30 minutes	<2 gross body movements
	Fetal tone	≥1 episode of flexion/extension	No flexion/extension
Chronic stress	Amniotic fluid volume	≥1 pocket 1 × 1 cm	No pocket >1 cm

Fetal Movement Counts
Fetus should be noted to move by mother at least 10 times per 12-hr period
Have mother count number of movements felt during a 60-minute recumbent
period 2 hours after main meal. Three to 10 or more movements is normal
Excess movement is not alarming

Modified from Manning FA, et al: *Am J Obstet Gynecol* 151:343, 1985.
*NST = nonstress test. See Table 6-42 for interpretation.
†NST may be nonreactive if infant sleeping. Try retest after giving orange juice to mother
and tapping on her abdomen to interrupt fetal sleep period.

TABLE 6-42.—INTERPRETING NONSTRESS TEST (NST) AND CONTRACTION STRESS
TEST (CST)

Indications for NST/CST

Chronic hypertension	Pregnancy-induced hypertension
Diabetes mellitus	Collagen vascular disorder
Chronic renal disease	Prolonged (>42 weeks) pregnancy
Oligohydramnios	Intrauterine growth retardation
Cyanotic heart disease	Hemoglobinopathy
Prior fetal demise	Cigarette smoking
Isoimmunization	Hyperthyroidism
Discordant twin growth	Maternal perception of decreased fetal movements

TEST RESULT	INTERPRETATION
NST	
Reactive	Two or more fetal heart rate accelerations of 15 beats/min above baseline, lasting at least 15 seconds within a 20-minute period, with or without maternal perception of movement
Nonreactive	Criteria for "reactive" are not met. Monitor for at least 40 minutes; acoustic stimulation may be used to shorten observation period
Equivocal	Only one acceleration occurs over any 10-minute period
Unsatisfactory	Poor quality tracing, unable to interpret
CST*	
Negative	No late decelerations; contractions are occurring at least three times in 10 minutes and are lasting 40-60 seconds
Positive	Late decelerations following ≥50% of contractions even if the contraction frequency is less than 3 in 10 minutes
Equivocal	Intermittent late or significant variable decelerations
Unsatisfactory	Poor quality tracing, unable to interpret; unable to attain contraction frequency of 3 in 10 minutes

Modified from Roussis P, Troiano NH, Shah DM: Fetal assessment part I: nonstress and contraction stress testing. *The Female Patient* 15:33, 1990; ACOG Technical Bulletin #188, January 1994.

*Fetal respirations can aid interpretation of CST. Normal fetal respirations are 30-70 breaths/min, episodic, and occur 50%-90% of the time. If CST is positive, and fetal respirations are normal, there is an 87% chance that it is a false positive. If there are no breathing movements, it is true positive.

TABLE 6-43.—Fᴇᴛᴀʟ Hᴇᴀʀᴛ Rᴀᴛᴇ Mᴏɴɪᴛᴏʀɪɴɢ

Baseline Features (between contractions)
Rate
120-160 beats/min (normal)
<120 beats/min bradycardia (heart block, drugs, hypothermia, hypoxia)
>160 beats/min tachycardia (catecholamines, asphyxia, infection, fever, drugs, tachydysrhythmia, thyrotoxicosis, prematurity)
Variability
Short-term or beat-to-beat type, differing serial or adjacent beats
  Requires fetal scalp lead for reliable interpretation
Long-term or sine wave type, >6 beats/min of wavy oscillation; 3-6 cycles/min
Variability normal or decreased (hypoxia, anencephaly, drugs, complete heart block)

Periodic Changes
Acceleration (normal with contractions)
Decelerations (see Fig. 6-13)
Early: Transient hypoxia, noncompromised fetus
Late: Maternal hypotension if normal FHR variability. With absent FHR variability, suspect hypoxia and decompensation.
Variables: Abrupt drop of 60 beats/min with quick recovery. Usually reassuring to see "shoulders" of acceleration at onset and end
Ominous severe variables: >60 beats/min drop, >60 beats/min baseline, >60 seconds long
"W" wave type of deceleration: Nuchal cord with compression

Patterns
Reassuring
All parameters normal
Acute stress
Normal or abnormal rate, >6 beats/min variability, late or variable decelerations
Prolonged stress
Normal or abnormal note, <6 beats/min variability, late or variable decelerations or absent periodicity
Sinister
Normal or abnormal rate, absent variability, severe late or variable decelerations or absent periodicity
Sinusoidal
Monotonously regular, smooth, sine wave baseline with frequency of 3-6/min and range of amplitude up to 30 beats/min (Rh-isoimmunized fetus, acid-base abnormality, or oxytocin administration)
Saltatory
Excessive variability, bizarre pattern like venous tachycardia in appearance (drug use, brief hypoxia)

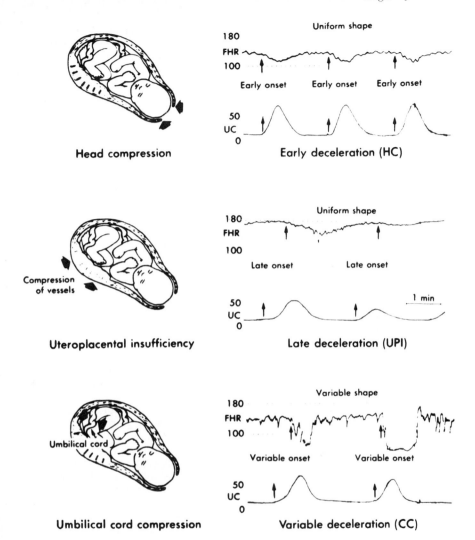

FIG 6-13.
Changes in fetal heart rate patterns due to various causes. (From Hon EH: *An atlas of fetal heart rate patterns,* New Haven, Conn, 1968, Harty Press.)

TABLE 6-44.—Fᴇᴛᴀʟ Sᴄᴀʟᴘ Bʟᴏᴏᴅ Sᴀᴍᴘʟɪɴɢ

When an abnormal FHR pattern is detected, fetal scalp blood should be sampled:

Cervix is dilated to at least 2 cm with the patient in the dorsal lithotomy position. *Contraindications:* bleeding disorder, amnionitis.

Endoscope is passed through the cervix and the fetal scalp visualized.

Fetal scalp is swabbed with ethyl chloride to achieve reactive hyperemia, and then with silicon to facilitate blood collection.

A deep puncture, 2-3 mm, is made with a small scalp blade.

Blood is drawn into heparinized pipette or capillary tube. Analyze immediately. pH requires 50 µl, base deficit 120 µl.

Scalp pH of 7.25-7.35 is acceptable; a progressive decline, or scalp pH <7.2 is ominous.

A difference of 0.15 to 0.19 in maternal-fetal pH is preacidemic.

A pH difference of >0.2 indicates fetal acidemia.

Fetal Po_2 is normally 20-25 torr, indicating 50% saturation.

Fetal Pco_2 is normally 41-51 torr.

TABLE 6-45.—Iɴᴛʀᴀᴜᴛᴇʀɪɴᴇ Rᴇsᴜsᴄɪᴛᴀᴛɪᴏɴ ᴏꜰ Dɪsᴛʀᴇssᴇᴅ Iɴꜰᴀɴᴛ

Place patient in lateral decubitus position.

Start O_2 by mask.

Start IV with D_5W solution; infuse at a rate of 125 ml/hr after 200-ml bolus.

Do vaginal examination to check for prolapse of cord, and, if found, decompress cord if possible.

Arrest labor if possible; administer a single 250-µg dose of terbutaline by bolus IV injection. If oxytocin is being administered, discontinue it.

Place intrauterine pressure catheter and fetal scalp electrode; discontinue external Doppler tracing.

Administer amnioinfusion 250-500 ml of sterile normal saline solution through an intrauterine catheter over a 20-minute period. Set infusion at 180 ml/hr.

Monitor intrauterine pressure to guard against hypertonia or hyperstimulation.

LABOR AND DELIVERY

TABLE 6-46.—Assessment at Onset of Labor

History: Bleeding; membranes ruptured; green color to fluid; recent illness; headache; nausea or epigastric pain; recent weight gain

Physical examination: Maternal BP, pulse, temperature; FHTs; breasts; heart sounds; lungs; reflexes; edema; veins of the legs; abdominal examination; costovertebral percussion. *Vaginal examination:* presenting part; dilation of cervix; descent; membrane intact or ruptured

Laboratory: If prenatal care, none needed. Otherwise, do CBC, VDRL, typing and Rh sensitivity, catheterized urinalysis. Consider fetal vital signs

---

TABLE 6-47.—Cervical Dilation: Translating Fingers into Centimeters

FINGERS	CENTIMETERS
1 (tight)	1
1 (loose)	2
2 (tight)	3
2 (loose to slightly spread)	4
2 (spread)	5-7
1 fingerbreadth of lateral cervix	8
½ fingerbreadth of lateral cervix remaining on each side	9
Only anterior cervix palpable	9+ (anterior lip)
No palpable cervix	10 (complete dilation)

From Iffy L, Kaminetzky H: *Principles and practice of obstetrics and perinatology,* New York, 1981, John Wiley & Sons, vol 2, p. 818.

TABLE 6-48.—Stages of Labor

| PHASE OF LABOR | DEFINITION | DURATION/RATE | |
		NULLIPARAS	MULTIPARAS
First stage (onset of labor to complete dilation)			
Latent	Slow dilation	21 hours, ≤0.5 cm/hr	14 hours, ≤0.5 cm/hr
Active			
Acceleration	Usually begins at 4-5 cm	0.6-1.0 cm/hr	0.6-1.0 cm/hr
Maximum slope	Cervix ≥5 cm	1.2 cm/hr (average, 3.0)	1.5 cm/hr (average, 5.7)
Deceleration	Cervix ≥9 cm, but not complete	Descent 1.0 cm/hr (average, 3.3)	Descent 2.1 cm/hr (average, 6.6)
Second stage (complete dilation to delivery)		2 hr (average, 33 min)	45 min (average, 8.5 min)
Third stage (from delivery of fetus to placenta)		10 min or less	10 min or less
Total labor (onset of labor to delivery of placenta)		25.8 hours (mean, 10.0)	19.5 hours (mean, 6.2)

Modified from Iffy L, Kaminetzky H: *Principles and practice of obstetrics and perinatology.* New York, 1981, John Wiley & Sons, vol 2, pp. 818-820.

TABLE 6-49.—Dysfunctional Labors: Diagnosis and Management

Latent Phase Disorders (before 4 cm of Cervical Dilation)
Dx: Prolonged latent phase is >20 hours in nulliparas; >14 hours in multiparas
  Causes

Unripe cervix 18%	Sedation 19%	Unknown 17%
False labor 10%	Anesthesia 7%	
Uterine inertia 9%	CPD rare	

  Rx
    False labor observed (10%): Discharge
    Observed to progress: Expect NSVD or cesarean
    Fail to progress (5%): Oxytocin stimulation

Active Phase Disorders (from ≥4-5 cm of Cervical Dilation)
Dx: Primary dysfunctional labor is <1.2 cm/hr nullipara; <1.5 cm/hr multipara
  Causes

CPD 28%	Sedation 42%
Malposition 74%	Anesthesia 14%

  Rx
    CPD: Cesarean delivery
    Other causes: Observed and two out of three progress to vaginal delivery
    If cervical dilation not progressing and you suspect uterine inertia, try oxytocin stimulation
Dx: Secondary arrest of labor is in active phase but without full dilation
  Causes

CPD 45%	Malposition 73%	Exhaustion
Sedation 63%	Anesthesia 19%	

  Rx
    CPD: Cesarean delivery
    Other causes: Try oxytocin; many will require cesarean delivery
NOTE: All dysfunctional labors should be monitored with internal fetal scalp electrode and uterine pressure catheter as soon as insertion is possible.

Modified from Friedman EA, et al: *Obstet Gynecol* 25:845, 1965.

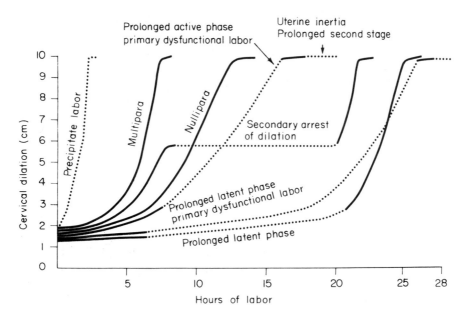

FIG 6-14.
Friedman labor curves typifying various normal and abnormal patterns of cervical dilation. (From Vorherr H: Disorders of uterine function during pregnancy. In Assali NS, ed: *Pathophysiology of gestation,* New York, 1972, Academic Press, p. 191.)

Montevideo Units

Montevideo units can be used to determine the existence of sufficient uterine expulsive forces to accomplish delivery. A minimum of 200-225 Montevideo units should be sought before cesarean delivery is considered for presumed uterine inertia or cephalopelvic disproportion.

An intrauterine pressure catheter must be placed:

1. Count the number of contractions in 10 minutes
2. Determine baseline uterine tone (usually 10-20 mm)
3. Sum the intensities of all contractions over a 10-minute period (to find intensity, subtract baseline from peak reading of each contraction).
4. This determination can be repeated several times in an hour and averaged. For example, 5 contractions occurring over 10 minutes have a mean intensity of 45 mm over baseline and supply 225 Montevideo units.

Pelvimetry

X-ray pelvimetry is thought to be rarely indicated. CT pelvimetry is preferable (see Table 6-39), but when it is unavailable, and when lack of adequate progress is accompanied by moderate to forceful uterine contractions as documented by electronic monitoring, particularly in a primipara, plain film pelvimetry may be indicated.

TABLE 6-50.—Pelvimetry

Mengert's Pelvimetry Rules:

Inlet:	AP (~11 cm) × transverse (~13 cm) = ~145*
Midplane:	AP (~11.5 cm) × transverse (~10.5 cm) = ~125*

*Values less than these imply narrow pelvis.

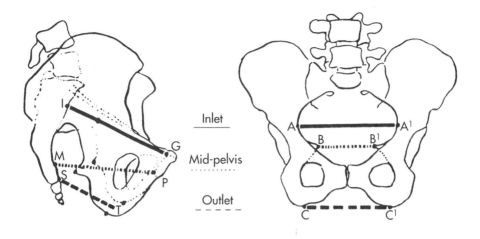

Diameters			Average normal	Average total	Low normal
Actual inlet	Anteroposterior	1 to G	12.5	25.5	22.0
	Transverse	A to A¹	13.0		
Mid-pelvis	Anteroposterior	M to P	11.5	22.0	20.0
	Transverse (bispinous)	B to B¹	10.5		
Outlet	Anteroposterior (post. sagittal)	S to T	7.5	18.0	16.0
	Transverse (bituberal)	C to C¹	10.5		

FIG 6-15.

Standard pelvic diameters. Three levels embody all salient bony landmarks of the true pelvis. (Courtesy Mercy Hospital x-ray department, Iowa City, Ia.)

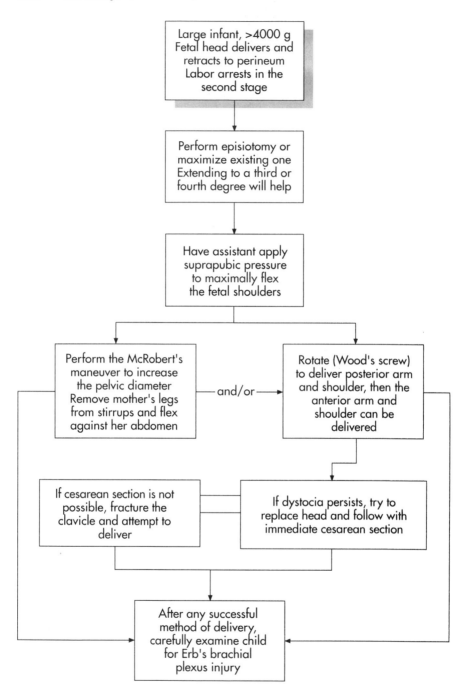

FIG 6-16.
Management of shoulder dystocia.

Delivery Methods

TABLE 6-51.—GUIDELINES FOR USE OF FORCEPS

Use in the Event of the Following:
Cervix dilated to 10 cm, membranes ruptured
Fetal head on or just above pelvic floor (below interspinous plane), e.g., low or outlet forceps
Vertex or face presentation, or aftercoming head of breech

Indications
Obliterated perineal reflex, as with conduction anesthesia
Maternal heart disease, hypertension, neurological disorder, vascular anomaly
Abruptio placentae or vasa previa
Second stage fails to progress (>2 hours) and head is well into pelvis, maternal exhaustion
Rotatory arrest
Some cases of fetal distress
Breech and delivery of aftercoming head

Technique
Use Simpson's, DeWeese, or Tarnier's forceps for primipara with fetus with long, molded head
 Elliot (fenestrated) or Tucker-McLean (nonfenestrated) forceps for multipara with rounded fetal head
 Kielland's forceps (no pelvic curve) for rotation
 Piper forceps (long blades with deep curve) for breech
Wash genitalia, empty bladder by straight catheterization
Assess position of head, sutures, and fontanelles
Give adequate anesthetic (pudendal, conduction, general)
Insert left blade (lies to your right) first, then right, keeping hand between maternal tissue and blade
Close forceps and check position by palpation of fetal head, maternal vaginal and cervical tissues
Cut generous episiotomy
Gently test pull, then pull for effect in a downward and outward axis, moving to almost vertical upward as head emerges, then remove forceps

---

TABLE 6-52.—USE OF THE VACUUM EXTRACTOR FOR PROLONGED SECOND STAGE OF LABOR

Use of Mityvac device or Silastic cup:

Indications
 Fetal distress (if delivery imminent)
 Prolonged second stage of labor
 Maternal exhaustion, weak uterine expulsive force

Contraindications
 Malpresentation (breech, face, brow); must be vertex
 Premature infant
 Intact membranes
 Incomplete cervical dilation; head not engaged
 Presenting part requires rotation
 Cephalopelvic disproportion
 Prior fetal scalp sampling

Technique
 Connect cup to pump
 Ascertain fetal head in normal vertex position and well engaged; remove
  scalp electrode if present
 Spread labia, fold cup, and insert into position over posterior fontanelle
 Sweep finger around edge to check for entrapped maternal tissue
 Reduce pressure to −100 mm Hg (10-20 cm of water)
 With next contraction rapidly reduce pressure to −380-580 mm Hg (maxi-
  mum 65 cm of water), and begin traction in line with the pelvic axis
 When contraction subsides, take pressure up to −100 mm Hg.
 Recheck with finger sweep
 Episiotomy may be needed
 Once head delivered, remove cup. Cephalohematoma occurs in about 15%
  of cases

Discontinue Under the Following Circumstances:
 Delivery not accomplished after 10 minutes at maximum pressure or 30 min-
  utes from start of procedure
 Cup disengages three times
 No progress after three consecutive pulls
 Fetal scalp traumatized by extractor

Complications
 Injury to maternal tissue (cervix, vaginal wall)
 Fourth-degree extension of episiotomy
 Cephalohematoma (red or blue circular scalp discoloration)
 Skin swelling, petechiae, or injury of fetal scalp
 Failure to extract promptly

Modified from Epperly TD, Breitinger ER: *Am Fam Physician* 38:205, 1988.

APGAR Scoring

TABLE 6-53.—APGAR SCORING

PARAMETER	SCORE		
	0	1	2
Heart rate	Absent	Less than 100 beats/min	100 beats/min or greater
Respiratory effort	Absent	Shallow or irregular breathing	Lusty breathing, crying
Reflex irritability*	No response	Little response	Normal response
Muscle tone	Limp	Intermediate	Spontaneously flexed extremities that resist extension
Color	Entirely cyanotic	Partly cyanotic	Entirely pink

*A perfect score is 10. Scores of 6 or less are currently interpreted as significant depression. Any form of stimulation may be used. Commonly, Dr. Apgar evaluated coughing, gagging, or sneezing in response to suctioning of the mouth or nose.

TABLE 6-54.—CLINICAL RESPIRATORY DISTRESS SCORING (RDS) SYSTEM

PARAMETER	SCORE		
	0	1	2
Respiratory rate (breaths/minute)	60	60-80	>80 or apneic episodes
Cyanosis	None	In air	In 40% O_2
Retractions	None	Mild	Moderate to severe
Grunting	None	Audible with stethoscope	Audible without stethoscope
Air entry (crying)*	Clear	Delayed or decreased	Barely audible

From Downes JJ, et al.: *Clin Pediatr* 9:325, 1970.
*Air entry represents the quality of inspiratory breath sounds as heard in the midaxillary line.
The RDS score is the sum of the individual scores for each of the five observations.
RDS score: 0-3, give oxygen by hood; 4-5, continuous positive pressure breathing; ≥6, mechanical ventilation required.

ESTIMATION OF GESTATIONAL AGE BY MATURITY RATING   Side 1

Symbols: X - 1st Exam   O - 2nd Exam

Scoring system: Ballard JL, *et al:* A Simplified Assessment of Gestational Age. Pediatr Res 11:374, 1977. Figures adapted from "Classification of the Low-Birth-Weight Infant" by AY Sweet in Care of the High-Risk Infant by MH Klaus and AA Fanaroff, WB Saunders Co, Philadelphia, 1977, p. 47.

NEUROMUSCULAR MATURITY

	0	1	2	3	4	5
Posture						
Square Window (Wrist)	90°	60°	45°	30°	0°	
Arm Recoil	180°	100°-180°	90°-100°	< 90°		
Popliteal Angle	180°	160°	130°	110°	90°	< 90°
Scarf Sign						
Heel to Ear						

PHYSICAL MATURITY

	0	1	2	3	4	5
SKIN	gelatinous red, transparent	smooth pink, visible veins	superficial peeling &/or rash, few veins	cracking pale area, rare veins	parchment, deep cracking, no vessels	leathery, cracked, wrinkled
LANUGO	none	abundant	thinning	bald areas	mostly bald	
PLANTAR CREASES	no crease	faint red marks	anterior transverse crease only	creases ant. 2/3	creases cover entire sole	
BREAST	barely percept.	flat areola, no bud	stippled areola, 1—2 mm bud	raised areola, 3—4 mm bud	full areola, 5—10 mm bud	
EAR	pinna flat, stays folded	sl. curved pinna, soft with slow recoil	well-curv. pinna, soft but ready recoil	formed & firm with instant recoil	thick cartilage, ear stiff	
GENITALS Male	scrotum empty, no rugae		testes descending, few rugae	testes down, good rugae	testes pendulous, deep rugae	
GENITALS Female	prominent clitoris & labia minora		majora & minora equally prominent	majora large, minora small	clitoris & minora completely covered	

Gestation by Dates _____ wks

Birth Date _____ Hour _____ am / pm

APGAR _____ 1 min _____ 5 min

MATURITY RATING

Score	Wks
5	26
10	28
15	30
20	32
25	34
30	36
35	38
40	40
45	42
50	44

SCORING SECTION

	1st Exam=X	2nd Exam=O
Estimating Gest Age by Maturity Rating	_____ Weeks	_____ Weeks
Time of Exam	Date _____ Hour ____pm am	Date _____ Hour ____pm am
Age at Exam	_____ Hours	_____ Hours
Signature of Examiner	M.D.	M.D.

FIG 6-17.

Newborn maturity rating and classification. Estimation of gestational age by maturity rating. *X,* First examination; *O,* Second examination. (Scoring system from Ballard JL, et al: A simplified assessment of gestational age, *Pediatr Res* 11:374, 1977. Figures modified from Sweet AY: Classification of the low-birth-weight infant. In Klaus MH: *Care of the high-risk neonate,* Philadelphia, 1986, WB Saunders, p. 47.)

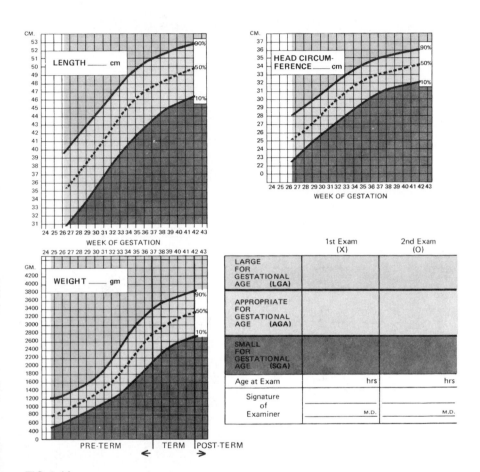

FIG 6-18.
Classification of newborns based on maturity and intrauterine growth. *X,* First examination; *O,* Second examination. (From Lubchenco LC, Hansman C, Boyd E: *Pediatrics* 37:403, 1966; Battaglia FC, Lubchenco LC: *J Pediatr* 71:159, 1967.)

Indications for a Cesarean Section

TABLE 6-55.—MATERNAL AND FETAL INDICATIONS FOR CESAREAN SECTION

MATERNAL OR FETAL CONDITION	ABSOLUTE INDICATION	STRONG INDICATION	MODERATE INDICATION	WEAK INDICATION	CONTRAINDICATION
Prolapsed cord	Undeliverable		Deliverable		
High-risk pregnancy (e.g., diabetes)		Positive stress test		Questionable stress test	
Abnormal monitoring patterns		Definite		Equivocal	
Hypertensive disease		Fetal distress	Patient not severely ill		Very ill patient, unfit for immediate surgery
Abruptio placentae	Severe abruption	Severe abruption Fetus undeliverable		Mild abruption (marginal—no indication)	Clotting disorder Fetus deliverable
Cephalopelvic disproportion	Severe		Mild		
Instead of midforceps delivery		Small pelvis		Epidural anesthetic	
Breech	Size-position progress			Frank, average size Good progress	
Multiple birth	Viable triplets		Twins		
Premature breech		Viable			
Placenta previa	Total or partial	Lateral	Low lying		

	Transverse Face-posterior	Transverse Face-posterior		Brow Face-anterior	Severe infection (special operation)
Abnormal presentation of fetus	Transverse, Face-posterior			Brow, Face-anterior	
Maternal infection		Herpes; fetus not infected			Severe infection (special operation)
Cervix unfavorable				Attempt induction	
Dead fetus					No indication
Nonviable fetus					No indication
Obstruction of birth canal	Pelvic mass or tumor				
Vascular disease			Previous cerebral hemorrhage from aneurysm		
Cervical neoplasia	Invasive carcinoma			Noninvasive carcinoma in situ	
Cardiac disease		Obstetrical indications only			Not indicated per se
Previous pelvic injury					
Fistula	Vesicovaginal				
Cesarean section	Recurring indication (e.g., CPD)	Nonrecurring indication (e.g., previa)			

Modified from Iffy L, Kaminetzky H: *Principles and practice of obstetrics and perinatology*, New York, 1981, John Wiley & Sons, vol 2, pp. 1536, 1537.

POSTPARTUM MATERNAL CARE

TABLE 6-56.—Postpartum Maternal Care

General
Control uterine atony
Estimated blood loss should be 250-500 ml
Postpartum hemorrhage is defined as 500 ml or more
Inspect cervix, vagina, and perineum; provide hemostasis and repair (3%-5% incidence of significant lacerations with normal delivery; 10%-15% incidence after forceps use)

Retained Placenta
If not delivered after 30 minutes, mix 10 IU of oxytocin in 20 ml of sterile normal saline and inject into umbilical vein
Manual extraction with sedation and analgesics

Uterine Atony/Postpartum Hemorrhage
Abdominal uterine massage, repeat every 15 minutes
Bimanual compression; express clots
Give oxytocin, 10 units IM (after placenta delivery to avoid entrapment)
Start IV, add 20 units of oxytocin to 1000 ml and give 20-50 mU/min
Ergot drugs may be added if no hypertension: methylergonovine, 0.2 mg PO or IM
15-methyl prostaglandin $F_{2\alpha}$ 0.25 mg IM every 15 minutes (maximum of 2 mg)
If uterine hemorrhage continues, explore uterine cavity under anesthetic for retained placenta and give volume expanders, oxygen, and blood replacement. Consider coagulopathy
MAST garment may be used on legs as therapy for shock

Routine Postpartum Orders
Observe vital signs, fundus, and perineum for hemorrhage every 15 minutes for 2 hours, then every 30 minutes for 2 hours, then every 60 minutes for 4 hours, then every 8 hours if stable. Patient's temperature should be checked at least daily
Uterine massage every 15 minutes for 2 hours and as needed thereafter
Patient may ambulate as possible, at first with assistance. Encourage activity
If patient is unable to void within 6 hours following delivery, may be catheterized
Prescribe general lactating diet (increased protein and fluids)
Prescribe tight breast binder and ice to breasts for engorgement symptoms if patient is not nursing
If patient is breast-feeding on demand of infant, begin as soon as possible after delivery
Perineal care: Ice bags to perineum for first 12 hours, followed by warm sitz baths as needed. Perineal pads used with Tucks applied to anal area and perineum

---

TABLE 6-56.—Postpartum Maternal Care—cont'd

Stool softener and laxatives used as needed

Analgesics as needed (acetaminophen with or without codeine). The appearance of fever may be masked.

If mother is Rh negative, check infant cord blood for type, Rh, and direct Coombs' test. If infant is Rh positive, administer appropriate dose of RhoGAM to mother

Recheck hemoglobin and hematocrit on second postpartum day; may need to begin iron replacement

Ensure appropriate bonding and interaction of parents with newborn

Appointments made for follow-up of infant (2 and 4 weeks) and mother (4 weeks)

Discharge on third postpartum day (or before) if no contraindications; instruct in contraception, infant care, danger signals of puerperium

TABLE 6-57.—Protocol for the Administration of RhoGAM

OFFICE	BLOOD BANK
Initial Visit	
Draw clotted blood for ABO group, Rh type, and antibody screening test.	If patient is Rh negative, and antibody screen is negative for anti-Rh_o (D), report as candidate for RhoGAM at 28 weeks and at delivery
28 Weeks	
If patient is Rh negative:	If antibody screen is negative or antibody other than anti-Rh_o (D) is detected, report as candidate for RhoGAM at delivery if infant is not Rh negative
Draw clotted blood for antibody screen	
Inject RhoGAM, 300-μg dose	
Following Delivery	
Collect mother's blood and cord blood	Perform fetal cell screen on maternal sample using micro-D^u procedure
Inject RhoGAM, 300-μg dose	Type cord blood. If not Rh negative (D and D^u negative), issue appropriate amount of RhoGAM

Courtesy Johnson & Johnson, New Brunswick, New Jersey.

LACTATION

Milk production occurs in stages that may be recognized by the nutritional content of the milk. Colostrum, secreted from 0 to 5 days after birth, contains 55-60 kcal/100 g. Maturation of the milk occurs through transition milk (5-10 days), immature milk (10-30 days), to mature milk (>30 days), which contains 65-75 kcal/100 g.

TABLE 6-58.—LACTATION

Milk Letdown may be Encouraged by the Following:
Increased amount of fluid intake
Heat to the breasts
Relaxation exercises (e.g., yoga, Lamaze) and quiet rest
Gentle breast massage or caress
Increased frequency of suckling
Syntocinon nasal spray (one spray in each nostril, 2-3 minutes before nursing)

TABLE 6-59.—MANAGING COMMON BREAST-FEEDING PROBLEMS

CONDITION	SYMPTOMS	RECOMMENDATIONS
Sore nipples	Cracking, bruising, bleeding, and soreness	Beginning 35 weeks, use nipple rolling to prepare them and prevent soreness; proper positioning of infant's mouth
Inhibited letdown	Difficulty with the letdown reflex; no uterine cramping or breast tingling	Comfort, rest, adequate privacy, and proper positioning; local heat and oxytocin nasal spray
Engorgement	Occurs third or fourth postpartum day; breast large and hard	Hand expression or pumping before nursing to soften the breast
Blocked ducts	Smooth, tender lump in breast that does not decrease after nursing	Local heat, massage lump toward the nipple, frequent nursing
Mastitis	Infection with *S. aureus, E. coli,* or streptococcus species causes warm, red, tender wedge-shaped area	Frequent nursing, rest, fluids, pain medication and dicloxacillin for 10 days
Breast abscess	Tender, hard mass with overlying erythema	Needle aspiration for culture, incise and drain, give antibiotics
Candida infection	Intense, burning nipple pain; papules	Topical nystatin
Return to work	Missed feedings; the infant is also using bottle and formula	On-site feeding, breast pump, can refrigerate milk for up to 48 hours or freeze for 6 months
Poor infant gain	Sluggish feeder, poor suckling	May use supplemental lactation device (Lact-Aid)
Infant jaundice	Bilirubin is ≥15 after third day of life	Interrupt breast-feeding for 24 hours for bili to fall
Medications	Drug is prescribed	See Table 6-61

TABLE 6-60.—MANAGEMENT OF BREAST-FEEDING IN THE PRESENCE
OF MATERNAL INFECTION

ORGANISM	CONDITION	ISOLATE FROM MOTHER
Bacteria	Premature rupture of membranes; >24 hours without fever:	
	Full-term infant	No
	Premature infant	No
	Maternal fever >38° C twice, 4 hours apart, 24 hours before to 24 hours after delivery, or endometritis; full-term or premature infant	Yes, until mother is afebrile for 24 hours
Salmonella, Shigella, Staphylococcus, group B β-hemolytic streptococci	Mother with possible cervical culture but otherwise negative obstetrical history	No No No
	Mother with possible cervical culture and obstetrical history of fever, premature rupture of membranes >24 hours, fetal distress, meconium, low Apgar score, any symptoms of prematurity	No
	Infant with surface colonizing:	
	Negative history and physical examination	No
	With PROM or maternal infection	No
Group A streptococci	Mother with infection	Yes
Gonorrhea	Mother with positive smear or culture; infant well	No
	Infant with conjunctivitis	No

MOTHER CAN VISIT NURSERY	MOTHER CAN BREAST-FEED	IMMEDIATE TREATMENT	CONTACT WITH PREGNANT WOMEN ALLOWED
Yes	Yes	Observe	Yes
Yes	Yes	Treat with ampicillin and kanamycin	Yes
No, until mother is afebrile for 24 hours	No, until mother is afebrile for 24 hours	Treat with ampicillin and kanamycin	Yes
Yes, if culture negative	Yes, if culture is negative	In most cases	Yes
Yes	Yes	Yes	Yes
Yes	Yes		Yes
Yes	Yes, after treatment	Treat with ampicillin and kanamycin	Yes
Yes	Yes	Observe	Yes
Yes	Yes	Treat with penicillin	Yes
Not in acute stage	Not in acute stage, after 24 hours treatment	Prophylactic penicillin for 10 days	Yes
Yes, after treatment	Yes, after treatment	AgNO$_3$ to the eyes, once in delivery room and once in nursery	Yes
Yes, after treatment	Yes, after treatment	Penicillin IM or IV, plus chloramphenicol drops topically	Yes

Continued.

TABLE 6-60.—MANAGEMENT OF BREAST-FEEDING IN THE PRESENCE
OF MATERNAL INFECTION—cont'd

ORGANISM	CONDITION	ISOLATE FROM MOTHER
Syphilis	Mother with positive VDRL test or clinical disease not treated	Only if mother has second-degree disease or with skin lesions
	Mother treated	No
Tuberculosis	Mother with inactive disease	No
Hepatitis	Mother had in first trimester, well at delivery	No
	Mother with active hepatitis at delivery or in third trimester	No, may room-in after good handwashing technique followed
	Mother is chronic carrier	No
Protozoa		
Toxoplasma	Toxoplasmosis	No

MOTHER CAN VISIT NURSERY	MOTHER CAN BREAST-FEED	IMMEDIATE TREATMENT	CONTACT WITH PREGNANT WOMEN ALLOWED
No, if skin lesions; yes otherwise	Yes	Penicillin IM or IV after workup done; follow-up after discharge	Yes
Yes	Yes		Yes
Yes	Yes	Consider BCG vaccine if follow-up in doubt	Yes
Yes	Yes		
			Yes
No	No	Pooled globulin or hyperimmune if available	Yes
Yes, but do not kiss other infants	Ask for infectious disease opinion		Yes
Yes	Yes		No

TABLE 6-61.—Effects of Drugs that Mothers Ingest while Nursing Infants

DRUGS	CONTRAINDICATED	EFFECTS ON INFANT	SAFE	UNCERTAIN: USE WITH CAUTION	EFFECTS ON INFANT
Analgesics			Acetaminophen, propoxyphene, morphine, codeine; meperidine; aspirin in small doses	Aspirin in large doses	May cause bleeding problems
Anticoagulants	Ethyl biscoumacetate, phenindione	May cause bleeding problems	Warfarin sodium, heparin (not excreted in breast milk)		
Antidiabetics			Insulin		
Antihistamines			All		
Antihypertensives	Reserpine	May cause lethargy, diarrhea, nasal congestion	Guanethidine, pronolol		
Antiinfectives				Antibiotics Sulfonamides, chloramphenicol, nalidixic acid	May cause methemoglobinemia or hypnotic effects May cause hemolytic anemia; may affect infant's bone marrow

Category				
Antimicrobials	Isoniazid	May cause peripheral neuropathy, hepatitis, vomiting	Tetracyclines, metronidazole, streptomycin	Could cause teeth staining and bone retardation
Antineoplastics			All	Inconclusive results; experts disagree
Antithyroid drugs	Radioactive iodine	May be destructive to the infant's thyroid synthesis and release	Propylthiouracil	
Autonomic drugs	Atropine, benztropine mesylate, trihexyphenidyl	May cause constipation and inhibit lactation		
Cathartics	Anthroquinone derivatives	May affect GI tracts of mother and infant	Most cathartics are not absorbed	
Diuretics			Chlorothiazide	Could cause thrombocytopenia
Hypnotics			Chloral hydrate, flurazepam	
Oral contraceptives	Estrogens	May reduce lactation; some cause fetal gynecomastia		
Psychotropic agents	Lithium carbonate	May cause hypotonia, hypothermia, and episodes of cyanosis	Chlordiazepoxide, chlorpromazine	Haloperidol / Marijuana, theophylline, reserpine — Occasionally causes restlessness

Modified from *Guidelines to professional pharmacy.*

Continued.

TABLE 6-61.—EFFECTS OF DRUGS THAT MOTHERS INGEST WHILE NURSING INFANTS—cont'd

DRUGS	CONTRAINDICATED	EFFECTS ON INFANT	SAFE	UNCERTAIN: USE WITH CAUTION	EFFECTS ON INFANT
Sedative hypnotics	Diazepam (regular use)	May cause lethargy, weight loss, changes in EEG	Diazepam (occasional use)		
	Meprobamate				
Steroids	All except low doses (see "safe")	May suppress growth and interfere with endogenous corticosteroid production	Prednisone, prednisolone (in low doses)		
Miscellaneous	Dihydrotachysterol	May cause renal calcification			
	Ergot alkaloids (in migraine preparations)	May cause symptoms of ergotism			
	Gold thioglucose	May cause rashes, nephritis, hepatitis, hematological alterations			

Modified from *Guidelines to professional pharmacy.*

7 The Heart and Vascular System

Edward T. Bope

EVALUATION OF THE HEART

Heart Murmurs

Murmurs should be identified by their length, intensity (grade), the area in which they are best heard, and the area toward which they radiate (Table 7-2).

TABLE 7-1.—Auscultation

Each heart sound should be evaluated separately. Begin with S_1 and S_2 and evaluate the splitting of S_2. Fig. 7-1 illustrates the patterns of splitting and their diagnostic significance.

There are several other diastolic filling sounds with which you should be familiar and be able to identify because of their pathological significance. The following description refers to Fig. 7-2:

a. An atrial sound *(A)* occurs in presystole in patients with hypertension, coronary artery disease, and long P-R intervals.

b. A filling sound may occur in early diastole in children and young adults, but it disappears with age. This sound is called a *normal third heart sound.* When it is heard in middle age, it is called a *ventricular gallop* and indicates myocardial failure or AV valve incompetence.

c. In constrictive pericarditis, a sound occurs in early diastole *(K),* which is earlier, louder, and higher-pitched than the usual ventricular gallop but is, in fact, an accelerated form of this filling sound.

d. If both an atrial *(A)* and ventricular *(V)* gallop are present, a quadruple rhythm results.

e. At faster heart rates these sounds occurring in rapid succession may give the illusion of a middiastolic rumble.

f. When the heart rate is sufficiently fast, the two rapid phases of ventricular filling reinforce each other and a very loud summation gallop (SG) may appear. This sound may be louder than the other two heart sounds.

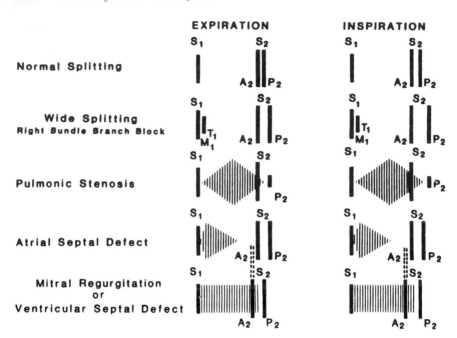

FIG 7-1.

Patterns of splitting of S_2 and their significance. (From *Examination of the heart,* Part 4: Ausculation. Dallas, 1990, American Heart Association.)

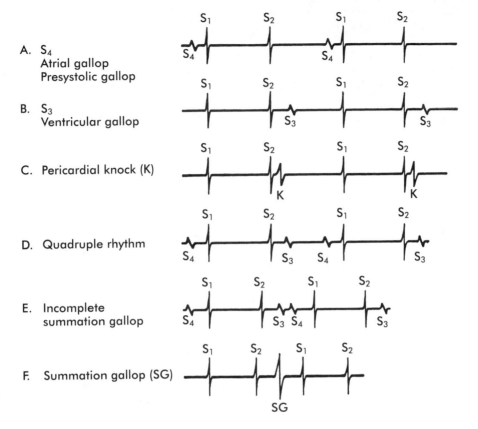

FIG 7-2.
Diastolic filling sounds. **A,** Fourth heart sound *(S₄)* occurs in presystole and is frequently called atrial or presystolic gallop. **B,** Third heart sound *(S₃)* occurs during rapid phase of ventricular filling. It is normal and commonly heard in children and young adults, disappearing with increasing age. In middle age, it is called *pathological S₃,* or *ventricular gallop,* and indicates ventricular dysfunction or atrioventricular valve incompetence. **C,** In constrictive pericarditis, sound in early diastole *(K)* is earlier, louder, and higher pitched than usual pathological S₃. **D,** Quadruple rhythm results if both S₄ and S₃ are present. **E,** At faster heart rates, these sounds occurring in rapid succession may give the illusion of mid-diastolic rumble. **F,** When the hear rate is sufficiently fast, two rapid phases of ventricular filling reinforce each other and loud summation gallop *(SG)* may appear; this may be louder than either S₃ or S₄ alone. S₁, first heart sound; S₂, second heart sound. (From *Examination of the heart, Part IV: Auscultation of the heart,* 1990, American Heart Association.)

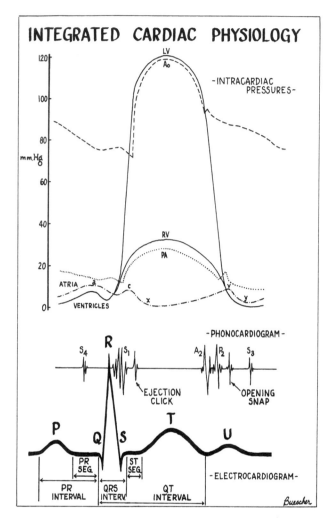

FIG 7-3.
Integrated cardiac physiology. (From Johnson K, ed: *The Harriet Lane handbook,* ed 13, Chicago, 1993, Mosby.)

TABLE 7-2.—GRADING HEART MURMURS

Grading of Murmurs (classification of Freeman and Levine)

Grade 1—Murmur very difficult to hear and not immediately apparent
2—Faintest murmur immediately heard
3—Intermediate intensity
4—Intermediate intensity with thrill
5—Loudest murmur heard with rim of stethoscope touching skin
6—Murmur audible with stethoscope removed from chest wall

Nonorganic (Innocent)

Systolic: Usually heard at the pulmonic area, second left interspace or at the left border of the sternum or in the mitral area. It is not transmitted and is unaccompanied by hypertrophy of the heart or any other evidence of abnormality. It is usually heard only in the sitting position and changes with position

Organic

Mitral regurgitation: Systolic; maximum intensity at apex, transmitted to axilla, heard behind at angle of scapula. Accentuation of pulmonic second sound
Aortic stenosis: Systolic; maximum intensity at right second interspace close to sternum. Transmitted upward into great vessels of the neck
Aortic regurgitation: Diastolic; replaces or follows the second sound. Maximum intensity at second right interspace, radiating to third and downward
Mitral stenosis: Presystolic, running into snapping first sound. Heart in mitral area. Not transmitted. Usually accompanied by a thrill along left margin of heart area

TABLE 7-3.—HEART MURMURS AND MANEUVERS TO DIFFERENTIATE THEM

MANEUVER	AS	IHSS	MR	MVP
Isometric—squeeze hands	Decrease	Decrease	Increase	No change
Valsalva's—causes decreased ventricular filling	Decrease	Increase	Decrease	Increase
Squatting—increases venous return and arteriolar resistance	No change	Decrease	Increase	Decrease
Standing—decreases heart size	Increase	Increase	Decrease	Increase
Amyl nitrite—decrease in left ventricular volume and pressure	Increase	Increase	Decrease	Increase

*Idiopathic hypertrophic subaortic stenosis

TABLE 7-4.—Helpful Points in Differential Diagnosis of Mitral Regurgitation, Ventricular Septal Defect, Tricuspid Regurgitation, and Aortic Stenosis

PHYSICAL, ROENTGENOGRAPHIC, OR ELECTROCARDIOGRAPHIC FEATURE	MITRAL REGURGITATION	VENTRICULAR SEPTAL DEFECT	TRICUSPID REGURGITATION	AORTIC STENOSIS
Systolic murmur	Harsh and pansystolic	Harsh and pansystolic	Pansystolic	Ejection, crescendo-decrescendo
Primary location of murmur	Apex	Left sternal border	Left sternal border	Base of heart; occasionally apical
Radiation of murmur	Axilla; occasionally base and neck	Left precordium	Little	Carotids
Thrill	Occasionally present at apex	Usually present at left sternal border	Rare	Occasionally present at base
Murmur with inspiration	No change	No change	Increases	No change
Valsalva's maneuver	May increase	Increases or no change	No change	Decreases
Venous pressure	Often normal	Slightly elevated with prominent A and V waves	Elevated, with very prominent V waves	Usually normal
Pulsatile liver	No	No	Yes	No
Pulmonary component of S_2	Normal; occasionally increased	Normal or loud; usually delayed	Usually increased	Normal
Apical impulse	Hyperkinetic; occasional heaving	Hyperkinetic	Weak or normal	Forceful and sustained
ECG	Left ventricular hypertrophy; left atrial hypertrophy	Biventricular hypertrophy (Katz-Wachtel phenomenon)	Right ventricular hypertrophy, occasional right atrial hypertrophy	Left ventricular hypertrophy with associated ST-T changes
Chest roentgenogram	Moderately enlarged heart, marked left atrial enlargement	Enlarged left and right ventricle	Enlarged right ventricle	Often normal heart size or left ventricular hypertrophy

From Haffajee CI: Chronic mitral regurgitation. In Dalen JE, Alpert JS: *Valvular heart disease*, ed 2, Boston, 1987, Little, Brown and Company, p. 141.

ELECTROCARDIOGRAPHY

Electrocardiography (ECG) is a noninvasive procedure that provides information about heart rate, rhythm, state of the myocardium, the presence or absence of hypertrophy, ischemia, necrosis, or abnormalities of conduction (Table 7-5).

TABLE 7-5.—ELECTROCARDIOGRAPHY

Rate

The cardiac rate can be determined in the following two ways: (1) Count the number of dark EKG lines between R waves and divide this number into 300. (2) Many use the method illustrated in Fig. 7-4 and memorize the underlined land marks for quick reference (e.g., 300, 150, 100, 75, 60, 50, 43).

Rhythm

Is the rhythm regular or irregular?

Rhythm	P Wave
Sinus arrhythmia	Identical
Wandering pacemaker	Different shapes
Atrial fibrillation	No P waves discernible

# of small squares	Rate/min.	# of small squares	Rate/min.	# of small squares	Rate/min.
5	300	20	75	35	43
6	250	21	71	36	42
7	214	22	68	37	41
8	187	23	65	38	39
9	167	24	62	39	38
10	150	25	60	40	37
11	136	26	58	41	37
12	125	27	56	42	36
13	175	28	54	43	35
14	107	29	52	44	34
15	100	30	50	45	33
16	94	31	48	46	33
17	88	32	47	47	32
18	83	33	45	48	31
19	79	34	44	49	31
				50	30

FIG 7-4.

Guide for determining ECG rate. Count the number of small squares between R waves, and use this table to convert to heart rate per minute.

TABLE 7-6.—ELECTRICAL EVENTS

Evaluate each electrical component of the ECG using the following tables of normal values.

P Wave
Upright in I, II, and aV$_F$
Inverted in III, aV$_R$
Amplitude should not exceed 2 or 3 mm

PR Interval
Becomes shorter as the rate rises

Age	Average Interval
1 year	0.11 seconds
6 years	0.13 seconds
12 years	0.14 seconds
Adult	0.12-0.20 seconds

QRS Complex
Normal: 0.04-0.10 seconds
Normal variant or conduction delay: 0.10-0.12 seconds
Right or left bundle-branch block: 0.12 seconds
If the QRS is greater than 0.12 seconds and occurs before the expected sinus beat, the following may be helpful in diagnosis:

Feature	RBBB Morphology	QRS	Direction of Initial 0.02 seconds of QRS
Ventricular ectopy	60%-70%	Monophasic in V$_1$ or triphasic R > R'	Different from normal beats
Supraventricular beat with aberrancy	90%	Triphasic R < R'	Same as normal beat

PR Prolongations

A PR interval prolongation is a delay or interruption in conduction between the atria and ventricles. First degree AV block has a PR interval greater
than 0.20 seconds.

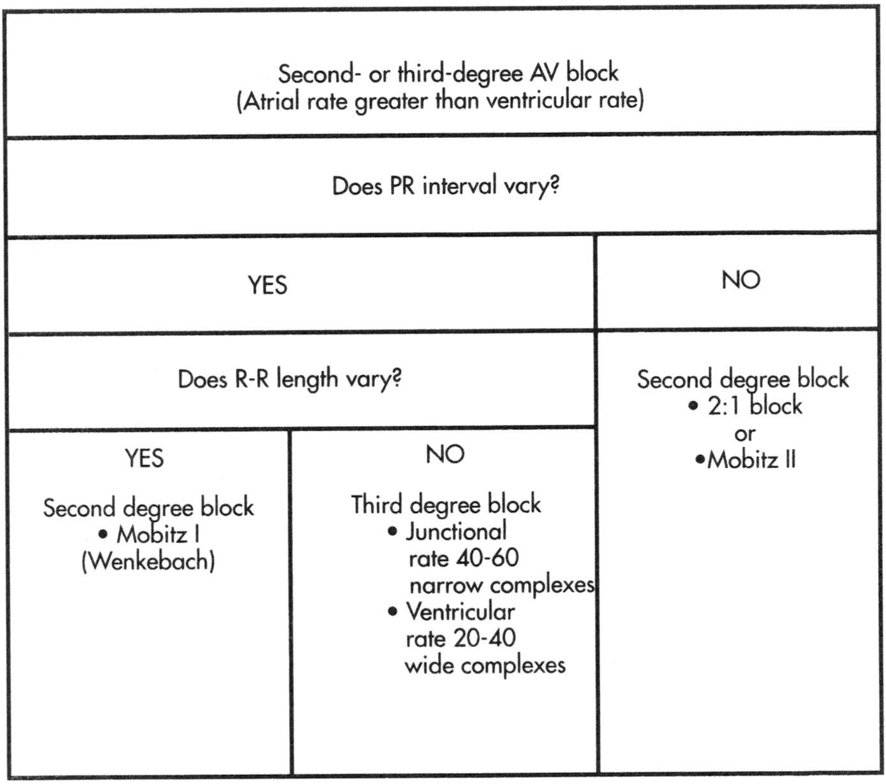

Second- or third-degree AV block (Atrial rate greater than ventricular rate)		
Does PR interval vary?		
YES		NO
Does R-R length vary?		Second degree block • 2:1 block or •Mobitz II
YES	NO	
Second degree block • Mobitz I (Wenkebach)	Third degree block • Junctional rate 40-60 narrow complexes • Ventricular rate 20-40 wide complexes	

FIG 7-5.
AV block.

TABLE 7-7.—DRUGS THAT WILL AFFECT THE ECG

DRUG	EFFECT	TOXICITY
Disopyramide	Prolongation of QT Widened QRS	AV block Ventricular dysrhythmia
Quinidine	Prolonged QT Widened QRS	Intraventricular block Ventricular dysrhythmia
Procainamide	Prolonged QT Widened QRS	Intraventricular block Ventricular dysrhythmia
Digitalis	Depression of ST segment	PVCs, PAT, AV block 1, 2, 3
Tricyclic antidepressants	Prolonged conduction time	Dysrhythmia, tachycardia
Encainide	Widened QRS Unchanged or prolonged QT	Ventricular dysrhythmia AV block
Flecainide	Widened QRS Prolonged PR Unchanged or prolonged QT	Ventricular dysrhythmia First-degree AV block Intraventricular block
Amiodarone	Prolonged PR Prolonged QT	Ventricular dysrhythmia SA node dysfunction AV block Intraventricular block

TABLE 7-8.—DEFECTS IN CONDUCTION: QRS PROLONGATION

Right Bundle-Branch Block (RBBB)
QRS > 0.12 seconds
V_1—Late intrinsicoid, M-shaped QRS
V_6—Early intrinsicoid
I—Wide S wave

Incomplete RBBB
Same as above except QRS < 0.12

Left Bundle-Branch Block (LBBB)
QRS > 0.12
V_1—Early intrinsicoid
V_6—Late intrinsicoid, no Q wave
I—Monophasic R

Left Anterior Hemiblock
Normal QRS duration
Left axis deviation
Small Q in I, and R in III

Left Posterior Hemiblock
Normal QRS duration
Right axis deviation
Small R in I and Q in III
No evidence of right ventricular hypertrophy

Right and Left Bundle-Branch Block are Associated with the Following:
Coronary artery disease
Hypertensive cardiovascular disease
Rheumatic heart disease
Cardiomyopathy
Myocarditis
Nonspecific fibrosis
Trauma

RBBB Only	LBBB Only
Congenital heart disease	Aortic valvular disease
Pulmonary embolism	Short left main coronary artery
Cor pulmonale	

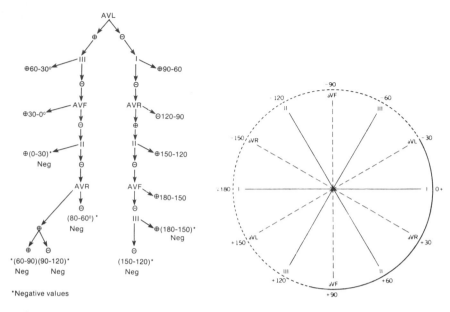

FIG 7-6.
Vector flowsheet and axis diagram.

TABLE 7-9.—DETERMINATION OF AXIS

To determine the axis, proceed through the vector flow sheet shown in Fig. 7-6, *A* looking at each QRS complex on the ECG to decide if it is positive or negative. Start with the QRS in aV$_L$. Work through each QRS in the limb of the flowsheet until a range is identified, then go to the axis diagram (Fig. 7-6, *B*) to find the area of the range you have determined.

Look at each lead on the ECG bounding that range to determine which has the QRS of greatest magnitude. The vector is in the direction closest to that lead.

Example:
Range: −60 to −90
aV$_F$'s QRS is greater in magnitude than III's → vector is −90.

Interpretation of axis
−30 to +90   Normal axis
−30 to −90   Left axis deviation
+90 to +180   Right axis deviation
−90 to +180   Marked right axis deviation

TABLE 7-10.—Cause of Axis Deviation

RIGHT	LEFT
Normal variation	Normal variation
Mechanical shifts: inspiration, emphysema	Mechanical shifts: expiration, high diaphragm (e.g., pregnancy)
Right bundle-branch block	
Right ventricular hypertrophy	Left anterior hemiblock
Left posterior hemiblock	Left bundle-branch block
Dextrocardia	Congenital lesions
Left ventricular ectopic rhythms	Wolff-Parkinson-White syndrome
Some right ventricular ectopic rhythms	Emphysema, hyperkalemia, right ventricular ectopic beats

TABLE 7-11.—Normal Orientation of T Wave

AGE	V_1, V_2	AV_F	I, V_5, V_6
Birth to 1 day	Either	Positive	Either
1-4 days	Either	Positive	Positive
4 days to 12 years	Negative	Positive	Positive
Adult	Positive	Positive	Positive

Modified from Johnson K, ed: *The Harriet Lane handbook,* ed 13, Chicago. 1993, Mosby.

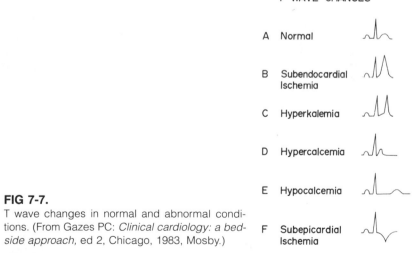

T WAVE CHANGES

A Normal

B Subendocardial Ischemia

C Hyperkalemia

D Hypercalcemia

E Hypocalcemia

F Subepicardial Ischemia

FIG 7-7.
T wave changes in normal and abnormal conditions. (From Gazes PC: *Clinical cardiology: a bedside approach,* ed 2, Chicago, 1983, Mosby.)

ST - T CHANGES

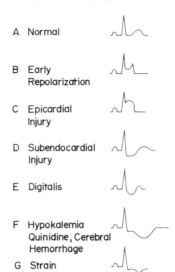

A Normal

B Early
   Repolarization

C Epicardial
   Injury

D Subendocardial
   Injury

E Digitalis

F Hypokalemia
   Quinidine, Cerebral
   Hemorrhage

G Strain

FIG 7-8.
ST-T wave changes in normal and abnormal conditions. (From Gazes PC: *Clinical cardiology: a bedside approach*, ed. 2, Chicago, 1983, Mosby.)

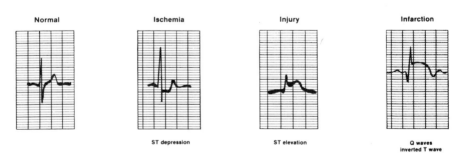

Normal	Ischemia	Injury	Infarction
	ST depression	ST elevation	Q waves inverted T wave

FIG 7-9.
Progression of ST-T wave in infarction.

TABLE 7-12.—QT INTERVAL

HEART RATE PER MINUTE	MEN AND CHILDREN (SECONDS)	WOMEN (SECONDS)	UPPER LIMITS OF THE NORMAL	
			MEN AND CHILDREN (SECONDS)	WOMEN (SECONDS)
40.0	0.449	0.461	0.491	0.503
43.0	0.438	0.450	0.479	0.491
46.0	0.426	0.438	0.466	0.478
48.0	0.420	0.432	0.460	0.471
50.0	0.414	0.425	0.453	0.464
52.0	0.407	0.418	0.445	0.456
54.5	0.400	0.411	0.438	0.449
57.0	0.393	0.404	0.430	0.441
60.0	0.386	0.396	0.422	0.432
63.0	0.378	0.388	0.413	0.423
66.5	0.370	0.380	0.404	0.414
70.5	0.361	0.371	0.395	0.405
75.0	0.352	0.362	0.384	0.394
80.0	0.342	0.352	0.374	0.384
86.0	0.332	0.341	0.363	0.372
92.5	0.321	0.330	0.351	0.360
100.0	0.310	0.318	0.338	0.347
109.0	0.297	0.305	0.325	0.333
120.0	0.283	0.291	0.310	0.317
133.0	0.268	0.276	0.294	0.301
150.0	0.252	0.258	0.275	0.282
172.0	0.234	0.240	0.255	0.262

Modified from Ashman R, Hull E: *Essentials of electrocardiography*, New York, 1945, Macmillan.

TABLE 7-13.—FUNCTIONAL CLASSIFICATION OF CARDIAC DISEASE

Cardiac Status
Class 1 Uncompromised
Class 2 Angina with moderate exertion
Class 3 Angina with mild exertion
Class 4 Angina at rest

Prognosis
Class 1 Good
Class 2 Good with therapy
Class 3 Fair with therapy
Class 4 Guarded despite therapy

MANAGING AMBULATORY ANGINA

TABLE 7-14.—Antianginal Drug Therapy: Selected Nitrates Products

DRUG	FORMULATION AND NAME	ONSET (MINUTES)	DURATION	INITIAL DOSE
Nitroglycerin	IV (Nitrobid IV and others)	1-2	3-5 min	5 μg/min
	Sublingual tablets (Nitrostat)	1-3	30-60 min	0.4 mg sublingual
	Translingual spray (Nitrolingual)	2	30-60 min	1-2 sprays (0.4-0.8 mg) sublingual
	Transmucosal tablet (Nitrogard)	1-2	3-5 hrs	1 mg buccally every 3-5 hrs while awake
	Sustained release tablets and capsules (Nitrobid and others)	30-45	3-6 hrs	2.5 or 2.6 mg 3 times daily
	Ointment (Nitrobid, Nitrol and others)	30-60	2-8 hrs	1-2 in every 8 hrs
	Patches	30-60	12 hrs	0.2-0.4 mg/hr. Place patch on in the morning and remove at bedtime
Isosorbide dinitrate	Tablets (Isordil titradose and others)	30-40	4-5 hrs	5-20 mg 2-3 times daily
	Sustained release tablets (Isordil tembids and others)	2-4 hrs	4-6 hrs	40 mg once or twice daily
Isosorbide mononitrate	Tablets (ISMO)	30-60	Up to 8 hrs	20 mg twice daily. First dose on awakening, second dose 7 hrs later

TABLE 7-15.—ANTIANGINAL DRUG THERAPY: β-BLOCKERS

DRUG AND RECEPTORS BLOCKED	USUAL DOSAGE RANGE	COST†	COMMENTS
Nonselective Agents			
Nadolol (Corgard)	20-240 mg once daily*	$49	β_1 selective agents will inhibit β_2 in higher doses
Propranolol (Inderal and generic)	40-120 mg twice daily	$10	
Propranolol long-acting (Inderal and generic)	60-240 mg once daily	$29	All may aggravate asthma, COPD, CHF, and block symptoms of hypoglycemia in insulin-dependent diabetics; avoid using
Timolol (Blocadren and generic)	10-20 mg twice daily	$28	
Cardioselective Agents			
Atenolol (Tenormin and generic)	25-100 mg once daily*	$20	Reduce dose over 1-2 weeks when discontinuing
Betaxolol (Kerlone)	5-40 mg once daily	$30	
Bisoprolol (Zebeta)	5-20 mg once daily*	NA	
Metoprolol (Lopressor)	100-200 mg once or 50-100 mg twice daily	$14	No clear advantage for agents with intrinsic sympathemimetic activity, and these agents are not cardioprotective after MI
Metoprolol extended release (Toprol XL)	50-200 mg once daily	$19	
Agents with Intrinsic Sympathomimetic Activity			
Acebutolol (Sectral)	200-600 mg twice daily*	$64	↑Incidence of bradycardia and conduction disturbances when used with verapamil and diltiazem
Carteolol (Cartrol)	2.5-10 mg once daily*	$26	
Penbutolol (Levatol)	20-80 mg once daily*	$51	
Pindolol (Visken and generic)	10-60 mg once daily*	$72	

*Dosage reductions or increased dosing intervals are required in renal impairment because these are renally eliminated.
†Approximate cost for one month of therapy at the middosage range listed. Generic prices are used when available.

TABLE 7-16.—Antianginal Drug Therapy: Calcium Channel Antagonists

DRUG	USUAL DOSAGE RANGE	COST*	COMMENTS
Diltiazem (Cardizem and generic)	30-120 mg three times daily	$68	Verapamil and diltiazem may reduce heart rate and/or cause heart block. Use caution in patients with congestive heart failure
Diltiazem extended release (Cardizem CD)	180-300 mg once daily	$49	
Verapamil (generic)	80-240 mg twice daily	$18	
Verapamil long-acting	120-240 mg once daily to 240 mg twice daily	$34	
Dihydropyridines			Dihydropyridines are more potent vasodilators and cause more dizziness, headache, flushing, peripheral edema, and tachycardia
Amlodipine (Norvasc)	2.5-10 mg once daily	$33	
Felodipine (Plendil)	5-20 mg once daily	$45	
Isradipine (DynaCirc)	2.5-5 mg twice daily	$29	
Nicardipine sustained release (Cardene SR)	30-60 mg twice daily	$58	
Nifedipine (generic)	10-40 mg three times daily	$71	
Nifedipine sustained release (Procardia XL, Adalat CC)	30-90 mg once daily	$48	

Approximate cost for 1 month of therapy at the middosage range listed.

TABLE 7-17.—Angiotensin Converting Enzyme (ACE) Inhibitors

DRUG	USUAL DOSAGE RANGE (MG PER DAY)	DOSING FREQUENCY	COST†	COMMENTS
Benazepril (Lotensin)	10-40*	1-2	$19	Diuretic doses should be reduced or discontinued before starting ACE inhibitors to prevent hypotension.
Captopril (Capoten)	12.5-150*	2-3	$48	May cause hyperkalemia in patients with renal impairment or in those receiving potassium-sparing agents.
Enalapril (Vasotec)	2.5-40*	1-2	$38	Can cause acute renal failure in patients with severe bilateral renal artery stenosis.
Fosinopril (Monopril)	10-40	1-2	$23	Contraindicated in pregnancy, renal artery stenosis.
Lisinopril (Prinivil, Zestril)	5-40*	1-2	$35	Side effects include cough, rash, taste disturbance, hypotension, neutropenia, angioedema.
Quinapril (Accupril)	5-80*	1-2	$45	
Ramipril (Altace)	1.25-20*	1-2	$26	

*Dosage reductions or increased dosing intervals are required in renal impairment because these are renally eliminated.
†Approximate cost for 1 month of therapy at the middosage range listed.

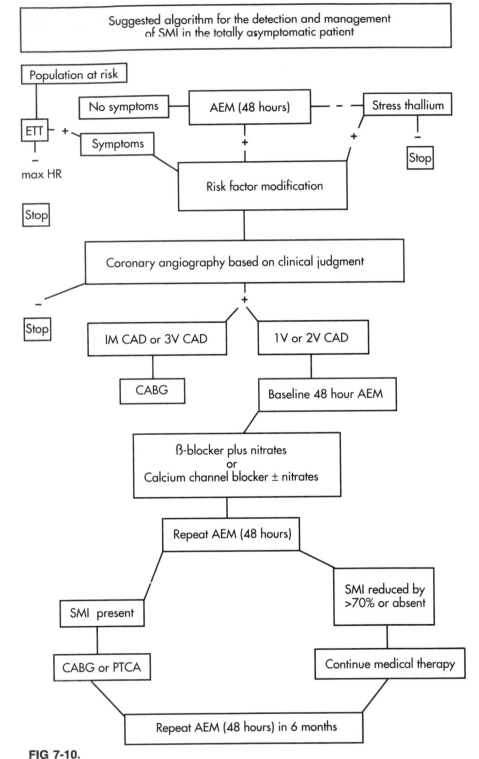

FIG 7-10.
Suggested algorithm for the detection and management of silent myocardial ischemia in the totally asymptomatic patient. *AEM,* Ambulatory electrocardiographic monitoring; *MAX HR,* maximum heart rate; *ETT,* exercise thallium testing; *SMI,* silent myocardial ischemia.

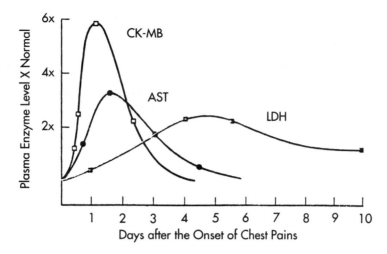

FIG 7-11.
Changes in cardiac enzyme levels following an acute myocardial infarction. (From Braunwald, E: *Heart disease,* ed 4, Philadelphia, W.B. Saunders, p. 1218.)

MYOCARDIAL INFARCTION

Myocardial infarction (MI) requires an accurate diagnosis and careful management. One of the most important parts of management is the prevention or treatment of complications (Table 7-18).

TABLE 7-18.—DIAGNOSIS AND MANAGEMENT OF MI

Diagnosis Requires at Least Two of the Following:
History of typical chest pain
ECG changes evolving with Q waves appearing.
Elevated CPK, SGOT, and LDH levels (Fig. 7-10).
Other aids in diagnosis: Myocardial imaging (pyrophosphate Tc99) is positive
   within 24 hours and until 7 days. This test is most useful to establish the di-
   agnosis in a patient a few days after the infarction.
Think about the following differential for chest pain
   Myocardial infarction
   Aneurysm
   Pericarditis
   Pulmonary embolus
   Pneumothorax

Management
Admit and monitor
Maintain IV
Provide rest; sedate if needed
Control pain with the following:
   Morphine 1-4 mg IV
   NTG SL or IV and/or β-blocker (see Tables 7-14 and 7-15)
Administer oxygen by nasal cannula at 2-3 L/min. Keep Po$_2$ above 70 mm Hg
Restrict diet to low salt, easily chewed and digested foods, no caffeine
Prevent constipation by administering a stool softener
Watch for and treat common complications, such as premature ventricular con-
   tractions, congestive heart failure, dysrhythmias, heart block, papillary muscle
   dysfunction, VSD, aneurysm, pericarditis
Maintain normal blood pressure

Percutaneous Transluminal Angioplasty (PCTA)
   PCTA (balloon angioplasty) has proven to be an effective new therapeutic
modality for patients with single and, in some cases, multivessel coronary artery
disease. Stretching of the stenotic coronary artery can be done in patients with
unstable angina or early in MI to limit infarct size.
   Thrombolytic Therapy
   There is good evidence that administration of streptokinase within the first
4-6 hours of MI will reduce the infarct size and also reduce mortality. Tissue
plasminogen activator (TPA) is given only intravenously and has been shown to
limit both infarct size and mortality. Contraindications include recent trauma (including CPR) and active bleeding in the CNS or GI tract, uncontrolled hypertension, pregnancy, diabetic retinopathy with hemorrhage, recent cardiovascular
arrest, and allergy to the medication. They may be used in conjunction with
PCTA in the acute MI setting. Most hospitals have a protocol for the administration of these medications.

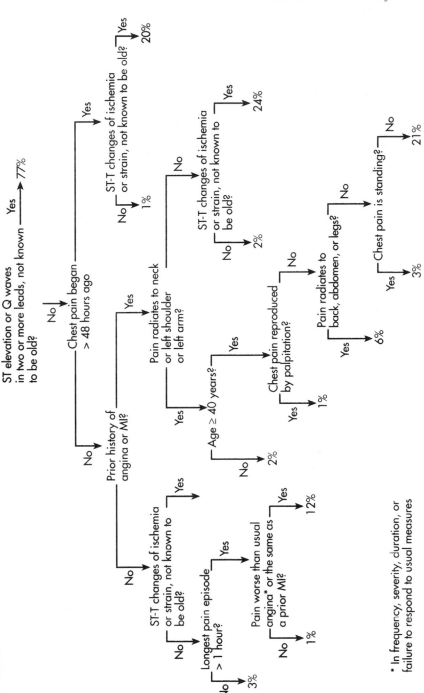

FIG 7-12.
Probability of myocardial infarction in emergency room patients with acute chest pain. (From Lee TH, Lee R: *Cardiology problems in primary care*, Oradell, New Jersey, 1990, Medical Economics Books.)

* In frequency, severity, duration, or failure to respond to usual measures

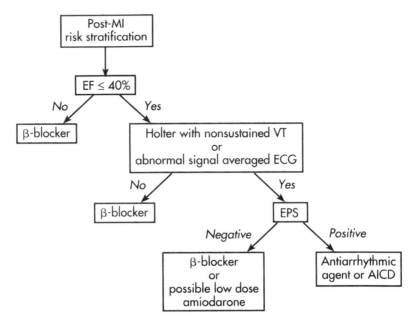

FIG 7-13.
Post-MI. *EF,* Ejection fraction; *EPS,* electrophysiologic study; *AICD,* automatic internal cardiac defibrillator.

TABLE 7-19.—LIDOCAINE FOR VENTRICULAR ECTOPY

Indication
Pathological ventricular ectopy

Dosage
Normal liver and cardiac function:
   100-mg (1-1.5 mg/kg) bolus, then 3-4 boluses of 25-50 mg every 5 minutes, then infusion at 2-4 mg/min
With liver disease:
   100-mg bolus, followed by infusion at 1-2 mg/min (50% reduction)
With congestive heart failure:
   50-mg bolus (50% reduction), followed by infusion at 1-2 mg/min (50% reduction)
To increase levels when at steady state, give a new bolus of 25-50 mg and increase the infusion rate

TABLE 7-20.—LOCALIZATION OF MYOCARDIAL ISCHEMIA/INFARCTION

AREA OF ISCHEMIA	ECG CHANGES	CORONARY ARTERY
Anteroseptal	Chest leads V1-V4	Left anterior descending
Anterior	Chest leads V3-V5	Proximal left anterior descending
Inferior wall	II, III, aVF	Right coronary 80% Left circumflex 20%
Inferior wall with posterior involvement	II, III, aVF and Prominent R in V1	More likely to be left circumflex
Apical	Chest leads V2-V5 and II, III, aVF	Distal anterior descending
Lateral wall	No characteristic ECG abnormalities	Nondominant circumflex branches

Modified from myocardial infarction: electrocardiography, *Sci Am*, April 1995 (CD-ROM version).

DYSRHYTHMIAS AND RESUSCITATION

Cardiac Rhythm Review

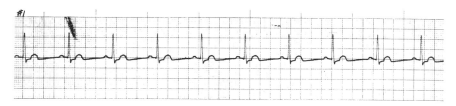

FIG 7-14.
Normal sinus rhythm.
Criteria:
  Rate: 60-100 beats/min
  Rhythm: Regular
  P waves: Upright in leads I, II, aV$_F$

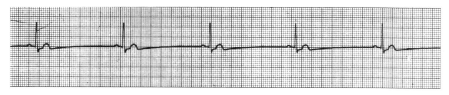

FIG 7-15.
Sinus bradycardia.
Criteria:
  Rate: <60 beats/min
  Rhythm: Regular
  P waves: Upright in leads I, II, aV$_F$

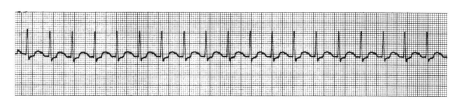

FIG 7-16.
Sinus tachycardia.
Criteria:
  Rate: >100 beats/min
  Rhythm: Regular
  P waves: Upright in leads I, II, aV$_F$

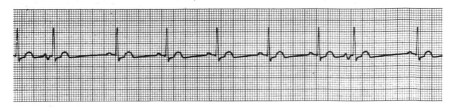

FIG 7-17.

Premature atrial contractions. PACs illustrated by second and eighth complexes.
Criteria:
Rhythm: Irregular
P waves: Differ in morphology because they are from different foci. PP interval varies.
PR interval: Normal or prolonged
QRS: Normal or prolonged

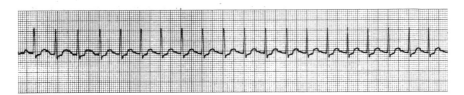

FIG 7-18.

Paroxysmal atrial tachycardia.
Criteria:
Rate: 160-220 beats/min
Rhythm: atrial, regular; ventricular, may have block (2:1, 3:1, or 4:1)
P waves: Hard to see, different from sinus P waves
PR interval: Normal or prolonged
QRS: Normal or prolonged

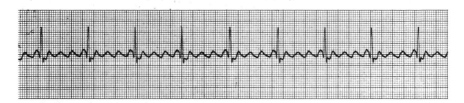

FIG 7-19.

Atrial flutter.
Criteria:
Rate: Usually 300 beats/min (range, 220-350 beats/min)
Rhythm: atrial, regular; ventricular, varying block (2:1, 3:1)
P waves: Sawtooth pattern seen in II, III, aV$_F$
PR interval: Regular
QRS: Usually normal, perhaps aberrant

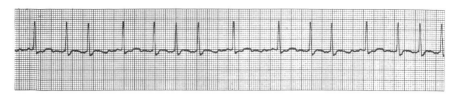

FIG 7-20.
Atrial fibrillation.
Criteria:
   Rate: atrial, 400-700 beats/min; ventricular, 160-180 beats/min
   Rhythm: Irregular
   P waves: No P waves
   QRS: Usually normal, perhaps aberrant

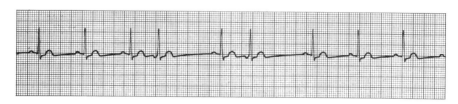

FIG 7-21.
Premature junctional complexes.
Criteria:
   Rhythm: Irregular
   P waves: Negative in leads II, III, aV$_F$
   PR interval: If P wave is before the QRS, the PR interval is less than 0.12 seconds. PR
interval may be prolonged or show complete block
   QRS: Normal or widened

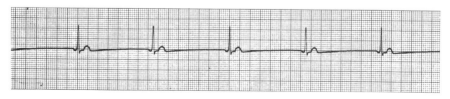

FIG 7-22.
Junctional escape complexes.
Criteria:
   Rate: 40-60 beats/min
   Rhythm: Complexes may or may not occur regularly
   P waves: Negative in II, III, aV$_F$, may precede, coincide with, or follow QRS
   PR interval: Variable
   QRS: Normal

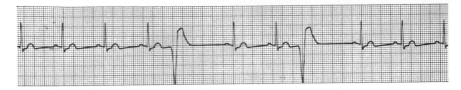

FIG 7-23.
Premature ventricular complexes.
Criteria:
   Rhythm: Irregular
   P waves: Often hidden by QRS of PVC
   QRS: >0.12 seconds; bizarre morphology
   ST segment and T wave: Opposite in polarity to the QRS
   Full compensatory pause

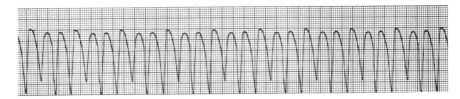

FIG 7-24.
Ventricular tachycardia.
Criteria:
   Rate: 100-220 beats/min
   Rhythm: Usually regular
   P waves: May not be seen
   QRS: Wide
   ST segment and T wave: Opposite in polarity to the QRS

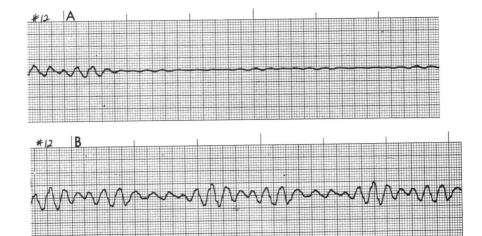

FIG 7-25.
A and **B,** Ventricular fibrillation.
Criteria:
   Rate: Very rapid, cannot count
   Rhythm: Irregular
   No P wave, QRS, ST segment, or T wave

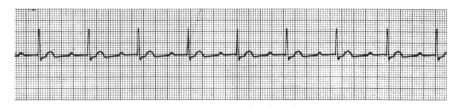

FIG 7-26.
First-degree AV block.
Criteria:
  Rhythm: Regular
  P waves: Followed by QRS
  PR interval: >0.20 seconds

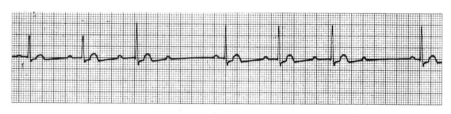

FIG 7-27.
Second-degree AV block, Mobitz type I (Wenckebach).
Criteria:
  Rate: Atrial, normal; ventricular, less than atrial
  Rhythm: Atrial, regular; ventricular, irregular; progressive shortening of RR interval until QRS is dropped
  P waves: Normal
  PR interval: Progressive increase until one P wave is blocked
  QRS: Normal

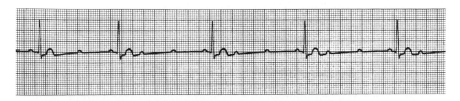

FIG 7-28.
Mobitz type II.
Criteria:
 Rate: Atrial, normal; ventricular, less than atrial
 Rhythm: Atrial, regular; ventricular, regular or irregular with pauses at nonconducted beats
 P waves: Normal except for blocked one
 PR interval: Normal or prolonged
 QRS: Normal or wide

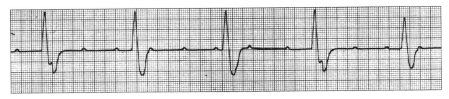

FIG 7-29.
Third-degree AV block.
Criteria:
 Rate: Atria and ventricles at different rates; ventricles slower than atria
 Rhythm: Atrial, usually regular; ventricular, regular
 P waves: Normal
 PR interval: Varies
 QRS: Normal or wide
 PR interval: Progressive increase until one P wave is blocked
 QRS: Normal

Wolff-Parkinson-White (WPW) Syndrome

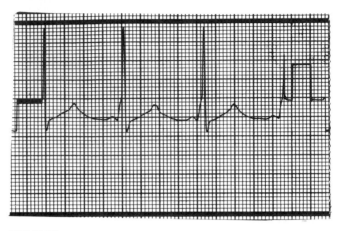

FIG 7-30.
Wolff-Parkinson-White (WPW) syndrome.
ECG
   PR: 0.12 seconds
   QRS: 0.11 seconds
   Delta wave
   These changes may be intermittent

Complications: This syndrome may lead to atrial fibrillation or supraventricular tachycardia that resembles ventricular tachycardia caused by wide, rapid QRS complexes.

Therapy: Digitalis is not used in atrial fibrillation and WPW syndrome since it may speed conduction and lead to rapid ventricular response. Procainamide and propranolol are indicated for acute management. Lidocaine is safe when ventricular tachycardia cannot be distinguished from supraventricular tachycardia with aberrancy. Radio frequency ablation is an alternate, effective cure for this syndrome.

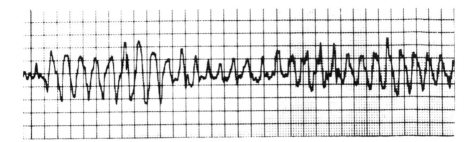

FIG 7-31.

Torsades de Pointes. Torsades de Pointes is a ventricular dysrhythmia resulting from QT interval prolongation. Causes of this included severe bradycardia and drug effects (group IA antidysrhythymics).

Other Dysrhythmias

TABLE 7-21.—SUMMARY OF TREATMENT OF DYSRHYTHMIAS

DYSRHYTHMIA	CHARACTER	TREATMENT*
Sinus bradycardia	Rate: <60/min	*Atropine:* treat if patient is symptomatic; pacemaker may be necessary
Sinus tachycardia	Rate: >100/min Transient slowing with carotid massage	*None* if stable Treat underlying cause: fever, sepsis, Po_2, volume, pain
Premature atrial	PR intervals Contractions vary; P waves different	*None* if stable Treat underlying cause
Junctional rhythm	Rate: 40-70/min, or 130-150/min No p waves	*None* if rate is adequate; consider digitalis toxicity If rapid, treat as PAT
Paroxysmal atrial tachycardia (PAT)	Rate: 160-220/min Normal P waves May have aberrant QRS If block present, consider digitalis toxicity	*Carotid massage,* adenosine, *verapamil,* Valsalva's maneuver, phenylephrine, edrophonium, cardioversion, digitalization, β-blockers, procainamide, lidocaine
Tachybrady dysrhythmia	Bradycardic events predominate	*Pacemaker*
Atrial flutter	Rate: 220-350/min "Sawtooth pattern"	*Verapamil,* digitalization, or cardioversion
Atrial fibrillation	Atrial rate: 400-700/min; ventricular rate: 160-180/min Irregularly irregular	*Digitalization,* verapamil, cardioversion, consider anticoagulation
PVC and ventricular tachycardia	No P wave Wide QRS Compensatory pause Rate: 100-220/min	*Lidocaine bolus* and *infusion,* then procainamide or bretylium; treat hypotension and chest pain if present
Ventricular fibrillation	Emergency No organized rhythm	*CPR, defibrillation, lidocaine,* bretylium
Asystole	Emergency condition, no electrical activity	*CPR, epinephrine, atropine,* isoproterenol
First-degree AV block	Prolonged PR interval	*None;* check for digitalis toxicity
Second-degree AV block	Type I Wenckebach Type II Mobitz	*None* *Pacemaker*
Third-degree AV block	Atria, ventricles	*Atropine* or *pacemaker*

*Treatment of choice is italicized. See Table 7-22 for dosages.

TABLE 7-22.—Drugs for Resuscitation and Dysrhythmias in Adults

DRUG	INITIAL DOSE	THERAPEUTIC LEVEL	FREQUENCY	ACTION	INDICATION	SIDE EFFECTS
Quinidine	200-300 mg	2-8 µg/ml	4 mg/kg/6 hr	Depresses phase 0 depolarization, slow conduction, prolongs phases 2 and 3, decreases phase 4	Atrial fibrillation, ventricular ectopy, reentry, WPW syndrome, automaticity	Dysrhythmias, tinnitus, increased QT, diarrhea
Procain-amide	100 mg over 5 minutes, repeat until up to 1 gm is given	4-12 µg/ml	7 mg/kg/4 hr			Decreased BP, SLE, dysrhythmias
Disopyramide	200-300 mg	2-7 µg/ml	400-800/day divide every 6 hrs			Negative inotrope, CHF, increased QT, anticholinergic
Lidocaine	See Table 7-19	2-6 µg/ml	Infusion of 2-4 mg/min	Speeds conduction, decreases resting potential	Acute VT	Paresthesias, seizures, rash, dysrhythmia
Phenytoin	100 mg q 5-10 min, up to 1 gm	10-20 µg/ml	1.5-2 mg/kg/6 hr		Digitalis-induced SVT and VT	CNS, rash, sedation
Propranolol	0.1 mg/kg; 1 mg IV over 5 min		10-120 mg qid	Inhibits sympathetic activity	SVT	Negative inotrope, bronchospasm, AV block, hypotension

Continued.

TABLE 7-22.—DRUGS FOR RESUSCITATION AND DYSRHYTHMIAS IN ADULTS—cont'd

DRUG	INITIAL DOSE	THERAPEUTIC LEVEL	FREQUENCY	ACTION	INDICATION	SIDE EFFECTS
Bretylium	5 mg/kg IV push over 2 minutes, up to 30 mg/kg	1.5	5-10 mg/kg/6 hr	Prolongs duration of action potential	Resistant VT and ventricular fibrillation	Parotid pain, hypotension, nausea and vomiting, bradydysrhythmia
Verapamil	5 mg IV over 1-2 minutes		Give 10 mg in 15-30 minutes if needed	Slows AV conduction	PAT, SVT	HA, flushing, constipation, hypotension, bradycardia, AV block, asystole
Adenosine	6 mg rapid IV bolus		Give 12 mg in 1-2 minutes; if not effective give additional 12 mg	Slows AV conduction	Paroxysmal supraventricular tachycardia	Facial flushing, headache, dyspnea, chest pressure, light headedness, nausea

Drug	Dose	Volume	Action	Indication	Complications
Epinephrine 1:10,000	0.5-1.0 mg	(5-10 ml)	Adrenergic cardiac stimulation	Asystole, fine ventricular fibrillation	Dysrhythmias, hypertension, myocardial ischemia
$NaHCO_3$	1 mEq/kg	(8-16 ml)	Increases pH	Acidosis	Alkalosis, sodium overload
Atropine	0.5	(5 ml)	Increases SA and AV nodal conduction	Bradycardia asystole	Anticholinergic, tachycardia
$CaCl_2$	500 mg	(2.5-50 ml)	Improves or stimulates conduction	Electromechanical dissociation, asystole	Arrest if the heart is beating
Morphine	2-5 mg		Reduced afterload analgesia, venous capacitance	Acute MI Pulmonary edema	Sedation Respiratory depression

TABLE 7-22 cont.—Drugs for Resuscitation and Dysrhythmias in Adults

DRUG	AVAILABLE	INFUSION DOSE	ACTION	INDICATION	SIDE EFFECTS
Dopamine	400 mg/5 ml	400 mg in 250 ml D$_5$W = 1600 μg/ml; infuse 2-4 μg/kg/min	α-, β- and dopamine-receptor stimulation	Cardiogenic shock	Tachydysrhythmias, ectopy, nausea, vomiting, peripheral ischemia
Dobutamine	250 mg/20 ml	250 mg in 1 L infuse 2.5-10 μg/kg/min	Inotropic β-receptor stimulation	Refractory heart failure	↑HR, BP, PVCs
Isoproterenol	1 mg	1 mg in 500 ml D$_5$W = 2 μg/ml; infuse 2-10 μg/min	Inotropic, chronotropic	Bradycardia caused by heart block	↑PVCs, cardiac output
Amrinone		0.75 mg/kg dose over 2-3 minutes, followed by 5-10 μg/kg/min	Inotropic, vasodilation	CHF	May exacerbate MI
Sodium nitroprusside		0.5-10 μg/kg/min	Peripheral vasodila-tor, cardiac output	CHF, hypertension	↑Cardiac output

TABLE 7-23.—Pediatric Resuscitation Medications

MEDICATION	DOSAGE*	COMMENTS	INDICATIONS
Atropine sulfate 1 mg/10 ml	0.02 mg/kg IV, IO, ET (0.2 ml/kg)	Min 0.1 mg (1 ml) every 5 minutes up to max if needed; max child-dose 1 mg (10 ml)	Asystole and bradycardia
(0.1 mg/ml)	Adolescents: total dose = 1-2 mg	Max adolescent dose = 2 mg (20 ml)	
Bretylium 500 mg/10 ml Continue CPR for 2 minutes before attempting defibrillation	5 mg/kg (0.1 ml/kg) IV, IO	Initial dose	Ventricular fibrillation and tachycardia
	10 mg/kg (0.2 ml/kg)	If VF persists	
Bicarbonate sodium 1 mEq/ml (8.4%)	1 mEq/kg IV, IO (1 ml/kg) (2 mEq/kg raises pH 0.1 unit) Adolescents: 50-100 mEq	Administer slowly; monitor subsequent doses determined by ABG values (Use only 0.5 mEq/ml solution for infants)	Severe metabolic acidosis (pH < 7.20), prolonged (>10 minutes) cardiac arrest, and hyperkalemia
For Rx acidosis:	0.3 × kg × BE (24-CO^2) = mEq	Use only if ventilation is established	
For Rx hyperkalemia:	1 mEq/kg	Administer over at least 10 minutes	
Calcium chloride 10% (100 mg/ml) (1.35 mEq/ml)	20 mg/kg IV, IO (0.2 ml/kg) max dose 1 g	Give slowly: <1 ml/min with ECG and BP monitoring; use extreme caution with digitalis. Use only for indications	Hypocalcemia, hyperkalemia, hypermagnesemia, calcium channel blocker over dose

From Hoekelman, Robert A: *Primary pediatric care*, ed 2, p. 1692, St. Louis, 1992, Mosby.
ABG, Arterial blood gas; *BE*, base excess; *BP*, blood pressure; *CPR*, cardiopulmonary resuscitation; CO_2, carbon dioxide; *ECG*, electrocardiogram; *ET*, endotracheal; *IO*, intraosseous; *IV*, intravenous; *max*, maximum; *min*, minimum; *Rx*, therapy; *VF*, ventricular fibrillation.
*It is useful to have precalculated dose schedules for resuscitative medications. Some pediatric intensive care units are using "megadoses of epinephrine—10 times the usual concentration by using a 1:1000 dilution (1 mg/ml, but the same volume (0.1 ml/kg).

Continued.

TABLE 7-23.—Pediatric Resuscitation Medications—cont'd

MEDICATION	DOSAGE*	COMMENTS	INDICATIONS
Defibrillation	2 J/kg	Double the dose if first shock fails	Absent pulse, ventricular tachycardia and ventricular fibrillation
Cardioversion	0.5-1 J/kg		Ventricular tachycardia with pulses and supraventricular tachycardia
Dextrose 50% 25 g/50 ml	0.5-1 g/kg IV, IO 10% <1 year (4 ml/kg)	Dilute $D_{50}W$ 1:4 = 10%	Hypoglycemia and hypokalemia
Rx hypoglycemia:	25% >1 year (2 ml/kg) 50% adolescents or adults (1-2 ml/kg IV, IO)	A large dose given too rapidly may cause insulin release	
Rx hyperkalemia:	0.5-1 g/kg administered over at least 30 minutes	Monitor blood glucose	
Epinephrine 1:10,000 (0.1 mg/ml)	0.01 mg/kg/dose IV, IO, ET (0.1 ml/kg/dose) Adolescents: total dose, 0.5-1 mg (5-10 ml)	Every 5 minutes if needed; ET dose = 0.2-0.3 ml/kg 0.5 ml, max total dose = 10 ml	Asystole and ventricular fibrillation
Fluid Challenge: Ringer's lactate or 0.9% saline	20 ml/kg IV, IO in 30-60 minutes		Volume expansion
Shock: Ringer's lactate or 0.9% saline Dextrose: see above	20 ml/kg IV bolus and reassess		
Lidocaine 1% 10 mg/ml 2% 20 mg/ml	1 mg/kg IV, IO, ET (0.1 ml/kg 1%) (0.05 ml/kg 2%)	Every 5-10 minutes if needed, max dose = 3-4 mg/kg/hr Toxicity: Seizures, myocardial depression	Ventricular tachycardia and fibrillation

SELECTED DRUG CATEGORIES

TABLE 7-24.—ANTIARRHYTHMIC AGENTS*

DRUG/HOW SUPPLIED	DOSAGE	ADVERSE REACTIONS	COMMENTS
1 Agent (unclassified) Moricizine (Ethmozine) Tabs: 200, 250, 300 mg	*Initial:* 200 mg every 8 hours. Slowly titrate up to 300 mg daily (should be started in the hospital)	May cause proarrhythmias, CHF, palpitations, dizziness, CNS, dyspnea, nausea. Proarrhythmia and mortality was more common in elderly patients.	*Contraindications:* Second- or third-degree AV block, bifascicular block, cardiogenic shock.
1A Agents Quinidine sulfate (various) Tabs, caps: 100, 200, 300 mg Tabs (sustained-release) (Quinidex): 300 mg Inj: 200 mg/ml Quinidine gluconate (Duraquine, Quinaglute) Tabs: 324, 330 mg (sustained-release)	200-300 mg 3-4 times daily, then individualize Sustained-release: 300-600 mg every 8-12 hours (max 1800 mg/day) Parenteral: 300-600 mg IM or IV; inject IV *slowly* (1 ml/min of diluted solution) Therapeutic range: 2-6 µg/ml (should be started in the hospital)	Nausea, diarrhea, cinchonism (tinnitus, headache, vertigo), hypotension, syncope, thrombocytopenia, fever, dysrhythmias, angioedema, asthma	Monitor BP, ECG, QT prolongation, serum levels Sulfate = 83% quinidine; gluconate = 62% quinidine *Interactions:* Quinidine↑digoxin levels, warfarin response; ↓quinidine effect with phenobarbital, phenytoin, rifampin, thiazides, urinary alkalinization; ↑quinidine effect with cimetidine *Warnings:* Digitalize first in patients with atrial fibrillation/flutter; avoid IV administration; caution with heart block *Contraindications:* Digoxin toxicity, severe conduction defects, CHF, poor renal function

*<small>NOTE:</small> Because of the proarrhythmic potential of many antiarrythmic drugs, these agents should only be initiated in the hospital setting by an individual experienced with their use. Antiarrhythmic drugs (other than β-blockers post MI) have not been shown to lower mortality.

Continued.

TABLE 7-24.—ANTIARRHYTHMIC AGENTS*—cont'd

DRUG/HOW SUPPLIED	DOSAGE	ADVERSE REACTIONS	COMMENTS
1C Agents			
Encainide (Enkaid) Caps: 25, 35, 50 mg	25 mg every 8 hours, increase in 3-5 days if necessary to 50 mg every 8 hours (recommend that drug be started in the hospital)	Proarrhythmias, dizziness, tremor, headache, GI disturbances, CHF	Complex kinetics are phenotypically determined *Contraindications:* Second- or third-degree block *Caution:* CHF, sick sinus syndrome
Flecainide (Tambocor) Tabs: 100 mg	*Initial:* 100 mg every 12 hours (max 600 mg/day) (recommend that drug be started in the hospital)	CNS common, proarrhythmias, CHF, heart block, rash, blood dyscrasias (rare)	*Contraindications:* Second- or third-degree block *Caution:* CHF, liver disease, SSS, propranolol, verapamil There are many drug interactions (see product labeling)
Propafenone (Rythmol) Tabs: 150, 300 mg	*Initial:* 150 mg every 8 hours. May increase at 3-4 day intervals to 225-300 mg every 8 hours. Reduced doses may be necessary with hepatic or renal insufficiency or in the elderly (drug should be started in the hospital)	Angina, heart block, CHF, palpitations, proarrhythmia, headache, constipation, nausea/vomiting, blurred vision, dyspnea	*Contraindications:* Uncontrolled CHF, cardiogenic shock, sick sinus syndrome or AV block, bradycardia, hypotension, asthma
II Agents			
Propranolol Tabs: 10,20,40,60,80, 90 mg; Caps (long acting): 60,80,120,160 mg	See Table 7-15	See Table 7-15	See Table 7-15
Esmolol (Brevibloc) Inj: 10, 250 mg/ml	*Initial:* For SVT, see product labeling dose is 500 µg/kg/min for 1 minute followed by a 4 minute maintenance infusion of 50 µg/kg/min. Dosage titration is then based on response and weight	See Table 7-15	The use of infusions for up to 24 hours is well documented, and it has been used for up to 48 hours For other comments see Table 7-15

Drug	Dosage	Side Effects	Comments
Acebutolol (Sectral) Capsules: 200, 400 mg	*Initial:* 200 mg bid up to 400-600 mg bid	See Table 7-15	Indicated for management of ventricular premature beats. For other comments see Table 7-15
III Agents			
Bretylium (Bretylol) Inj: 50 mg/ml	5-10 mg/kg IV, repeat if needed; *Maintenance:* 1-2 mg/min	Hypotension, nausea, vomiting, proarrhythmias	Monitor BP, arrythmias
Sotalol (Betapace) Tabs: 80, 160, 240 mg	*Initial:* 80 mg bid. Usual dose is 120-160 mg bid but some require up to 320 mg bid. *Renal insufficiency:* Lengthen the dosing interval as follows: CrCl 30-60: q 24 hours CrCl 10-30: q 36-48 hours	May cause proarrhythmic effects, otherwise, see Table 7-15	Only indicated for life-threatening ventricular arrhythmias caused by its proarrhythmic potential. For other comments see Table 7-15
Amiodarone (Cordarone) Tabs: 200 mg	*Loading dose:* 800-1600 mg daily for 1-3 weeks. *Adjustment dosage:* 600-800 mg daily for the next 3-4 weeks. *Maintenance:* 400 mg daily	Pulmonary infiltrates or fibrosis, PSVT, CHF, increased liver function studies, CNS, visual disturbances, corneal deposits, photosensitivity, solar dermatitis, hypothyroidism, hyperthyroidism	Because of the complex pharmacokinetics, drug interactions, and adverse effects, the drug should only be managed by those with experience with this agent
IV Agents Verapamil	See calcium channel blocker Table 7-22		
Digoxin	See Table 7-22		
Adenosine (Adenocard) Inj: 6 mg/2 ml	*Initial:* 6 mg rapid IV bolus. If not effective within 1-2 minutes give 12 mg rapid IV bolus which can be repeated once	Facial flushing, headache, dyspnea, chest pressure, lightheadedness, nausea	Half-life is <10 seconds, so the effects rapidly disappear. *Contraindications:* Second- or third-degree AV block, sick sinus syndrome, atrial fibrillation/flutter, ventricular tachycardia

TABLE 7-24 cont.—ANTIARRHYTHMIC AGENTS*

DRUG/HOW SUPPLIED	DOSAGE	ADVERSE REACTIONS	COMMENTS
1B Agents			
Lidocaine (Xylocaine, various) Inj: various Cream, solution, jelly	120 mg (3 ml of 5% clextrose in water, 1200 µg/ml. Then 1 ml/kg/hr delivers 20 µg/kg/min	Numbness, twitching, euphoria, dysphoria, drowsiness, convulsions, bradycardia, hypotension, rash, urticaria	*Contraindications:* Hypersensitivity, Adams-Stokes disease, WPW syndrome, severe nodal block ↓Metabolism in CHF and liver disease ↑Levels with propranolol and cimetidine (Tagamet) Additive effects with procainamide Levels↑after 24 hours following acute MI
Phenytoin IM/IV 50 mg/ml	100 mg IV q5min until arrhythmia controlled, max dose 1000 mg	Nystagmus, ataxia, drowsiness, stupor, coma, hypotension	Of limited value; many drug-drug interactions; monitor levels
Tocainide (Tonocard) Tabs: 400, 600 mg	400 mg every q8h, range (1200-1800 mg) well controlled patients q12h (should be started in the hospital)	Up to 50% of patients have nausea, vomiting, dizziness, tremor, confusion, paresthesia, and other CNS reactions, such as pulmonary fibrosis, blood dyscrasia; increase rate in atrial fibrillation/flutter	*Cautions:* CHF, heart block *Monitor:* CBC Food may decrease side effects
Mexiletine (Mexitil) Caps: 150, 200, 250 mg	*Load:* 400 mg: maintenance: 200 mg q8h (max 1200 mg day); some controlled every 12 h; reduce dose with liver disease or severe CHF (should be started in the hospital)	High percentage nausea, vomiting, dizziness, tremor, increased LFTs, rash, seizures	*Cautions:* Conduction disturbance, liver damage *Contraindications:* Second- or third-degree heart block

Drug	Dose	Side Effects	Comments
Disopyramide (Norpace and various) Caps: 100 mg, 150 mg Controlled release (Norpace CR): 100, 150 mg	*Load:* 300 mg (200 mg if <50 kg); maintenance: 400-800 mg/day in 4 doses (q12h with sustained release) *Children:* <1 yr, 10-30 mg/kg/day, 1-4 yr, 10-20; 4-12 yr, 10-15; 12-18 yr, 6-15 mg/kg/day *Renal Impairment:* CrCl: 30-40 ml/min, 100 mg q8h; 15-30, 100 mg q12h; <15, 100 mg q24h (should be started in hospital)	Dry mouth, urinary retention, constipation, blurred vision, congestive heart failure, enhanced AV conduction, heart block, ventricular arrhythmias	Capsule contents can be mixed in cherry syrup High anticholinergic Avoid in patients with history of CHF, WPW syndrome, bundle-branch block, or those taking β-blockers or verapamil *Contraindications:* Shock, sick sinus syndrome, AV block Digitalize before using in atrial fibrillation Monitor ECG for QRS or QT prolongation, discontinue or lower dose if >25%-30% widening; monitor serum levels
Procainamide (Procan, Pronestyl, various) Tabs, caps: 250, 375, 500 mg Tabs (sustained): 250, 500, 750, 1000 mg Inj: 100, 500 mg/ml	*Oral:* load 1 gm, maintenance dose is 50 mg/kg/day (given 3gh), then adjust (q6h for sustained release) *IV bolus:* 100 mg q5min (slowly at 50 mg/min), up to 1 gm or suppression of dysrhythmia or toxicity *IV infusion:* 20-25 mg/min for 30 min, then 2-5 mg/min (should be started in hospital)	Anorexia, nausea, urticaria, SLE syndrome, blood dyscrasia, QRS and QT interval prolongation, dysrhythmia, fever, neutropenia, hypotension	Monitor BP, ECG, QT interval, procainamide and NAPA serum levels, ANA *Contraindications:* procainamide, allergy, second- or third-degree AV block, myasthenia gravis Procan SR or Pronestyl SR given every 6 hours—wax matrix may be found in stool but no drug remains

DEFIBRILLATION AND SYNCHRONIZED CARDIOVERSION

Defibrillation is used in ventricular fibrillation and ventricular tachycardia in an unconscious patient with no circulation. *Synchronized cardioversion* is countershock delivered during QRS. Used to convert ventricular and supraventricular tachydysrhythmias in settings where rapid conversion is needed (Table 7-25).

TABLE 7-25.—GUIDELINES FOR DEFIBRILLATION AND SYNCHRONIZED CARDIOVERSION

Technique
Defibrillation
Charge paddles: 200 J for first charge, 300 J for second charge, and 360 J for third charge
Place paddles: One to right of upper sternum, below clavicle; second to left of left nipple in anterior axillary line
Recheck rhythm on monitor
Clear area around patient. Make sure no one is in contact with patient or bed
Firmly press paddles against chest wall
Deliver countershock; simultaneously depress paddle buttons
Synchronized cardioversion
Sedate patient. Use diazepam 5-10 mg IV
Check QRS: Must be upright on monitor
Activate synchronizer circuit
Charge paddle:
    Atrial fibrillation
        100 J for first charge
        200 J for second charge, if needed
        360 J for third charge, if needed
    Paroxysmal atrial tachycardia
        75-100 J
    Ventricular tachycardia
        50 J, then 100 J, then 200 J, then 360 J
    Atrial flutter
        25 J
Place paddle: as above
Clear area: as above
Press against chest wall, simultaneously depress paddle button, and hold until countershock is delivered

Contraindications
Atrial fibrillation with slow ventricular response and coronary artery disease
Digitalis toxicity
Sick sinus syndrome
Long-standing atrial fibrillation
Atrial fibrillation secondary to hyperthyroidism

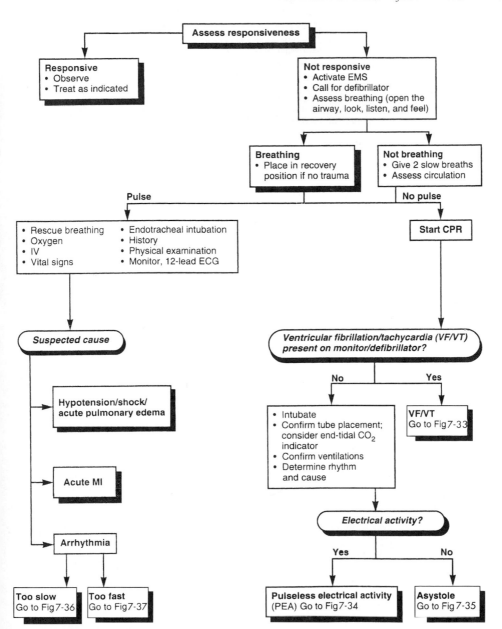

FIG 7-32.
Universal algorithm for adult (From *JAMA* 268:2199, 1992.)

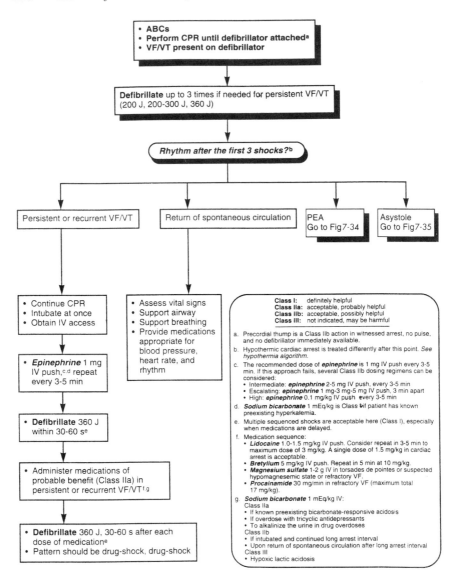

FIG 7-33.
Ventricular fibrillation/pulseless ventricular tachycardia (VF/VT) algorithm (From *JAMA* 268:2199, 1992.)

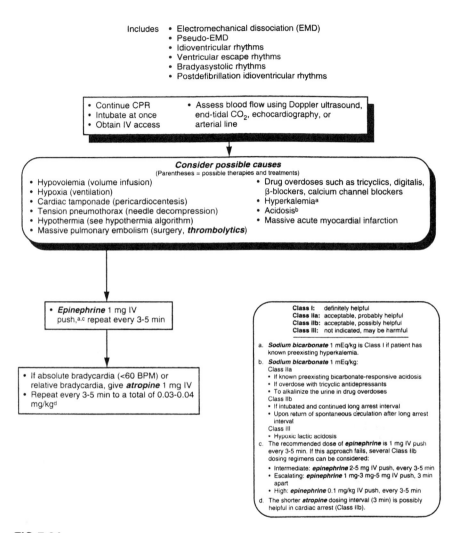

Includes
- Electromechanical dissociation (EMD)
- Pseudo-EMD
- Idioventricular rhythms
- Ventricular escape rhythms
- Bradyasystolic rhythms
- Postdefibrillation idioventricular rhythms

- Continue CPR
- Intubate at once
- Obtain IV access
- Assess blood flow using Doppler ultrasound, end-tidal CO_2, echocardiography, or arterial line

---

Consider possible causes
(Parentheses = possible therapies and treatments)

- Hypovolemia (volume infusion)
- Hypoxia (ventilation)
- Cardiac tamponade (pericardiocentesis)
- Tension pneumothorax (needle decompression)
- Hypothermia (see hypothermia algorithm)
- Massive pulmonary embolism (surgery, *thrombolytics*)
- Drug overdoses such as tricyclics, digitalis, β-blockers, calcium channel blockers
- Hyperkalemia[a]
- Acidosis[b]
- Massive acute myocardial infarction

- *Epinephrine* 1 mg IV push,[a,c] repeat every 3-5 min

- If absolute bradycardia (<60 BPM) or relative bradycardia, give *atropine* 1 mg IV
- Repeat every 3-5 min to a total of 0.03-0.04 mg/kg[d]

Class I: definitely helpful
Class IIa: acceptable, probably helpful
Class IIb: acceptable, possibly helpful
Class III: not indicated, may be harmful

a. *Sodium bicarbonate* 1 mEq/kg is Class I if patient has known preexisting hyperkalemia.
b. *Sodium bicarbonate* 1 mEq/kg:
   Class IIa
   - If known preexisting bicarbonate-responsive acidosis
   - If overdose with tricyclic antidepressants
   - To alkalinize the urine in drug overdoses
   Class IIb
   - If intubated and continued long arrest interval
   - Upon return of spontaneous circulation after long arrest interval
   Class III
   - Hypoxic lactic acidosis
c. The recommended dose of *epinephrine* is 1 mg IV push every 3-5 min. If this approach fails, several Class IIb dosing regimens can be considered:
   - Intermediate: *epinephrine* 2-5 mg IV push, every 3-5 min
   - Escalating: *epinephrine* 1 mg-3 mg-5 mg IV push, 3 min apart
   - High: *epinephrine* 0.1 mg/kg IV push, every 3-5 min
d. The shorter *atropine* dosing interval (3 min) is possibly helpful in cardiac arrest (Class IIb).

FIG 7-34.
Pulseless electrical activity (PEA) algorithm (From *JAMA* 268:2199, 1992.)

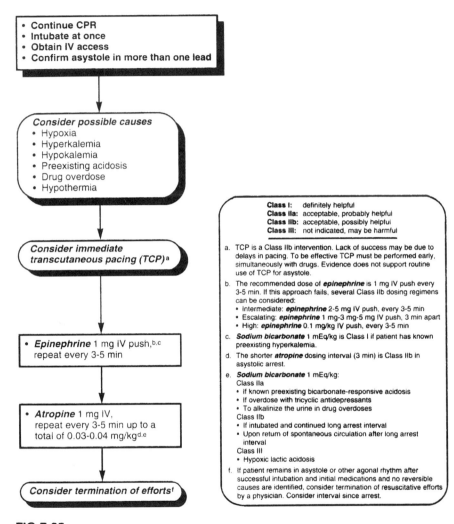

FIG 7-35.
Asystole treatment algorithm (From *JAMA* 268:2199, 1992.)

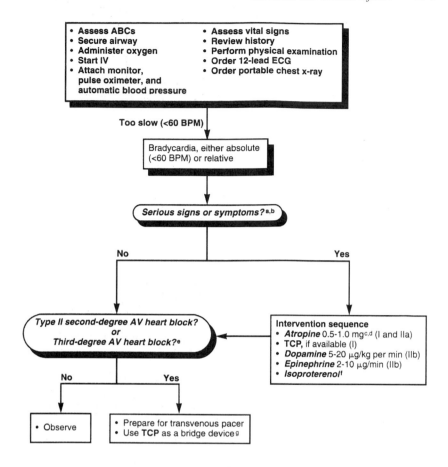

- Assess ABCs
- Secure airway
- Administer oxygen
- Start IV
- Attach monitor, pulse oximeter, and automatic blood pressure

- Assess vital signs
- Review history
- Perform physical examination
- Order 12-lead ECG
- Order portable chest x-ray

Too slow (<60 BPM)

Bradycardia, either absolute (<60 BPM) or relative

Serious signs or symptoms? [a,b]

No   Yes

Type II second-degree AV heart block?
or
Third-degree AV heart block? [e]

No   Yes

- Observe

- Prepare for transvenous pacer
- Use **TCP** as a bridge device [g]

Intervention sequence
- *Atropine* 0.5-1.0 mg[c,d] (I and IIa)
- **TCP**, if available (I)
- *Dopamine* 5-20 μg/kg per min (IIb)
- *Epinephrine* 2-10 μg/min (IIb)
- *Isoproterenol*[f]

a. Serious signs or symptoms must be related to the slow rate. Clinical manifestations include
   - Symptoms (chest pain, shortness of breath, decreased level of consciousness)
   - Signs (low BP, shock, pulmonary congestion, CHF, acute MI)
b. Do not delay TCP while awaiting IV access or for *atropine* to take effect if patient is symptomatic.
c. Denervated transplanted hearts will not respond to *atropine*. Go at once to pacing, *catecholamine* infusion, or both.
d. *Atropine* should be given in repeat doses every 3-5 min up to total of 0.03-0.04 mg/kg. Use the shorter dosing interval (3 min) in severe clinical conditions. It has been suggested that *atropine* should be used with caution in atrioventricular (AV) block at the His-Purkinje level (type II AV block and new third-degree block with wide QRS complexes) (Class IIb).
e. Never treat third-degree heart block plus ventricular escape beats with *lidocaine*.
f. *Isoproterenol* should be used, if at all, with extreme caution. At low doses it is Class IIb (possibly helpful); at higher doses it is Class III (harmful).
g. Verify patient tolerance and mechanical capture. Use analgesia and sedation as needed.

FIG 7-36.
Bradycardia (From *JAMA* 268:2199, 1992.)

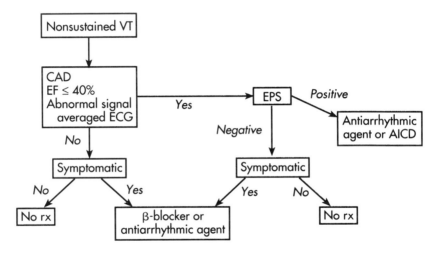

FIG 7-37.
Algorithm for electrophysiological study (EPS) evaluation and management of nonsustained ventricular tachycardia.

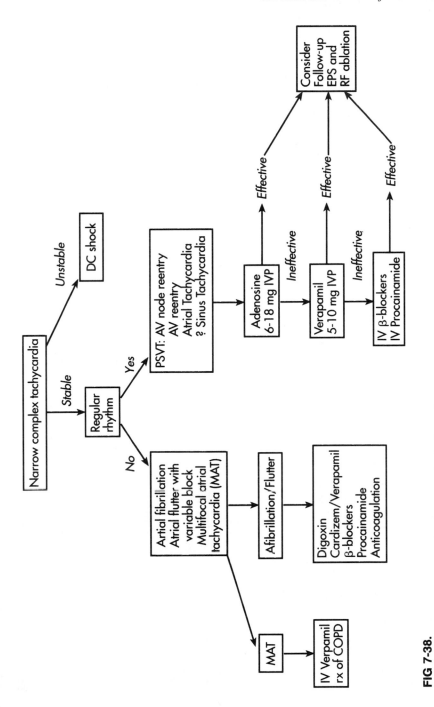

FIG 7-38.
Evaluation and management of narrow complex tachycardia.

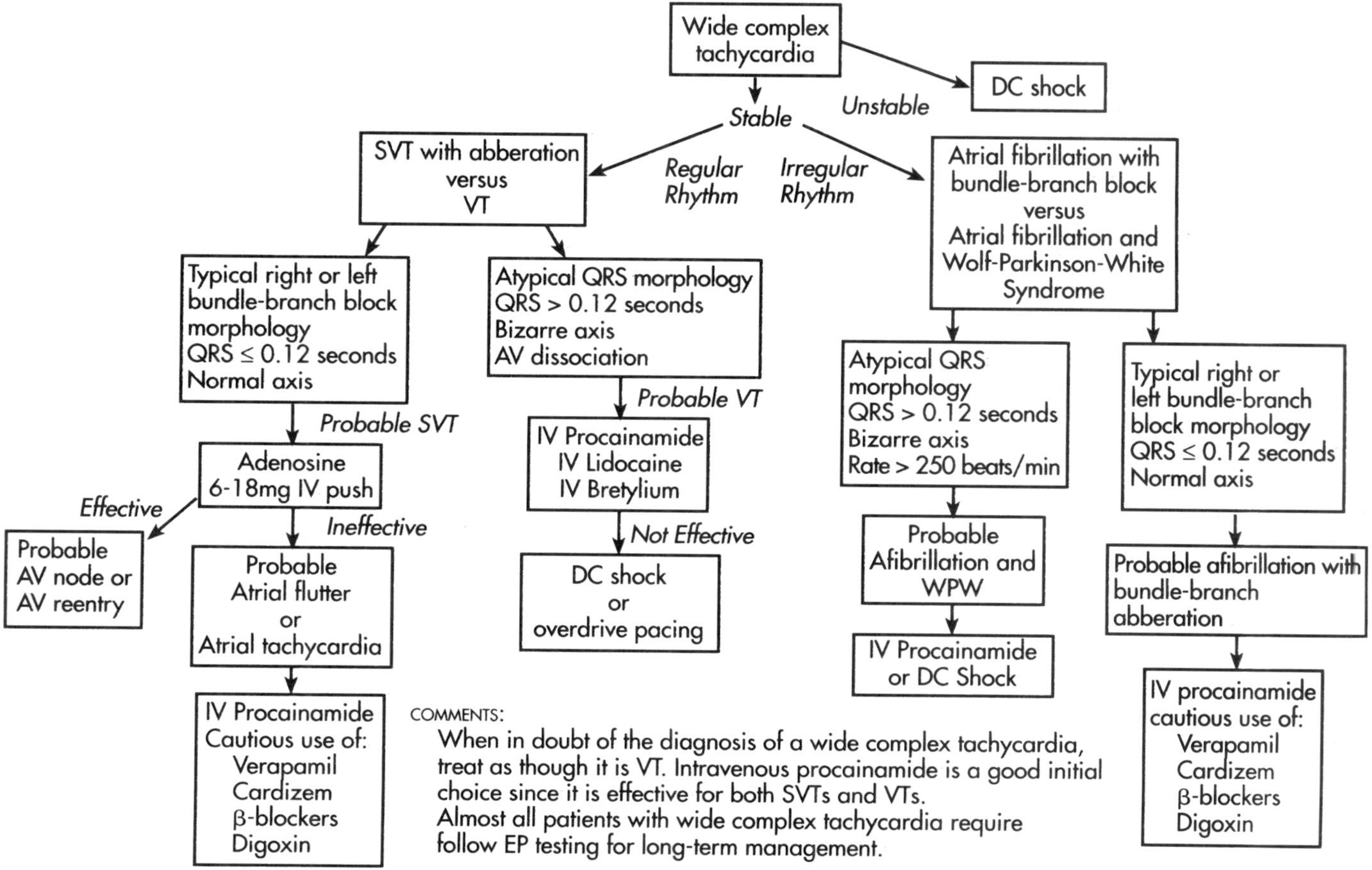
Wide complex tachycardia
Unstable
DC shock
Stable
Regular Rhythm
Irregular Rhythm
SVT with abberation versus VT
Typical right or left bundle-branch block morphology QRS ≤ 0.12 seconds Normal axis
Probable SVT
Adenosine 6-18mg IV push
Effective
Probable AV node or AV reentry
Ineffective
Probable Atrial flutter or Atrial tachycardia
IV Procainamide Cautious use of: Verapamil Cardizem β-blockers Digoxin
Atypical QRS morphology QRS > 0.12 seconds Bizarre axis AV dissociation
Probable VT
IV Procainamide IV Lidocaine IV Bretylium
Not Effective
DC shock or overdrive pacing
Atrial fibrillation with bundle-branch block versus Atrial fibrillation and Wolf-Parkinson-White Syndrome
Atypical QRS morphology QRS > 0.12 seconds Bizarre axis Rate > 250 beats/min
Probable Afibrillation and WPW
IV Procainamide or DC Shock
Typical right or left bundle-branch block morphology QRS ≤ 0.12 seconds Normal axis
Probable afibrillation with bundle-branch abberation
IV procainamide cautious use of: Verapamil Cardizem β-blockers Digoxin
COMMENTS:
When in doubt of the diagnosis of a wide complex tachycardia, treat as though it is VT. Intravenous procainamide is a good initial choice since it is effective for both SVTs and VTs.
Almost all patients with wide complex tachycardia require follow EP testing for long-term management.

FIG 7-39.
Algorithm for evaluation and management of wide complex tachycardia.

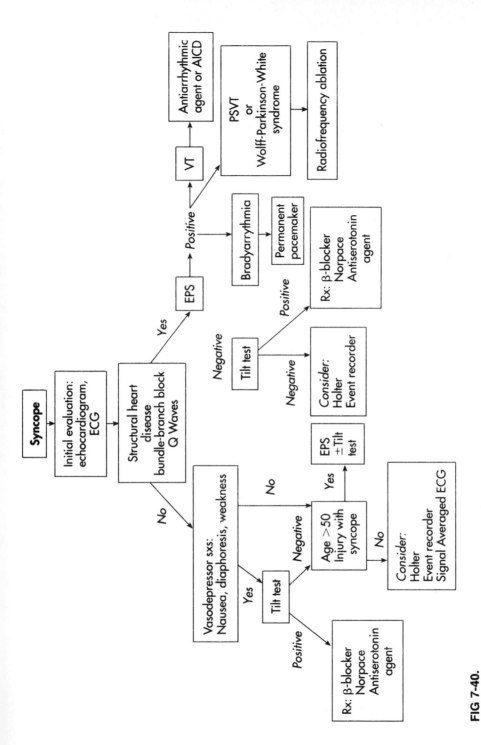

FIG 7-40.
Algorithm for evaluation and management of syncope.

CONGESTIVE HEART FAILURE (CHF)

TABLE 7-26.—CONGESTIVE HEART FAILURE

Establish the Diagnosis

SYMPTOMS	SIGNS	X-RAY
Orthopnea	Rales	Cardiomegaly
Dyspnea on exertion	S_3 gallop	Base to apex redistri-
Fatigue	Peripheral edema	bution of pulmonary
		vasculature
		Interstitial edema

Think about Precipitating Causes

Alcoholism

Anemia

Arrhythmias

Emotional strain

Hypothyroidism

Hyperthyroidism

Medications, such as sodium retain-
ing, disopyramide, or propranolol

Myocardial infarction

Physical exertion, particularly in hot,
humid weather

Pregnancy

Pulmonary embolus

Sodium intake excess

Stopping medications, particularly
cardiac stimulants and afterload
reducers

Five Goals of Therapy

1. *Reduce cardiac work:* The need for hospitalization is determined by the acuteness and severity of symptoms, the precipitating cause, and an evaluation of the home care providers. Put the patient at bed rest in a relaxed atmosphere with legs and head elevated slightly.
2. *ACE Inhibitor reduces mortality of CHF and should be used as initial treatment.* They include captopril and enalapril.
3. *Improve myocardial contractility:*
   a. Digitalis should be administered after obtaining baseline ECG to rule out AV block or dysrhythmia. ECG may define valve disease or IHSS; checking renal function and potassium.
   b. Other inotropic agents include dopamine, amrinone, dobutamine, and milrinone.
4. *Reduce afterload:*
   Vasodilating agents are used for CHF not responding to digitalis and diuretics. Examples of vasodilators include isosorbide dinitrate, sublingual nitroglycerin, nitroglycerin paste, hydralazine (arteriolar dilation), prazosin (arteriolar and venous), and nitroprusside (arteriolar and venous).
5. *Reduce excess fluid:*
   2-4 g sodium chloride diet and diuretics.

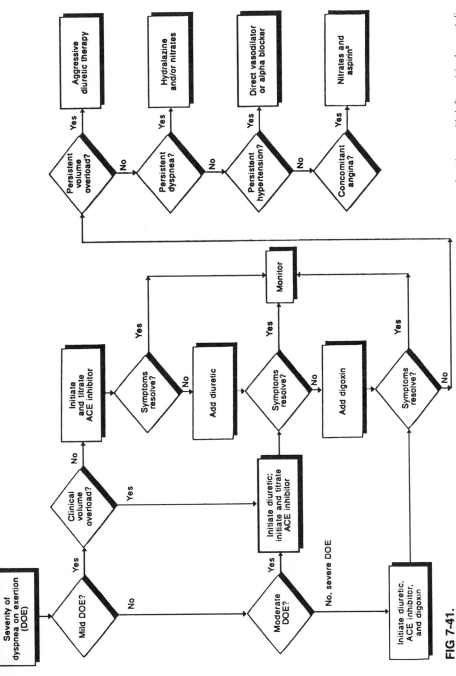

FIG 7-41.

Algorithm for pharmacological treatment of heart failure. (From Heart Failure: *Evaluation and care of patients with left-ventricular systolic dysfunction.* Clinical practice guideline no. 11. Rockville, Maryland, June 1994, Agency for Health Care Policy and Research, Public Health Service, U.S. Department of Health and Human Services, AHCPR publication no. 94-0612.)

TABLE 7-27.—DIGITALIZATION

Complete familiarity with one preparation is desirable. Since digoxin is the most widely used, it will be used as the model. Digitoxin is not affected as extensively as digoxin by renal function, so it might be used also.

Digoxin
Rapid IV route for acute, severe, unstable CHF: 0.25-0.50 mg IV over 5 minutes, followed by 0.125-0.25 mg IV every 4-6 hours until total dose of 0.5-1.0 mg has been administered, then daily dose of 0.125-0.25 mg IV
24-hour digitalization: 0.5-0.75 mg orally followed by 0.25-.25 mg IV every 6-8 hr until total dose of 1.0-1.5 mg has been administered, then daily dose of 0.125 mg-0.375 mg
One-week digitalization: 0.125-0.25 mg PO daily

Digoxin Calculations for Maintenance Dose Estimation

$$\text{Maintenance dose} = (\text{Loading dose}) \times (\% \text{ daily loss})$$
$$\text{Loading dose} = 8\text{-}10 \ \mu\text{g/kg in CHF}$$
$$= 13\text{-}15 \ \mu\text{g/kg in atrial fibrillation}$$
$$\text{Percentage of daily loss} = 14\% + \frac{\text{Creatinine clearance}}{5}$$
$$\frac{\text{Estimated}}{\text{Creatinine clearance}^*} = \frac{(140 - \text{Age})(\text{Weight in kg})}{\text{Serum creatinine} \times 72} \times (0.85 \text{ for females})$$

Oral tablet is only 80% absorbed, so:

$$\text{Tablet} = \frac{\text{IV dose (or Lanoxicap)}}{0.8}$$

Modified from Cockroft DW, Gault MH: *Nephron* 16:31, 1976.

TABLE 7-28.—Estimated Digoxin Dose

SERUM CREATININE	DAILY MAINTENANCE DOSE AS PERCENTAGE OF LOADING DOSE
100	34
75	29
60	26
50	24
30	20
15	17
10	16
5	15
0	14

Serum levels should be measured 8-12 hours after maintenance dose is given. Therapeutic level is 8-18 μg/kg.

TABLE 7-29.—Digitalis Intoxication

SYMPTOMS	ECG CHANGES
Anorexia	PVCs
Nausea and vomiting	AV block
Abdominal discomfort	PAT with block
Hazy or colored vision	Wenckebach second-degree
Photophobia	Complete heart block
Hallucinations	Sinus bradycardia
Drowsiness	Accelerated junctional rhythm
Disorientation	

Treatment: Discontinue digitalis; monitor cardiac rhythm and treat as needed; measure digitalis level (toxicity may occur at therapeutic levels). Consider charcoal lavage; see chapter 16.

OTHER CARDIAC DISEASE

TABLE 7-30.—BACTERIAL ENDOCARDITIS*

SIGNS	SYMPTOMS	LAB
Elevated temperature (cyclic)	Weakness	Leukocytosis
Patient appears very ill	Fatigability	ESR increased
Cardiac failure	Weight loss	Positive blood cultures
Petechiae of mucous membranes, retina, skin, nails	Feverishness	Echocardiogram—impaired valve
Emboli to large arteries causing ischemia and gangrene	Night sweats	excursion or vegetations
New murmur, primarily diastolic	Anorexia	
Splenomegaly	Arthralgia	
Arthritis		
Subacute: Insidious onset, usually in an abnormal heart		
Acute: Fulminant, rapid, usually in normal heart		

Treatment
Blood Cultures
Antibiotics
Crystalline penicillin G initially 10-30 million units per day, with gentamicin 3-5 mg/kg/day in three doses
Adjust antimicrobial dose as indicated by blood culture sensitivities and minimum bactericidal concentration (MBC)
Penicillin allergic, use vancomycin alone, 30 mg/kg/day in four doses
Surgery
May be indicated when organism is resistant or prosthetic valve is infected; should be accomplished before intractable heart failure occurs

ENDOCARDITIS PROPHYLAXIS RECOMMENDED	ENDOCARDITIS PROPHYLAXIS NOT RECOMMENDED§
Cardiac Conditions*	
Prosthetic cardiac valves, including bioprosthetic and homograft valves	Isolated secundum atrial septal defect
	Surgical repair without residua beyond 6 months of se-

Previous bacterial endocarditis, even in the absence of heart disease
Most congenital cardiac malformations
Rheumatic and other acquired valvular dysfunction, even after valvular surgery
Hypertrophic cardiomyopathy
Mitral valve prolapse with valvular regurgitation

cundum atrial septal defect, ventricular septal defect, or patent ductus arteriosus
Previous coronary artery bypass graft surgery
Mitral valve prolapse without valvular regurgitation†
Physiological, functional, or innocent heart murmurs
Previous Kawasaki disease without valvular dysfunction
Cardiac pacemakers and implanted defibrillators

Selected Dental or Surgical Procedures*

Dental procedures known to induce gingival or mucosal bleeding, including professional cleaning
Tonsillectomy and/or adenoidectomy
Surgical operations that involve intestinal or respiratory mucosa
Bronchoscopy with a rigid bronchoscope
Sclerotherapy for esophageal varices
Esophageal dilation
Gallbladder surgery
Cystoscopy
Urethral dilation
Urethral catheterization if urinary tract infection is present‡
Prostatic surgery
Incision and drainage of infected tissue‡
Vaginal hysterectomy
Vaginal delivery in the presence of infection‡

Dental procedures not likely to induce gingival bleeding, such as simple adjustment of orthodontic appliances or fillings above the gum line
Injection of local intraoral anesthetic (except intraligamentary injections)
Shedding of primary teeth
Tympanostomy tube insertion
Endotracheal intubation
Bronchoscopy with or without gastrointestinal biopsy
Cesarean section
In the absence of infection for urethral catheterization, D & C, uncomplicated vaginal delivery, therapeutic abortion, sterilization procedures, or insertion or removal of intrauterine devices

Modified from *JAMA* 264:2919, 1990.

*This table lists selected procedures and conditions only and is not meant to be all-inclusive.

†Individuals with a mitral valve prolapse associated with thickening and/or redundancy of the valve leaflets may be at increased risk for bacterial endocarditis, particularly men who are 45 years of age or older.

‡In addition to prophylactic regimen for genitourinary procedures, antibiotic therapy should be directed against the most likely bacterial pathogen.

§In patients who have prosthetic heart valves, a previous history of endocarditis, or surgically constructed systemic-pulmonary shunts or conduits, physicians may choose to administer prophylactic antibiotics even for low-risk procedures.

TABLE 7-31.—Recommended Prophylactic Regimens for Patients At Risk For Endocarditis[a]

	ADULTS	CHILDREN[b]
Dental, Oral, and Upper Respiratory Tract Procedures		
Oral[c] (Standard Regimen)		
Amoxicillin	3 g 1 hour before procedure and 1.5 g 6 hours after	50 mg/kg 1 hour before the procedure and 25 mg/kg follow-up dose (not to exceed adult dosage)
Patients allergic to penicillin		
Erythromycin	Erythromycin ethylsuccinate, 800 mg, or erythromycin stearate, 1.0 g, orally 2 hours before procedure; then half the dose 6 hours after initial dose	Erythromycin ethylsuccinate or erythromycin stearate 20 mg/kg; then one half the initial dose as follow-up
Clindamycin	300 mg orally 1 hour before procedure and 150 mg 6 hours after initial dose	10 mg/kg with follow-up dose one half the initial dose
Parenteral (patients unable to take oral)		
Ampicillin	2 g IM or IV 30 minutes before; then 1 g IV or IM 6 hours after initial dose, or substitute 1.5 g amoxicillin orally 6 hours after initial dose	50 mg/kg IM or IV 30 minutes before procedure; with follow-up dose one half the initial dose
High-risk patients are not candidates for standard regimen		
Ampicillin, *plus* gentamicin and amoxicillin[d,e]	2 g ampicillin plus 1.5 mg/kg gentamicin (not to exceed 80 mg), IV or IM 30 minutes before procedure; followed by amoxicillin, 1.5 g PO 6 hours after initial dose, alternatively the parenteral regimen may be repeated 8 hours after initial dose	50 mg/kg ampicillin plus 2 mg/kg gentamicin IM or IV 30 minutes before procedure; 25 mg/kg amoxicillin orally as follow-up, or repeat parenteral regimen, one half the initial dose as follow-up
Penicillin allergy		
Unable to take oral medication		
Vancomycin[d]	1 g IV infused *slowly* over 1 hour before procedure; no follow-up dose necessary	20 mg/kg infused *slowly* over 1 hour before procedure; no follow-up dose necessary

	Adults	Children
Clindamycin	300 mg IV 30 minutes before procedure; then 150 mg IV or oral 6 hours after initial dose	10 mg/kg IV 30 minutes before procedure, then one half initial dose as follow-up

Gastrointestinal and Genitourinary Procedures

	Adults	Children
Parenteral		
Ampicillin *plus* gentamicin and amoxicillin[c]	2 g ampicillin plus 1.5 mg/kg gentamicin (not to exceed 80 mg), IV or IM 30 min before procedure; followed by amoxicillin, 1.5 g orally 6 hours after initial dose, alternatively the parenteral regimen may be repeated 8 hours after initial dose	50 mg/kg ampicillin plus 2 mg/kg gentamicin IM or IV 30 minutes before procedure; 25 mg/kg amoxicillin orally as follow-up, or repeat parenteral regimen, one half the initial dose as follow-up
Patients allergic to penicillin		
Vancomycin *plus* gentamicin	1 g vancomycin IV infused *slowly* over 1 hour beginning 1 hour before procedure, *plus* 1.5 mg/kg gentamicin IV or IM (not to exceed 80 mg) 1 hour before procedure; may be repeated once 8 hours after initial dose	20 mg/kg vancomycin IV infused *slowly* over 1 hour beginning 1 hr before procedure, *plus* 1.5 mg/kg gentamicin IV or IM (not to exceed 80 mg) 1 hour before procedure; may be repeated once 8 hours after initial dose
Alternate regimen, low risk amoxicillin	3 g orally 1 hour before procedure and 1.5 g 6 hours later	50 mg/kg 1 hour before procedure then one half initial dose as follow-up

Dajan AS, Bisno AL, Chung KJ, Prevention of bacterial endocarditis: Recommendation of the American Heart Association, JAMA 1990; 214:2919-22.

[a]For patients with valvular heart disease, prosthetic heart valves, most forms of congenital heart disease (but not uncomplicated secundum atrial septal defect), idiopathic hypertrophic subaortic stenosis, and mitral valve prolapse with regurgitation.
[b]Total pediatric dose should not exceed adult dose.
[c]Oral regimens are more convenient and safer. Parenteral regimens are more likely to be effective; they are recommended especially for patients with prosthetic heart valves, those who have had endocarditis previously, or those taking continuous oral penicillin for rheumatic fever prophylaxis.
[d]For patients considered at very high risk.
[e]No initial dose of amoxicillin is recommended.

Continued.

TABLE 7-31.—Recommended Prophylactic Regimens for Patients At Risk For Endocarditis[a]—cont'd

ADULTS	CHILDREN[b]

Cardiac Surgery with Placement of Foreign Material

Cefazolin *plus* gentamicin — 2 g IV immediately preoperatively and every 6 hours for 24-28 hours *plus* gentamicin 1.7 mg/kg IV immediately, preoperatively, and every 8 hours for 24 hours

In institutions with a high incidence of methicillin-resistant staphylococci

Vancomycin *plus* gentamicin — 15 mg/kg IV over 1 hour beginning 1 hour before procedure, followed by 10 mg/kg IV immediately after cardiolpulmonary bypass surgery plus gentamicin 1.7 mg/kg IV immediately, preoperatively, and every 8 hours for 24 hours

TABLE 7-32.—OTHER CARDIAC DISEASES AND MISCELLANEOUS CONDITIONS

Acute Pericarditis
  Signs
  Pericardial friction rub: May be three-component rub
  Pericardial effusion: Best diagnosed with echocardiogram
  Pulsus paradoxus
  ECG changes: ST elevation in all leads except aV_R and only rarely in V_1
    Treatment
  Watch for effusion; consider antiinflammatory drugs

Cardiomyopathy
  Either primary myocardial disease or secondary to systemic disease, causing
    poor function of heart muscle
  Three major classifications:
    Congestive
  Signs
    Congestive heart failure, arrhythmias, cardiac chamber dilation, mitral and
      tricuspid valve regurgitation
  Treatment
    Bed rest, digitalis, diuretics, afterload and preload reduction, consider antico-
      agulation
    Restrictive
  Signs
    Dependent edema, elevated jugular venous pulse, ascites, enlarged heart,
      enlarged liver, ECG changes
  Treatment
    Transvenous biopsy; treat CHF
    Hypertrophic (Idiopathic Hypertrophic Subaortic Stenosis)
  Signs
    Hypertrophy of left ventricle, murmur
  Treatment
    β-blockers; surgical excision of hypertrophy; avoid inotropic agents and limit
      exercise

Secondary Hypertension

Causes	Screening Test
Coarctation	Chest PA and left lateral x-ray films
Cushing's syndrome	Plasma control after 1 mg dexameth- asone suppression
Drugs	Blood and urine screens
Amphetamines, cocaine, oral con- traceptives, estrogens, steroid or thyroid excess	
Increased intracranial pressure	CT scan
Pheochromocytoma	Urine metanephrine or VMA clonidine suppression test

Continued.

TABLE 7-32.—OTHER CARDIAC DISEASES AND MISCELLANEOUS CONDITIONS—cont'd

Primary aldosteronism	Serum potassium
Conn's syndrome	Stimulated plasma renin activity
Idiopathic hyperaldosteronism	Urine potassium
Renovascular disease	Screening tests, different for each
Renal parenchymal disease	disease
Chronic pyelonephritis	
Congenital renal disease	
Diabetic nephropathy	
Glomerulonephritis	
Gout	
Interstitial nephropathy	
Obstructive uropathy	
Polycystic disease	
Renin-secreting tumors	
Vasculitis	
Renovascular hypertension	IVP
	Suppressed or stimulated plasma
	renin activity

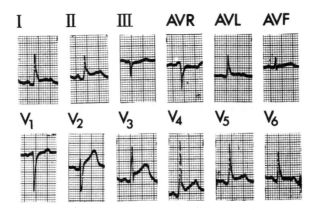

FIG 7-42.
Acute pericarditis. (From Gazes PC: *Clinical cardiology: a bedside approach,* ed 2, Chicago, 1983, Mosby.)

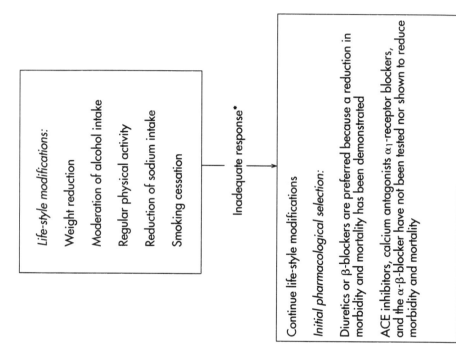

Life-style modifications:

Weight reduction

Moderation of alcohol intake

Regular physical activity

Reduction of sodium intake

Smoking cessation

Inadequate response*

Continue life-style modifications

Initial pharmacological selection:

Diuretics or β-blockers are preferred because a reduction in morbidity and mortality has been demonstrated

ACE inhibitors, calcium antagonists α₁-receptor blockers, and the α-β-blocker have not been tested nor shown to reduce morbidity and mortality

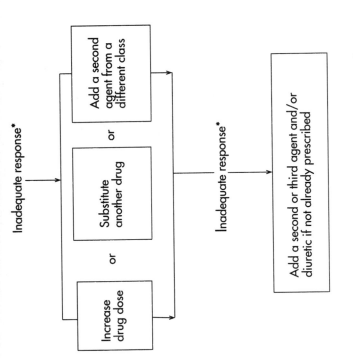

* Response means achieved goal blood pressure, or patient is making considerable progress towards this goal.

FIG 7-43.
Hypertension treatment algorithm. (From The Fifth Report of the Joint National Committee on Detection, Evaluation and Treatment of High Blood Pressure, *Arch Intern Med* 153:154, 1993.)

TABLE 7-33.—THE RELATIONSHIP OF RENIN AND ALDOSTERONE IN DISEASE

DISEASE	RENIN	ALDOSTERONE	DIAGNOSIS
Low renin state	Low	Low	Diabetes, renal insufficiency, fluid overload, and normal sodium
Pseudohypo-aldosteronism	Very high	Very high	Salt wasting with acidosis, hyperkalemia in infants
Gordon's syndrome	Reduced	Reduced	Hyperkalemia, acidosis in the absence of renal insufficiency
Pseudohyper-aldosteronism	Elevated	Elevated	Licorice ingestion
Renovascular hypertension	Elevated or normal	Elevated or normal	Abnormal IVP, renal vein renins differ
Primary aldosteronism	None	Elevated	Hyperkalemia, hypertension
Renal tumor/cyst	Elevated	Elevated	Abnormal IVP or ultrasound

Modified from Stein JH, ed: *Internal medicine*, ed 4, 1994, Mosby.

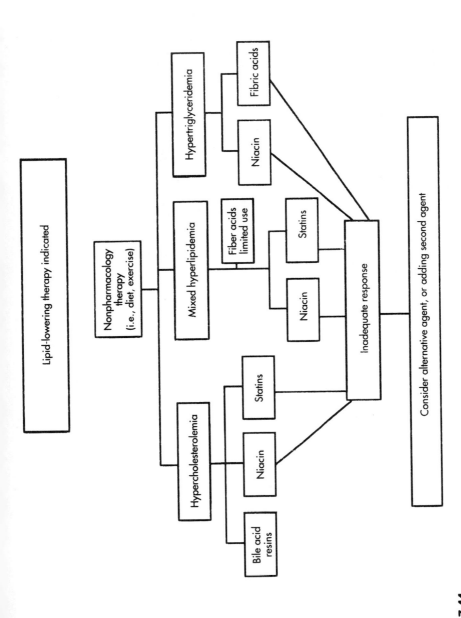

FIG 7-44.
Treatment algorithm for hyperlipidemia. (From Expert Panel on Detection, Evaluation and Treatment of High Blood Cholesterol in Adults, *JAMA* 269:3015, 1993.)

PROCEDURES

TABLE 7-34.—Pacemaker Insertion

Indications
Symptomatic bradydysrhythmias
Prophylactic pacing in acute MI
   Inferior MI: Mobitz I, no pacemaker
               Mobitz II, pacemaker
   Anterior MI: Mobitz I or II, pacemaker
Overdrive pacing of atria or ventricles in face of a tachydysrhythmia resistant to
   medications
   Method
Choose either a 3F or 5F balloon-tipped catheter, a 3F or 4F semifloating cath-
   eter, or a 6F or 7F regular pacing catheter
Choose site of insertion: subclavian, antecubital, internal jugular, or femoral vein
Use aseptic technique
Monitor ECG with IV in place
Insert catheter and advance while monitoring ECG for position; a large QRS
   indicates right ventricular position; proper positioning is against the wall,
   which causes marked ST elevation
Secure the catheter and set the rate above the intrinsic cardiac rate or the de-
   sired rate
Determine the threshold by decreasing the output until the capture is lost; set at
   two to three times the threshold
Put pacemaker in the demand mode to avoid arrhythmias caused by competi-
   tion with the intrinsic rate
Obtain chest x-ray radiograph to confirm correct placement and exclude pneumothorax; catheter tip should point anteriorly on the lateral x-ray film

---

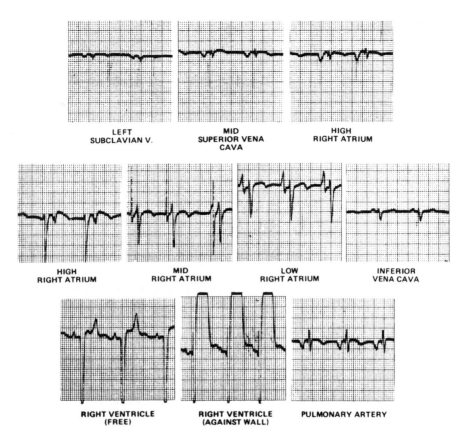

LEFT
SUBCLAVIAN V.

MID
SUPERIOR VENA
CAVA

HIGH
RIGHT ATRIUM

HIGH
RIGHT ATRIUM

MID
RIGHT ATRIUM

LOW
RIGHT ATRIUM

INFERIOR
VENA CAVA

RIGHT VENTRICLE
(FREE)

RIGHT VENTRICLE
(AGAINST WALL)

PULMONARY ARTERY

FIG 7-45.
Pacemaker location by ECG. (From Bing OHL: *N Engl J Med* 287:651, 1972.)

TABLE 7-35.—Exercise Stress Testing

Objectives

To diagnose ischemic heart disease

To measure functional capacity for working, sports participation, or rehabilitation potential

Method

Observe patient and ECG before and after to see baseline

Exercise by treadmill or bicycle to 80%-90% of predicted maximum heart rate (see Table 7-36) or beyond if no symptoms occur

Discontinue testing if symptoms occur

Evaluation

To be positive the ST segment must be a flat depression of at least 1.5 mm below the baseline, lasting at least 0.08 seconds; if 0.5 mm is used, there will be more false positives and fewer false negatives

Common causes of false positive exercise stress tests include anemia, digitalis, hypertension, hypoxia, left bundle-branch block, left ventricular hypertrophy, Lown-Ganong-Levine syndrome, pectus excavatum, ST changes at rest, valvular heart disease, vasoregulatory asthenia.

Many centers now do low-level exercise testing before post-MI patients are discharged to determine homegoing exercise prescriptions.

TABLE 7-36.—Target Heart Rate for Graded Exercise Test Based on Age and Activity

	AGE (YEARS)										
GROUP	20	25	30	35	40	45	50	55	60	65	70
Untrained											
MHR*	197	195	193	191	189	187	184	182	180	178	176
90% MHR	177	175	173	172	170	168	166	164	162	160	158
Trained											
MHR	190	188	186	184	182	180	177	175	173	171	169
90% MHR	171	169	167	166	164	162	159	158	156	154	152

Data from Sheffield, et al: *J S C Med Assoc* 65:18, 1969.

MHR, Maximum heart rate.

TABLE 7-37.—Screening for Coronary Artery Disease

RISK*	EXAMPLE	TEST
Very low < 10%	Female <60 years of age, male <40 years of age with nonanginal chest pain Female <40 years of age with atypical angina	None (Some may wish to do exercise ECG to confirm suspicion of low risk.)
Low 10%- 25%	Female 60-69 years of age, male 40-59 years of age with non-anginal chest pain Female 40-49 years of age, male 30-39 years of age with atypical angina	Exercise ECG
Moderate 25%- 68%	Male >60 years of age with non-anginal chest pain Female >50 years of age, male >40 years of age with atypical angina Female <50 years of age with typical angina	Stress thallium or stress MUGA
High 68%- 100%	Female >50 years of age, male >30 years of age with typical angina	Cardiac catheterization

Courtesy Mary Thoesen Coleman, M.D., Ph.D.; Donna Hosmer, M.D., Riverside Methodist Hospital, Columbus, Ohio.
*Pretest probability of coronary artery disease.

TABLE 7-38.—Cardiac Rehabilitation and Exercise

Cardiac rehabilitation with at least educational activities should begin in the coronary care unit. When the patient has left the coronary care unit, a program of progressive exercise should be started, including bathroom privileges, walking in the room, and progressively lengthy walks in the hallway.

Heart rate and blood pressure should be measured before and after exercise. Symptoms should be monitored and activity kept to a symptom-free level. In some centers a low-level exercise test is done to determine homegoing activity level. In general a patient, on discharge, should be able to do the following:

Walk 15 minutes per day at 80 steps per minute, 1 week after discharge.

In second week after discharge, walk same amount 2 and 3 times a day.

In third week, increase duration of walk until it reaches 1 hour twice a day, then increase rate to 100 steps per minute.

At 6 weeks the patient should undergo a symptom-limited exercise test.

In general, the patient is able to begin driving the car, resume sexual intercourse, and enter a routine exercise program that raises the heart rate to an exercise target heart rate (ETHR), which is 70% of maximal oxygen uptake. For this exercise formula, maximum heart rate (MHR) is found from Table 7-36. The resting heart rate is the pulse: ETHR = 0.7 MHR + 0.3 RHR. If this rate is fatiguing, 0.5 may be substituted for 0.7.

At 8 to 12 weeks the patient may return to work.

Modified from Hartley HL: *Cardiovasc Med* January 1983.

TABLE 7-39.—PULMONARY ARTERY CATHETERIZATION

Indications
Measurement of right atrial, pulmonary arterial, and pulmonary capillary wedge
  pressure
Measurement of cardiac output by either thermodilution or dye dilution
Sampling of right atrial and pulmonary arterial blood

Technique
Choose a 5F or 7F pulmonary artery catheter. To measure cardiac output, use a
  7F thermodilution catheter
Have an IV line in place to treat arrhythmias that may arise
Prepare a sterile field around the chosen insertion site: antecubital venous cut-
  down, subclavian, or internal jugular vein
Test balloon with air and deflate
Insert catheter through an adequate-sized introducer
Inflate balloon halfway when catheter approaches central circulation. Catheter
  measurement markers will assist in knowing the approximate position of the
  catheter
  R antecubital fossa to right atrium = 40 cm
  L antecubital fossa to right atrium = 50 cm
  Internal jugular and subclavian to right atrium = 15-20 cm
  Femoral vein to right atrium = 70 cm
Watch the monitor for waveforms similar to those shown in Fig. 7-46 to deter-
  mine site of catheter. Vena caval pressures are low and can be increased by
  asking the patient to cough
Once inside the right atrium, inflate balloon to full volume
Secure catheter in a position where the balloon can be slowly inflated to obtain
  a wedge pressure

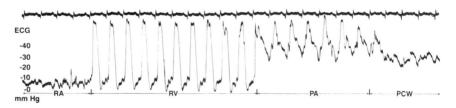

FIG 7-46.
Pressure waveforms recorded as pulmonary artery catheter is advanced through right
atrium *(RA)* and right ventricle *(RV)* into pulmonary artery *(PA)* and to wedge *(PCW)* position. (From *Textbook of advanced cardiac life support,* Dallas; 1994, American Heart Association.)

TABLE 7-40.—PERICARDIOCENTESIS

Indications
Diagnostic fluid
Relieve cardiac tamponade
   Causes of cardiac tamponade include trauma, infection, and neoplasm
   Signs of cardiac tamponade include pulsus paradoxus and elevated central
      venous pressure

Methods
Perform echocardiography to demonstrate the fluid
Use aseptic technique while monitoring ECG with IV line in place
Use atropine as premedication to avoid hypotension with puncture of pericar-
   dium
Attach ECG V-lead to needle. If ST changes occur, the ventricle has been
   touched
Choose site: Subxiphoid is preferred over apex and left sternal border in the
   fifth intercostal space
Place patient in 20- to 30-degree supine position and infiltrate the site with lido-
   caine
Insert large-bore needle 1 cm to left of xiphoid
Advance needle with constant aspiration at a 20- to 30-degree angle to frontal
   plane
Test aspirated fluid to see if it clots (pericardial fluid will not) or if it leaves a
   central dark red stain with peripheral clearing on a gauze pad (pericardial
   fluid will)

Intracardiac Injections
Indications
For injection of epinephrine and calcium when IV and ET routes are unavailable
Method
The technique is basically the same as it is for pericardiocentesis except that
   the blood returned usually indicates an intracardiac position. If the needle is
   fully inserted with no blood return (an 18-gauge 3½-inch needle is used),
   withdraw slowly while aspirating
Stop when blood returns and inject the medicines

Modified from *Textbook of advanced cardiac life support,* Dallas, American Heart Association, 1994.

TABLE 7-41.—Pediatric Heart Defects: Signs and Diagnostic Aids

DEFECT	CYANOSIS	CHAMBER ENLARGEMENT	P_1	MURMUR	CHEST FILM	ECG	ECHOCARDIOGRAM
Valvular pulmonic stenosis	0	Right ventricle	Lessened intensity Wide split	Ejection murmur in pulmonic area Ejection click	Right ventricular enlargement Normal pulmonary blood flow Poststenotic dilation	Right axis deviation Right ventricular enlargement	Right ventricular enlargement; if severe, increased *a* wave on the pulmonic valve
Ebstein's anomaly	20%	Quiet precordium	Single	Tricuspid insufficiency	Globular heart Clear lungs Large right atrium	Wolff-Parkinson-White syndrome (25%) Right atrial enlargement Atypical right bundle-branch block	Tricuspid valve displaced and abnormal
Atrial septal defect (primum)	0	Right and possibly left ventricle enlargement	Wide and fixed	Flow murmur, left sternal border Mitral regurgitation murmur	Increased pulmonary blood flow Enlargement of pulmonary artery, right ventricle, and atrium Enlargement of left atrium and ventricle	Incomplete right bundle-branch block Left axis deviation	Defect in the atrioventricular valves Paradoxical septal motion

Atrial septal defect (secundum)	0	Right ventricular lift	Wide and fixed	Flow murmur, left sternal border	Increased pulmonary artery size Increased pulmonary blood flow Right ventricular and right atrial enlargement	Incomplete right bundle branch block	Right ventricular enlargement Paradoxical septal motion
Ventricular septal defect	0	Thrill, left sternal border Left ventricle enlargement	Variable	Regurgitant murmur, left sternal border	Increased pulmonary blood flow Enlargement of right and left ventricles	Biatrial and biventricular enlargement	Increased left atrium size Left ventricular dilation Septal defect visualized at times
Patent ductus arteriosus	0	Wide pulse pressure Left ventricle enlargement	Variable	Continuous murmur, "machinery murmur"	Increased pulmonary blood flow Left ventricular and left atrial enlargement	Left ventricular enlargement	Increased left atrium size Left ventricular dilation
Tetralogy	+	Right ventricle enlargement	Lessened intensity	Ejection murmur	Decreased pulmonary artery size Decreased pulmonary blood flow No specific chamber enlargement Boot-shaped heart	Right ventricular enlargement	Overriding of the aorta Right ventricular enlargement

From Eich RH: *Introduction to cardiology,* New York, 1980, Harper & Row.

8 The Respiratory System

Charles W. Smith, Jr.

NORMAL PHYSIOLOGY AND PULMONARY FUNCTION TESTS

Table 8-1 provides short descriptions of commonly ordered pulmonary function tests. Vital capacity, inspiratory capacity, expiratory reserve volume, tidal volume, forced expiratory volume, forced midexpiratory flow rate, and maxi-

TABLE 8-1.—PULMONARY FUNCTION TESTS*

1. *Vital capacity (VC):* The maximum volume of gas that can be exhaled from the lung following a maximal inspiration. A combination of inspiratory reserve volume, tidal volume, and expiratory reserve volume (4 L).

2. *Inspiratory capacity (IC):* The maximum amount of air that can be inspired from the expiratory position of normal breathing. A combination of tidal volume and inspiratory reserve volume (3.37 L).

3. *Expiratory reserve volume (ERV):* The maximum amount of air that can be expired from the end-expiratory position of a normal breath (0.7 L).

4. *Tidal volume (TV):* The volume of inspired or expired air during each respiratory cycle (0.5 L).

5. *Functional residual capacity (FRC):* The amount of air remaining in the lungs at the expiratory position of normal breathing. A combination of ERV and RV (2 L).

6. *Residual volume (RV):* The volume of gas remaining in the lungs at the end of a maximal expiration (1.3 L).

7. *Total lung capacity (TLC):* The amount of air remaining in the lungs at the end of a maximal inspiration. A combination of the four lung volumes (5.37 L).

8. *Forced expiratory volume, 1 sec and 3 sec, (FEV$_1$, FEV$_3$):* The maximum amount of air that can be expired in 1 (3) seconds (FEV$_1$ = 3.7 L).

9. *Forced midexpiratory flow (FEF$_{25-75}$):* The flow rate of air measured during midexpiration (from spirometry, during 25% and 75% of the forced vital capacity) (2.8 L).

10. *Maximal breathing capacity (MBC):* The total volume of air a patient can move with maximum effort during a given period (also known as *maximal voluntary ventilation, MVV*) (158 L/min).

*Normal values are listed in parentheses.

mal breathing capacity are measured by routine spirometry. Functional residual capacity, residual volume, and total lung capacity require measurement
of lung volumes by gas diffusion studies.

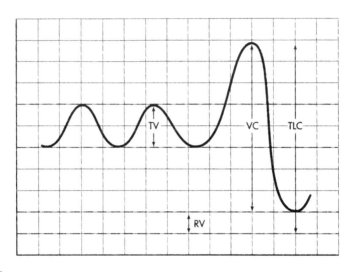

FIG 8-1.
Lung volumes and capacities. *TLC,* total lung capacity, total volume of air in the lung after
a maximal inspiration; *RV,* residual volume, total volume of air in the lung after a maximal
expiration. This volume never leaves the lung and thus cannot be measured by spirometry
(which only measures volumes and flows of inhaled and exhaled gases). Because the RV
is contained in the TLC and FRC, these latter measurements cannot be measured by spirometry either; *VC,* vital capacity, the maximal volume expired after a maximal inspiration
or maximal volume inspired after a maximal expiration; *TV,* tidal volume, the volume of air
inhaled or exhaled during normal comfortable breaths. (From Wachtel TJ, Stein MD: *Practical guide to the care of the ambulatory patient,* 1995, Mosby.

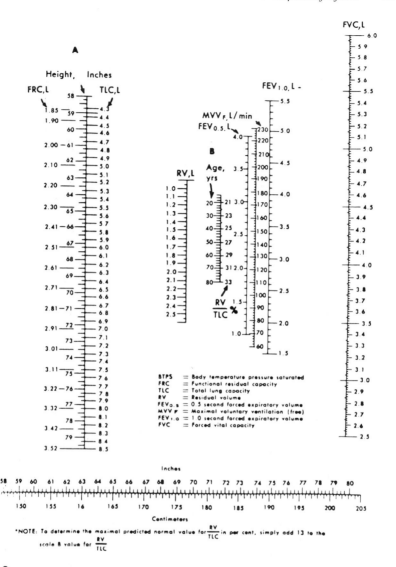

FIG 8-2.

Nomogram for predicting pulmonary function in men. The predicted FRC and TLC can be read directly from the left-hand scale **(A)** based on the patient's height. The horizontal scale at the bottom is for convenience in converting centimeters to inches. The RV/TLC % may be read directly from the age scale **(B)**. For other predicted values, lay a straight edge between the patient's height (scale A) and age (scale B). Predicted normal values can be read directly from the points where the straight edge crosses the *RV, FEV$_{0.5}$, MVV, FEV$_1$,* and *FVC* scales. (From Slonim NB, Hamilton LH: *Respiratory physiology,* ed 4. St. Louis, 1981, Mosby.)

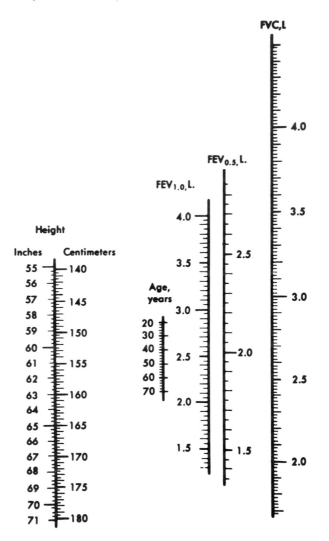

FIG 8-3.

Nomogram for predicting pulmonary function in women. To use this nomogram, lay a straight edge between the patient's height as read on the height scale and her age as it appears on the age scale. Predicted normal values for *FEV₁* and *FVC* can be read directly from the points where the straight edge crosses the two right-hand axes. (From Kory RA, Callahan R: Unpublished work. In Slonim NB, Hamilton LH: *Respiratory physiology,* ed 4. St. Louis, 1981, Mosby.)

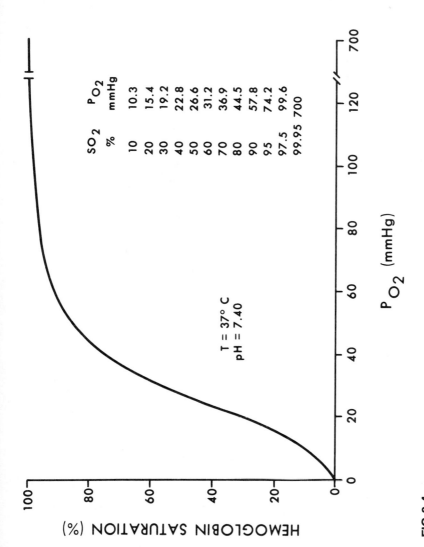

SO$_2$	P$_{O_2}$
%	mmHg
10	10.3
20	15.4
30	19.2
40	22.8
50	26.6
60	31.2
70	36.9
80	44.5
90	57.8
95	74.2
97.5	99.6
99.95	700

T = 37° C
pH = 7.40

HEMOGLOBIN SATURATION (%)

P$_{O_2}$ (mmHg)

FIG 8-4.
The normal oxyhemoglobin dissociation curves for men. Values for hemoglobin saturation (S$_{O_2}$) at different P$_{O_2}$ values, under standard conditions of temperature and pH, are indicated (data from Severinghaus). (From Murray JF: *The normal lung*, Philadelphia, 1976, WB Saunders, p. 162.)

RESPIRATORY INFECTIONS

TABLE 8-2.—Drugs of Choice for Common Respiratory Tract Infections

INFECTING ORGANISM	DRUG OF CHOICE	ALTERNATE DRUG
Gram-Positive Organisms		
Streptococcus pyogenes (β-streptococcus)	Penicillin	Erythromycin or cephalosporin
Staphylococcus aureus	Penicillinase-resistant penicillin	Cephalosporin or amoxicillin-clavulanic acid
Streptococcus pneumoniae (pneumococcus)	Penicillin*	Erythromycin or cephalosporin
Gram-Negative Organisms		
Bacteroides		
Oropharyngeal	Penicillin G	Clindamycin or metronidazole
Gastrointestinal	Clindamycin or metronidazole	Cefoxitin, piperacillin, or Imipenem
Escherichia coli	Ampicillin with or without gentamicin or tobramycin	Mezlocillin or piperacillin or cephalosporin
Klebsiella pneumoniae	A cephalosporin	Gentamicin, tobramycin, or amoxicillin-clavulanic acid
Haemophilus influenzae	Ampicillin or amoxicillin	Trimethoprim-sulfamethoxazole, amoxicillin-clavulanic acid cefaclor, or ceftriaxone
Legionella pneumophila	Erythromycin with or without rifampin	Trimethoprim-sulfamethoxazole
Pseudomonas aeruginosa	Carbenicillin or ticarcillin plus gentamicin or tobramycin	Gentamicin with ceftazidime or ciprofloxacin
Chlamydia organisms		
Chlamydia trachomatis	Tetracycline	Sulfonamide or erythromycin
Mycoplasma organisms		
Mycoplasma pneumoniae	Erythromycin	Tetracycline

*Some streptococcal strains show increasing resistance to penicillin.
Modified from *Med Lett* 30:30, 1988.

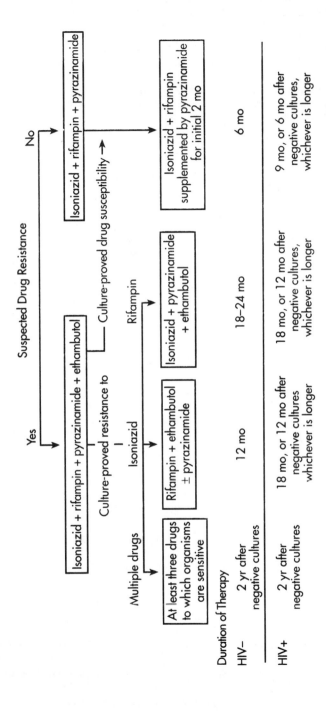

FIG 8-5.
Guidelines for the treatment of tuberculosis. (From Weinberger: Medical progress, *N Engl J Med* 328(20):1465, 1993.

TABLE 8-3.—Treatment of Tuberculosis (TB)

Guidelines for Preventive Therapy*
1. Treat patients with HIV or other immunosuppression, recent conversion of tuberculin skin test, patients in close contact with known infected persons.
2. Give isoniazid, 300 mg/day for adults (10 mg/kg up to 300 mg for children) for 6 to 12 months.
3. Don't give to patients over the age of 35 years unless conditions suggest a high-risk situation (known recent conversion, evidence of TB on x-ray examination, or immunosuppression).

*Modified from Drugs for tuberculosis, *Med Lett* 35(908):99, 1993.

TABLE 8-4.—Antituberculous Drugs

DRUG	DAILY ADULT DOSE	DAILY PEDIATRIC DOSE	ADVERSE EFFECTS
Isoniazid	300 mg PO*	10-20 mg/kg*	Hepatic toxicity, neurological
Rifampin	600 mg PO	10-20 mg/kg	Hepatic toxicity, flulike syndrome, hematological
Pyrazinamide	1 to 2 g PO	20-30 mg/kg	Hepatic toxicity, hyperuricemia
Ethambutol	15-25 mg/kg PO	Same as adult	Optic neuritis
Streptomycin	7-15 mg/kg IM	20-40 mg/kg	Vestibular (eighth nerve) toxicity, nephrotoxicity
Other Drugs Used Less Commonly			
Capreomycin	15 mg/kg IM	15 mg/kg IM	Auditory and vestibular (eighth nerve) toxicity, nephrotoxicity
Kanamycin	15 mg/kg IM, IV	7.5-15 mg/kg	Same as streptomycin
Amikacin	15 mg/kg IM, IV	7.5-15 mg/kg	Same as streptomycin
Cycloserine	250-500 mg bid PO	10-20 mg/kg	Psych sxs, seizures
Ethionamide	250-500 mg bid PO	15-20 mg/kg	GI and hepatic toxicity
Ciprofloxacin	500-750 mg bid PO	Contraindicated	Nausea, abdominal pain
Ofloxacin	300-400 mg every 12 hours or 600-800 mg/day PO	Contraindicated	Same as ciprofloxacin
Para-aminosalicylic acid	6-8 g bid PO	75-100 mg/kg bid	GI disturbance
Clofazimine	100-200 mg PO	1 mg/kg	GI disturbance, icthyosis, pigmentation of cornea, retina, and skin

*Some therapies have been used on a twice-weekly basis. Consult with an infectious disease specialist if necessary.
Modified from Drugs for tuberculosis, *Med Lett* 35(908):99, 1993.

TABLE 8-5.—Characteristics of Pneumonia Caused by Pyogenic Bacteria Versus Viruses, Chlamydiae, Rickettsiae, and Mycoplasmas

CLINICAL FINDINGS	PYOGENIC BACTERIA	VIRUSES, CHLAMYDIAE, RICKETTSIAE, AND MYCOPLASMAS
Onset	Often sudden	Usually gradual
Myalgia, headache, and photophobia	Not prominent	Often prominent
Fever	>104° F (40° C)	<104° F (40° C)
Rigors	Common, often multiple	Rare, except in influenza and usually single
Toxicity	Marked	Mild to moderate
Cough	Productive—purulent, bloody sputum	Nonproductive or only scant mucoid sputum
Physical findings	Consolidation	Often minimal
Roentgenographic findings	Agree with physical examination; localized	Involvement in excess of physical findings; often multiple sites
Leukocyte count	>15,000/mm³, marked shift to the left	<15,000/mm³, possible lymphocytosis

Modified from Hinshaw HC, Murray JF: *Diseases of the chest,* Philadelphia, 1980, WB Saunders, p. 212.

TABLE 8-6.—Characteristics of Pulmonary Mycoses

	BLASTOMYCOSIS	COCCIDIOIDOMYCOSIS	HISTOPLASMOSIS
Chest Roentgenogram			
Acute disease	Focal alveolar infiltrates	Focal alveolar infiltrates Pleural effusions Hilar adenopathy	Focal alveolar infiltrates Diffuse nodules Hilar adenopathy
Chronic disease	Cavities Masses	Thin-walled cavities	Cavities Parenchymal calcifications Fibrosing mediastinitis
Sites of Dissemination	Skin Bone Male genital tract	Skin Bone Meninges	Liver and spleen Mucosal surfaces Adrenal glands
Diagnostic Studies			
Skin test	No value	Excellent epidemiological tool	Limited value
Serological tests	No value	Diagnostic and prognostic value	Limited value

Modified from Whitcomb ME: *The lung,* St Louis, 1982, Mosby, p. 332.

ASTHMA AND CHRONIC OBSTRUCTIVE PULMONARY DISEASE (COPD)

Asthma results in recurrent attacks of wheezing dyspnea with coughing and sputum production. It affects 1 out of 25 people. Attacks are caused by an allergic reaction in atopic patients. Nonallergic asthma (intrinsic) is caused by air pollutants, cold, humid air, exercise, respiratory tract infection, drugs, or tension.

TABLE 8-7.—PATIENT INTERVIEW CHECKLIST FOR ASSESSING THE POSSIBLE ROLE OF ALLERGY IN ASTHMA

Is asthma worse in certain months? If so, are there symptoms at the same time of allergic rhinitis—sneezing, itching, nose runny and obstructed at the same time? (pollens and outdoor molds)*

Do symptoms appear when visiting a house where there are indoor pets? (animal dander)

If there are pets in the patient's home, do symptoms improve when the patient is away from home for a week or longer? Do nasal, eye, and chest symptoms improve? Do the symptoms become worse the first 24 hours after returning home? (animal dander)

Do eyes itch and become red after handling the pet? If the pet licks the patient, does a red, itchy welt develop? (animal dander)

Do symptoms appear in a room where carpets are being vacuumed? (animal dander or mites)

Does making a bed cause symptoms? (mites)

Do symptoms develop around hay or in a barn or stable? (molds and mites)

Do symptoms develop when the patient goes into a damp basement or a vacation cottage that has been closed up for a period of time? (molds)

Do symptoms develop related to certain job activities, either at work or after leaving work?

If symptoms develop at work, do they improve when away from work for a few days?

*Possible causes of symptoms are enclosed in parentheses.

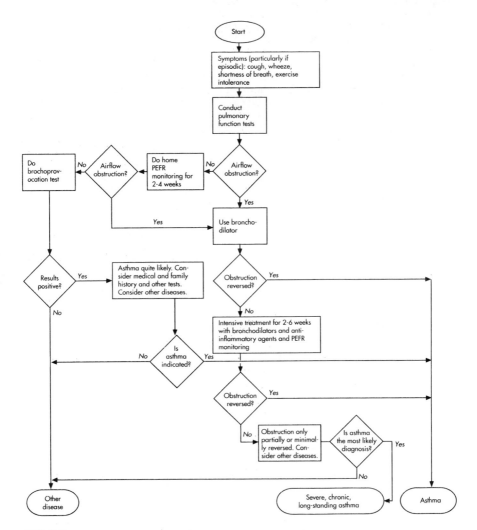

FIG 8-6.
Algorithm for diagnosing asthma. (From National Asthma Education Program Expert Panel Report: Guidelines for the diagnosis and management of asthma, Pub No 91-3042, 1991, Office of Prevention, Education, and Control, National Heart, Lung, and Blood Institute, Bethesda, MD, US Department of Health and Human Services, Public Health Service, NIH.)

TABLE 8-8.—GUIDELINES FOR MEASURING PEAK EXPIRATORY FLOW RATE*

At Home
All patients with asthma aged 5 years or older should monitor their peak flow:
    Twice daily and after bronchodilator therapy until asthma is well controlled
    Daily at the same time of day when asthma is well controlled
    Twice daily, two or three times a week if daily measurements cannot be obtained
    Before and after exposure to allergens or irritants
    During acute exacerbations to monitor course of attack and response to therapy

In Clinician's Office or Emergency Department
For patients with chronic asthma, measure peak flow:
    At each office visit, to guide therapeutic decisions (in all patients 5 years or older)
    To confirm exercise-induced bronchospasm
For patients with acute exacerbations, measure peak flow:
    During all acute exacerbations (in all patients 5 years or older)
    After β_2-agonist inhalation, to judge response
    Just before discharge from emergency department

Interpretation†
    70%-90% predicted or baseline = Mild exacerbation
    50%-70% predicted or baseline = Moderate exacerbation
    <50% predicted or baseline = Severe exacerbation

*Modified from the *National Asthma Education Program Expert Panel Report* 1991. *Guidelines for the Diagnosis and Management of Asthma,* U.S. Department of Health and Human Services publication No. 91-3042, Bethesda, Md, 1991.
†From *J Resp Dis* 15(95):S7, Sept. 1994.

FIG 8-7.
Stepwise approach to asthma management. *PEF,* Peak expiratory flow; *PEFB,* peak expiratory flow rate; *FEV₁,* forced expiratory volume in 1 second; *SR,* sustained release.
Step up: Progression to the next step is indicated when control cannot be achieved at the current step and there is assurance that medication is being used correctly. If PEFR ≤ 60% predicted or personal best, consider a burst of oral corticosteroids and then proceed. *Step down:* Reduction in therapy is considered when the outcome for therapy has been achieved and sustained for several weeks or even months at the current step. Reduction in therapy is also needed to identify the minimum therapy required to maintain control.
*All therapy must include patient education about prevention (including environmental control where appropriate), as well as control of symptoms.
†Obtain specialist consultation when considering inhaled steroid dosage > 1000 μg/d.
‡One or more features may be present to be assigned a grade of severity; a patient should usually be assigned to the most severe grade in which any feature occurs. (From the National Heart, Lung, and Blood Institute: *International Consensus Report on Diagnosis and Treatment of Asthma,* U.S. Dept of Health and Human Services publication No. 92-3091, Bethesda, Md, 1992.)

Outcome: Control of asthma

- Minimal or no chronic symptoms (including nocturnal)
- Infrequent episodes
- No emergency visits
- Minimal need for prn β_2-agonist
- No limitation on activity, including exercise
- PEF circadian variation < 20%
- Near normal PEF
- Minimal or no adverse effects from medicine

Outcome: Best possible results

- Least symptoms
- Least need for prn β_2-agonist
- Least limitation of activity
- Least PEFR circadian variation
- Best PEFR
- Least adverse effects from medicine

Therapy*

- Short–acting inhaled β_2–agonist prn not more than 3 times per week
- Short–acting inhaled β_2–agonist or cromolyn before exercise or exposure to antigen

Therapy*

- Inhaled anti–inflammatory daily
  Initally:
  Inhaled steroid, 200–500 μg/d, cromolyn, or nedocromil
  If necessary:
  Inhaled steroid, 400–750 μg/d (alternatively, particularly for nocturnal symptoms, proceed to Step 3 with additional long–acting bronchodilator)
  and
- Short–acting inhaled β_2–agonist prn, not to exceed 3 to 4 times daily

Therapy*

- Inhaled steroid 800–1,000 μg/d[†]
  and
- SR theophylline, oral β_2–agonist, or long-acting inhaled β_2–agonist, especially for nocturnal symptoms; may consider inhaled anti–cholinergics
  and
- Short–acting inhaled β_2–agonist prn, not to exceed 3 to 4 times daily

Therapy*

- Inhaled steroid 800–1,000 μg/d[†]
  and
- SR theophylline and /or oralβ_2–agonist, or long-acting inhaled β_2–agonist, especially for nocturnal symptoms
  with or without
- Short–acting inhaled β_2–agonist once a day; may consider inhaled anticholinergic
  and
- Oral steroid (alternate day or single daily dose)
  and
- Short–acting inhaled β_2–agonist prn, up to 3 to 4 times daily

Step down

- Once control is reached at any step, and sustained, a step down (reduction in therapy) may be carefully considered and is needed to identify the minimum therapy required to maintain control.
- Advise patients of signs of worsening asthma and actions to control it.

Clinical features pretreatment [†]

- Intermittent, brief symptoms < 1 or 2 times per week
- Nocturnal asthma symptoms < 1 or 2 times per month
- Asymptomatic between exacerbations
- PEFR or FEV$_1$ > 80% expected, variability <20%

Clinical features pretreatment [†]

- Exacerbations > 1 to 2 times per week
- Exacerbations may affect activity and sleep
- Nocturnal asthma symptoms > 2 times per month
- Chronic symptoms requiring short–acting β_2–agonist almost daily
- PEFR or FEV$_1$ 60% to 80% expected, variability 20% to 30%

Clinical features pretreatment [†]

- Frequent exacerbations
- Continuous symptoms
- Frequent nocturnal asthma symptoms
- Physical activities limited by asthma
- PEFR or FEV < 60% expected, variability > 30%

| STEP 1: MILD | STEP 2: MODERATE | STEP 3: MODERATE | STEP 4: SEVERE | |

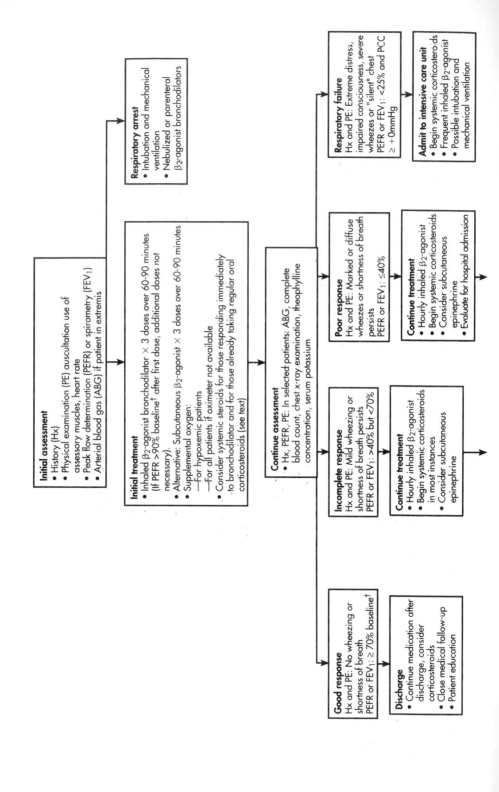

Initial assessment
- History (Hx)
- Physical examination (PE) auscultation use of assessory muscles, heart rate
- Peak flow determination (PEFR) or spirometry (FEV₁)
- Arterial blood gas (ABG) if patient in extremis

Initial treatment
- Inhaled β₂-agonist bronchodilator × 3 doses over 60-90 minutes (If PEFR >90% baseline† after first dose, additional doses not necessary).
- Alternative: Subcutaneous β₂-agonist × 3 doses over 60-90 minutes
- Supplemental oxygen:
  —For hypoxemic patients
  —For all patients if oximeter not available
- Consider systemic steroids for those responding immediately to bronchodilator and for those already taking regular oral corticosteroids (see text)

Respiratory arrest
- Intubation and mechanical ventilation
- Nebulized or parenteral β₂-agonist bronchodilators

Continue assessment
- Hx, PEFR, PE: In selected patients: ABG, complete blood count, chest x-ray examination, theophylline concentration, serum potassium

Respiratory failure
Hx and PE: Extreme distress, impaired consciousness, severe wheezes or "silent" chest PEFR or FEV₁: <25% and P꜀꜀ ≥ +0mmHg

Admit to intensive care unit
- Begin systemic corticosteroids
- Frequent inhaled β₂-agonist
- Possible intubation and mechanical ventilation

Poor response
Hx and PE: Marked or diffuse wheezes or shortness of breath persists
PEFR or FEV₁: ≤40%

Continue treatment
- Hourly inhaled β₂-agonist
- Begin systemic corticosteroids
- Consider subcutaneous epinephrine
- Evaluate for hospital admission

Incomplete response
Hx and PE: Mild wheezing or shortness of breath persists
PEFR or FEV₁: >40% but <70%

Continue treatment
- Hourly inhaled β₂-agonist
- Begin systemic corticosteroids in most instances
- Consider subcutaneous epinephrine

Good response
Hx and PE: No wheezing or shortness of breath
PEFR or FEV₁: ≥ 70% baseline†

Discharge
- Continue medication after discharge, consider corticosteroids
- Close medical follow-up
- Patient education

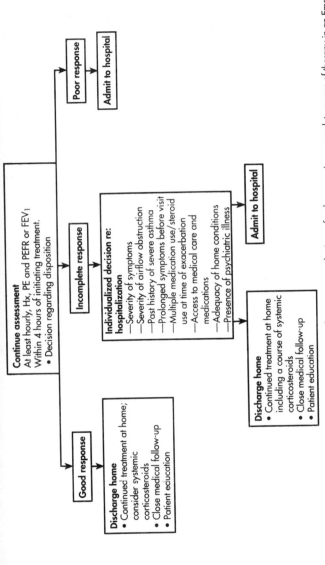

Continue assessment
At least hourly, Hx, PE and PEFR or FEV₁
Within 4 hours of initiating treatment.
• Decision regarding disposition

Good response

Incomplete response

Poor response

Admit to hospital

Discharge home
• Continued treatment at home; consider systemic corticosteroids
• Close medical follow-up
• Patient ecucation

Individualized decision re: hospitalization
—Severity of symptoms
—Severity of airflow obstruction
—Past history of severe asthma
—Prolonged symptoms before visit
—Multiple medication use/steroid use at time of exacerbation
—Access to medical care and medications
—Adequacy of home conditions
—Presence of psychiatric illness

Admit to hospital

Discharge home
• Continued treatment at home including a course of systemic corticosteroids
• Close medical follow-up
• Patient education

*Therapies are often available in a physician's office. However, most acutely severe exacerbations of asthma require a complete course of therapy in an Emergency Department
†PEFR % baseline refers to the norm for the individual, established by the physician. This may be of standardized norms or % patient's personal best.

FIG 8-8.

Emergency department management of acute exacerbations of asthma in adults. (From National Asthma Education Program, Office of prevention, education, and control; National Heart, Blood, and Lung Institute, NIH Publication No. 91-3042-A, June 1991, *Guidelines for diagnosis and management of asthma.*)

TABLE 8-9.—THEOPHYLLINE DOSING FOR ASTHMA*

1. *For patients currently receiving theophylline (within 24 hours):*
   Obtain stat serum level
   For each 1 μg/ml desired increase in serum level, give 0.6 mg/kg of amin-
   ophylline as loading infusion over 30 minutes
2. *For patients not receiving theophylline:*
   Loading dose of aminophylline is 6 mg/kg (equivalent to 5 mg/kg of anhy-
   drous theophylline) over 30 minutes
   Following infusion, obtain stat level
   Begin infusion listed in Table 8-10
   Measure level 4-6 hours after starting infusion
   Adjust infusion
   Obtain serum level 12-24 hours later.

*Acute management of asthma requires β-agonists and steroids. Theophylline may not be completely effective in the acute situation; aminophylline = theophylline/0.8 mg/kg.

TABLE 8-10.—INITIAL AMINOPHYLLINE MAINTENANCE INFUSIONS*

GROUP	AGE	AMINOPHYLLINE INFUSION (MG/KG/HR)
Neonates	<24 days	1.3 mg/kg/12 hr
	>24 days	1.9 mg/kg/12 hr
Infants	6 weeks to 1 year	mg/kg/hr = (0.008) (age in weeks) + 0.21
Children	1-9 years	1.0 mg/kg/hr
	9-12 years	0.9 mg/kg/hr
Adolescents (cigarette or marijuana smokers)	12-16 years	0.9 mg/kg/hr
Adolescents (nonsmokers)	12-16 years	0.6 mg/kg/hr
Adults (healthy cigarette or marijuana smokers)	16-50 years	0.6 mg/kg/hr
Adults (healthy nonsmokers)	16 years	0.5 mg/kg/hr
Cardiac decompensation, cor pulmonale, or liver disease	16 years	0.3 mg/kg/hr

Modified from Hendeles L, Weinberg M: *Am J Hosp Pharm* 39:249, 1982.
*Infusion is designed to achieve 10 μg/ml serum level. Anhydrous theophylline = aminophylline × 0.8.

TABLE 8-11.—DRUG TREATMENT OF ASTHMA

DRUG	FORMULATION	INITIAL ADULT DOSAGE	INITIAL PEDIATRIC DOSAGE
Corticosteroids			
Beclomethasone (Beclovent, Vanceril)	Metered dose inhaler	2 puffs qid or 4 puffs qid	2 puffs qid or 4 puffs bid
Budesonide	Metered dose inhaler (200 μg/puff)	400-2400 μg in two to four doses	200-400 μg bid
Flunisolide (AeroBid)	Metered dose inhaler (250 μg/puff)	2-4 puffs bid	2 puffs bid
Triamcinolone acetonide (Azmacort)	Metered dose inhaler (100 μg/puff)	2 puffs tid-qid or 4 puffs bid	2 puffs tid-qid or 4 puffs bid
Prednisone	Oral tabs (5, 10, 20 mg)	Acute: up to 80 mg/day for 7 to 14 days Chronic: up to 40 mg qod	Acute: 10-30 mg bid for 7 to 14 days Chronic: 20-40 mg qod
Cromolyn	Spinhaler, powder (20 mg/capsule)	1 cap qid	1 cap qid
	Metered dose inhaler (800 μg/puff)	2-4 puffs qid	2 puffs bid
	Nebulized solution (10 mg/ml)	20 mg qid	20 mg qid
β₂-Selective Adrenergic Drugs			
Albuterol (Proventil, Ventolin)	Metered dose inhaler (90 μg/puff)	2 puffs every 4-6 hours prn	2 puffs every 4-6 hours prn
	Syrup or tabs	2 to 4 mg tid or qid prn	0.1 mg/kg (maximum 2 mg) every 6-8 hours prn
	Extended release tabs (4 mg)	4-8 mg every 12 hours	0.1-0.2 mg/kg every 12 hours
Bitolterol mesylate (Tornalate)	Metered dose inhaler (370 μg/puff)	2-3 puffs every 4-6 hours prn	2 puffs every 4-6 hours prn

From Drugs for ambulatory asthma, *Med Lett* 35(889):11.

Continued.

TABLE 8-11.—D<small>RUG</small> T<small>REATMENT OF</small> A<small>STHMA</small>—cont'd

DRUG	FORMULATION	INITIAL ADULT DOSAGE	INITIAL PEDIATRIC DOSAGE
Pirbuterol (Maxair)	Nebulized solution (10 mg/ml)	20 mg qld	20 mg qld
	Metered dose inhaler (200 μg/puff)	2 puffs every 4-6 hours prn	2 puffs every 4-6 hours prn
Terbutaline (Brethine)	Subcutaneous (1 mg/ml)	0.25 mg (rep × 1 after 15-30 minutes; maximum 0.5 mg in 4 hours)	0.01 mg/kg, up to 0.25 mg (may rep × 1 after 15-30 minutes)
	Tablets	2.5-5 mg tid	1.25-2.5 mg tid
(Brethaire)	metered dose inhaler (200 μg/puff)	2-3 puffs every 4-6 hours prn	2-3 puffs every 4-6 hours prn
Theophylline	Extended release capsules or tablets (Theo-Dur, others)	300-600 mg/day	Less than 1 yr: mg/kg/day = (0.2) (age, weeks) + 5 1-9 years: 12-20 mg/kg/day 10-12 years: 12-18 mg/kg/day 13-16 years: 12-16 mg/kg/day

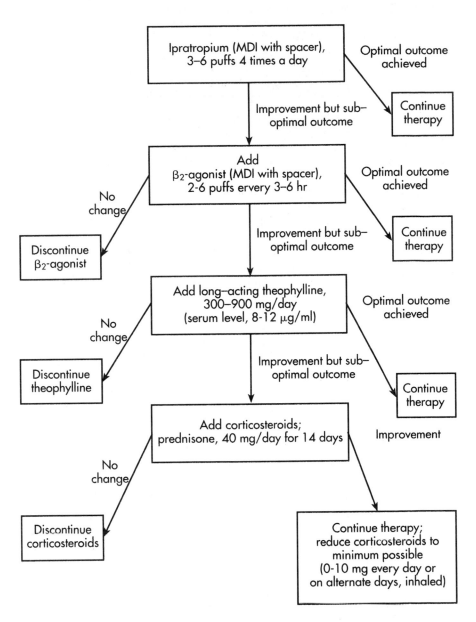

FIG 8-9.
Typical regimen for treating COPD. (From Ferguson, Cherniack: Current concepts, *N Engl J Med* 328(14):1019, 1993.)

TABLE 8-12.—INDICATIONS FOR ANTIINFLAMMATORY THERAPY IN ASTHMA MANAGEMENT

β-agonists are used >2 times/week
Exacerbations >1 or 2 times/week
Nocturnal awakenings >2 times/month
Activities are limited by asthma
Abnormal pulmonary function tests

TABLE 8-13.—RECOMMENDED DOSING SCHEDULE OF TRANSDERMAL NICOTINE FOR HEALTHY PATIENTS

	DURATION	
DOSE	PER STRENGTH OF PATCH	ENTIRE COURSE OF THERAPY
Habitrol[1]		
21 mg/day	First 6 weeks	
14 mg/day	Next 2 weeks[2]	8 to 12 weeks
7 mg/day	Last 2 weeks[3]	
Nicoderm[1]		
21 mg/day	First 6 weeks	
14 mg/day	Next 2 weeks[2]	8 to 12 weeks
7 mg/day	Last 2 weeks	
Nicotrol		
15 mg/day	First 12 weeks	
10 mg/day	Next 2 weeks[2]	14 to 20 weeks
5 mg/day	Last 2 weeks	
Prostep[3]		
22 mg/day	4 to 8 weeks	6 to 12 weeks
11 mg/day[4]	2 to 4 weeks	

From Facts and Comparisons, March 1993.
[1]Start with 14 mg/day for 6 weeks for patients who have cardiovascular disease, weigh <100 lb, or smoke < a half a pack of cigarettes a day. Decrease dose to 7 mg/day for the final 2 to 4 weeks.
[2]Patients who have successfully abstained from smoking should have their dose reduced after each 2 to 4 weeks of treatment until the 7 mg/day dose *(Habitrol; Nicoderm)* or 5 mg/day dose *(Nicotrol)* has been used for 2 to 4 weeks.
[3]Start with 22 mg/day except for patients who weigh <100 lb; they may start with 11 mg/day with the dose increased as appropriate.
[4]Optional weaning dose.

TABLE 8-14.—Pulmonary Function in Patients with Asthma, Chronic Bronchitis, and Emphysema

TEST*	ASTHMA†	CHRONIC SEVERE BRONCHITIS	EMPHYSEMA
Vital capacity	Decreased	Decreased	Normal or decreased
Residual volume	Increased	Increased	Increased
Total lung capacity	Normal	Normal	Increased
RV/TLC	Increased	Increased	Increased
FEV_1/FVC	Decreased	Decreased	Decreased
MMFR	Decreased	Decreased	Decreased
Single-breath O_2	Increased	Increased	Increased
Diffusing capacity	Normal or slightly increased	Normal	Decreased
Response to bronchodilators	Improvement	No change	No change
Arterial P_{O_2}	Decreased	Decreased	Slight decrease
Arterial P_{CO_2}	Decreased	Increased	Normal
Hematocrit	Normal	Increased	Normal

Modified from Hinshaw HC, Murray JF: *Diseases of the chest,* Philadelphia, 1980, WB Saunders, p. 94.
*RV/TLC, Residual volume to total lung capacity ratio; FEV_1/FVC, forced expiratory volume in 1 second to forced vital capacity ratio; MMFR, maximal midexpiratory flow rate.
†During an attack; values should approach or be normal when properly treated.

RESPIRATORY FAILURE, ARDS, AND VENTILATORS

Respiratory failure is the sudden reduction in oxygen tension to less than 50 mm Hg.

TABLE 8-15.—Principles of Management of Respiratory Failure

1. If patient is apneic or nearly apneic, intubate immediately.
2. Consider narcotic as a cause and give 0.4 mg of naloxone IV, IM, or SQ (0.01 mg/kg in children).
3. Measure blood gases and begin 24% oxygen.
4. Attempt to maintain P_{O_2} at about 50 mm Hg if patient has physical signs of COPD.
5. If pH is less than 7.20, give 44 mEq (1 ampule) sodium bicarbonate. Measure blood gases again, check electrolytes, and calculate anion gap.
6. Intubate and ventilate the patient if:
a. Patient cannot be adequately oxygenated without increasing CO_2 retention and acidosis.
b. There are respiratory depressant drugs "on board" or there is mechanical interference with chest wall function.
7. Look aggressively for the cause of the decompensation (CHF, pneumonia, pneumothorax).
8. Use bronchodilators to improve ventilation.
9. Give frequent chest physical therapy, even if patient is being mechanically ventilated.

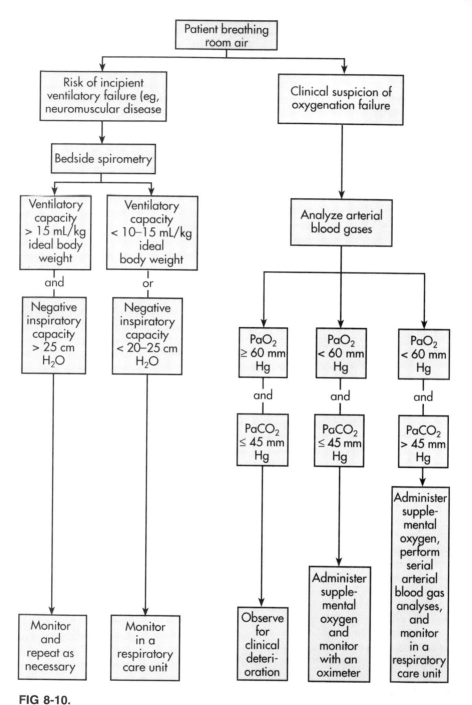

FIG 8-10.
Diagnostic algorithm for respiratory failure. (From Bukowski DM, Peters JI: Acute respiratory failure: diagnosis and management, *Hosp Med* 30:52, 1994.)

TABLE 8-16.—DEVICES FOR OXYGEN DELIVERY

DEVICE	FLOW (L/MIN)	RANGE (% Fio_2)
Nasal cannula	1-2	23-28
	3-4	28-38
	5-6	32-45
	Advantages:	*Disadvantages:*
	Inexpensive	Poor humidification
	Comfortable	Drying of mucosa
	Allows eating and exercise	Uncertain Fio_2
		Limited maximum Fio_2
Simple mask	3-4	25-30
	5-6	30-45
	7-8	40-60
	Advantages:	*Disadvantages:*
	Inexpensive	Bothersome
	Higher maximum Fio_2	Possible CO_2 collection
		Requires tight seal
Nonrebreathing mask	8	70-100
	Advantages:	*Disadvantages:*
	Useful for severely hypoxemic, normocapnic patients	Bothersome
		Requires tight seal
		Not tolerated for long
Rebreathing mask	8	50-60
	Advantages:	*Disadvantages:*
	Useful for hypoxemic, hypocapnic patients	Possible hypercapnia
		Bothersome
		Requires tight seal
Face tent or aerosol mask	8	30-100
	Advantages:	*Disadvantages:*
	Versatile	Requires frequent drainage of tubing and filling reservoir
	High humidity	Contamination with gram-negative bacteria
	Good CO_2 washout	Noisy
Venturi mask	4	24
	4	28
	6	31
	8	35
	8	40
	Advantages:	*Disadvantages:*
	Comfortable, cool	More expensive
	Accurate air flow	Not tolerated for long

TABLE 8-17.—INDICATIONS FOR HOME OXYGEN THERAPY

1. Documentation of persistent Po_2 < 55 mm Hg or
2. Presence of Po_2 between 55 and 59 mm Hg accompanied by one or more of the following:
   Cor pulmonale
   Evidence of pulmonary hypertension on physical examination, chest x-ray film, or ECG
   Hematocrit >55%
   Decreased mental function, improved by O_2 trial
   Markedly decreased exercise tolerance, improved by O_2 trial (requires documentation of worsening oxygenation after exercise)

TABLE 8-18.—CHECKLIST FOR PATIENTS USING A VENTILATOR

1. Use ≥7.5-mm tube for adults with a high compliance cuff.
2. Keep the cuff pressure <30 mm Hg.
3. Check the tube position with a portable chest x-ray film.
4. Keep the tidal volume at 10-13 ml/kg body weight.
5. Set the rate initially at a minute ventilation of 5-10 L (12-16 breaths/min), but adjust to keep blood gases optimal.
6. Set initial mode at assist/control.
7. Set sensitivity so that patient will trigger an inspiration at about −2 or −3 cm H_2O inspiratory force.
8. Select a flow rate that provides an inspiratory/expiratory flow of about 1:3 (usually about 40-60 L/min).
9. Set alarm at about 10 cm H_2O above pressure required to deliver the selected tidal volume, keep in continuous use, and check daily.
10. Set initial O_2 concentration at 100%, and adjust to keep arterial blood gases at about this level: Po_2 60-90 mm Hg; pH 7.35-7.50. NOTE: Ear oximetry, when calibrated against arterial blood gases, is adequate for monitoring oxygen saturation, provided there is no need to know $Paco_2$ or pH.
11. If inadequate oxygenation persists despite 100% O_2, add positive endexpiratory pressure (PEEP). Start with 4 cm H_2O and add increments of 2-4 cm H_2O every 15-30 minutes, monitoring blood gases before each change. Also consider PEEP if a Pao_2 ≥ 50 mm Hg cannot be maintained with an inspired O_2 concentration of ≤ 50%.
12. Monitor vital signs frequently, and look for a cause for sudden tachycardia or low blood pressure.
13. Continuously monitor cardiac rhythm.
14. Frequently monitor mentation and urine output.

Modified from Mitchell RL: *Synopsis of clinical pulmonary disease,* ed 2. St. Louis, 1978, Mosby; Popovich J: *Postgrad Med* 79:217, 1986.

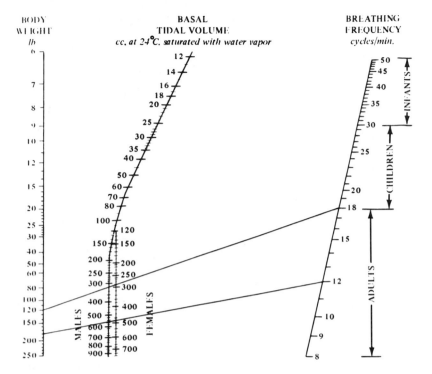

FIG 8-11.

Nomogram for predicting normal tidal volumes at different rates of breathing according to body weight. The values given represent minimum values in most clinical situations below which underventilation can be considered to have occurred. A spirometer or ventilation meter is necessary for the application of this nomogram. Correction of these values can be made in the following manner: Add 10% for daily activity and eating; add 5% for each degree of fever (° F) above rectal normal, 99° F, and 5% for each 2000 feet of residence above sea level. (From Crews ER, Lapuerta L: *A manual of respiratory failure*, Springfield, Ill, Charles C Thomas, p. 79.)

TABLE 8-19.—WEANING PATIENTS FROM VENTILATORS

---

1. Make sure alveolar-arterial oxygen tension difference on 100% O_2 is less than 300-350 mm Hg.
2. Make sure vital capacity is 10-15 ml/kg body weight.
3. Maximum inspiratory force should be >-20 ml H_2O.
4. Ratio of dead space to tidal volume (VD/VT) should be <0.6 for "difficult to wean" patients.
5. Place patient in a sitting position.
6. Reduce Fio_2 to 25%-30%.
7. Reduce tidal volume to about 500 ml.
8. Place ventilator on assist.
9. Take patient off all respiratory depressant drugs.
10. Ensure that patient has FVC 2 to 3 times normal tidal volume (about 1000 ml).
11. Try off ventilator for 15 minutes with O_2 increased by 5%-10% over baseline.
12. If Po_2 remains above 50 mm Hg and pH is above 7.25, keep off ventilator for 15 minutes of every hour. Otherwise, postpone weaning.
13. Check blood gases regularly.
14. Place back on ventilator for sleeping, first night.
15. Next day increase time off ventilator to 30 minutes per hour until morning of third day.
16. Third day allow off ventilator for 45 minutes every hour.
17. Increase time off to 1¾ hours off, 15 minutes on.
18. If tolerated, consider extubation at this point.
19. Administer IPPB treatment every 4-6 hours and continue to monitor blood gases and clinical status closely. Monitor vital signs every 5-10 minutes in first hour, then every 15-20 minutes; blood gases about every hour.

NOTE: Intermittent mandatory ventilation is an alternative weaning procedure that allows a gradual decrease in the number of ventilator-delivered breaths per minute. The criteria and monitoring are otherwise the same as for the traditional approach.

Modified from Berte JB: *Pulmonary emergencies,* Philadelphia, 1977, JB Lippincott, p. 86; Feely TW, Hedley-Whyte J: *N Engl J Med* 292:903, 1975.

LUNG TUMORS AND PULMONARY NODULES

TABLE 8-20.—CONTRAINDICATIONS TO RESECTIONAL SURGERY IN PATIENTS WITH LUNG CANCER

Absolute Contraindications
1. Extrathoracic metastases
2. Involvement of the trachea, carina, or proximal mainstem bronchus
3. Obstruction of the superior vena cava
4. Involvement of the recurrent laryngeal nerve
5. Malignant effusion
6. Positive mediastinoscopy; positive contralateral nodes
7. Phrenic nerve, pericardial, or esophageal involvement
8. Undifferentiated small cell (oat cell)
9. Inadequate pulmonary function to tolerate surgery

Relative Contraindications
1. Age 70 or older
2. Local chest wall involvement
3. Pancoast's tumor
4. Positive mediastinoscopy; ipsilateral nodes
5. Pleural effusion with negative cytology

TABLE 8-21.—THE SOLITARY PULMONARY NODULE

Lesion more Likely Benign if:
Previous x-ray examination documents no growth
It is totally calcified
It has target, "popcorn," or lamellated calcification (suggests inflammatory lesion)
It is small (<1.5 cm)
It is near an interlobular fissure (characteristic of granuloma)

Lesion more Likely Malignant if:
It has grown in the past year
It has no calcification (or only a "fleck")
It has spicular radiations at the peripheral edge
It has a lobular appearance
It is in the center of a lobule
It is a large lesion

TABLE 8-22.—INITIAL APPROACH TO EVALUATING HEMOPTYSIS

1. Determine whether sputum is blood-streaked or whether gross blood is present
2. Look at a Gram stain
3. Obtain a chest x-ray radiograph
4. Apply a tuberculin test
5. Obtain sputum cytology
6. Further testing or referral, depending on results of above

TABLE 8-23.—DIFFERENTIAL DIAGNOSIS OF HEMOPTYSIS*

GROSS HEMOPTYSIS	BLOOD-STREAKED SPUTUM
Tuberculosis	Upper respiratory tract infection
Bronchiectasis	Chronic bronchitis
Bronchial adenoma	Sarcoidosis
Bronchogenic carcinoma	Bronchogenic carcinoma
Aspergilloma	Tuberculosis
Necrotizing pneumonia	Pulmonary infarction
Lung abscess	Pulmonary edema
Pulmonary contusion	Mitral stenosis
Arteriovenous malformation	Idiopathic pulmonary hemosiderosis
Bleeding disorder or excessive anti-coagulant therapy	
Mitral stenosis	

*Modified from Goroll AH, May LA, Mulley AG: *Primary care medicine,* Philadelphia, 1981, JB Lippincott.

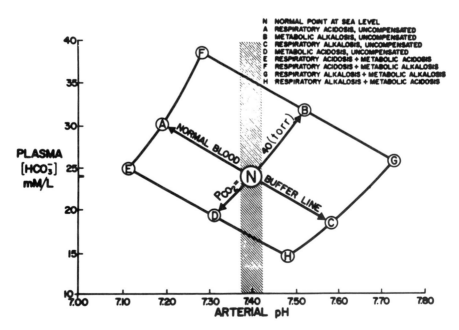

FIG 8-12.
Curve for acidosis and alkalosis. (From Davenport: *The ABC of acid-base chemistry,* ed 4, The University of Chicago Press.

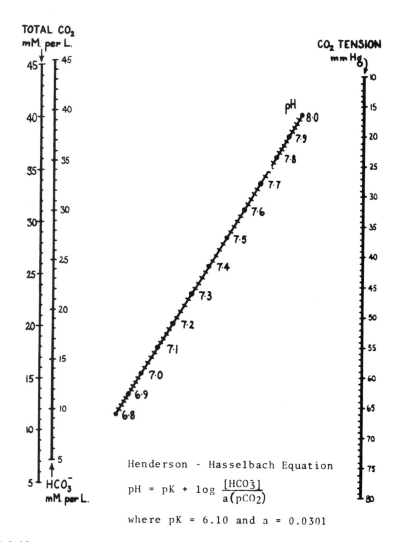

TOTAL CO$_2$
mM. per L.

CO$_2$ TENSION
mm Hg

pH

Henderson - Hasselbach Equation

$$pH = pK + \log \frac{[HCO_3^-]}{a(pCO_2)}$$

where pK = 6.10 and a = 0.0301

FIG 8-13.
Henderson-Hasselbalch equation: acid-base nomogram. (From Biller JA, Yeager AM: *The Harriet Lane handbook,* ed 9, Chicago, 1981, Mosby, p. 256.)

TABLE 8-24.—Acid-Base Balance

ANION GAP = $(Na^+ + K^+) - (Cl^- + HCO_3^- + Prot^-, Phos^-, Sulfate^-)$
Normally this value should not exceed 12 mmol/L. If it does, consider the following:
  Renal failure
  Diabetic ketoacidosis
  Alcoholic ketoacidosis
  Lactic acidosis
  Salicylate poisoning
  Ethylene glycol poisoning
  Methyl alcohol poisoning
(NOTE: $Prot^-$, $Phos^-$, $Sulfate^-$ is estimated by a constant = 20 mEq/L)

Modified from Levinsky N: Acidosis and alkalosis. In Isselbacher K, et al, eds: *Harrison's principles of internal medicine*, ed 11, New York, 1980, McGraw-Hill.

TABLE 8-25.—Calculation of Anion Gap

	POSITIVE CHARGES (MEQ/L)		NEGATIVE CHARGES (MEQ/L)		ANION GAP
Normal	Na^+	140	Cl^-	100	
	K^+	5	HCO_3^-	25	145 − 145 = 0 mEq/L
			$Protein^-$, phosphate$^-$,		
	Positive charges	145	and sulfate$^-$	20	
			Negative charges	145	
Organic (lactic acidosis)	Na^+	140	Cl^-	95	
	K^+	5	HCO_3^-	10	145 − 125 = 20 mEq/L
			$Protein^-$, phosphate$^-$,		
	Positive charges	145	and sulfate$^-$	20	
			Negative charges	125	

From Robin EG: Respiratory medicine. In Rubenstein E, Federman D, eds: *Scientific american medicine*, New York, 1984, Scientific American Co, vol 2, Chap 14, pp. 1-10.

INTERSTITIAL LUNG DISEASE

TABLE 8-26.—DRUGS THAT CAUSE INTERSTITIAL LUNG DISEASE*

Acute Infiltrations	Chronic Infiltrations
WITH EOSINOPHILIA	DIFFUSE INTERSTITIAL FIBROSIS
Aurothioglucose (Solganal)	*Bleomycin*
Chlorpropamide (Diabinese)	*Busulfan (Myleran)*
Disodium cromoglycate (Cromolyn)	Carmustine (BiCNU)
Imipramine (Tofranil)	*Cyclophosphamide (Cytoxan)*
Isoniazid	Gold sodium thiomalate (Myochrysine)
Mephenesin carbamate	Hexamethonium
Methotrexate	Mecamylamine (Inversine)
Nitrofurantoin (Furadantin)	Melphalan (Alkeran)
Paraaminosalicylic acid	Methysergide (Sansert)
Penicillin	*Nitrofurantoin (Furadantin)*
Pituitary snuff	*Oxygen*
Sulfonamides	Pentolinium tartrate (Ansolysen)
WITHOUT EOSINOPHILIA	Pituitary snuff
Amitriptyline (Elavil)	*Radiation*
Azathioprine (Imuran)	WITH LUPUS ERYTHEMATOSUS-LIKE
Procarbazine (Matulane)	SYNDROME
	Digitalis
	Gold salts
	Griseofulvin
	Hydantoin (Dilantin)
	Hydralazine (Apresoline)
	Isoniazid
	Mephenytoin (Mesantoin)
	Methyldopa (Aldomet)
	Methylthiouracil
	Oral contraceptives
	Penicillin
	Phenylbutazone (Butazolidin)
	Procainamide (Pronestyl)
	Propylthiouracil
	Reserpine
	Streptomycin
	Sulfonamides
	Tetracyclines
	Thiazides

From Hinshaw HC, Murray JF: *Diseases of the chest,* Philadelphia, 1980, WB Saunders, p. 573.

*Those indicated in italics are of particular clinical importance; the others are rarely encountered.

TABLE 8-27.—Chest Radiographic Findings of the Interstitial Lung Diseases

Pleural Disease
Lymphangitic carcinomatosis
Lymphangiolieomyomatosis
  Chylous pleural effusion
Drug induced: Nitrofurantoin
Sarcoidosis
Radiation pneumonitis
Asbestosis: effusion, pleural thickening, calcified pleural plaques, mesothelioma
Collagen vascular disease (excluding polymyositis)

Hilar or Mediastinal Lymphadenopathy
Common: sarcoidosis, lymphoma, lymphangitic carcinomatosis
Uncommon: lymphocytic interstitial pneumonia, amyloidosis, Gaucher's disease, berylliosis

Hilar Nodal Eggshell Calcification
Silicosis
Sarcoidosis

Kerley B Lines
Chronic left ventricular failure
Lymphangitic carcinomatosis
Lymphoma
Lymphangiolieomyomatosis
Pulmonary veno-occlusive disease

Pneumothorax
Eosinophilic granuloma
Lymphangiolieomyomatosis
Tuberous sclerosis
Neurofibromatosis

Increased Lung Volumes
Lymphangiolieomyomatosis
Tuberous sclerosis
Sarcoidosis (type 3)
Eosinophilic granuloma (chronic)
Neurofibromatosis
Chronic hypersensitivitiy pneumonitis
Interstitial lung disease superimposed upon COPD

Subcutaneous Calcinosis
Scleroderma
Polymyositis-dermatomyositis

From Schwarz MI: *Clinical overview of interstitial lung disease.* In MI Schwarz and TE King, eds: *Interstitital lung disease,* 1993, Mosby.

CHEST X-RAY FILMS

TABLE 8-28.—Short Guide to Reading Chest X-ray Films

1. Check exposure technique for lightness or darkness.
2. Verify left and right by looking at stomach bubble and heart shape.
3. Check for rotation: Does the thoracic spine shadow align in the center of the sternum between the clavicles?
4. Make sure the x-ray is taken in full inspiration (10 posterior or 6 anterior ribs should be visible).
5. Is the film a portable, anteroposterior, or posteroanterior film? (The heart size cannot be accurately judged from an AP film.)
6. Check the soft tissues for foreign bodies or subcutaneous emphysema.
7. Check all visible bones and joints for osteoporosis, old fractures, metastatic lesions, rib notching, or presence of cervical ribs.
8. Look at diaphragm for tenting, free air, and position.
9. Check hilar and mediastinal areas for the following: size and shape of aorta, presence of hilar nodes, prominence of hilar blood vessels, elevation of vessels (left normally slightly higher)
10. Look at heart for size, shape, calcified valves, and enlarged atria.
11. Check costophrenic angles for fluid or pleural scarring.
12. Check pulmonary parenchyma for infiltrates, increased interstitial markings, masses, absence of normal margins, air bronchograms, or increased vascularity, and "silhouette" signs.
13. Look at lateral film for the following: confirmation and position of questionable masses or infiltrates, size of retrosternal air space, anteroposterior chest diameter, vertebral bodies for bony lesions or overlying infiltrates, posterior costophrenic angle for small effusion

PLEURAL EFFUSIONS

TABLE 8-29.—PLEURAL FLUID TRANSUDATES AND EXUDATES

CHARACTER OF PLEURAL EFFUSION	RELATED DISORDERS
Transudate	
Protein less than 2.5 g/dl	Cardiac, renal, or hepatic failure
Clear, yellow; specific gravity less than 1.016	Myxedema (protein content increased)
	Severe anemia
Fluid/serum protein ratio < 0.5	Nephrotic state
Fluid/serum LDH ratio < 0.6	Hypoproteinemic states
Fluid LDH $< 2/3$ upper limit of nl for serum LDH	Pancreatic disease
	Liver disease (cirrhosis)
	Meig's tumor
	Superior vena cava obstruction
Exudate	
Protein greater than 3 g/dl	Bacterial infections
Cloudy; specific gravity greater than 1.016	Viral infections
	Tuberculosis
At least one of the following:	Thoracic neoplasms
Fluid/serum protein ratio > 0.5	Rheumatic fever
Fluid/serum LDH ratio > 0.6	Septicemia
Fluid LDH $> 2/3$ upper limit of nl for serum LDH	Postmyocardial infarction
	Infectious mononucleosis
	Pulmonary infarct
	Rheumatoid arthritis
	SLE (lupus erythematosus, systemic)
Increased Eosinophils	
	Hydatid cyst
	Löffler's syndrome
	Tropical eosinophilia
	Polyarteritis nodosa
	Hodgkin's disease
	Carcinoma
	Pulmonary infarct
Decreased Pleural Glucose	
	SLE
	TBC (tuberculosis)
(as low as 6 mg/dl)	RA (rheumatoid arthritis)

Modified from Berte JB: *Pulmonary emergencies,* New York, 1977, JB Lippincott, p. 149; Sahn SA: *Hosp Med* 24(8):77, 1988.

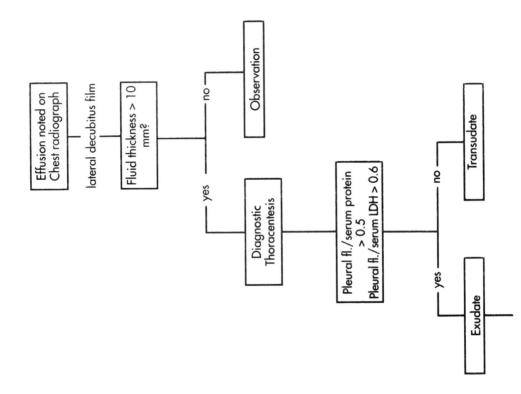

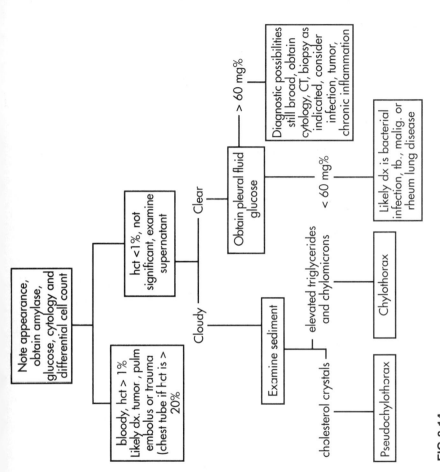

FIG 8-14.
Evaluation of patient with pleural effusion.

COMMON PULMONARY DIAGNOSTIC PROCEDURES

TABLE 8-30.—THORACENTESIS

Materials
Antiseptic solution and swabs
Sterile field
Small and large syringes
25-gauge needle and 1% Xylocaine
15- to 18-gauge needle
Three-way stopcock
Sterile specimen containers

Procedure
1. Determine puncture site by x-ray examination and percussion.
2. Entry site should be directly above the rib (nerve and vessels are under the rib surface).
3. Raise a skin wheal and inject 1-2 ml along the rib periosteum.
4. Inject 3-5 ml near the pleural surface.
5. Use a large syringe and needle with three-way stopcock and draw off fluid as needed. An intracath or angiocath can be used to minimize the risk of lung puncture.
6. When attempting to draw all the fluid off, stop when aspiration begins to block further drainage (the pleura is being drawn into the end of the needle at this point).
7. Send fluid for all needed studies. Routinely these should include cell count and differential, protein, glucose, LDH, routine culture, Gram stain, and specific gravity. If indicated, include cytology, AFB, and fungal cultures.
8. A posttap chest x-ray film should be obtained to rule out traumatic pneumothorax.

Modified from Fishman NH: *Thoracic drainage: a manual of procedures,* Chicago, 1983, Mosby, pp. 27-32.

TABLE 8-31.—Placement of Chest Tube

Materials
Applicators for antiseptic
Antiseptic (Iodophor)
Sterile gloves
Lidocaine, 1% without epinephrine
Syringes, 10 ml and 30 ml
Needles: ½-inch, 25-gauge; 1½-inch, 22-gauge
Scalpel with no. 11 and no. 15 blades
Suture, 2-0 silk or synthetic with cutting skin needle
Hemostats, one sharp pointed "mosquito," one Kelly or Mayo clamp
Scissors, preferably pointed
Connectors, two "five-in-one" double-tapered
Test tubes for laboratory specimens
Dressings, four 4 × 4 inches
Chest tubes (usually kept separately): 12 F Trocarcath; 20 or 36 F multifenes-
   trated vinyl tube
Suction/underwater seal apparatus, (e.g., Pleurevac [kept separately])
Tubing, to connect apparatus to vacuum source

Procedure (See Corresponding Letters in Fig. 8-14)
 1. Prepare patient in the appropriate area.
 2. Anesthetize skin, periosteum, and pleura as for thoracentesis. Insert needle
    and aspirate to confirm presence of air or fluid *(A)*.
 3. Make a 1-1½-inch transverse incision just above the rib in the appropriate
    interspace. The incision should be carried through the dermis *(B)*.
 4. Work a closed Kelly clamp through the subcutaneous tissue, intercostal
    muscles, and into the pleural space. Turn the clamp with a "screwlike" mo-
    tion, but maintain control of the clamp. Entering the pleura may require ad-
    ditional pressure and will probably be accompanied by a sudden "popping"
    into the space *(C)*.
 5. Enlarge the opening in the chest wall and pleura by spreading the clamp in
    several different planes.
 6. Insert a 12 F trocar along same path. After the tube is through the pleura,
    withdraw stylet a few mm *(D)*, *(E)*.
 7. Insert the tube into the opening and advance until it is suitably placed
    within the pleural space, withdrawing stylet as you go *(F)*. Clamp the tube
    to avoid entry of air into the chest.
 8. Attach the tubing to the bottle with an underwater seal.
 9. Secure the chest tube to the chest wall with a skin suture *(inset)*.
10. Further secure and protect the tube by taping.

Modified from Fishman NH: *Thoracic drainage: a manual of procedures,* Chicago, 1983,
Mosby, pp. 32-37.

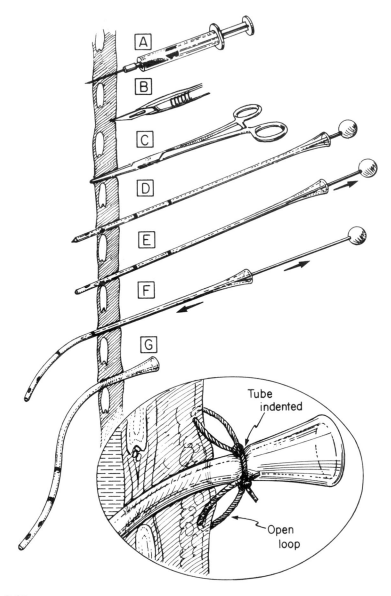

FIG 8-15.
Technique of chest tube placement (see text). (From Fishman NH: *Thoracic drainage: a manual of procedures,* Chicago, 1983, Mosby, p. 34.)

TABLE 8-32.—Making and Interpreting Gram Stains

Materials
Gram's iodine
Crystal violet
Acetone or 95% ethyl alcohol
Safranin

Procedure
1. Spread sputum in thin layer over slide. Use another slide to obtain good uniformity. Do not use cotton swab.
2. Fix slide with match, burner, or by placing in incubator for 3-5 minutes.
3. Flood slide with crystal violet for 15-30 seconds, and rinse with tap water.
4. Flood slide with Gram's iodine for 15-30 seconds, and rinse with tap water.
5. Decolorize with acetone or alcohol by rinsing just until the blue color disappears.
6. Counterstain for 15 seconds with safranin.
7. Dry by leaving in open air, placing in incubator, or by carefully blotting with soft, absorbent paper.

Tips on Interpretation
1. Obtain the sputum yourself if you feel it is important to have accurate information.
2. Check for the presence of epithelial cells, and, if large numbers are present, obtain another specimen. The one you have is not sputum, it is saliva.
3. If there are five or more polymorphonuclear cells per high power field, it is probably an infectious or inflammatory process.
4. There will almost always be various kinds of organisms on the slide; look for the predominant one.
5. Look especially for intracellular organisms. They are a certain indicator of the infecting process.
6. Even if the slide is not technically ideal, look for an interpretable area (e.g., not overdecolorized, few or no epithelial cells, numerous polys).

TABLE 8-33.—Arterial Puncture

Materials
10-ml glass syringe
Heparin 1:1000 dilution
22- to 25-gauge needle
Rubber stopper or other occlusive device for needle
Ice

Procedure
1. Line the glass syringe with heparin by aspirating 1 ml, pumping the plunger twice, and squirting out all but what remains in the hub and the needle.
2. Palpate the pulse with two or three fingers to "map" the course of the vessel.
3. Prepare the area with an alcohol swab.
4. Insert the needle at about 90 degrees (45 degrees for radial samples).
5. A short, quick, downward motion will be more likely to enter the artery. The depth of insertion depends on the site of the puncture (2 cm for brachial and 3-4 cm for femoral punctures).
6. Allow the arterial pressure to fill the syringe to about 3 ml volume.
7. If the first insertion is not successful, gently and slowly withdraw the needle, since the artery may have been overshot on the way in.
8. If still unsuccessful, repalpate pulse, redirect needle, and reinsert.
9. Do not aspirate except as a last resort. If aspiration is necessary to get the specimen, it is much more likely to contain venous blood.
10. Place pressure over the puncture with a dry gauze pad for at least 5 minutes.
11. Occlude the needle, and transport the specimen to the lab in ice.

9 *The Gastrointestinal Tract*

Charles W. Smith, Jr.

REFLUX ESOPHAGITIS

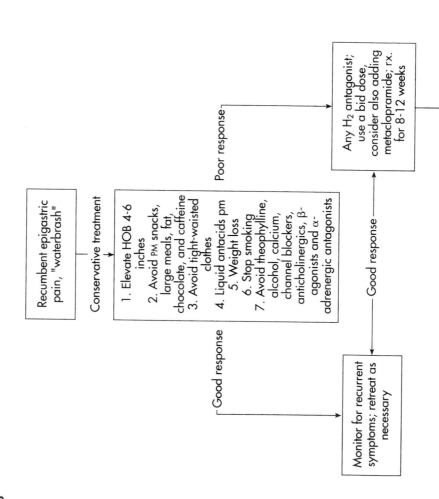

Recumbent epigastric pain, "waterbrash"

Conservative treatment

1. Elevate HOB 4-6 inches
2. Avoid PM snacks, large meals, fat, chocolate, and caffeine
3. Avoid tight-waisted clothes
4. Liquid antacids pm
5. Weight loss
6. Stop smoking
7. Avoid theophylline, alcohol, calcium, channel blockers, anticholinergics, β-agonists and α-adrenergic antagonists

Poor response

Good response

Any H_2 antagonist; use a bid dose, consider also adding metaclopramide; rx. for 8-12 weeks

Good response

Monitor for recurrent symptoms; retreat as necessary

348

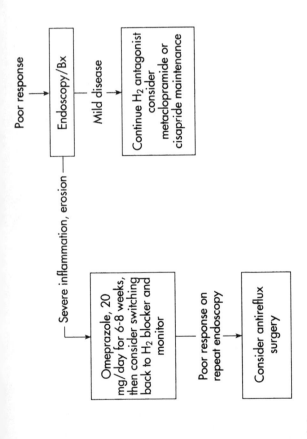

FIG 9-1.

Gastroesophageal reflux disease. (From Feldman M, Maton PN, McCallum RW, McCarthy DM: Treating ulcers and reflux: what's new? *Patient care,* 53, 1994.)

PEPTIC ULCER DISEASE

TABLE 9-1.—Differential Features of Peptic Ulcer*

TYPE OF LESION	INCIDENCE	PATHOPHYSIOLOGY	CLINICAL FEATURES	COURSE
Duodenal ulcer	M:F ratio, 3:1 Peak incidence, fifth and sixth decades Prevalence, 10%–12%	Normal to increased parietal cell mass Normal to increased gastric acid secretion Normal to mildly elevated circulating gastrin levels Excessive gastrin response to meals, excessive parietal cell sensitivity Genetic factors: familial tendency, frequent blood group O, nonsecretor Positive associations: chronic obstructive pulmonary disease, hepatic cirrhosis, pancreatic insufficiency, hyperparathyroidism Located in duodenal bulb, pyloric channel, postbulbar area *H. Pylori* infection in 95%–100% of patients Ingestion of NSAIDs	Pain: rhythmic, periodic, chronic Pain-food-relief-pain pattern	Remissions and exacerbations for 10-25 years after onset. "Once an ulcer, always an ulcer", seasonal trend (spring and fall)

| Gastric ulcer | M:F ratio, 3-4:1
Peak incidence, sixth and seventh decades
Duodenal ulcer: gastric ulcer, 4:1 | Normal to decreased parietal cell mass
Normal to decreased gastric acid secretion (not achlorhydria)
Normal to elevated circulating gastrin level
Presence of gastritis
Abnormal gastric mucosal barrier
Abnormal pyloric function, bile reflux
Ulcerogenic drugs
H. Pylori infection in 70%-90% of patients | Pain-food-relief-pain pattern, or food-pain pattern
Weight loss, anorexia | Remissions and exacerbations less than in duodenal ulcer: high recurrence rate: no seasonal trend |
| Gastric erosions or stress ulcer | No sex difference
Related to severe stress, sepsis, burns, trauma, head injuries | Head injuries; marked gastric acid hypersecretion
Others: gastric mucosal ischemia, acid back-diffusion, acute gastritis | Bleeding frequent in recognized cases; may be severe, persistent (actual frequency unknown) | Half of those who bleed require surgery |

*Modified from Greenberger NJ: *Gastrointestinal disorders,* ed 2, Chicago, 1981, Mosby, p. 72.

TABLE 9-2.—COMPARISON OF H$_2$-RECEPTOR ANTAGONISTS

	CIMETIDINE (TAGAMET, GENERIC)	RANITIDINE (ZANTAC)	NIZATIDINE (AXID)	FAMOTIDINE (PEPCID)
Drug interactions	++++	+	±	±
Adverse reactions	++	+	+	+
Dosage for duodenal ulcer*	300 mg qid or 400 mg bid or 800 mg hs	150 mg bid or 300 mg hs	150 mg bid or 300 mg hs	40 mg hs
Maintenance dosage*	400 mg hs	150 mg hs	150 mg hs	20 mg hs
Dosage for gastric ulcer*	300 mg qid or 400 mg bid or 800 mg hs	150 mg bid	150 mg bid or 300 mg hs	40 mg hs
Dosage for gastroesophageal reflux*	400 mg qid or 800 mg bid	150 mg bid	150 mg bid	20 mg bid
Cost†	$96‡	$115	$113	$112

*Dosage must be reduced with renal insufficiency. See product labeling.
†Cost based on Average Wholesale Price (AWP 1993 Redbook) for a 6-week course using the bedtime dose for duodenal ulcer.
‡Less expensive generic preparations are now available.

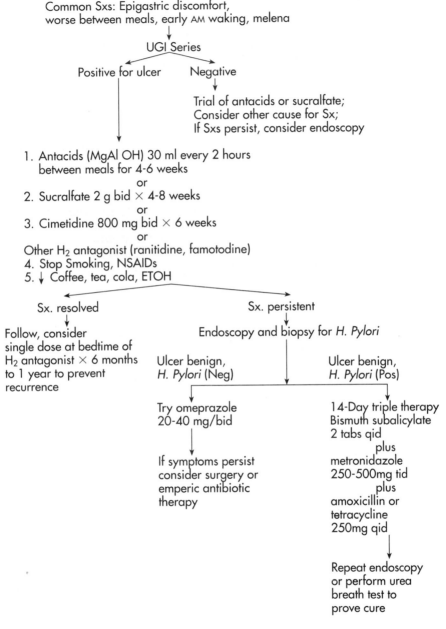

FIG 9-2.
Evaluation and treatment of peptic ulcer disease.

UPPER AND LOWER GI BLEEDING

TABLE 9-3.—Sources of Gastrointestinal Tract Bleeding

CATEGORY	UPPER GI TRACT	LOWER GI TRACT
Inflammatory	Peptic ulcer*	Ulcerative colitis*
	Esophagitis*	Crohn's disease*
	Gastritis*	Diverticulitis
	Stress ulcer	Enterocolitis; tuberculosis bac-
	Pancreatitis	terial, toxic, radiation
Mechanical	Hiatal hernia	Diverticulosis*
	Mallory-Weiss syndrome*	Anal fissure*
	Hematobilia	
Vascular	Esophageal or gastric varices*	Hemorrhoids*
	Mesenteric vascular occlusion	Mesenteric vascular occlusion
	Aortoduodenal fistula	Aortointestinal fistula
	Malformations: hemangioma,	Aortic aneurysm
	Osler-Weber-Rendu dis-	Malformations: hemangioma,
	ease, blue nevus bleb	Osler-Weber-Rendu dis-
		ease, blue nevus bleb, an-
		giodysplasia
Neoplastic	Carcinoma	Carcinoma*
	Polyps; single, multiple, Peutz-	Polyps*; adenomatous and
	Jeghers syndrome	villous, familial polyposis,
	Leiomyoma	Peutz-Jeghers syndrome
	Carcinoid	Leiomyoma
	Leukemia	Carcinoid
	Sarcoma	Leukemia
	Metastatic (e.g., melanoma)	Sarcoma
		Metastatic (e.g., melanoma)
Systemic	Blood dyscrasias and clotting	Blood dyscrasias and clotting
	abnormalities	abnormalities
	Collagen diseases	Collagen diseases
	Uremia	Uremia
Anomalies	Gastric and duodenal diver-	Meckel's diverticulum
	ticula	

Modified from Greenberger NJ, Norton J: *Gastrointestinal disorders,* ed 2, Chicago, 1981, Mosby.
*Most common disorders.

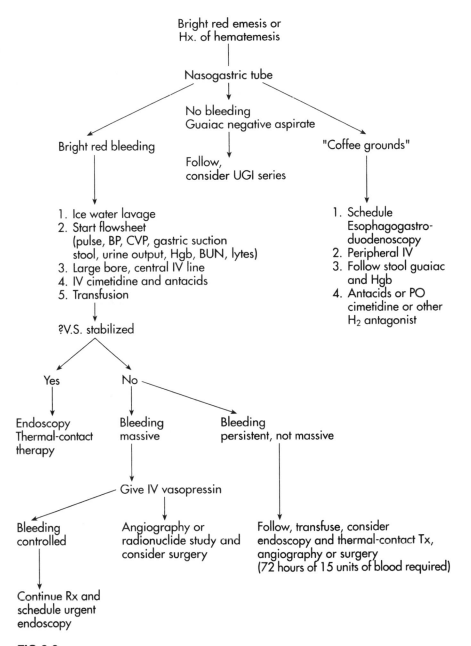

FIG 9-3.
Evaluation and treatment of upper gastrointestinal tract bleeding.

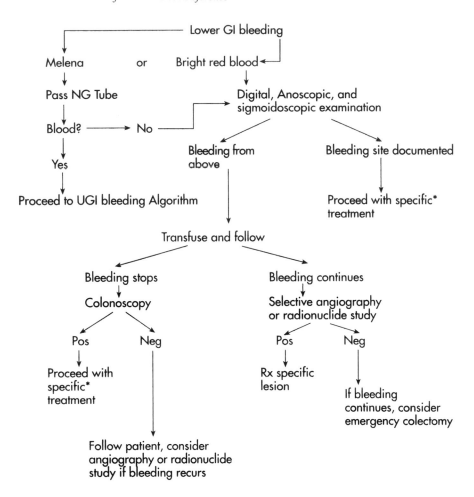

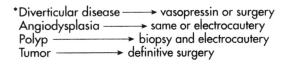

*Diverticular disease ⟶ vasopressin or surgery
Angiodysplasia ⟶ same or electrocautery
Polyp ⟶ biopsy and electrocautery
Tumor ⟶ definitive surgery

FIG 9-4.
Management of lower gastrointestinal tract bleeding. (Modified from Bope ET: *Prim Care* 15:93, 1988.)

ABDOMINAL PAIN

TABLE 9-4.—EVALUATION OF ACUTE ABDOMINAL PAIN

TEST	METHOD	INTERPRETATION	SIGNIFICANCE
Rebound tenderness	Gentle, deep pressure over abdomen, quick release	Severe pain on release indicates positive test	Localized or generalized peritonitis
Guarding (rigidity)	Careful gentle pressure on abdominal wall	Patient resists palpation; may be voluntary or involuntary	May be positive in some normal patients; consider nervous state of patient; "board-like" indicates perforated viscus
Hyperesthesia	Lightly stroke abdominal wall with point of a pin at slight angle	Stroke feels sharper in positive area	Positive along dermatome affected or in distribution of affected peripheral nerve
Iliopsoas sign	Place patient on side opposite pain; extend and hyperextend thigh	Causes pain or patient resists maneuver because of psoas spasm	Caused by direct or indirect psoas (retroperitoneal) irritation
Obturator sign (thigh rotation test)	Flex knee and thigh on affected side; rotate lower leg medially and thigh laterally	Positive test causes lower quadrant pain	Positive when focus in contact with obturator internus (e.g., perforated appendix)

DIARRHEA AND MALABSORPTION

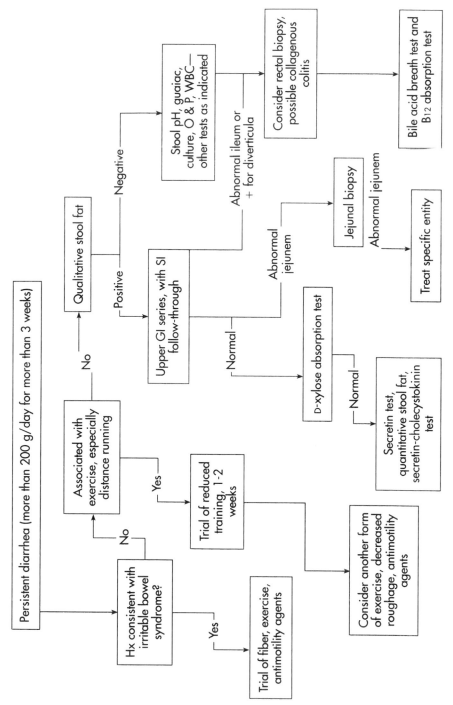

FIG 9-5.
Evaluation of chronic diarrhea.

TABLE 9-5.—PREVENTION AND MANAGEMENT OF TRAVELER'S DIARRHEA

I. Dietary Precautions to Prevent Traveler's Diarrhea
Fluids to Avoid
Tap water, even for brushing teeth
Bottled water, unless the traveler is the one who breaks the seal
Ice made from contaminated water
Unpasteurized milk or dairy products
Fluids that are Safe to Drink
Carbonated soft drinks
Hot drinks, such as tea or coffee, as long as the water was boiled in preparing
   the drink
Carbonated or noncarbonated bottled water, as long as the traveler is the one
   who breaks the seal
Foods to Avoid*
Raw fruits or vegetables, unless they can be peeled and the traveler is the one
   who peels them
Lettuce and other leafy vegetables
Cut-up fruit salad
Raw or rare meat and fish
Meat or shellfish that is not hot when it is served
All food from street vendors

II. Summary of the Recommended Measures for Preventing Traveler's Diarrhea
1. Food and water precautions should be followed.
2. Consider antibiotic prophylaxis if the trip is to last less than 2 weeks and one
   or more of the following are present:
   Patient has potentially reduced gastric acidity
   Patient is elderly
   Patient is receiving chronic histamine H_2-receptor antagonist therapy
   Patient has had gastric surgery
   Patient has a chronic illness, such as diabetes, renal disease, cancer or
      an immunosuppressive disorder (e.g., acquired immunodeficiency syn-
      drome)
   Patient is taking a critically important trip or a trip that would be severely
      affected if the patient developed traveler's diarrhea
3. If prophylactic therapy is selected, one of the following may be used in adult
   patients:
   Ciprofloxacin (Cipro), one 500-mg tablet or two 250-mg tablets per day
   Norfloxacin (Noroxin), one 400-mg tablet per day
   Trimethoprim-sulfamethoxazole, double strength (Bactrim DS, Cotrim DS,
      Septra DS), one tablet per day
   Bismuth subsalicylate (Pepto-Bismol), two tablets four times daily

Continued.

TABLE 9-5.—Prevention and Management of Traveler's Diarrhea—cont'd

---

III. Empiric Therapy for Adults with Traveler's Diarrhea
Fluid and Electrolyte Replacement
Oral rehydration solution, if available; if appropriate solutions are not available, the adult traveler with diarrhea should drink fruit juice, caffeine-free soft drinks or bottled water and should eat salted crackers
Antibiotics†
Ciprofloxacin (Cipro), one 500-mg tablet or two 250-mg tablets twice daily for 3 days
or
Norfloxacin (Noroxin), one 400-mg tablet twice daily for 3 days
or
Trimethoprim-sulfamethoxazole, double strength (Bactrim DS, Cotrim DS, Septra DS), one tablet twice daily for 3 days
Antimotility Medications
Loperamide (Imodium), two 2-mg tablets after the first loose stool, then one tablet after each loose stool, for a maximum of 16 mg in 24 hours
or
Diphenoxylate with atropine (Lomotil), two 2.5-mg tablets four times daily for loose stools

IV. Empiric Therapy for Children with Traveler's Diarrhea
Fluid and Electrolyte Replacement‡
Oral rehydration solutions, if available; if appropriate solutions are not available, the child should drink fruit juices, caffeine-free soft drinks, or bottled water and should eat salted crackers.
Loperamide (Imodium)§
For a child weighing 27.3 to 43.2 kg (60 to 95 lb), the initial dose is 2 tsp, with 1 tsp given after each subsequent loose stool, for a maximum of 6 tsp in 24 hours
For a child weighing 21.8 to 26.8 kg (48 to 59 lb), the initial dose is 2 tsp, with 1 tsp given after each subsequent loose stool, for a maximum of 4 tsp in 24 hours
For a child weighing 10.9 to 21.4 kg (24 to 47 lb), the initial dose is 1 tsp, with 1 tsp given after each subsequent loose stool, for a maximum of 3 tsp in 24 hours
Do not use loperamide in a child weighing less than 10.9 kg (24 lb)
Antibiotics‖
Trimethoprim-sulfamethoxazole (Bactrim, Cotrim, Septra), 4 mg of trimethoprim per kg and 20 mg of sulfamethoxazole per kg twice daily for 3 days

From *Am Fam Physician* 48(5):795, Oct. 1993.
*Foods other than those listed are considered safe to eat.
†Antibiotics may be used in combination with antimotility medications.
‡Fluid and electrolyte replacement is critically important in all children with traveler's diarrhea.
§Loperamide can be used only if there is no blood in the stools and the child's temperature is less than 38.3° C (101° F).
‖Antibiotic therapy may be used if loperamide is not effective or as an alternative to initial therapy.

TABLE 9-6.—TESTS FOR MALABSORPTION

TEST	NORMAL VALUES	MALABSORPTION (NONTROPICAL SPRUE)	MALDIGESTION (PANCREATIC INSUFFICIENCY)	COMMENT
Quantitative determination of stool fat	<6 g/24 hr; >95% coefficient of fat absorption	>6 g/24 hr	>6 g/24 hr	Best test for establishing presence of steatorrhea
D-Xylose absorption (25 g oral dose)	5-hr urinary excretion >4.5 g; peak blood level >30 mg/dl	↓	Normal	A good screening test for carbohydrate absorption
X-ray examination of small intestine		Malabsorption pattern	Normal or minimal malabsorption pattern; occasionally pancreatic calcification	Moulage sign and other abnormalities may be present in several disorders
Mucosal biopsy of small intestine		Abnormal	Normal	A specific diagnosis can be established in a small number of disorders
Schilling test for vitamin B_{12} absorption	>8% urinary excretion in 48 hours	Frequently↓	Frequently↓	Useful in determining whether vitamin B_{12} malabsorption is due to gastric or small intestinal disorders
Secretin test	Volume >1.8 (ml/kg)/hr Bicarbonate concentration >80 mEq/L	Normal	Abnormal	
Serum calcium	9-11 mg/dl	Frequently↓	Usually normal	Decreased levels of both serum albumin and globulins should raise the question of protein-losing enteropathy
Serum albumin	3.5-5.5 g/dl	Frequently↓	Usually normal	

Modified from MacDonald WC, Rubin CE: Gastric tumors, gastritis, and other gastric diseases. In Braunwald E, ed: *Harrison's principles of internal medicine*, ed 11, New York, 1987, McGraw-Hill, p. 64.

Continued.

TABLE 9-6.—Tests for Malabsorption—cont'd

TEST	NORMAL VALUES	MALABSORPTION (NONTROPICAL SPRUE)	MALDIGESTION (PANCREATIC INSUFFICIENCY)	COMMENT
Serum cholesterol	150–250 mg/dl	→	Frequently↓	Usually decreased in disorders associated with significant steatorrhea
Serum iron	80–150 µg/dl	Frequently↓	Normal	Low values may reflect decreased body iron stores
Serum carotenes	>100 IU/dl	→	Usually↓	Fairly satisfactory screening tests for malabsorption
Serum vitamin A	>100 IU/dl	→	Frequently↓	
Prothrombin time	70%–100%; 12–15 seconds	Frequently↓		
Urine 5-hydroxyindoleacetic acid (5-HIAA)	2–9 mg/24 hr	↑	Normal	Slightly increased level (12–16 mg/24 hr) characteristically found in nontropical sprue
Breath H₂ (after 50 g lactose)	Minimal breath H₂	May be↑	Normal	Secondary to lactase deficiency
Duodenal fluid analysis: Conjugated bile salts	>2 mmole/ml	Normal	Normal	May be decreased with bacterial overgrowth, ileal resection, or ileal inflammatory disease

Test	Normal			Comments
Unconjugated bile salts	Not present	Normal	Normal	Increased with bacterial overgrowth
Micellar lipid	>50% ingested lipid in micellar phase	Normal or decreased	Decreased	Decreased with a deficiency of conjugated bile salts or pancreatic lipase
Bacteria (culture)	$<10^3$ organisms/ml	Normal	Normal	$>10^5$ organisms/ml indicates bacterial overgrowth
Glycocholic acid metabolism (oral glycine-1-[14C]glycocholate)	<1% of dose excreted as $^{14}CO_2$ in 4 hours	Normal	Normal	Increased $^{14}CO_2$ excretion with bacterial overgrowth or bile acid malabsorption (caused by ileal resection or inflammatory disease)
	<4% of dose excreted in stools	Normal	Normal	Increased fecal excretion of ^{14}C in bile acid malabsorption
[14C]Triolein absorption (breath test)	>3.5% of dose as breath $^{14}CO_2$ per hour	Decreased	Decreased	Correlates well with chemical stool fat; recently introduced test

INFLAMMATORY BOWEL DISEASE

TABLE 9-7.—DIAGNOSIS OF ACUTE COLITIS/PROCTITIS

DIAGNOSIS	ENDOSCOPIC APPEARANCE	BARIUM ENEMA	RECTAL BIOPSY
Ulcerative colitis	Diffuse erythema and ulceration (no normal mucosa)	Pseudopolyposis; loss of haustra; involvement from rectum proximally	Goblet cell depletion, pseudopolyps
Crohn's disease	Diffuse erythema and ulceration (some normal mucosa)	"Skip" lesions (thickening and luminal narrowing with areas of normal bowel between)	Crypt abscesses, epithelioid granulomas
Salmonella, Shigella, or *Campylobacter*	Same as ulcerative colitis	Usually normal	Crypt abscesses
Amebiasis	Diffuse inflammation, ulceration	Usually normal	Trophozoite in ulcer base
Antibiotic-associated colitis	Multiple, discrete yellow plaques	Usually normal	Fibrinous pseudomembrane over inflammation
Gonorrheal proctitis	Erythema and ulceration, limited to rectum	Normal	Intracellular diplococci
Lymphogranuloma venereum	Same as gonorrhea	Normal	Nonspecific inflammation

Modified from Lewis JH, et al: *Postgrad Med* 70(4):145-162, 1981.

TABLE 9-8.—CLINICAL DISTINCTIONS BETWEEN CROHN'S DISEASE AND ULCERATIVE COLITIS

FEATURE	CROHN'S DISEASE	ULCERATIVE COLITIS
In the Intestine		
Rectal bleeding	Uncommon	Very common
Sigmoidoscopic findings	Normal or spotty lesions	Diffusely abnormal
Spontaneous fistulas	Common	Never occurs
Perianal disease	Common	Uncommon
Abdominal pain	Very common	Uncommon
Abdominal mass	Common	Only with cancers
Strictures	Common	Rare, suspect cancer
Distribution	Discontinuous, entire GI tract	Continuous, colon and rectum
Shortening from incidence of cancer	Fibrosis increased	Muscle thickening greatly increased
Extraintestinal Manifestations		
Arthritis	Occurs	Occurs
Dermatitis	Occurs	Occurs
Episcleritis and uveitis	Occurs	Occurs
Hydronephrosis	Occurs	Occurs
Liver disease	Occurs	Occurs
Metabolic Manifestations		
Amyloidosis	Incidence increased	Rare
Anemia	Common	Common
Fever	Occurs	Occurs
Gallstones	Incidence increased	Incidence normal
Growth retardation	Occurs	Occurs
Kidney stones	Occurs	Occurs

From Sessions T, Jr: *Viewpoints Dig Dis* Sept. 7, 1975.

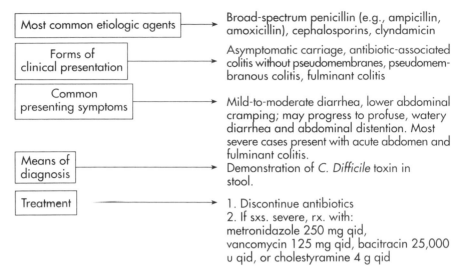

| Most common etiologic agents | → | Broad-spectrum penicillin (e.g., ampicillin, amoxicillin), cephalosporins, clyndamicin |

| Forms of clinical presentation | → | Asymptomatic carriage, antibiotic-associated colitis without pseudomembranes, pseudomembranous colitis, fulminant colitis |

| Common presenting symptoms | → | Mild-to-moderate diarrhea, lower abdominal cramping; may progress to profuse, watery diarrhea and abdominal distention. Most severe cases present with acute abdomen and fulminant colitis. |

| Means of diagnosis | → | Demonstration of C. Difficile toxin in stool. |

| Treatment | → | 1. Discontinue antibiotics
2. If sxs. severe, rx. with:
metronidazole 250 mg qid,
vancomycin 125 mg qid, bacitracin 25,000 u qid, or cholestyramine 4 g qid |

FIG 9-6.
Clostridium difficile (antibiotic–associated) colitis. (From Kelly CP, Pothoulakis C, LaMont JT: *Clostridium difficile* colitis, *N Engl J Med* 330 (4):257, 1994.)

TABLE 9-9.—TREATMENT OF IRRITABLE BOWEL SYNDROME

General Measures

MODALITY	COMMENT
Establish good doctor-patient relationship	Nonjudgemental, realistic expectations, involvement of patient benign nature of the
Patient education about illness	illness, excellent long-term prognosis
Dietary modification	Eliminate dairy products, gas-forming foods, fiber supplementation

Drug Treatment

MEDICATION	DOSAGE	INDICATION
Fiber Supplementation		
Wheat bran	½ cup to 1 bowl a day	If constipation is predominant symptom;
Psyllium	½ to 1 tbsp 1 or 2 times a day	use as trial for all
Antispasmodic Agents		
Belladonna	5-10 qtts 3 times a day ac	If pain is predominant symptom; use to prevent postprandial pain
Dicyclomine	10-20 mg 3-4 times a day	
Antidiarrheal Agents		
Diphenoxylate	2.5-5 mg 4 times a day	If diarrhea is predominant symptom; may help some patients' abdominal pain
Loperamide	2 mg, 2 times a day	
Cholestyramine	½-1 packet 1 or 2 times a day	
Tricyclic Antidepressants		
Desipramine	50 mg at bedtime	If pain is the predominant symptom; may be useful in patients who have chronic pain syndrome
Amitriptyline	10-25 mg at bedtime	

From Lynn RB, Friedman LS: Irritable bowel syndrome, *N Engl J Med* 329(26):1943, 1993.

MALIGNANCIES

TABLE 9-10.—APPROACH FOR DETECTING COLONIC NEOPLASMS

SCREENING TEST	ASYMPTOMATIC	HIGH RISK	POSTSPLENECTOMY	POSTRESECTION FOR CARCINOMA
Fecal occult blood	Annually	Annually (except in ulcerative colitis)	Annually	Annually plus annual CEA*
Proctosigmoidoscopy	Annually for 2 years after age 50, then every 5 years	Annually	Every 2-3 years when necessary to supplement colonoscopy	Annually
Air contrast barium enema (ACBE)	Only for positive findings	ACBE; frequency depends on underlying risk factors	ACBE every 2-3 years	ACBE annually for 2 years then every 2-3 years
Colonoscopy	Only for positive findings	May be required annually in certain diseases (e.g., ulcerative colitis after 10 years)	Every 2-3 years	Every 2-3 years

Modified from Stouffer JQ: Polypoid tumors of the colon. In Sleisenger MH, Fordtran JS, eds: *Gastrointestinal disease*, ed 2, Philadelphia, 1981, WB Saunders, p. 1780.
*CEA, carcinoembryonic antigen.

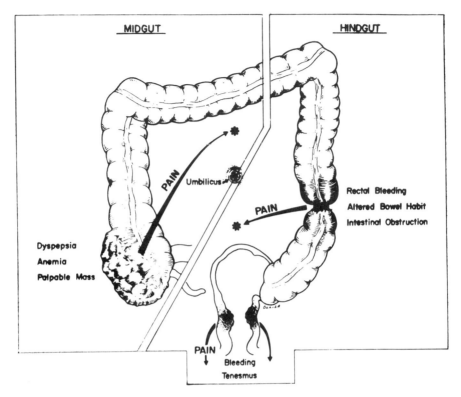

FIG 9-7.
Symptoms of carcinoma of the colon. (From Cohn I, Nance FC: Intermediate or precancerous lesions and malignant lesions. In Sabiston DC, ed: *Textbook of surgery,* ed 12, Philadelphia, 1981, WB Saunders, p. 1098.)

LIVER DISEASE

TABLE 9-11.—Passive Immunization Recommendations for Hepatitis A with Immune Serum Globulin

STATUS	COMMENT
Preexposure prophylaxis recommended	
International travelers	Recommended for travel to developing countries*
Postexposure prophylaxis recommended	
Close personal contact	For household and sexual contacts
Day-care centers	Day-care centers should be evaluated on an individual basis, recognizing that diapered children present a higher risk of transmission to parents and staff. Contact appropriate local or state health department for assistance.
Institutions	For residents and staff of prisons and facilities for custodial care for the developmentally disabled, when an outbreak occurs
Common-source exposure	IG might be effective in preventing foodborne hepatitis A if recognized in time. IG is recommended if all of the following conditions exist: (1) source is directly involved in handling (without gloves) food that will not be cooked before being eaten; (2) the hygienic practices of source area are deficient or a food handler had diarrhea; and (3) patrons can be identified and treated within 2 weeks of exposure
Postexposure prophylaxis not routinely recommended	
Schools	IG is usually not indicated for pupils and teachers in contact with a patient
Hospitals	IG is not recommended for either roommates or staff caring for a patient with hepatitis A
Offices and factories	IG is not indicated under the usual conditions for those exposed to a fellow worker with hepatitis A

IMMUNE GLOBULIN DOSE FOR PROTECTION AGAINST VIRAL HEPATITIS A

BODY WEIGHT	DOSE VOLUME FOR INTRAMUSCULAR INJECTION
Under 50 lb	0.5 ml
50-100 lb	1.0 ml
Over 100 lb	2.0 ml

From Centers for Disease Control and Prevention: *Iowa Dis Bull* 17(1):4, 1994, Iowa Department of Public Health.

*Hepatitis A vaccination is preferred since vaccine licensure is February of 1995.

TABLE 9-12.—RECOMMENDATIONS FOR VACCINATION AND IMMUNOPROPHYLAXIS OF HEPATITIS B

Recommended Doses of Currently Licensed Hepatitis B Vaccines

GROUP	RECOMBIVAX HB* DOSE (MG)	(ML)	ENGERIX-B* DOSE (µG)	(ML)
Infants of HB$_s$Ag negative mothers and children <11 years	2.5	(0.5)	10	(0.5)
Infants of HB$_s$Ag positive mothers; prevention of perinatal infection	5	(0.5)	10	(0.5)
Children and adolescents 11-19 years	5	(0.5)	20	(1.0)
Adults ≥ 20 years	10	(1.0)	20	(1.0)
Dialysis patients and other immunocompromised persons	40	(1.0)†	40	(2.0)‡

Recommendations for Hepatitis B Prophylaxis Following Percutaneous or Permucosal Exposure

EXPOSED PERSON	TREATMENT WHEN SOURCE IS FOUND TO BE:		
	HB$_s$AG POSITIVE	HB$_s$AG NEGATIVE	SOURCE NOT TESTED OR UNKNOWN
Unvaccinated	HBIG × 1§ and initiate HB Vaccine	Initiate HB vaccine	Initiate HB vaccine
Previously vaccinated: Known responder	Test exposed person for anti-HBs 1. If adequate,‖ give no treatment 2. If inadequate, give HB vaccine booster dose	No treatment	No treatment
Known nonresponder	HBIG × 2 or HBIG × 1 plus 1 dose of HB vaccine	No treatment	If a known high-risk source, may treat as if source were HB$_s$Ag positive
Response unknown	Test exposed person for anti-HBs 1. If inadequate,‖ give HBIG × 1 plus HB vaccine booster dose 2. If adequate, give no treatment	No treatment	Test exposed person for anti-HBs 1. If inadequate,‖ give HB vaccine booster dose 2. If adequate, give no treatment

From Centers for Disease Control and Prevention: *Iowa Dis Bull* 17(1):8, 1994, Iowa Department of Public Health.
*Both vaccines are routinely administered in a three-dose series. Engerix-B has also been licensed for a four-dose series administered at 0, 1, 2, and 12 months.
†Special formulation.
‡Two 1.0-ml doses administered at one site, in a four-dose schedule at 0, 1, 2, and 6 months.
§HBIG dose 0.06 ml/kg given intramuscularly.
‖Adequate anti-HBs is ≥ 10 SRU by RIA or positive by EIA.

TABLE 9-13.—Recommendations for Hepatitis B Vaccination and Immunoprophylaxis of Infants

Recommendations to Prevent Perinatal Transmission of Hepatitis B Virus Infection
Infant Born to Mother Known to be HB$_s$Ag[a] Positive

Vaccine Dose[b]	Age of Infant
First	Birth (within 12 hours)
HBIG[c]	Birth (within 12 hours)
Second	1 month
Third	6 months[d]

Infant Born to Mother not Screened for HB$_s$Ag

Vaccine Dose[e]	Age of Infant
First	Birth (within 12 hours)
HBIG[c]	If mother is found to be HB$_s$Ag positive, administer dose to infant as soon as possible, but not later than 1 week after birth
Second	1-2 months
Third	6 months[d]

Recommendations for Infants Born to HB$_s$Ag Negative Mothers

HEPATITIS B VACCINE	AGE OF INFANT
Option 1 (2.5 µg each dose)	
Dose 1	Birth—before hospital discharge
Dose 2	1-2 months[g]
Dose 3	6-18 months[g]
Option 2 (2.5 µg each dose)	
Dose 1	1-2 months[g]
Dose 2	4 months[g]
Dose 3	6-18 months[g]

Modified from Centers for Disease Control and Prevention: *Iowa Dis Bull* 17(1):9, 1994, Iowa Department of Public Health.

[a]*HB$_s$Ag*, Hepatitis B surface antigen.

[b]0.5 mL (5 µg) of hepatitis B vaccine recombinant.

[c]Hepatitis B immune globulin (HBIG)—0.5 ml administered intramuscularly at a site different from that used for the vaccine.

[d]If four-dose schedule (Engerix-B) is used, the third dose is administered at 2 months of age and the fourth dose at 12-18 months.

[e]First dose is a dose for infant of HB$_s$Ag positive mother (5 µg). If mother is found to be HB$_s$Ag positive, continue that dose; if mother is found to be HB$_s$Ag negative, use appropriate 3-dose schedule of 0.25 mL (2.5 µg).

[f]Infants of women who are HB$_s$Ag negative can be vaccinated at 2 months of age.

[g]Hepatitis B vaccine can be administered simultaneously with diphtheria-tetanus-pertussis, *Haemophilus influenzae* type b conjugate, measles-mumps-rubella, and oral polio vaccines.

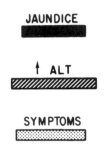

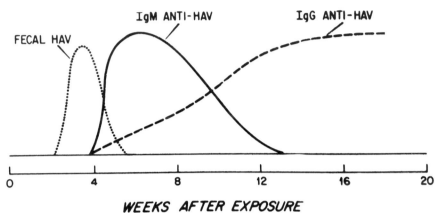

FIG 9-8.

Clinical and virological events during acute type A hepatitis. (From Dienstag JL, Wands JR, Koff RS: Acute hepatitis. In Petersdorf RG, ed: *Harrison's principles of internal medicine,* ed 10, New York, 1981, McGraw-Hill, p. 1792.)

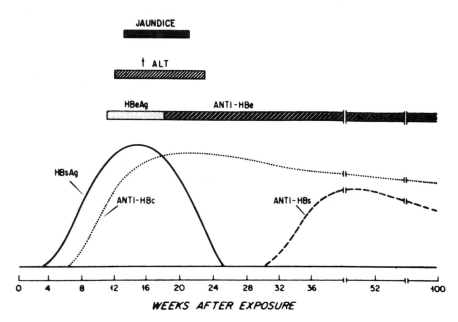

FIG 9-9.
Clinical and virological events during a typical self-limiting episode of acute viral hepatitis type B. (From Dienstag JL, Wands JR, Koff RS: Acute hepatitis. In Petersdorf RG, ed: *Harrison's principles of internal medicine,* ed 10, New York, 1981, McGraw-Hill, p. 1793.)

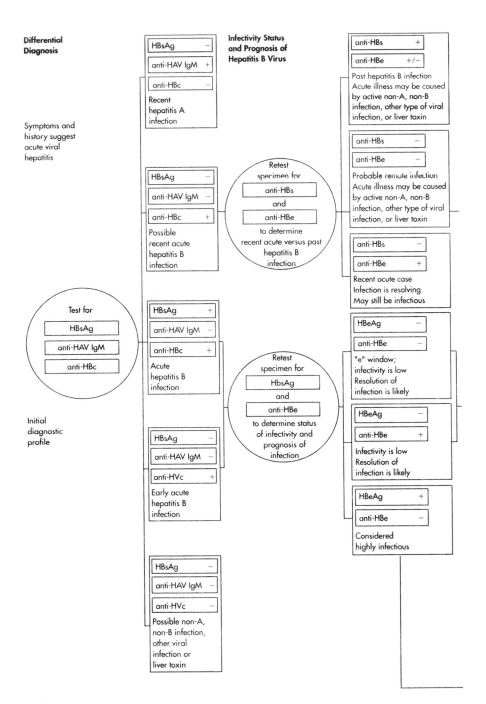

FIG 9-10.
Laboratory evaluation of acute hepatitis. *HB$_s$Ag,* Hepatitis B surface antigen; *anti-HAV IgM,* hepatitis A antibody; *anti-HB$_c$,* hepatitis B "core" antigen; *anti-HB$_s$,* hepatitis B surface antibody; *anti-HB$_e$,* hepatitis B "E" antibody; *HB$_e$Ag,* hepatitis B "E" antigen. (Modified from *Perspectives on viral hepatitis,* New York, Biomedical Information Corp.)

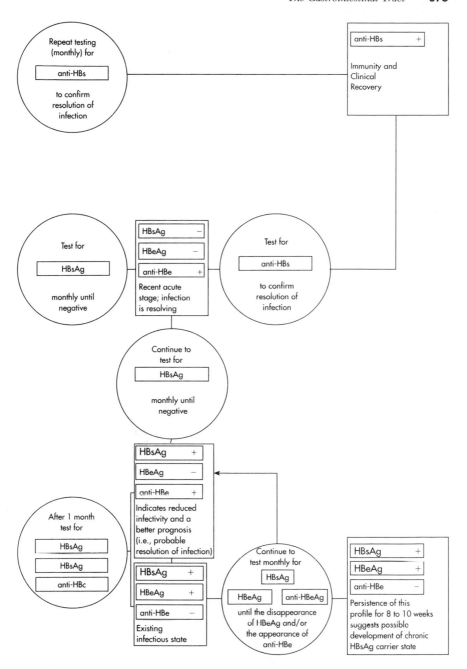

FIG 9-10, cont'd
For legend see opposite page.

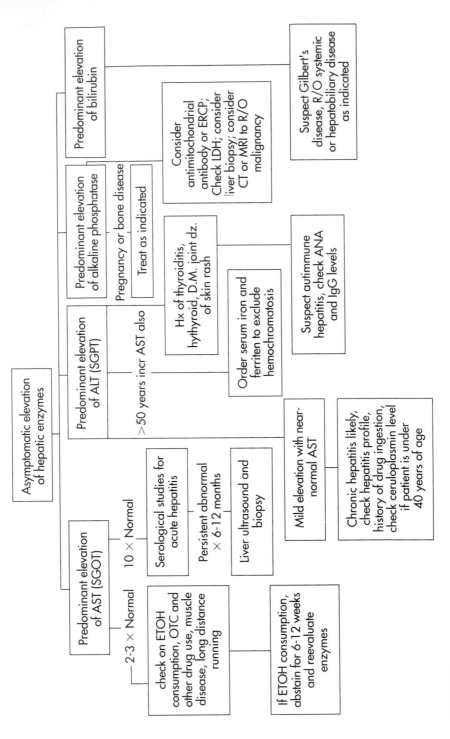

FIG 9-11.

Evaluation of liver function tests. (From Jensen D, Koff RS: Abnormal liver tests: what next? *Patient Care* Aug. 15, 1994, p. 143.)

PROCEDURES

TABLE 9-14.—PROCEDURES IN THE GASTROINTESTINAL TRACT

Flexible Sigmoidoscopy*
1. The patient should administer 2 Fleet's enemas on the morning of the procedure. If patient has chronic constipation, preparation of the bowel requires 3 bisacodyl (Dulcolax) tablets the afternoon before the test in addition to the enemas on the morning of the procedure.
2. Place patient in left lateral decubitus position.
3. Perform digital examination and anoscopy first.
4. Hold shaft of instrument in right hand and control head of endoscope with left hand.
5. Apply water-soluble lubricant to endoscope shaft.
6. Guide scope into rectum with finger.
7. Advance scope, always with lumen in view.
8. Insufflate air periodically to distend collapsed bowel.
9. Aspirate liquid with suction control as needed.
10. Extra care is required to negotiate the angle at the rectosigmoid junction.
11. If colonic spasm occurs, pull back 3-4 cm and reinsert.
12. Examine mucosa on withdrawal of scope.
13. Biopsy suspicious lesions on withdrawal.

Diagnostic Paracentesis†
1. Turn patient on left side for 5 minutes.
2. After the bladder has been emptied, insert a 19-gauge, short, beveled spinal needle halfway between the umbilicus and pubis at the left lateral edge of the rectus sheath.
3. Do *not* use local anesthesia (pain signals entering peritoneum).
4. Apply gentle suction with 15-20 ml syringe.
5. If no fluid is obtained, repeat on the right side.

Alternate Method
1. Use intracath.
2. Insert in lower abdominal midline, 1 inch below umbilicus.
3. Pass catheter and withdraw needle; apply gentle suction.
4. If no fluid is obtained, infuse 500 ml of sterile saline over 10-15 minutes.
5. Aspirate and check fluid for pH, bile, amylase, WBCs, RBCs, cytology, and cultures, as indicated.

String Test (for Localization of Chronic GI Blood Loss)‡
This procedure is indicated to evaluate guaiac-positive stools when barium studies and colonoscopy are negative.
1. Pass weighted umbilical tape with radiopaque markers (available from Advanced Laboratory Associates, New Brunswick, N.J.) orally. It will advance by peristalsis through the small bowel over 2-3 hours.
2. Document the position of the tape with abdominal x-ray radiograph.
3. Inject 20 ml of fluorescein IV over 2-3 minutes.
4. Withdraw tape and examine under fluorescent light and with guaiac reagent.
5. Correlate presence of blood with position on x-ray film.

Continued.

TABLE 9-14.—PROCEDURES IN THE GASTROINTESTINAL TRACT—cont'd

Bedside Test for Gastric Outlet Obstruction (Saline Load Test)‡
1. Empty stomach and irrigate with normal saline until clear through a No. 30 Ewald tube.
2. Insert soft nasogastric tube to 65 cm.
3. Infuse 750 ml of normal saline over 3-5 minutes.
4. Aspirate after 30 minutes with patient in supine, upright, and both right and left decubitus positions.
5. A residual of 400 ml or more indicates probable obstruction; 300-400 ml is suggestive.
6. Repeat daily to assess results of medical therapy; if positive after 72 hours of suction, surgery will usually be required.

Insertion of Nasogastric Tube
1. Measure from the xiphoid to either ear lobe. This is the distance the tube should be passed.
2. The tube should be placed in ice or refrigerated before insertion to facilitate passage through the pharynx.
3. Insert gently through the nose to the posterior pharynx.
4. Ask the patient to swallow, or have patient drink sips of water. Tube should be passed synchronous with swallowing.
5. Aspiration of gastric contents and/or auscultation of borborygmi with air insertion confirms proper placement in the stomach.
6. Tube should be carefully taped to the nose, avoiding excessive pressure of the tube on the nares.

Routine Stool Examination
Observe for odor, color, consistency, mucus, blood, concretions, adult parasites, pus, and fat (a puttylike appearance).

Qualitative Stool Examination for Fat (Sudan Stain)
1. Emulsify a small portion of stool with normal saline.
2. Add 1 drop of glacial acetic acid.
3. Add 1 drop of Sudan III or IV stain.
4. Place a drop on a slide, cover with a cover slip, and examine for fat droplets.
5. Neutral fat appears as deep orange or red drops.

Ova and Parasites
1. Obtain a fresh, preferably warm stool specimen.
2. Emulsify a 1-2 mm portion of fecal material with normal saline using an applicator stick.
3. Emulsify a second specimen as above, but add 2-3 drops of Gram's iodine.
4. Make two thin wet preparations and cover each with a cover slip.
5. Look for trophozoites in the saline prep.
6. Look for cysts in the iodine solution (will stain light brown).

White Blood Cells in Stool
1. Emulsify stool in normal saline as above.
2. Add one drop of methylene blue.
3. Place a drop on a slide and cover with a cover slip.
4. Observe under high dry. White cell nuclei will stain blue. More than five WBCs per high-power field suggests inflammation.

*Flexible sigmoidoscopy procedure modified from Quan M, Rodney WM, Johnson RA: *Postgrad Med* 72:151, 1982; Rodney WM, Felmar E: *Your patient and cancer* Feb. 1984.

†Diagnostic paracentesis procedure modified from Baker RJ: Differential diagnosis of abdominal pain. In Condon RE, Nyhus LM, eds: *Manual of surgical therapeutics,* ed 2, Boston, 1972, Little, Brown, p. 286.

‡String test and bedside test for gastric outlet obstruction modified from Boedeker EC: Gastrointestinal disease. In Boedeker EC, Dauber JH, eds: *Manual of medical therapeutics,* ed 21, Boston, 1974, Little, Brown, p. 256.

GALLBLADDER DISEASE

TABLE 9-15.—TREATMENT OF GALLBLADDER DISEASE

Indications for Cholecystectomy
Acute cholecystitis, if medically possible (generally open)
Bile duct obstruction, common duct stones (generally open)
Recurrent biliary colic (generally laparascopic)
Asymptomatic gallstones, sickle cell disease, and children

Indications for Oral Dissolution Therapy
(If available, contact dissolution therapy may be attempted for same group of
 patients)
Gallstones must be noncalcified and small
Cystic duct patent
Patient refuses surgery or is a poor risk

Guidelines for Initiation of Chenodiol Therapy
1. Begin at 250 mg bid for 2 weeks. Divide dose between morning and evening
   meals.
2. Increase the dose gradually to about 15 mg/kg/day in two divided doses or
   until symptoms such as diarrhea and flatulence become unacceptable.
3. Monitor liver hepatocellular enzymes periodically (about once per month) for
   the first 12 months of therapy.
4. Perform gallbladder ultrasound at 6- to 9-month intervals to monitor dissolution rate.
5. If reduction in stone size is not obvious by 16 months, therapy should be
   discontinued.
NOTE: Only about 15%-30% of patients have experienced complete dissolution
 over 2 years of therapy.

ANORECTAL DISORDERS

TABLE 9-16.—ANORECTAL DISORDERS

Hemorrhoids
Thrombosed External Hemorrhoids
Pain is prominent, and bleeding is infrequent
Examination reveals a bluish perianal mass just below the mucocutaneous junction
Treatment consists of sitz baths and stool softeners
Pain usually disappears within 1 week, and the mass disappears within 2 weeks
Residual skin tags are common and do not indicate chronic hemorrhoidal disease
If acutely painful, overlying skin may be anesthetized with 1% lidocaine, incised, and the clot removed with resultant immediate pain relief
Internal Hemorrhoids
Symptoms usually limited to bright red bleeding, almost always *painless*
Large hemorrhoids may prolapse out of the rectum at bowel movement
Digital examination is often negative; diagnosis requires anoscope with a good light source
Even if hemorrhoids are present on examination, other sources of bleeding such as colon cancer must be excluded
Small, minimally symptomatic lesions may be treated with observation and a high-fiber diet
Larger lesions may be treated with sclerotherapy with injection of 5% phenol solution in oil into the submucosal area. (Care must be exercised not to inject into the vein)
Very large, prolapsing lesions are best treated by rubber band ligature technique
Anal Fissure
Characterized by pain associated with a hard bowel movement with minor bleeding on the toilet tissue
Patients usually mistake them for hemorrhoids
Mucosal tears are demonstrable, usually at 6 o'clock or 12 o'clock, by everting the buttocks; will often be missed unless specifically sought
Treat with sitz baths, stool softeners, high-fiber diet, and hydrocortisone suppositories
Chronic, recalcitrant cases may require sphincterotomy and/or fissurectomy
Pruritus Ani
Causes are multiple and poorly understood but include poor perianal hygiene, trauma from scratching or excessive cleaning or wiping, excessive moisture, yeast infections, hypersensitivity reactions to local or systemic agents, dietary irritants such as jalapeno peppers, or personality or psychological factors
Once started, a vicious cycle occurs and is hard to break
Treatment approaches should include the following:
1. Correct all predisposing anatomical conditions (e.g., hemorrhoids)
2. Direct attention to meticulous perianal hygiene; use water, not soap. If sitz bath is unavailable, use premoistened towelettes.
3. Avoid scratching; use oral Vistaril, Phenergan, or Benadryl as antipruritic, if necessary.
4. Keep the area dry with loose clothing; consider tucking gauze into the buttocks; cornstarch or other drying powder may help.
5. Medications should be minimized; topical steroids are contraindicated except for a short, initial course; avoid local anesthetic such as benzocaine, which is highly sensitizing. Yeast infections are often secondary and should be treated with nystatin or miconazole cream.
6. Efforts should be directed toward complete normalization of stool patterns. Overly soft stool may be as irritating as constipated stool.
7. Consider the importance of psychological factors.

10 *The Genitourinary System*

Charles E. Driscoll

TABLE 10-1.—Urine Collection from Infants

Catheterization

For female infants, use sterile technique and insert a lubricated no. 5 or 8 French polyethylene pediatric feeding tube through the urethra into the bladder.

Bladder Aspiration

To obtain an uncontaminated urine specimen from an infant or child younger than 4 years of age, wait at least 1 hour after the last voiding.

Give liquids to ensure a full bladder.

Place child supine in a frogleg position with an assistant providing gentle restraint if needed.

Cleanse the suprapubic area above the symphysis with povidine-iodine solution.

With a sterile gloved finger, palpate symphysis, which is usually at or just above the fat crease.

Use a 10-ml syringe with a 1½-inch 23-gauge needle and insert in the midline just above the palpating finger. Aim the needle toward the infant's coccyx and advance while applying negative pressure until urine appears in the syringe.

If the needle is advanced to its hub without urine entering the syringe, assume a dry tap and withdraw the needle to just under the skin surface before redirecting.

Urination can be prevented during the procedure by applying light pressure to the urethral opening.

Apply a Band-Aid over the needle insertion site.

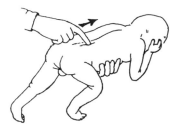 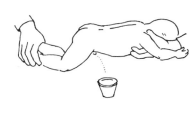

FIG 10-1.

Collection of urine from children may be done noninvasively in the male by stimulating the Perez reflex. Holding the infant in ventral suspension, stroke along the midline cephalad. As the infant's back is arched, position the infant over a sterile collection cup. (From Kuhlberg A: *Top Emerg Med* 1983; 5:50.)

TABLE 10-2.—Substances in Urine that May Change Urine Color*

SUBSTANCE	COLORS PRODUCED IN URINE
Acetanilid	Yellow to red
Acetophenetidin (metabolite)	Yellow (dark brown to wine color)
Alcohol	Lightens color
Aloin	Red-brown to yellow-pink (alkaline urine), yellow-brown (acid urine)
Aminopyrine	Red-brown
Aminosalicylic acid (paraaminosalicylic acid)	Discoloration (no distinctive color)
Amitriptyline	Blue-green
Anisindione	Orange (alkaline urine), pink to red brown
Anthraqulnone laxatives	Reddish (alkaline urine)
Antipyrine	Yellow to red-brown
Azuresin	Blue or green
Beets	Red
Benzene	Red-brown
Biliverdin	Yellow-green
Carbon tetrachloride	Red-brown
Carrots	Yellow
Cascara	Yellow-brown (acid urine), yellow-pink (alkaline urine), darkens to brown to black on standing
Chloroquine	Rust-yellow to brown
Chlorzoxazone	Orange to purple-red
Cinchophen	Red-brown
Creosote	Dark green
Cresol	Dark color on standing
Danthron	Pink to red
Deferoxamine mesylate	Reddish
Dihydroxyanthraquinone	Pink to orange (alkaline urine)
Dinitrophenol	Red-brown
Diphenylhydantoin (see phenytoin)	
Dithiazanine hydrochloride	Blue
Doan's kidney pills	Greenish blue
Doxorubicin	Red-brown
Emodin (in cascara)	Pink to red to red-brown (alkaline urine)
Ethoxazene	Orange to red
Ferrous salts	Black
Fluorescein (intravenous)	Yellow-orange
Furazolidone (metabolite)	Brownish or rust-yellow
Ibuprofen	Red or pink
Indanediones	Orange (alkaline urine)
Indomethacin	Green (biliverdinemia)
Iron sorbitex	Dark to black on standing
Lead	Red-brown
Levodopa	Dark red-brown
Melanin	Black-brown
Mercury	Red-brown
Methocarbamol	Dark brown, black or green on standing
Methyldopa	Dark (red to black) on standing
Methylene blue	Greenish yellow to blue
Metronidazole	Dark brown in acidic urine

Modified from Martin EW: *Hazards of medication*, Philadelphia, JB Lippincott. Raymond JR, Yarger WE: *South Med J* 81:837, 1988.

TABLE 10-2.—Substances in Urine that May Change Urine Color*—cont'd

SUBSTANCE	COLORS PRODUCED IN URINE
Naphthol	Dark color on standing
Nitrobenzene	Dark color on standing
Nitrofurantoin and derivatives	Brown or rust-yellow
Oxamniquine	Red-orange
Pamaquine naphthoate	Rust-yellow or brown
Phenacetin (see acetophenetidin)	
Phenazopyridine	Orange-red to red brown (HNO_3 turns orange to pink)
Phenindione	Reddish brown to pink, orange in alkaline urine
Phenolphthalein	Pink to red to magenta (alkaline urine), yellow-brown (acid urine)
Phenolsulfonphthalein	Red (alkaline urine)
Phenols	Dark green to brownish black (darkens on standing)
Phenothiazines	Pink to red-brown
Phensuximide	Pink to red to red-brown
Phenyl salicylate	Dark green
Phenytoin	Pink to red to reddish brown
Picric acid	Yellow to red-brown
Porphyrins	Burgundy red, darkens on standing
Primaquine phosphate	Rust-yellow to brown
Pyocyanin	Blue-green
Pyrogallol	Brown to black (darkens on standing)
Quinacrine hydrochloride	Yellow (deep yellow on acidification)
Quinine and derivatives	Brown to black
Resorcinol	Dark green to green-blue, darkens on standing
Rhubarb	Yellow-brown (acid urine), yellow-pink (alkaline urine), darkens to brown to black on standing
Riboflavin	Yellow
Rifampin	Red to orange
Salicylazosulfapyridine	Orange-yellow (alkaline urine)
Salol	Dark color on standing
Santonin	Bright yellow (NaOH changes to pink or scarlet)
Senna	Yellow-brown (acid urine), yellow-pink (alkaline urine), darkens on standing
Sulfonamides	Rust-yellow or brown
Sulfonethylmethane	Red
Sulfonmethane	Red-brown
Tetralin (tetrahydronaphthalene)	Greenish blue
Thiazosulfone	Pink to red
Thymol	Greenish blue
TNT (trinitrotoluene)	Red-brown
Tolonium (Blutene)	Blue-Green
Triamterene	Bluish color (pale blue fluorescence)
Warfarin sodium	Orange

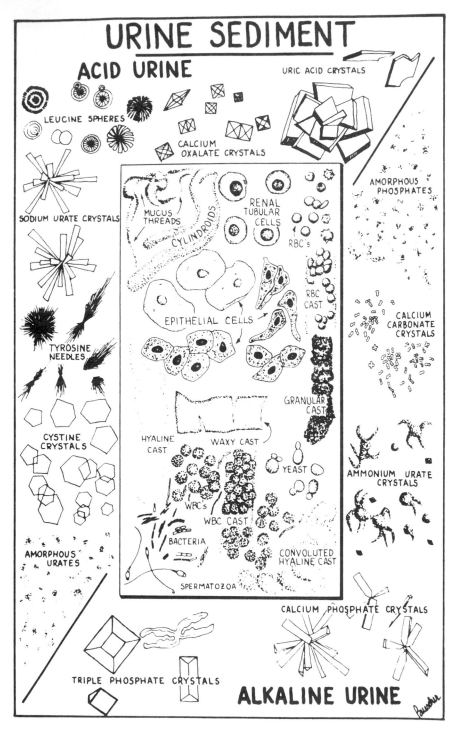

FIG 10-2.
Microscopic appearance of urine sediment. (From Biller JA, Yeager AM, eds: *The Harriet Lane handbook,* ed 10, Chicago, 1984, Mosby.)

RENAL FUNCTION

TABLE 10-3.—Creatinine Clearance Dosing Interval Estimates*

Cockroft-Gault Equation:

$$CrCl = \frac{(140 - Age) \times Weight\ (kg)}{72 \times S_{cr}}$$

Multiply by 0.85 for females.

Weight: Lean weight in kg
   CrCl: Creatinine clearance
    S_{cr}: Serum creatinine
NOTE: A 75-year-old woman (60 kg/lean) who has a "normal" serum creatinine
  value of 1.0 may not have "normal" renal function:

$$\frac{(140 - 75) \times 60\ kg}{72(1.0)} \times 0.85 = 46\ ml/min$$

The following equation may be used for drugs that are primarily excreted by the
  kidney. The change in dosing interval is estimated by using the estimated creatinine clearance and the usual dosing interval in the following equation:

$$\frac{100}{Estimated\ creatinine\ clearance} \times Usual\ interval\ in\ hours$$

Modified from Cockroft DW, Gault MH: *Nephron* 1976; 16:31-41.
*In young healthy persons with stable renal function. May be less accurate in the elderly.

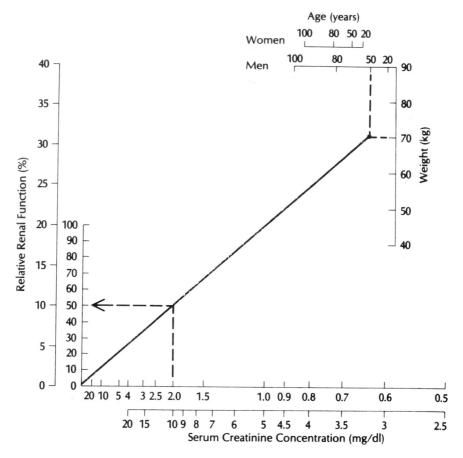

FIG 10-3.

Estimating relative renal function. Nomogram graphically depicts patient's relative renal function from the serum creatinine concentration. To prepare, a line is drawn from the point of intersection of individual's sex, age, and weight to the origin; the percent of renal function remaining for a given serum creatinine value is read on the ordinate, using the outer scales for serum creatinine values above 2.5 mg/dl. For example, renal function is 50% of normal in a 50-year-old man weighing 70 kg, with a serum creatinine of 2 mg/dl. (From Anderson R: *Hosp Pract* 18:155, 1983.)

ACID-BASE BALANCE

TABLE 10-4.—THE GOLDEN RULES OF ACID-BASE BALANCE

---

1. A change in $Paco_2$, either up or down, of 10 mm Hg is associated with an increase or decrease of pH by 0.08 unit (as $Paco_2$ increases pH falls).
2. A pH change of 0.15 is the result of a base change of 10 mEq/L.
3. Total body bicarbonate deficit equals =

$$\text{Base deficit (mEq/L)} \times \frac{[\text{Pt. weight (kg)}]}{4}$$

Use 100% correction for acute conditions (CPR) and 50% correction for subacute/chronic conditions.

Example: 70-kg man in cardiac arrest with $Paco_2$ of 52 mm Hg and pH of 7.17: Since $Paco_2$ is increased by 12 mm Hg, respiratory acidosis is present. Calculating pH from change in $Paco_2$ gives an expected pH of 7.30. There is an unexplained pH difference of 0.13 (7.30 − 7.17), which is attributed to metabolic acidosis.

Calculation of base deficit by rule 2 $\left(\dfrac{0.15}{10}\right) \times \left(\dfrac{0.13}{X}\right)$

Bicarbonate deficit $= 9 \times \dfrac{70}{4} = 157$ mEq.

The patient requires increased ventilation for respiratory acidosis and 157 mEq of sodium bicarbonate for metabolic acidosis.

URINARY INCONTINENCE

TABLE 10-5.—ENURESIS

The male to female prevalence is 2 : 1
Prevalence relative to age is:
    Age 5 years,   20%
    Age 10 years,   5%
    Age 15 years,   1%
Evaluate and treat when the problem threatens self-image.

Evaluation

Hx: Dysuria, never dry versus recent onset, occurs during the day as well as at night, urinary anomalies in patient or family, how often does it happen, developmental or maturational lags, family history of enuresis, associated sleep disorder, psychological factors

Px: Look for abdominal masses, anomalous genitalia, hypertension, neurological signs, fecal impaction if associated with encopresis

Lab: Urinalysis is usually all that is needed unless anomalous genitalia are noted, then do intravenous pyelogram

Treatment*

MODE	TIME TO RESPONSE, SUCCESS AND RELAPSE RATES
Reassurance	15% Spontaneous remission/year
Limit Fluids	Minimal help; better to empty bladder often
Alarm Systems	Takes 3-4 months to condition, 70% success, 30% relapse rate
Medications	
Imipramine	1-2 mg/kg (maximum 25-50 mg) at bedtime for 6-8 weeks, 40%-60% success, 30%-60% relapse
Ditropan	5 mg at bedtime for 6 weeks, variable success rates, relapse 50%-60%
Desmopressin (DDAVP)	20-40 μg (e.g., 1-2 puffs each nostril) at bedtime will give response in 2-3 weeks, 70% success rate, 30% relapse rate

*For additional information: Rosenfeld J, Jerkins GR: The bed-wetting child, *Postgrad Med* 89:(2)63, 1991.

A Capacity : Normal
  Proprioception (sense of fullness and desire to void at
  normal volume) : Intact
  Exteroception (normal voiding
  sensation) : Intact
  Motor Function : Voluntary
  control of normal voiding
  contraction
  Post-Void Residual : Negligible
  or increased in patients with
  true outlet obstruction (e.g. BPH)

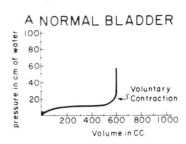

A NORMAL BLADDER

B Capacity : Reduced
  Proprioception : Present or absent
  Exteroception : Present or absent
  Motor Function : absent voluntary
  control
  Post-Void Residual : Variable

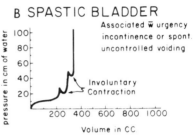

B SPASTIC BLADDER

C Capacity : Increased except when
  catheter has been indwelling
  Proprioception : Diminished or
  absent
  Exteroception : Present or absent
  Motor Function : Cannot initiate
  bladder contraction
  Post-Void Residual : Large

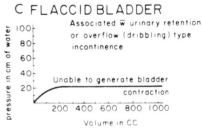

C FLACCID BLADDER

FIG 10-4.
Typical cystometrograms. Patients with pattern *A* may be expected to benefit from prostatectomy. Patients with pattern *B* deserve a more thorough urodynamic workup before surgery is considered. Although these patients have symptoms that mimic prostatic obstruction, they usually are not obstructed, and surgery may aggravate the problem. Patients
with pattern *C* may benefit from surgery. Although the neurogenically induced flaccid bladder is not relieved by prostatectomy, the procedure reduces the resistance to emptying
and thereby may improve function. (From Branch WT Jr: *Office practice of medicine,* Philadelphia, 1982, WB Saunders, p. 516.)

TABLE 10-6.—MNEMONICS FOR REMEMBERING CAUSES OF INCONTINENCE

Acute Incontinence
D—*D*elirium
R—*R*estricted mobility, (acute) retention
I — *I*nfection, inflammation, impaction
P—*P*harmaceuticals, polyuria

Or

D—*D*elirium
I — *I*nfection
A—*A*trophic urethritis/vaginitis
P—*P*harmaceuticals
P—*P*sychological
E—*E*ndocrine (hypercalcemia, hyperglycemia)
R—*R*estricted mobility
S—*S*tool impaction

Established Incontinence
S—*S*tress (sphincter)
O—*O*verflow
U—*U*rge (detrusor instability)
P—*P*sychological (functional)

TABLE 10-7.—DRUGS THAT MAY CAUSE URINARY INCONTINENCE

α-Adrenergic agonists (phenylpropanolamine, pseudoephedrine)
α-Adrenergic antagonists (doxazosin, prazosin, terazosin)
Analgesics
Antidepressants
Anticholinergics (propantheline, oxybutynin)
Antihistamines (includes over-the-counter cold medications)
Antipsychotics
Calcium channel blockers
Diuretics
Sedatives
Tranquilizers

TABLE 10-8.—Primary Treatments for Different Types of Geriatric
Urinary Incontinence

TYPE OF INCONTINENCE	PRIMARY TREATMENTS
Stress	Pelvic floor (Kegel's) exercises α-Adrenergic agonists (e.g., phenylpropanolamine or pseudoephedrine) Estrogen Biofeedback, behavioral training Surgical bladder neck suspension
Overflow	Surgical removal of obstruction Intermittent catheterization (if practical) Indwelling catheterization
Urge	Bladder relaxants (e.g., propantheline, flavoxate, or oxybutynin) Estrogen (if vaginal atrophy present) Training procedures (e.g., biofeedback, behavioral therapy Surgical removal of obstruction or other irritating pathological lesions
Psychological (functional)	Behavioral therapies (e.g., habit training, scheduled toileting) Environmental manipulations Incontinence undergarments and pads External collection devices Bladder relaxants (selected patients) Indwelling catheters (selected patients)

TABLE 10-9.—Simple Office Testing of Lower Urinary Tract Function

TEST	PROCEDURE	INTERPRETATION
1. Stress test	With full bladder, cough 3 times in standing position with filter paper at urethra	Urine leakage indicates stress incontinence
2. Normal voiding volume	Patient asked to empty bladder into measuring "hat"	Small volumes may indicate obstruction; check for straining, hesitancy; <200 ml = urge, 300-500 ml = stress, <200 ml or >600 ml = overflow
3. Residual urine	Pass sterile 14 F catheter into bladder after voiding	Obstruction is indicated by difficult passage; ≥100 ml urine indicates obstruction or contractility problem
4. Bladder filling	Fill bladder with sterile room temperature saline through 14 F catheter attached to 50-ml catheter tip syringe without piston. Pinch catheter while filling 50-ml measure to ensure accurate volumes	Note volume at first urge to void; note involuntary contractions and volume of urine lost. Severe urgency or urine involuntarily lost at ≤300 ml suggests urge incontinence; >600 ml suggests overflow

Modified from Ouslander JG, Leach GE, Staskin DR: *J Am Geriatr Soc* 37:706, 1989.

INDWELLING CATHETERS

TABLE 10-10.—INDICATIONS AND CARE OF INDWELLING CATHETERS

Indications
Urinary retention
Skin wounds, pressure sores
Terminally ill
Patient and caregiver preference

Technique for Care
Insert with careful aseptic technique, use 16-18 F size with 5-ml balloon
Secure catheter to leg to minimize urethral trauma
Cleanse perineum twice daily with Hibiclens antiseptic soap
Keep system closed; open only at bag
Irrigate only *after* infection is established (use 0.25% acetic acid solution)
Do not routinely use suppressive antibiotics
Obtain specimens for culture by sterile needle aspiration from distal catheter
   (after cleansing with antiseptic soap and sterile water)
Always place collection bag below bladder
Topical antibiotic ointment should be applied to meatus once daily
Change catheter only if obstructed or malfunctioning
Separate bacteriuric from nonbacteriuric patients
Discontinue use as soon as possible
Maintain at least 2 L of fluid intake daily
Symptomatic (temperature < 102° F and normotensive) beyond 24 hours, give
   broad-spectrum antibiotics. If serious (temperature > 102° F and hypoten-
   sive), obtain urine and blood cultures, hospitalize, prescribe parenteral
   antibiotics

Paraphimosis

When a phimotic foreskin of the uncircumcised male is retracted behind the glans penis, edema may develop and trap the prepuce so that it cannot be replaced. This condition occurs more frequently in small children and elderly, demented males. Most foreskin can be retracted by manipulation; some will require dorsal slit surgery (Table 10-11).

TABLE 10-11.—MANAGEMENT OF PARAPHIMOSIS

Retraction Techniques
Administer sedation; relieve pain
Lubricate the corona with K-Y jelly
Then
Grasp the penis, and apply firm pressure around the circumference of the swollen area. Maintain pressure for 5-10 minutes to reduce the swelling, then try to gently draw the incarcerated foreskin forward over the glans
Or
Apply pressure as above, then place the index and third fingers behind the edematous mass with the thumb on the meatus. Then apply opposing pressure to withdraw the foreskin back over the glans

Dorsal Slit Surgery
Prep with antibacterial soap such as povidine-iodine
Identify the opening of the prepuce, which appears as a constricting band within the edematous mass
Infiltrate this area with 1% lidocaine, used sparingly so as to not increase the edema
With a no. 15 blade, incise through the constricting band, extending the incision as necessary
Reduce the paraphimosis
Hemostasis is usually accomplished by a few minutes of pressure
Elective circumcision can be done when the dorsal slit is healed

INFECTIONS

TABLE 10-12.—Workup and Treatment of Urinary Tract Infections in Children

CAUSES	WORKUP
30%-50% have anomalies All boys and girls < 6 years of age and girls > 6 years of age with ≥ 2 UTIs should be worked up as soon as urine becomes sterile Vesicoureteral reflux should be considered a medical (antibiotic suppression) problem; 20%-30% resolve within a 2-year period; overall long-term disappearance rate is 80% Obstruction is a surgical problem	Renal sonogram and voiding cystogram; *isotope cystogram* is more sensitive for vesicoureteral reflux in girls; *contrast cystograms* are better to evaluate the urethra in boys ^{99m}Tc-DTPA renal scan for diagnosing obstruction* ^{99m}Tc-DMSA if reflux is detected to look for renal scarring or interstitial pyelonephritis

Treatment for Acute UTIs

Age Group	Drug	Dose
Infants	Amoxicillin	5-7 Days of 20 mg/kg/day given in three doses
Child > 3 months	Trimethoprim-sulfamethoxazole	5-7 Days of 8 mg of TMP and 40 mg of SMX/kg/day in two doses
Child with high fever, vomiting, sepsis, known vesicoureteral reflux	Parenteral antibiotics	Ampicillin + aminoglycoside until afebrile for 48 hours; then oral antibiotic specific to culture (for 4-6 weeks)

Modified from O'Brien WM, Gibbons MD: *Am Fam Physician* 1988; 38(1)101-112.
*NOTE: Radionuclide scanning is now preferred over IV urogram for children.

TABLE 10-13.—Selecting Patients for Single-Dose Therapy of Acute Cystitis

Selection
Patient is reliable female who will return for follow-up visits
Contraindications to single dose therapy include pregnancy, diabetes, renal disease, anatomical urinary anomaly, allergy to drug, symptoms for >6 days, immunocompromise, postmenopausal, urinary tract infection in the past 6 weeks, upper urinary tract infection

Treatment
Trimethoprim-sulfamethoxazole, two or three double-strength tablets PO or
Amoxicillin, 3 g PO or
Sulfisoxazole, 2 g PO or Trimethoprim (Proloprim), 400 mg PO

Follow-up Care
Culture 14 days after treatment

TABLE 10-14.—Overview of Outpatient Antimicrobial Therapy for Lower Urinary Tract Infections in Adults

INDICATIONS	ANTIMICROBIAL AGENT (ORAL ADMINISTRATION)	DOSE	INTERVAL	DURATION (DAYS)
Lower urinary tract infection	Amoxicillin, 250- or 500-mg capsule	6 × 500-mg capsules 1 or 2 × 250-mg capsules	Single dose Every 8 hours	— 3, 7, or 10
	Ciprofloxacin, 500-mg tablet	1 Tablet	Every 12 hours	7 or 10
	Nitrofurantoin macrocrystals (Macrodantin), 50 or 100-mg capsule	1 Capsule	Every 6 hours	3, 7, or 10
	Norfloxacin, 400-mg tablet	1 Tablet	Every 12 hours	3, 7, or 10
	Ofloxacin, 200-mg tablet	1 Tablet	Every 12 hours	7 or 10
	Sulfisoxazole, 500-mg tablet	4 Tablets 2 Tablets	Single dose Every 6 hours	— 7-10
	Trimethoprim, 100-mg tablet	1 Tablet	Every 12 hours	3, 7, or 10
	Trimethoprim-sulfamethoxazole, double-strength tablet*	2 Tablets 1 Tablet	Single dose Every 12 hours	— 3, 7, or 10

Acute urethral syndrome: initial therapy	Amoxicillin, 500-mg capsule	6 Capsules	Single dose	—
	Trimethoprim-sulfamethoxazole, double-strength tablet*	2 Tablets	Single dose	—
After failure	Doxycycline, 100-mg capsule	1 Capsule	Every 12 hours	10
Long-term prophylaxis against recurrent bacteriuria				
First-choice agents	Trimethoprim-sulfamethoxazole, single-strength tablet†	½ Tablet	Every evening	≥6 months
	Nitrofurantoin, 50-mg capsule	1 Capsule	Every evening	≥6 months
	Trimethoprim, 100-mg tablet	½ Tablet	Every evening	≥6 months

From Wilhelm MP, Edson RS: *Mayo Clin Proc* 62:1025, 1987.
*Each double-strength tablet consists of 160 mg of trimethoprim and 800 mg of sulfamethoxazole.
†Each single-strength table consists of 80 mg of trimethoprim and 400 mg of sulfamethoxazole.

TABLE 10-15.—ACUTE PYELONEPHRITIS

Definition
Upper urinary tract infection of the renal parenchyma. As many as one third of patients presumed to have only cystitis will also have "occult" pyelonephritis. This condition is defined clinically as fever, chills, flank pain, nausea, vomiting, myalgias, pyuria, WBC casts in the urine, and bacteriuria.

Risk Factors for Occult Pyelonephritis
Diabetes
History of >3 UTIs within 1 year
Hospital-acquired infection
Immunosuppression or immunoincompetency
Indwelling catheter
Lower socioeconomic status
Nephrolithiasis
Neurological disorder
Pregnancy
Prior history of pyelonephritis
Prior history of urinary infection before adolescence
Recent antibiotic use
Recent urological manipulation or surgery
Symptoms for > 1 week before seeking treatment

Causative Organisms
E. coli (80%-90%)
Proteus and *Klebsiella* (4%-10%)
Staphylococcus aureus or *Candida albicans* (hematogenous) (3%-8%)
Pseudomonas or Providencia (immunosuppressed) (1%)
Mycobacterium tuberculosis (5% of active TB patients) (<1%)
Torulopsis glabrata (diabetes) (<1%)

Imaging Studies
Do for: 1. A child under 5 years of age
        2. A female who fails to respond promptly to therapy
        3. All males
CT Scan: Shows renal enlargement, poor corticomedullary definition, perinephric abscess
IVP/US: Shows obstruction, perinephric abscess, urinary tract anomalies, urinary stones

Management (Fig. 10-5)

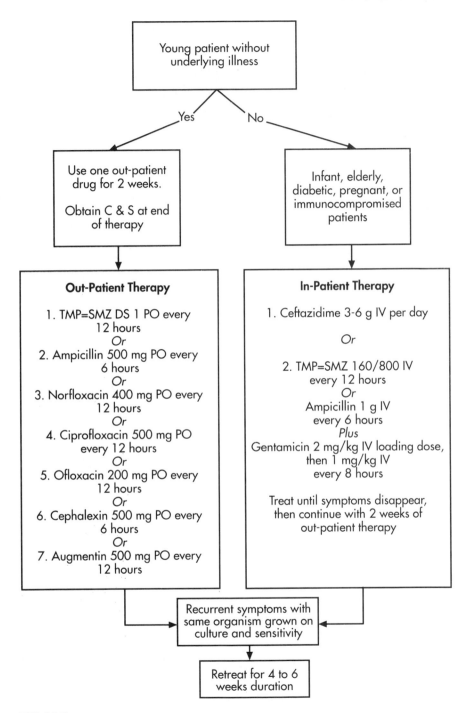

FIG 10-5.
Management of acute pyelonephritis.

TABLE 10-16.—Asymptomatic Bacteriuria

The Problem
The prevalence of asymptomatic bacteriuria as defined by 2 or more cultures
  yielding the same organism at $>10^5$ bacteria/ml is 15%-20%. Symptomatic
  urinary tract infection will develop in 40% of these patients

Indications for Therapy of Asymptomatic Bacteriuria
Before urinary tract instrumentation or surgery
In patients with diabetes
In immunocompromised patients

Prevention of Symptomatic Infections
Correct underlying pathology (e.g., prolapse, obstruction)
Estrogen replacement therapy
Increase mobility
Improve bladder emptying (e.g., reduce prolapse, discontinue anticholinergic
  drugs, use double-voiding technique, Créde's maneuver)
Improve perineal hygiene
Minimize instrumentation and catheter use
Prophylactic antibiotics if recurrent infections

TABLE 10-17.—TREATMENT OF SEXUALLY TRANSMITTED DISEASES

TYPE/CONDITION	RECOMMENDED REGIMEN	ALTERNATIVE
Gonorrhea		
Urethral, cervical, rectal, pharyngeal	Ceftriaxone 125 mg IM once *plus* doxycycline 100 mg PO bid for 7 days	Spectinomycin 2 g IM once *plus* erythromycin 500 mg PO QID for 7 days
Disseminated	Ceftriaxone 1 g IV every 24 hours for 7-10 days	Ceftizoxime 1 g IV every 8 hours for 2-3 days followed by Cefixime 400 mg PO bid to complete 7-10 days
Ophthalmic (adult)	Ceftriaxone 1 g IM once *plus* saline irrigation	Ceftriaxone 1 g IV daily for 5 days *plus* saline irrigation
Meningitis	Ceftriaxone 2 g IV daily for 10-14 days	Penicillin G 10 million U/day IV for 10 days
Endocarditis	Ceftriaxone 2 g IV daily for 4 weeks	
Children	If ≥ 45 kg, use adult regimen; if < 45 kg, ceftriaxone 125 mg IM once; and if ≥ 8 years of age, add doxycycline 100 mg PO bid for 7 days	
Syphilis		
Early	Benzathine penicillin G, 2.4 million U IM once	Doxycycline 100 mg PO bid for 2 weeks *or* erythromycin 500 mg PO qid for 2 weeks if compliance is assured
Late latent (>1 year)	Benzathine penicillin G, 2.4 million U 1 time/week for 3 doses (total 7.2 million U)	Doxycycline 100 mg PO bid for 4 weeks
Neurosyphilis	Aqueous crystalline penicillin G, 2-4 million U IV every 4 hours for 10-14 days (total 12-24 million U day)	Desensitize penicillin allergic patients
Congenital	Aqueous crystalline penicillin G 50,000 U/kg IV every 8-12 hours for 10-14 days (total 100,000-150,000 U)	

Modified from *Med Let Drugs Ther* 36(913):1-6, Jan. 7, 1994.

Continued.

TABLE 10-17.—Treatment of Sexually Transmitted Diseases—cont'd

TYPE/CONDITION	RECOMMENDED REGIMEN	ALTERNATIVE
Chancroid	Erythromycin 500 mg PO qid for 7 days *or* ceftriaxone 250 mg IM once	Azithromycin 1 g PO once *or* Cipro-floxacin 5C0 mg PO bid for 3 days
Lymphogranuloma Venereum	Doxycycline 100 mg PO bid for 21 days	Erythromycin 500 mg PO qid for 21 days
Genital Herpes Simplex		
First clinical episode	Acyclovir 400 mg PO 3 times a day for 7-10 days	Acyclovir 20C mg PO 5 times a day for 7-10 days
Severe disease	Acyclovir 5 mg/kg IV every 8 hours for 5-7 days	
Herpes proctitis	Acyclovir 800 mg PO 3 times a day for 7-10 days	
Recurrent	Acyclovir 400 mg PO 3 times a day for 5 days	
Daily suppressive	Acyclovir 400 mg PO 2 times a day	Acyclovir 200 mg PO 2-5 times a day
Genital Warts	Cryotherapy with liquid nitrogen or cryoprobe	10%-25% podophyllum *or* 80%-90% trichloracetic acid (TCA) or electro-desiccation
Chlamydial Infections		
Urethral, endocervical, or rectal	Azithromycin 1 g once or doxycycline 100 mg PO bid for 7 days	Erythromycin 500 mg PO qid for 7 days *or* ofloxacim 300 mg PO bid for 7 days
Pregnant	Erythromycin 500 mg PO qid for 7 days	Erythromycin 250 mg PO qid for 14 days or amoxicillin 500 mg PO tid for 10 days
Epididymitis	Ceftriaxone 250 mg IM once *plus* doxycycline 100 mg PO bid for 10 days	Ciprofloxacin 500 mg PO once plus doxycycline 100 mg PO bid for 10 days

Pelvic Inflammatory Disease

Outpatients (no concern for fertility)	Ceftriaxone 250 mg IM once *or* cefoxitin 2 g IM *plus* probenecid 1 g PO *plus* doxycycline 100 mg PO bid for 14 days	Ofloxacin 400 mg PO bid *plus* clindamycin 450 mg PO qid for 14 days
Inpatients	Cefoxitin 2 g IV every 6 hours *plus* doxycycline 100 mg IV bid until 48 hours after clinical improvement, then continue doxycycline dose orally for 10-14 days	Clindamycin 900 mg IV every 8 hours *plus* gentamycin 2 mg/kg loading dose (IM or IV) followed by 1.5 mg/kg every 8 hours; 48 hours after clinical improvement, continue doxycycline 100 mg PO bid for 10-14 days
Vaginal Trichomoniasis	Metronidazole 2 g PO in 1 dose *or* 500 mg PO bid for 7 days	
Vaginal Candidiasis	Miconazole nitrate 200 mg vaginal suppository qhs for 3 days *or* clotrimazole 200-mg vaginal tablet qhs for 3 days *or* terconazole 80 mg suppository *or* 0.4% cream vaginally qhs for 3 days	Fluconazole 150 mg PO once
Bacterial Vaginosis	Metronidazole 500 mg PO bid for 7 days	Clindamycin 300 mg PO bid for 7 days or topical metronidazole or clindamycin
Hepatitis B	Postexposure, hepatitis B immune globulin (HBIG) 0.06 ml/kg IM once *plus* immediately begin hepatitis B vaccine series	
Cytomegalovirus	No therapy exists	
Pediculosis and Scabies	1% Permethrin for pediculosis, 5% permethrin for scabies	

SEXUALLY TRANSMITTED DISEASES (STDs)

HPV types 16 and 18 are clearly associated with precancers and invasive cancers of the lower female genital tract. Since HPV is an STD, male partners of these women should be examined for subclinical infection that may be present in up to 80% of cases (Table 10-18).

TABLE 10-18.—ANDROSCOPY: DETECTION OF OCCULT PAPILLOMAVIRUS INFECTION

Indications
Men who have sexual partners with known HPV infection
Men who have had sex with prostitutes or $\geq$ 20 sexual partners
Men who have (or who have had) penile warts
Men who have bowenoid papillosis

Technique for Detection
An initial colposcopic examination should be made before staining to identify any lesions. The supine patient may be placed in stirrups in the lithotomy position, and if uncircumcised, foreskin should be withdrawn and held back by the patient for examination of the glans. Examine glans, shaft and scrotal skin, perineal body, and perianal tissues.
Soak gauze 4 × 4's in a 5% acetic acid solution and allow to remain in contact with the skin that needs to be examined for approximately 5 minutes. More dilute solutions (e.g., 3%) are less effective on the keratinized squamous epithelium; however, 3% acetic acid may be more comfortable for mucosal surfaces such as the glans of the uncircumcised male.
Carefully repeat the colposcope examination looking for acetowhite lesions.
Biopsy of acetowhite lesions may be performed using local anesthetic with 0.1 to 0.2 ml of 1% lidocaine inserted sublesionally. The lesion may be shaved with a scalpel blade and removed with conventional colposcopic biopsy forceps, or a skin biopsy may be taken using punch biopsy technique.
Accomplish hemostasis with topical styptic.
Biopsy specimens may be submitted in formalin for histological examination.

Aftercare
When biopsy report returns indicating HPV infection, lesions identified by their acetowhite change may be treated with topical application of 75% trichloroacetic acid, cryotherapy, or carbon dioxide laser fulguration. Recurrence rates may be as high as 10%-50%.

INTERSTITIAL CYSTITIS

TABLE 10-19.—INTERSTITIAL CYSTITIS

Underdiagnosed and difficult to treat condition of the bladder
Urinalysis results are usually normal; 10% of patients may have ≥ 5 RBCs/HPF; urine culture is sterile despite occasional pyuria
Patients must have all three of the following criteria:
1. Irritative voiding symptoms: urgency, frequency, suprapubic or pelvic pain relieved by voiding, dyspareunia
2. Absence of other urological disease; normal x-ray and cystometric studies
3. Cystoscopic evidence: focal ulceration, edema, perineural-perivascular infiltrates, increased mast cells in detrusor muscle biopsy specimens
Treatments vary from medical, surgical, to laser therapy with less than optimal success.

CALCULI

Urinary calculi are manifested by pain over the T12-L1 dermatomes, hematuria (10%-15% gross), and dysuria. Fever, urinary retention, and vomiting may be present.

TABLE 10-20.—URINARY CALCULI

Urinary Calculi Composition

Type	Incidence	X-ray
Calcium oxalate or phosphate	75% of stones	Opaque
Calcium phosphate with magnesium ammonia phosphate	15% of stones	Opaque
Uric acid	7% of stones	Lucent
Cystine	2% of stones	Opaque
Other types	1% of stones	? Opaque

Diagnosis
Family history, diet history (high calcium, vitamin D, inadequate fluid intake, drugs)
Complete physical examination to rule out malignancy and chronic disease
Urinalysis and C & S
pH > 7.5 = infection
pH < 5.5 = uric acid
Serum BUN and creatinine, creatinine clearance rates
Serum electrolytes, calcium, phosphorus, uric acid, glucose, alkaline phosphatase and total protein; serum parathormone if calcium is elevated
24-hour urine for uric acid, cystine, and oxalate
IVP with delayed films; retrograde pyelogram if obstruction
Stone analysis

Management
Increase urine volumes to >2 L/day to dilute urinary crystalloids
Vigorously treat any infection, consider prophylaxis
Rule out hyperparathyroidism
Stones caused by renal tubular acidosis (e.g., low potassium and carbon dioxide; high chloride); treat with alkalinization (citrate mixture of sodium bicarbonate).
Thiazide (hydrochlorthiazide 50 mg bid) diuretics to reduce urinary calcium for patients with renal leak hypercalciuria
Orthophosphates decrease urinary calcium and improve solubilizing effect
Low oxalate diet and pyridoxine to treat hyperoxaluria; cholestyramine to bind oxalate
Magnesium oxide (200 mg tid) plus pyridoxine (25 mg/day) for treatment of calcium oxalate stones
Methylene blue (65 mg tid) for recurrent calcium stones
Alkalinization of urine to pH 7.0 to prevent uric acid stone formation
Add allopurinol (300 mg/day) if serum uric acid is elevated
Potassium citrate 60 mEq/day for hyperuricosuria and to inhibit crystallization of calcium oxalate
Alkalinization of urine to pH of 7.8 or more, high fluid intake, low-calcium diet for cystine stones (low methionine diet raises cystine)
Add D-penicillamine and pyridoxine for large amounts of urinary cystine
Single stone, young and healthy, normal lab and IVP: increase fluid volumes only

TABLE 10-21.—WORKUP OF HYPERCALCIURIA AND NEPHROLITHIASIS*

| | PRIMARY HYPERPARATHYROIDISM | ABSORPTIVE HYPERCALCIURIAS | | HYPOPHOSPHATEMIC HYPERCALCIURIA | RENAL LEAK HYPERCALCIURIA | HYPEROXALURIA OF ENTERIC CAUSE | HYPERURICOSURIC CALCIUM OXALATE NEPHROLITHIASIS |
		TYPE I	TYPE II				
Percent of patients	5	24	20	7	6	3	7
Serum calcium	E	N	N	N	N	L/N	N
Serum phosphorus	L/N	N	N	L	N	L/N	N
Urinary calcium	E/N	E	N	E/N	E	L	N
Serum PTH†	E	L/N	L/N	L/N	E	E/N	N
Urinary cyclic AMP	E	L/N	L/N	L/N	E	E/N	N
Urinary uric acid	E/N	E/N	E/N	E/N	E/N	L	E
Urinary oxalate	E/N	E/N	E/N	E/N	E/N	E	N
Urinary citrate	N	L/N	L/N	L/N	L/N	L	L/N
Bone density‡	L/N	N	N	N	L/N	L/N	N
Fractional calcium absorption§	E/N	E	E/N	E/N	E/N	L	N
Urinary pH	N	N	N	N	N	L/N	L

*E, Elevated; N, normal; L, low.
†PTH, Parathyroid hormone.
‡Bone density in distal third of radius by phcton absorptiometry.
§Fractional calcium absorption-fecal recovery of radioactivity after oral ingestion of 100 mg radioactive calcium.

TABLE 10-22.—Extracorporeal Shock Wave Lithotripsy (ESWL)

Successful clearance in 3 months (50% 90%); kidney stone prognosis better than ureteral.

Contraindications to ESWL
Obstruction distal to stone
Coagulopathy, bleeding dyscrasia
Pregnancy
Marked obesity (>300 lb)

Postprocedure Problems; Monitor for Occurrence
Ureteral obstruction, 4%
Hemorrhage (usually inconsequential but up to ⅓ require transfusion), 20%-30%
Hypertension, 10% up to 1 yr
Cardiac dysrhythmias, 1%

Modified from Atala A, Steinbock GS: *Am J Surg* 157:350, 1989.

HEMATURIA AND PROTEINURIA

TABLE 10-23.—Differential Diagnosis of Asymptomatic Hematuria

AGE GROUP	DIAGNOSTIC POSSIBILITIES	CHARACTERISTICS
Neonates and toddlers	Nephroblastoma, renal vein thrombosis, polycystic kidney disease, obstructive uropathy, medullary sponge kidney, occult trauma, abuse, *infection,* coagulopathy, ischemic injury	Usually manifested by gross hematuria, invariably serious in nature; aggressive workup indicated
Children aged 5-15 years	Glomerulonephritis, sickle cell disease or trait, acute hemorrhagic cystitis, trauma, menstruation, hypercalciuria, drugs, infection	Usually benign disorders with a good prognosis; workup needs to exclude reduced renal function
Young adults (after puberty to age 40)	Honeymoon cystitis, schistosomiasis, exercise induced, associated with pregnancy, urinary calculi, inflammatory bladder conditions, bladder tumor, essential hematuria, urethritis	Rarely due to a life-threatening or surgical lesion; evaluation can usually stop after IVP and cystoscopy
Adults 40 and older	Renal or bladder neoplasm, urinary calculi, analgesic nephropathy, prostatic disease, anticoagulants	Suspect neoplastic disorder until proved otherwise; complete workup indicated

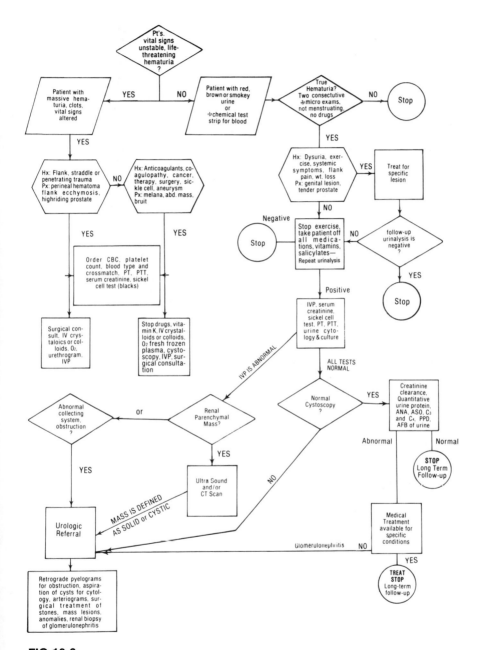

FIG 10-6.
Primary care of hematuria. (Modified from Driscoll CE: *Emerg Decisions* 1(4):35, 1985.)

TABLE 10-24.—Determining the Significance of Proteinuria

True Proteinuria
When urinalysis dipstick test is positive for protein you may perform the following sulfosalicylic acid (Exton's) test:
1. Collect fresh, concentrated urine by clean catch method.
2. Add 8 drops of 20% sulfosalicylic acid to 2 ml of urine.
Exton's test also detects nonalbumin proteins. Protein concentration is directly proportional to white turbidity.
+Dipstick/−Exton's → False positive dipstick
+Dipstick/++Exton's → Suspect nonalbumin protein
+Dipstick/+Exton's → Confirms presence of protein

Orthostatic Proteinuria
Caused by upright body posture; prognosis probably benign. Instruct patient to do the following:
Void at 7 AM and discard urine
Collect all urine 7 AM to 9 PM in container no. 1
Assume recumbent position from 9 PM until 7 AM
Void 11 PM urine into container no. 1
Collect all urines 11 PM to and including 7 AM voiding in container no. 2
Determine urinary protein and creatinine for both containers
Orthostatic proteinuria: Total 24-hour protein greater than 150 mg with less than 75 mg excreted over 8 hours in recumbent position

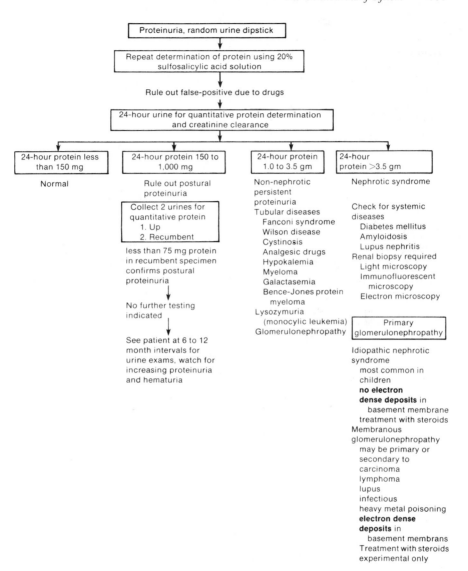

FIG 10-7.
Evaluation for asymptomatic proteinuria. (From Weber H Jr: *Contin Ed Fam Physician* 8:18, 1978.)

TABLE 10-25.—THE NEPHROTIC SYNDROME

Diagnosis
>3.5 g/day of proteinuria
Hypoalbuminemia
Edema
Hyperlipidemia
Lipiduria

Classification
Primary (idiopathic): Minimal change or membranous glomerulonephritis
Secondary: Associated with diabetes, cancer, amyloidosis, lupus erythemato-
   sus, drug induced

Laboratory Evidence Needed
On all patients: Serum multichemistry profile, CBC, UA, serum lipids, 24-hour
   urine collection for protein and creatinine clearance
On selected patients: ANA, rheumatoid factor, hepatitis B antigen, serum and
   urine protein electrophoresis, ESR

Treatment
For primary subtype: An empiric trial of prednisone can be given starting with 2
   mg/kg/day for 1 week, then qod for 7 weeks. About 80% of adults respond
   and are believed to have minimal change disease. If no response is evident,
   proceed to referral for renal biopsy.
For secondary subtype: Remove or treat the underlying cause. Restrict sodium;
   judiciously use loop diuretics to reduce edema; and give a trial of bed rest. A
   low dose of an ACE inhibitor or calcium channel blocker (verapamil or dil-
   tiazem but *not* nifedipine or other dihydropyridine) is indicated for patients
   with diabetes. Use lipid lowering agents if needed.

PROSTATE DISEASE

TABLE 10-30.—Recommendations for Use of Prostate-Specific Antigen (PSA)

PSA is positive (>4.0 ng/ml) in 16.1% of patients tested and 30.6% are true positives. The sensitivity of PSA is 78.4% and the specificity is 50.7%; the positive predictive value is 30.6.

Conditions to Consider when PSA is >4.0
Prostate cancer
Benign prostatic hyperplasia
Prostatitis
Prostatic manipulation

Improving the Accuracy of PSA
Use age-specific PSA norms
Age   40-49 = 0-2.5 ng/ml
      50-59 = 0-3.5 ng/ml
      60-69 = 0-4.5 ng/ml
      70-79 = 0-6.5 ng/ml
Use PSAΔ (PSA velocity)
Suspect cancer if PSA increases >20% or >0.75 ng/ml in 1 year.
Use PSAD (PSA density)
Suspect cancer if PSA is between 4.0-10.0 ng/ml and the PSAD is >0.58.

$$PSAD = \frac{\text{Serum PSA in ng/ml}}{\text{Volume of Prostate in ml by TRUS*}}$$

From Small EJ: Prostate cancer: who to screen, and what the results mean, *Geriatrics* 48:28, Dec. 1993; Hudson MA: Screening for prostate cancer: is it worthwhile? *Contemp Urol* p.37, March 1994; Ruckle HC, Klee GG, Oesterling JE: Prostate-specific antigen: critical issues for the practicing physician, *Mayo Clin Proc* 69:59, 1994.
TRUS, Transrectal ultrasound.

TABLE 10-27.—PROSTATIC DISEASES

CONDITION	SYMPTOMS	EXAMINATION	LAB STUDIES	TREATMENT
Benign hypertrophy	Nocturia, hesitancy, urge incontinence, dribbling, decreased urine flow, obstruction	Smooth, symmetrical enlargement	>150 ml postvoid residual, urinalysis, IVP, cystoscopy, urine flow studies, serum PSA	TURP, balloon dilation, α-blocker, finasteride
Acute bacterial prostatitis	Sudden onset of fever, chills, malaise, arthralgia, frequency, dysuria, pain in perineum	Tender and warm prostate, boggy enlargement (examine gingerly)	Urine culture, blood culture, avoid catheterization	IV antibiotics, analgesics, stool softeners, NSAIDs
Prostatic abscess	Acute bacterial prostatitis with spiking fevers and rectal pain, chills	Firm, tender, or fluctuant mass	Elevated blood glucose level, persistent leukocytosis despite antibiotics	Surgical drainage and antibiotics
Chronic bacterial prostatitis	Recurrent UTIs, irritative voiding symptoms, no systemic signs	Prostatic calculi, boggy enlargement	Persistent bacteria in prostatic fluid, hematospermia, split-voided urinalysis	4-6 weeks of antibiotic therapy, surgery if calculi
Nonbacterial prostatitis	Frequency, urgency, dysuria, testicular or penile pain; no systemic signs and no recurrent UTIs	Prostate may be normal on examination	≥10 WBCs/HPF in prostatic secretions, no bacteria, lipid-laden prostatic macrophages, cystoscopy to rule out interstitial cystitis	Oxybutynin 5 mg PO tid or propantheline 15 mg PO tid or diazepam 2 mg PO tid
Prostatodynia	Painful prostate, symptoms similar to chronic bacterial or nonbacterial prostatitis, history of sexual or marital difficulties	Normal prostate on examination, pelvic muscle tension	Prostatic secretions without WBCs	Prazosin 1 mg PO bid or baclofen 5-10 mg PO tid, warm sitz baths, psychosocial support

TABLE 10-28.—Prostatitis

Acute inflammation increases vascular permeability and antibiotics may gain easier access; chronic prostatic infection is "protected" from most antibiotics, which fail to diffuse into prostatic fluid.

Best antibiotics to use will:

Be lipid soluble

Have ionization potential (pKa) $\geq$ 8.6

Have gram-negative spectrum at pH of 6.6

Have low degree of protein binding

Type	Organisms	Drug	Duration
Acute infection	Gram-negative coliforms, enterococci	Aminoglycoside or ampicillin	7-10 days
Chronic infection	Gram-negative coliforms, *Chlamydia*	Trimethoprim-sulfamethoxazole, doxycycline, or erythromycin	2-3 months

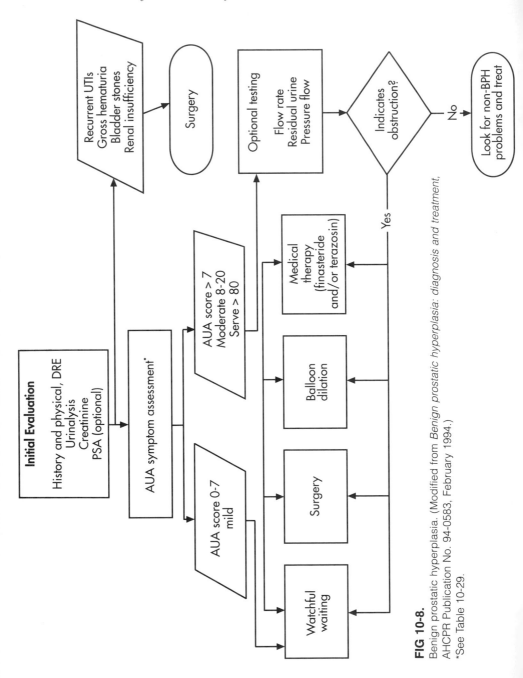

FIG 10-8.
Benign prostatic hyperplasia. (Modified from *Benign prostatic hyperplasia: diagnosis and treatment,*
AHCPR Publication No. 94-0583, February 1994.)
*See Table 10-29.

TABLE 10-29.—AUA Symptom Index

| QUESTIONS TO BE ANSWERED | AUA SYMPTOM SCORE (CIRCLE 1 NUMBER ON EACH LINE) | | | | | |
	NOT AT ALL	LESS THAN 1 TIME IN 5	LESS THAN HALF THE TIME	ABOUT HALF THE TIME	MORE THAN HALF THE TIME	ALMOST ALWAYS
1. Over the past month, how often have you had a sensation of not emptying your bladder completely after you finished urinating?	0	1	2	3	4	5
2. Over the past month, how often have you had to urinate again less than 2 hours after you finished urinating?	0	1	2	3	4	5
3. Over the past month, how often have you found you stopped and started again several times when you urinated?	0	1	2	3	4	5
4. Over the past month, how often have you found it difficult to postpone urination?	0	1	2	3	4	5
5. Over the past month, how often have you had a weak urinary stream?	0	1	2	3	4	5
6. Over the past month, how often have you had to push or strain to begin urination?	0	1	2	3	4	5
7. Over the past month, how many times did you most typically get up to urinate from the time you went to bed at night until the time you got up in the morning?	0 (None)	1 (1 time)	2 (2 times)	3 (3 times)	4 (4 times)	5 (5 times)

Sum of 7 circled numbers (AUA Symptom Score): _____

From Barry MJ, et al: The American Urological Association symptom index for benign prostatic hyperplasia, *J Urol* 148:1549, Nov. 1992.

TABLE 10-30.—Balance Sheet for Benign Prostatic Hyperplasia (BPH) Treatment Outcomes

DIRECT TREATMENT OUTCOMES	SURGICAL OPTIONS				NONSURGICAL OPTIONS		
	BALLOON DILATION	TUIP	OPEN SURGERY	TURP	WATCHFUL WAITING	α-BLOCKERS	FINASTERIDE
1. Chance for improvement of symptoms (90% confidence interval)	37%-76%	78%-83%	94%-99.8%	75%-96%	31%-55%	59%-86%	54%-78%
2. Degree of symptom improvement (percent reduction in symptom score)	51%	73%	79%	85%	Unknown	51%	31%
3. Morbidity/complications associated with surgical or medical treatment (90% confidence interval), about 20% of all complications assumed to be significant	1.78%-9.86%	2.2%-33.3%	6.98%-42.7%	5.2%-30.7%	1%-5% Complications from BPH progression	2.9%-43.3%	13.6%-18.8%
4. Chance of dying within 30-90 days	0.72%-9.78% (high-risk/	0.2%-1.5%	0.99%-4.56%	0.53%-3.31%	0.8% Chance of death ≤90 days for 67-year-old man		

	...of treatment (90% confidence interval) ...elderly patients)					Incontinence associated with aging
5. Risk of total urinary incontinence (90% confidence interval)	Unknown	0.06%-1.1%	0.34%-0.74%	0.68%-1.4%	0	
6. Need for operative treatment for surgical complications in future (90% confidence interval)	Unknown	1.34%-2.65%	0.6%-14.1%	0.65%-10.1%	0	0
7. Risk of impotence (90% confidence interval)	No long-term follow-up available	3.9%-24.5%	4.7%-39.2%	3.3%-34.8%	0	About 2% of men age 67 become impotent every year. Long-term data on α-blockers are not available.
8. Risk of retrograde ejaculation (percent of patients)	Unknown	6%-55%	36%-95%	25%-99%	4%-11%	2.5%-5.3% (also decreased volume of ejaculate)
9. Loss of work time (days)	4	7-21	21-28	7-21	1	1.5
10. Hospital stay (days)	1	1-3	5-10	3-5	0	0

McConnell JD, et al: Benign prostatic hyperplasia: diagnosis and treatment, *Clinical practice guideline*, Number 8, AHCPR Publication No. 94-0582, Rockville, MD, Agency for Health Care Policy and Research, Public Health Service, U.S. Department of Health and Human Services, February 1994, pp. 196-197.

Assessment of Treatment Outcomes for BPH

Explanation of Balance Sheet (Table 10-29)

Line 1: Likelihood that given patient will experience some symptom improvement; likelihood of improvement greater if pretreatment symptoms more severe

Line 2: Expected amount of improvement (for patients who improve)

Line 3: Likelihood that given patient will have treatment complications or adverse events

Line 4: Likelihood that given patient will die from any causes within 3 months of treatment

Line 5: Likelihood that a given patient will experience total incontinence caused by the treatment

Line 6: Likelihood that given patient will require surgical correction for a late complication of BPH treatment, such as bladder neck contracture or urethral stricture

Line 7: Likelihood that a patient who was potent before treatment will experience impotence following treatment

Line 8: Likelihood that a patient who was potent before treatment and still potent after treatment will experience retrograde ejaculation following treatment

Line 9: Estimated number of days a given patient may miss from work during first year of treatment

Line 10: Estimated number of days spent in the hospital

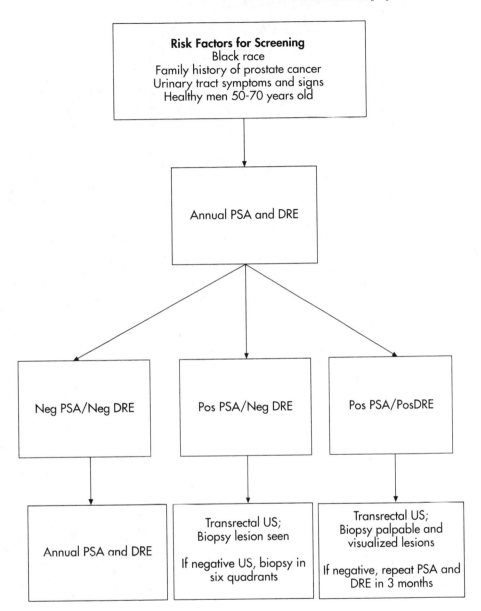

FIG 10-9.
Strategies for diagnosis of prostatic cancer.

ABNORMALITIES OF THE GENITALIA

TABLE 10-31.—Scrotal Problems

CONDITION	CLINICAL DIFFERENTIATION	DIAGNOSTIC STUDIES	TREATMENT
Cryptorchidism	Nonexistent testicle, asymptomatic	Chromosome studies if bilateral	Surgical exploration
Epididymo-orchitis	Gradual onset (hours-days), worsening incrementally; late adolescence to young adults; elevating scrotum decreases pain	Nuclear scan with technetium reveals increased blood flow; normal Doppler study; >10 WBCs/HPF in prostatic secretions	Bed rest, heat or cold to scrotum, NSAIDs, doxycycline. Use trimethoprim-sulfamethoxazole
Fournier's gangrene	History of trauma, UTI, rectal disease, diabetes, compromised immunity. Explosive onset. Edema, extreme pain, block necrotic skin, crepitance	Aspiration of skin yields purulent fluid with bacteria. Do sigmoidoscopy	Acute surgical emergency; debriding of necrotic tissue followed later by skin grafting. Broad-spectrum antibiotics
Hydrocele	Rule out hernia; irreducible painless mass, occurs in all age groups; may communicate intraabdominally	No bowel sounds on auscultation; transilluminates	Because of likelihood of associated hernia, surgically explore and repair if persists after 1 year of age
Spermatocele	Painless lump in spermatic cord following vasectomy	Does not transilluminate	Trial of NSAIDs; Surgical removal if large or cosmetically undesirable
Testicular cancer	Painless firm enlarging mass; often ignored for months	Ultrasonography; biopsy of mass	Exploratory surgery, removal and lymph node dissection
Torsion	Sudden onset, extreme pain; nausea, vomiting; young boys to early teens; elevating scrotum increases pain	Thicker ipsilateral spermatic cord; unequal Doppler flow; testicle higher in scrotum; no blood flow by nuclear scan; diagnostic ultrasound	Surgery within 6 hours
Trauma	Painful trauma, gross swelling with ecchymosis	Urethrography; ultrasonography	Exploratory surgery
Varicocele	"Bag of worms" or "spaghetti" of spermatic cord usually on left; be suspicious of serious problem if acute onset on right side	IVP or CT scan of retroperitoneal space if acute onset	Surgically remove if painful or infertility is a problem

TABLE 10-32.—Assessment and Treatment of Penile Curvature

Presentation
Congenital or acquired curvature noted during a spontaneous erection. May be associated with urethral stricture. In Peyronie's disease, patient palpates mass in shaft of penis.

Congenital	Acquired
With epispadias or hypospadias	Stricture of urethra
Chordee without hypospadias	Penile trauma
Penile torsion	Peyronie's disease

Clinical Evaluation
History, physical examination, and special studies are needed

History	Physical	Studies
Onset	Palpable plaque	At-home polaroid pictures of curvature with erection
Degree of curvature	Other penile abnormalities	X-ray or ultrasound of plaque
Pain		Evaluation for erectile failure (NPT, Rigiscan)
Erectile failure		Corporacavernosogram
Sexual difficulties		

Treatment
Treatment may be necessary if curvature is severe, problem has been stable over time, and it interferes with intercourse

Nonsurgical (for Peyronie's disease)	Surgical
None has been documented to be successful but may serve to show concern for patient's problem; the condition tends to abate somewhat over time; vitamin E, aminobenzoate potassium	Urethral repair
	Release of inelastic integument
	Nesbit plication of corpora
	Excision of plaque with skin graft if not impotent
	Impotent patients may have excision and prosthesis

Modified from Gregory JG, Purcell MH: *Med Aspects Hum Sexuality* 23:64, 1989.

TABLE 10-33.—EMERGENCY MANAGEMENT OF PRIAPISM

Since impotence is a known complication of priapism, this possibility should be explained to the patient early on; informed consent for an emergency procedure should be obtained.

Aspiration
Thoroughly cleanse penis with povidine-iodine to prep the skin.
Wearing sterile gloves, drape off surrounding area to create a sterile field.
Locate the 3 o'clock or 9 o'clock position on the shaft of the penis, approximately 1 inch proximal to the corona. Avoid the dorsal neurovascular bundle and the ventral urethral areas. Inject 0.5-1.0 ml of lidocaine to anesthetize skin over the aspiration site. Only one side of the penis needs to be aspirated because of the cross-flow of circulation.
Insert a 19-gauge butterfly needle into the corpora through the anesthetized skin and aspirate blood into a sterile 20-ml syringe. If blood gases on sludged penile blood are desired, use a 5-ml glass heparinized syringe to do the first aspiration, then change to the 20-ml syringe. If the condition has persisted for >36 hours and/or pH is <7.25, $Po_2 < 30$ and Pco_2 is > 60 mm Hg, a significant ischemic condition exists, and the patient should be referred for surgical shunt procedure.
Continue aspiration until all possible blood is obtained and the penis loses its rigidity. Squeezing, or "milking," of blood from the penis may help in removing blood.
When aspiration is no longer productive, move to the irrigation stage of the procedure.

Irrigation
Add 1 ml of epinephrine 1:1000 to a 1-L bag of sterile saline. Attach an IV administration set, run some fluid through the tubing, and fill a clean sterile 20-ml syringe from it.
Slowly inject epinephrine/saline solution into cavernosa and aspirate back into syringe and discard.
Repeat the step above until satisfactory detumescence has occurred and blood returned from the penis is bright red instead of dark and viscous. Then withdraw the butterfly needle from the penis, and cover the aspiration site with a sterile dressing. If no satisfactory results are obtained after 200 ml of irrigation, abandon the procedure and plan for surgical shunting.
Hospitalize the patient for 24 hours of observation to ensure that priapism does not recur. Success should be anticipated in ≥75% of the cases regardless of cause.

Modified from Driscoll CE: *Patient Care* 24(10):117, 1990.

SEXUAL PROBLEMS

TABLE 10-34.—Differentiation of Psychogenic and Organic Erectile Dysfunction*

FEATURE	PSYCHOGENIC	ORGANIC
History		
Onset	Usually abrupt with temporal relationship to specific stress	Usually gradual
Course	Selective, intermittent, episodic	Persistent, progressive
Severity	Variable, erection may occur with masturbation or with alternate partners; nocturnal or morning erections generally present	Unable to achieve erection in any setting; nocturnal erections absent or markedly reduced
Physical		
Nocturnal penile tumescence (NPT)	Normal	Absent or decreased in number, duration, or rigidity
Penile blood pressure	Penile index 0.90; systolic pressure no more than 20 mm Hg below brachial systolic	Penile index 0.60; systolic pressure 30 mm Hg below brachial systolic
Bulbocavernosus reflex latency	Normal (33.5-35 m/sec)	Prolonged (>40 m/sec)
Lab		
Serum-free testosterone	Normal	Low
Luteinizing hormone (if low testosterone)	Normal	Low (pituitary), high (testicular)
Serum prolactin	Normal	Elevated

Modified from Vliet LW, Meyer JK: *Johns Hopkins Med J* 151:246, 1982.
*Erectile dysfunction is defined as *erectile failure in 25% or more of attempts at intromission.*

TABLE 10-35.—ANABOLIC-ANDROGENIC STEROID SIDE EFFECTS

RATE OF OCCURRENCE (%)	CONDITION
Rare	Cholestatic jaundice, peliosis hepatis, hepatic carcinoma, infection or nerve trauma from injections, tendon pain
1-2	Intolerance reaction consisting of anorexia, burning tongue, nausea and vomiting, abdominal pressure, diarrhea
5-10	Increase in liver enzymes
20-30	↓ HDL, ↑ LDL, voice deepening, alopecia, acne, aggressiveness, gynecomastia
>60	Testicular atrophy, altered libido, virilization

Modified from Frankle MA: *J Musculoskeletal Med* pp 69-88, Nov. 1989.

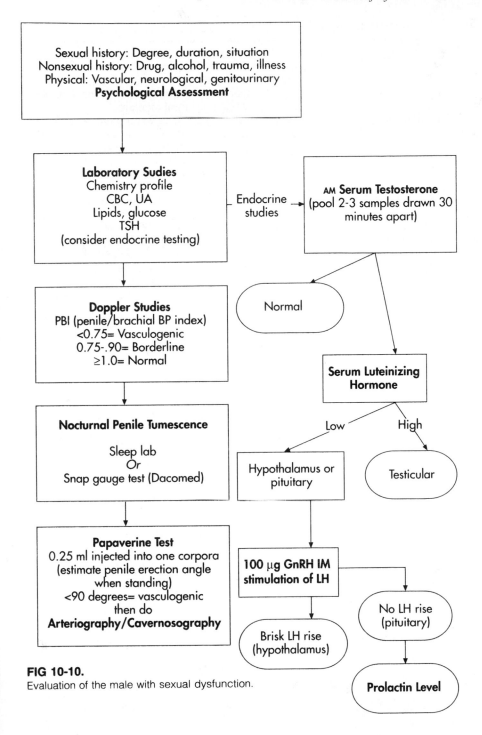

FIG 10-10.
Evaluation of the male with sexual dysfunction.

TABLE 10-36.—Possible Causes of Organic Erectile Dysfunction

Inflammatory	Urethritis, prostatitis, seminal vesiculitis, cystitis, gonorrhea, tuberculosis, elephantiasis, mumps
Mechanical	Congenital deformities, Peyronie's disease, morbid obesity, hydrocele, spermatocele, varicocele, phimosis, priapism, urethral stricture
Postoperative	Perineal prostatic biopsy, perineal prostatectomy, abdominal aortic aneurysmectomy, aortofemoral bypass, retroperitoneal lymphadenectomy, sympathectomy (lumbar, dorsal, pelvic), cystectomy, abdominoperineal resection, external spincterotomy
Occlusive-vascular	Atherosclerosis, arteritis, thrombosis, embolism, aneurism, Leriche's syndrome
Traumatic	Penectomy, urethral rupture, pelvic fracture
Endurance related	Myocardial failure, angina pectoris, related insufficiency, anemia, leukemia, systemic illness, renal or hepatic failure, sickle cell disease
Neurological	Myasthenia gravis, multiple sclerosis, parkinsonism, amyotrophic lateral sclerosis, stroke, cerebral tumors, temporal lobe, infections, head trauma, spinal cord trauma, spinal cord compression, tabes dorsalis, temporal lobe epilepsy, spina bifida, syringomyelia, subacute combined degeneration of the cord, peripheral neuropathy, cerebral palsy, electroconvulsive treatment (occasionally)
Chemical	Multiple pharmacological agents affect sexual function, notably antihypertensives, anticholinergics, antidepressants, sedatives, and narcotics
Endocrine	Acromegaly, chromophobe adenoma, craniopharyngioma, pituitary ablation, hyperprolactinemia, Addison's or Cushing's syndrome, hyperthyroidism, hypothyroidism, castration, postinflammatory fibrosis; exogenous estrogens; Klinefelter's syndrome, male Turner's syndrome, feminizing interstitial cell tumor, diabetes, Fröhlich's syndrome

Modified from Vliet LW, Meyer JK: *Johns Hopkins Med J* 151:246, 1982.

RENAL FAILURE

Acute Renal Failure

Diagnosis can be made if urine volume falls below 400 ml/24 hr with elevated serum BUN and creatinine. BUN rises 10-20 mg/day; creatinine rises 0.5-1.0 mg/day. Mortality is about 50% (Table 10-37).

TABLE 10-37.—RENAL FAILURE

Types of Renal Failure

Characteristic	Prerenal	Renal	Postrenal
Causes	Volume depletion, low cardiac output, reduced renal blood flow	Glomerular or tubular lesions	Urethral or ureteral obstruction
Urine osmolality (mOsm/kg H_2O)	>500	<350	Usually <350
Urine to serum osmolar ratio	>1.2	<1.1	<1.1
Urine sodium (mEq/L)	<20	>40	Variable
Urine to serum urea ratio	>8	<3	<3
Urine to serum creatinine ratio	>40	<20	<20
Serum BUN to serum creatinine ratio	>20:1	<20:1	<20:1

Causes of Renal Azotemia
Glomerular
Glomerulonephritis, lupus, allergic angiitis, polyarteritis nodosa, Wegener's granulomatosis, streptococcal disease
Tubular
Ischemic hypotension, contrast materials, antibiotics, heavy metals, methoxyflurane anesthesia, ethylene glycol, methanol, carbon tetrachloride, rhabdomyolysis, septic abortion, eclampsia, uric acid, sulfonamide, hypercalcemia, Bence Jones protein

TABLE 10-38.—POLYCYSTIC KIDNEY DISEASE (PCKD)

EXPECTED FINDINGS	PERCENT OF CASES*
Colonic diverticula	75-80
Proteinuria	75
Palpable kidneys	66
Abdominal or flank pain	66
Hypertension	50
Pyuria	50
Hematuria	50-80
Liver cysts	33-50
Renal insufficiency	33-45
Nephrolithiasis	10-20
Intracranial aneurysm†	5-10

Incidence is 1 in 500 at autopsy; typically a middle-aged patient with abdominal pain and hematuria
Infection is the most common complication
Hypertension and azotemia associated with eclampsia of pregnancy
Diagnose by ultrasound (or by IVP, renal CT, or MRI)
Aggressively treat hypertension to minimize risk of intracerebral hemorrhage; avoid manipulations of lower urinary tract

From Chester AC, Harris JP, Schreiner GE: *Am Fam Physician* 16:94, 1977; Gabow PA: Autosomal dominant polycystic kidney disease, *N Engl J Med* 329:332, 1993.
*Based on a number of large series.
†Responsible for 15% of deaths in patients with PCKD.

TABLE 10-39.—Clinical Management of Renal Failure

CONDITION	OBSERVATION	MANAGEMENT
Hyperkalemia	Serum K^+, ECGs	Kayexalate (oral or enema) 50 g in 200 ml of 20% sorbitol, repeat every 4 hours and/or dialysis
Acidosis	Serum pH, serum bicarbonate	Oral bicarbonate solutions if serum bicarbonate <15 mEq/L; guard against hypernatremia; dialysis
Protein/calorie malnutrition	Daily weights	Consider hyperalimentation; restrict Na^+, K^+, H_2O
Hypermagnesemia	Serum Mg	Avoid laxatives and antacids, dialysis
Hyperphosphatemia	Serum P	Aluminum-containing antacids
Hypocalcemia	Serum Ca^{2+}	Accompanied by rise in phosphorus; if Ca^{2+} < 7.5, administer replacement with 2 g/day; restrict dietary phosphate, bind phosphorus in gut with aluminum carbonate or hydroxide antacids
Fluid overload	Observe for loss of thirst response, serum sodium, urine specific gravity	At least 2 L of fluid daily, free water access; if dilutional hyponatremia occurs, restrict fluids; loop diuretics

Indications for Dialysis
Volume expansion with life-threatening CHF and pulmonary edema uncontrolled
Severe uncontrollable hypernatremia and/or hyperkalemia and/or metabolic acidosis (pH < 7.2)
When serum calcium × serum phosphate (mmol/dl) product is ≥ 6
Poisoning with salicylates, ethanol, methanol, short-acting barbiturates
Chronic renal failure with acute temporary decline
Terminal renal failure awaiting transplantation
Uremic pericarditis

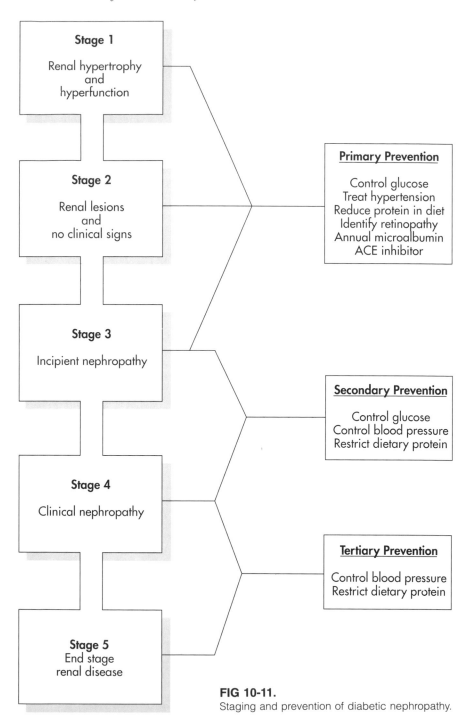

FIG 10-11.
Staging and prevention of diabetic nephropathy.

TABLE 10-40.—DRUG-RELATED RENAL SYNDROMES

RENAL SYNDROME	MECHANISM	CAUSATIVE AGENTS
Acute renal failure (acute tubular necrosis)	Direct tubular injury	Aminoglycosides; radio-contrast agents; cisplatin; amphotericin B; cephaloridine; heavy metals
Acute renal failure (interstitial nephritis)	Immunological, inflammatory	Penicillins; sulfonamides; cephalosporins; phenytoin; allopurinol; NSAIDs; diuretics; cimetidine; rifampin
Acute renal failure (myoglobinuric)	Myopathy	Lovastatin, gemfibrozil, heroin
Acute renal failure (obstruction)	Intratubular obstruction; retroperitoneal fibrosis	Methotrexate; acyclovir; radiocontrast agents; methysergide; sulfonamides
Acute renal failure (prerenal)	Decreased renal perfusion	NSAIDs*; converting enzyme inhibitors; radiocontrast agents; cyclosporine; interleukin-2
Chronic renal failure	Chronic tubulointerstitial nephritis	Analgesics; lead; nitrosoureas; lithium; cyclosporine
Hyperkalemia	Altered renal and extrarenal potassium homeostasis	β-Blockers; NSAIDs; captopril; thiazides; spironolactone; triamterine; calcium channel blockers; cyclosporine
Hypocalcemia	—	Cisplatin
Hypomagnesemia	Increased excretion	Aminoglycosides, cisplatin, amphotericin B
Hyponatremia	Decreased free-water excretion	NSAIDs; chlorpropamide; thiazides; clofibrate; vincristine; lithium; demeclocycline
Nephrogenic diabetes insipidus	—	Lithium
Nephrotic syndrome	Primary glomerulopathy	Gold; penicillamine; captopril; NSAIDs; heroin; interferon-α
Urolithiasis	Stone precipitation	Acetazolamide, allopurinol, triamterene

From Cooper K, Bennett WM: *Arch Intern Med* 147:1213, 1987; Farrugia E, Larson T: Drug-induced renal toxicity, *Postgrad Med* 90:241, 1991.
*NSAIDs, Nonsteroidal antiinflammatory drugs.

TABLE 10-41.—Characteristic Features of Renal Masses on Various Imaging Methods

RENAL MASSES	IV UROGRAPHY	ULTRASOUND	COMPUTED TOMOGRAPHY	ANGIOGRAPHY
Benign Masses				
Cyst	Sharp demarcation from surrounding renal parenchyma; pencil-thin wall	Thin, smooth wall; lack of internal echoes with through-transmission	Smooth, sharply marginated nonenhancing homogeneous lesion	Nonspecific avascular mass (this method rarely necessary)
Angiomyolipoma	Nonspecific renal mass	Increased echogenicity similar to that of renal sinus fat	Fat within tumor	
Adenoma (oncocytoma)	Nonspecific well-demarcated mass	Homogeneous well-encapsulated mass	Homogeneous mass with attenuation value similar to that of normal renal tissue; central fibrous scar	Quite vascular with sharp, smooth-rimmed homogeneous appearance ("spoke wheel," cortical pattern)
Malignant Masses				
Renal cell carcinoma*	Possible calcification, irregularity in renal contour, distortion of collecting system	Isoechoic mass with inhomogeneity caused by hemorrhage and necrosis	Solid mass that may be necrotic or have cystic components and variable contrast enhancement	Often hypervascular and neovascular
Metastasis	Often appears normal; if abnormal, solid contour-deforming mass is compressing collecting system	Possible multiple homogeneous hypoechoic masses that do not display through-transmission	Enhanced after administration of contrast medium but less than surrounding normal parenchyma	Hypovascular infiltrating mass with truncation and encasement of segmental renal arteries
Transitional cell carcinoma	Lucent filling defects with irregular surface	Low-echogenic mass in renal pelvis surrounded by normal, highly echogenic renal sinus	Flat or rounded solid intrapelvic mass outlined by contrast medium in renal pelvis	Mass that is hypovascular or avascular

Pseudoneoplasms

Xanthogranulomatous pyelonephritis	Nonspecific renal mass	Kidney appears enlarged with echogenic foci and acoustic shadowing if stone is present	Renal parenchyma is replaced by nonenhancing xanthogranulomatous deposit	
Hydronephrosis	Obstructed kidney may be enlarged with delayed nephrogram; visualization of collecting system delayed	Parenchyma is thin; loss of normal cortical medullary junction	Kidneys enlarged; renal parenchyma thinned	
Abscess	Focal enlargement of kidney	Mature abscess: anechoic mass with irregular margins; septations and floating debris may be present Chronic abscess: thick rim	Air-fluid level, fascial thickening, perirenal spread of infection	Chronic abscess: similar to renal neoplasm with stretched vessels and surrounding hyperemia
Hematoma	Mass distorts kidney	Localized fluid collections; focal low-attenuation mass with dispersed internal echoes	Nonenhancing mass	Distal renal branch or capsular artery may show site of active bleeding

From Graham TE, Rockey KE: *Postgrad Med* 87:111, 1990.
*Magnetic resonance imaging may also be used and shows intravascular tumor thrombus, perirenal adenopathy, and tumor extension.

11 *The Nervous System*
Charles W. Smith, Jr.

NEUROANATOMY AND NEUROLOGICAL EXAMINATION

TABLE 11-1.—PATHOLOGICAL REFLEXES*

REFLEX	STIMULUS	RESPONSE
Babinski's	Stroke outer edge of side of foot	Extension great toe, flexion small toes, spreading small toes
Chaddock's	Stroke lateral aspect of dorsum of foot and external malleolus	Extension great toe
Oppenheim's	Firm stroke, medial tibia	Extension great toe
Rossolimo's	Tap balls of toes	Plantar flexion of toes
Mendel-Bekhterev	Tap dorsum of foot on outer surface	Plantar flexion of toes
Palm-chin (palmomen-tal)	Stroke thenar emi-nence	Elevation of corner of mouth, contraction of chin
Thumb-adductor	Stroke hypothenar area	Adduction and flexion, thumb
Hoffmann's sign	Snap nail of middle fin-ger	Flexion of thumb and fingers
Gordon's sign	Compression of pisi-form bone	Extension of flexed fin-gers
Chaddock's sign	Pressure of palmaris longus tendon	Flexion of wrist; exten-sion of fingers

Modified from Mancall EL: *Essentials of the neurologic examination,* ed 2, Philadelphia, 1981, FA Davis, pp. 94-95.
*All pathological reflexes listed in the table are indicative of pyramidal tract disease.

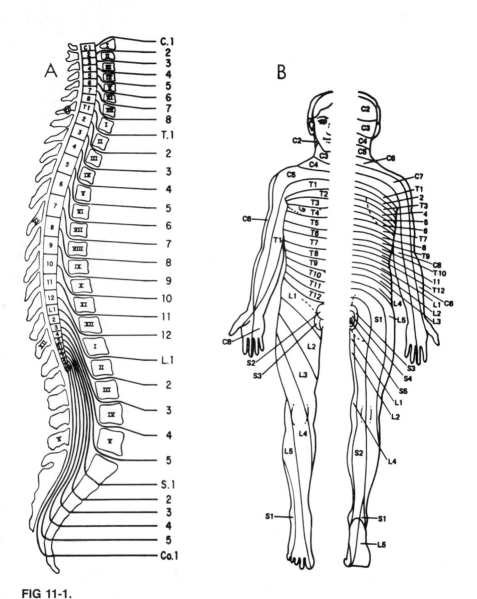

FIG 11-1.
Neuroanatomy. **A,** Relationship of spinal nerves to the vertebral column. **B,** Dermatome chart. (**A** From Van Allen MW, Rodnitzky RL: *Pictorial manual of neurologic tests,* ed 2, Chicago, 1981, Mosby, p. 80. Redrawn from Favill J: Outline of the Spinal Nerves. Springfield, Ill, Charles C Thomas, Publisher, 1946. **B** from Chaplin JP, Demers A: *Primer of neurology and neurophysiology,* New York, 1978, John Wiley & Sons, p. 57.)

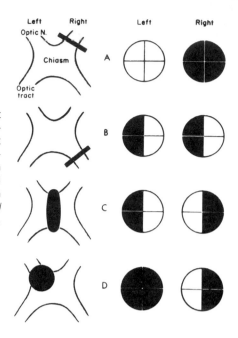

FIG 11-2.
Visual field defects. **A,** Transection of right optic nerve = ipsilateral monocular blindness. **B,** Lesion of right optic tract = left homonymous hemianopsia. **C,** Chiasmal lesion = bitemporal hemianopsia. **D,** Lesion of left optic nerve and chiasm = ipsilateral blindness and right temporal deficit. (From Van Allen MW, Rodnitzky RL: *Pictorial manual of neurologic tests.* Chicago, 1981, Mosby, p. 84.)

TABLE 11-2.—Effects of Autonomic Stimulation on Selected Body Organs

ORGAN	SYMPATHETIC EFFECTS	PARASYMPATHETIC EFFECTS
Eye		
Pupil	Dilation	Contraction
Ciliary process	None	Excitation
Gastrointestinal glands	Inhibition or no effect	Copious, serous, or watery secretion and enzymes
Salivary gland	Thick, viscous secretion	Serous or water secretion
Sweat glands	Copious secretion	None
Heart	Increase in rate and force of contraction	Decrease in rate and force of contraction
Lungs	Constricts blood vessels, dilates bronchi	Constricts bronchi
Gastrointestinal	Inhibits peristalsis, stimulates sphincters	Stimulates peristalsis, inhibits sphincters
Liver	Release of glucose	None
Genitalia	Ejaculation, orgasm	Erection, lubrication
Blood vessels	Constricts abdominal muscles, constricts or dilates other smooth muscles, depending on receptors in tissue	None
Bladder	Uncertain	Stimulates smooth muscle for emptying, contracts detrusor, relaxes internal sphincter

Modified from Chaplin JP, Demers A: *Primer of neurology and neurophysiology,* New York, 1978, John Wiley & Sons, p. 97.

TABLE 11-3.—Reflex Interpretation Chart

REFLEX	ELICITED BY	RESPONSE	SEGMENTAL LEVEL
Corneal	Touch cornea with cotton wisp	Contraction, orbicularis oculi	Pons
Pharyngeal	Touch posterior wall of pharynx	Contraction of pharynx	Medulla
Palatal	Touch soft palate	Elevation of palate	Medulla
Scapular	Stroke interscapular skin	Contraction of scapular muscles	C5 to T2
Epigastric	Stroke skin from nipples to epigastrium	Epigastrium "dimples" toward stroke	T7 to T9
Abdominal	Stroke skin along and under costal margins and inguinal ligaments	Contraction of abdominal muscles in quadrant stimulated	T8 to T12
Cremasteric	Stroke medial surface of upper thigh	Elevation of testicle, same side	L1 to L2
Gluteal	Stroke skin of buttock	Contraction of glutei	L4 to L5
Bulbocavernous	Pinch dorsum of glans	Contraction of bulbous urethra	S3 to S4
Anal	Prick perianal skin	Contraction of rectal sphincter	S5
Jaw jerk	Tap mandible, mouth open	Jaw closes	Pons
Triceps	Tap triceps tendon	Elbow extends	C7 to T1
Biceps	Tap biceps tendon	Elbow flexes	C5 to C6
Radial	Tap styloid process of radius	Supinator longus contracts	C5 to C6
Knee	Tap patellar tendon	Knee extends	L3 to L4
Ankle	Tap achilles tendon	Ankle extends	S1 to S3

Modified from Mancall EL: *Alper's and Mancall's essentials of the neurologic examination,* ed 2, Philadelphia, 1981, FA Davis, pp. 23, 25.

TABLE 11-4.—Clinical Features of Herniated Lumbosacral Disks

LEVEL OF HERNIATION	NERVE ROOT	PAIN PATTERN	NUMBNESS	WEAKNESS	REFLEXES
L3-L4	L4	Lower back, hip, posterolateral thigh, anterior leg	Anteromedial thigh and knee	Quadriceps	Knee jerk diminished
L4-L5	L5	Above sacroiliac joint, hip, lateral thigh and leg	Lateral leg, first three toes	Dorsiflexion great toe and foot; difficulty walking on heels; foot drop	Knee jerk and ankle jerk usually intact
L5-S1	S1	Above sacroiliac joint, hip, posterolateral thigh and leg, to heel	Back of calf, lateral heel, foot and toe	Plantar flexion of foot and (possibly) great toe; difficulty walking on toes	Ankle jerk diminished or absent

Modified from Gilmer HS, Papadopoulos SM, Tuite GF: Lumbar disk disease: pathophysiology, management and prevention, *Am Fam Physician* 47(5):1141, 1993.

TABLE 11-5.—Common Peripheral Nerve Lesions

NERVE	MANIFESTATION
Median (at wrist)	Weakness and atrophy of thumb and thenar eminence; sensory loss in palm and first three digits, palmar surface; paresthesia and pain in lateral hand and first three digits
Ulnar (at elbow)	Drooping fourth and fifth digits (hand of benediction); atrophy of hypothenar eminence; sensory loss of medial palm and fifth digit
Radial	Wrist drop; sensory loss in dorsal hand and thumb (variable)
Femoral	Loss of knee jerk; weakness of knee extension and hip flexion
Peroneal	Foot drop
Sciatic	Pain in lateral thigh; absent ankle jerk

Modified from Van Allen MW, Rodnitzky RL: *Pictorial manual of neurologic tests,* Chicago, 1981, Mosby, pp. 130-133; McKhann GM: Neurology. In Baughman KL, Green BM, eds: *Clinical diagnostic manual for the house officer,* Baltimore, 1981, Williams & Wilkins.

NEUROLOGICAL TESTS AND PROCEDURES

TABLE 11-6.—CEREBROSPINAL FLUID STUDIES IN MULTIPLE SCLEROSIS

TEST	INCIDENCE OF POSITIVE FINDINGS (%)	ABNORMAL VALUE	CAUSES OF FALSE POSITIVE RESULTS
γ-Globulins	60-75	>12% of protein	Neurosyphilis Guillain-Barré syndrome Systemic gammopathy
IgG index	80-90	>0.66	Viral encephalitis
Oligoclonal bands	85-95	>2 bands	Neurosyphilis Subacute sclerosing panencephalitis (SSPE) Guillain-Barré syndrome Chronic meningitis Optic neuritis
Myelin basic protein	70-90	Positive	Central pontine myelinolysis CNS lupus erythematosus Leukoencephalopathies Intrathecal chemotherapy Cranial irradiation Progressive multifocal leukoencephalopathy Encephalitis Anoxia Stroke

From Schwankhaus JD: *Am Fam Physician* 29:234, 1984.

TABLE 11-7.—MRI Compared with CT in Diagnosis of Neurological Disorders

	GENERAL	CEREBROVASCULAR	NEOPLASM	WHITE MATTER	INFECTIONS	EPILEPSY	SPINAL CORD
MRI	Better tissue contrast; multiple planes; vascular imaging	More sensitive in acute stroke; better for bleeds which are days old	Gadolinium-enhanced T_1 weighted preferred to detect tumors	MRI 95% to 99% specific in detection of MS	Abnormal in meningitis but not specific; good for herpes encephalitis and AIDS	Useful in detecting subtle CNS lesions that may cause seizures	Has almost eliminated need for myelogram Equal to CT for disk evaluation
CT	Shorter scanning time; useful for unstable and neurotic patients	Preferred for acute CNS bleeding because it is faster and easier to interpret	Double-dose, contrast-enhanced CT second choice to MRI	Not very helpful in diagnosis of white matter CNS lesions	Not very useful in detection of infections	Often negative in cases where MRI is positive	Still good for evaluation of herniated disk disease

Modified from Edelman RR, Warach S: Magnetic resonance imaging (first of two parts), *N Engl J Med* 328(10):708, 1993.

TABLE 11-8.—Technique of Lumbar Puncture*

1. Place patient on side on a firm mattress or padded examination table.
2. Flex patient with thighs on abdomen and neck moderately flexed.
3. Palpate L4 spinous process at level of iliac crest. Needle should be inserted into interspace either above (L3-L4) or below (L4-L5) this landmark.
4. Clean skin if necessary with soap and water.
5. Swab an area from the puncture site with an 8- to 10-inch radius with Merthiolate, iodine, or povidone solution.
6. Drape sterile towels over area, leaving an opening at the puncture site.
7. Use sterile gloves and inject 1-2 ml of local anesthetic (e.g., 1% Xylocaine) about 2 cm into the interspace.
8. Use a 20-gauge spinal needle with stylet, in the midline, angulated 5-15 degrees cephalad; advance slowly.
9. If needle meets bone, withdraw partially and redirect.
10. Withdraw stylet every 2-3 mm to see if CSF appears; usually a slight "click" will be felt on entering the subdural space.
11. When this occurs, advance the needle 2-3 mm more, and withdraw the stylet.
12. Determine opening pressure with manometer.
13. Withdraw 1 ml in each of four tubes, and send first tube for cultures and Gram stain, second for WBC and RBC, third for glucose and protein, and fourth for other indicated studies (e.g., viral titers or cultures, India ink prep, fungal cultures, VDRL, rickettsial titers, or cytologies).
14. Use same procedure for infant, except use a 22-gauge, 1½-inch spinal needle; have assistant hold patient in sitting position and obtain approximately 0.5 ml per tube.
15. If tap is bloody, centrifuge 1-2 ml. If supernatant is clear, the tap is probably traumatic; if it is xanthochromic, the blood was probably present before the tap.

*For normal values of CSF, see Appendix 18.

TABLE 11-9.—Electroencephalography

EEG TECHNIQUES	USEFULNESS
Resting EEG	Clinical evaluation of any CNS disorder
Hyperventilation 3 minutes	Alkalosis and vasoconstriction may activate seizure focus
Photic stimulation (1-20/sec strobe light)	May activate certain abnormal discharges
Sleep EEG	Activates some EEG abnormalities, especially temporal lobe seizures
Nasopharyngeal leads	May show lesion in temporal lobe or deep frontoparietal area

About 12%-18% of normal persons have nonspecific EEG abnormalities.
Localized EEG activity is always significant.
Focal abnormalities do not distinguish brain pathology.
Some 20%-40% of patients with seizures have normal EEGs.

Modified from Adams RD, Victor M: *Principles of neurology,* ed 2, New York, 1981, McGraw-Hill, p. 22.

TABLE 11-10.—Patterns of EEG Abnormalities

EEG ABNORMALITY	DIAGNOSTIC CONSIDERATIONS
Focal delta wave activity	Tumor, abscess, subdural hematoma, intracranial bleeding, cerebral infarct
Diffuse slow wave activity	Infratentorial tumor, cerebral edema, CNS hypoxia, meningitis, encephalitis, metabolic or toxic encephalopathy
Focal or generalized spike and wave activity	Petit mal epilepsy
Focal or generalized spike and slow wave complexes	Focal or generalized motor seizure disorder
No activity (flat line)	Brain death

Modified from Departments of neurology, physiology, and biophysics of the Mayo Clinic: *Clinical examinations in neurology,* ed 4, Philadelphia, 1976, WB Saunders, pp. 284-295.

TABLE 11-11.—EMG IN NEUROLOGICAL DIAGNOSIS

NEUROLOGICAL DEFICIT	CLINICAL EXAMPLE	EMG FINDINGS	DIAGNOSTIC USEFULNESS*
Normal	Hysteria/malingering	Irregular firing rhythm of action potentials	++++
Upper motor neuron lesions	Stroke	Diminished rate of action potential firing with contractions	0 to +
Myelopathy	Amyotrophic lateral sclerosis	Increased polyphasic potentials High amplitude and duration of action potentials	+++
Mononeuropathy	Carpal tunnel syndrome	Normal action potentials; diminished nerve conduction	+++ to ++++
Polyneuropathy	Diabetes	Same as mononeuropathy but in multiple sites	++++
Neuromuscular transmission defects	Myasthenia gravis	Increased polyphasic potentials; low amplitude and duration of potentials; progressive decline of action potentials	+++ to ++++
Myopathies	Polymyositis	Increased polyphasic potentials; decreased amplitude and duration of action potentials	++ to +++

Modified from Departments of neurology, physiology, and biophysics of the Mayo Clinic: *Clinical examinations in neurology,* ed 4, Philadelphia, 1976, WB Saunders, pp. 299-316.

0, Not useful; +, rarely useful; ++, occasionally useful; +++, usually helpful; ++++, always helpful.

SEIZURE DISORDERS

TABLE 11-12.—Classification of Epilepsies

Primary Generalized Epilepsies
  Absence
Classic absence of childhood with diffuse 3-Hz spike-and-wave complexes
Absence of juvenile myoclonic epilepsy: staring, with diffuse 3-Hz to 6-Hz
    multispike-and-wave complexes during adolescence
Juvenile absence with diffuse 8-Hz to 12-Hz rhythms
Myoclonic absence with diffuse 3-Hz to 6-Hz multispike-and-wave complexes
Myoclonic absence: staring, fragmentary myoclonus, automatisms, and diffuse
    12-Hz rhythms
  Myoclonic
Myoclonic seizures of early childhood, with 3-Hz to 6-Hz multispike-and-wave
    complexes without mental retardation (Doose syndrome)
Juvenile myoclonic seizures of Janz or benign myoclonic seizures of adoles-
    cence and late childhood, with diffuse 4-Hz to 6-Hz multispike-and-wave com-
    plexes
  Clonic-tonic-clonic (grand mal)
  Tonic-clonic (grand mal)

Partial Epilepsies
  Simple Partial
  Complex Partial
Simple partial at onset followed by impairment of consciousness and automa-
    tisms
Impairment of consciousness at onset
    Motionless stare and impaired consciousness followed by automatisms (tem-
        poral lobe epilepsy)
    Complex motor automatisms at start of impaired consciousness (frontal lobe,
        somatosensory, or occipital lobe epilepsy)
    Drop attack with impaired consciousness and automatisms (temporal lobe
        syncope)

Secondary Generalized Epilepsies
Simple partial evolving to tonic-clonic (secondary tonic-clonic)
Infantile spasms (propulsive petit mal, infantile myoclonic encephalopathy with
    dysarrhythmia or West syndrome)
Myoclonic astatic or atonic epilepsies (epileptic drop attacks of Lennox-Gastaut
    in children with mental retardation)
Progressive myoclonic epilepsies in adolescents and adults with dementia (my-
    oclonus epilepsies of Lafora, Lundborg, Hartung, Hunt, or Kuf)

Modified from Delgado-Escueta AV, Treiman DM, Walsh GO: *N Engl J Med* 308:1509, 1983.

TABLE 11-13.—COMMON ANTIEPILEPTIC DRUGS

| GENERIC NAME | TRADE NAME | USUAL DAILY DOSAGE | | PRINCIPAL THERAPEUTIC INDICATIONS | SERUM HALF-LIFE (hr) | EFFECTIVE BLOOD LEVEL (mg/ml) |
		CHILDREN	ADULTS (mg)			
Phenobarbital	Luminal	4-15 mg/kg (8 mg/kg infants)	60-300	Tonic-clonic seizures; simple and complex partial seizures; absence	96 ± 12	15-30
Phenytoin	Dilantin	4-7 mg/kg	300-400	Tonic-clonic seizures; simple and complex partial seizures	24 ± 12	10-20
Carbamazepine	Tegretol	20-30 mg/kg	400-1200	Tonic-clonic seizures; complex partial seizures	12 ± 3	4-12
Primidone	Mysoline	10-25 mg/kg	750-1500	Tonic-clonic seizures; simple and complex partial seizures	12 ± 6	6-12
Ethosuximide	Zarontin	20-30 mg/kg	750-1500	Absence	30 ± 6	40-100
Methsuximide	Celontin	10-20 mg/kg	500-1000	Absence	30 ± 6	40-100
Diazepam	Valium	0.15-0.25 mg/kg (IV)	10-150	Status epilepticus	30 ± 6	40-100
ACTH		40-60 U/day		Infantile spasms		
Valproic acid	Depakene Depakote	15-60 mg/kg	1000-3000	Absence; simple and complex partial seizures	8 ± 2	25-100
Clonazepam	Klonopin	0.01-0.2 mg/kg	1.5-20	Absence; myoclonus	18-50	0.01-0.07

Modified from Adams RD, Victor M: *Principles of neurology*, ed 2, New York, 1981, McGraw-Hill, p. 227.

TABLE 11-14.—A Suggested Timetable for the Treatment of Status Epilepticus*

TIME (min)	ACTION†
0-5	Diagnose status epilepticus by observing continued seizure activity or one additional seizure
	Give oxygen by nasal cannula or mask; position patient's head for optimal airway patency; consider intubation if respiratory assistance is needed
	Obtain and record vital signs at onset and periodically thereafter; control any abnormalities as necessary; initiate ECG monitoring
	Establish an IV; draw venous blood samples for glucose level, serum chemistries, hematology studies, toxicology screens, and determinations of antiepileptic drug levels
	Assess oxygenation with oximetry or periodic arterial blood gas determinations
6-9	If hypoglycemia is established or a blood glucose determination is unavailable, administer glucose; in adults, give 100 mg of thiamine first, followed by 50 ml of 50% glucose by direct push into the IV; in children, the dose of glucose is 2 ml/kg of 25% glucose
10-20	Administer either 0.1 mg/kg of lorazepam at 2 mg/min or 0.2 mg/kg of diazepam at 5 mg/min by IV; if diazepam is given, it can be repeated if seizures do not stop after 5 min; if diazepam is used to stop the status, phenytoin should be administered next to prevent recurrent status
21-60	If status persists, administer 15-20 mg/kg of phenytoin no faster than 50 mg/min in adults and 1 mg/kg per min in children by IV; monitor ECG and blood pressure during the infusion; phenytoin is incompatible with glucose-containing solutions—the IV should be purged with normal saline before the phenytoin infusion
>60	If status does not stop after 20 mg/kg of phenytoin, give additional doses of 5 mg/kg to a maximal dose of 30 mg/kg
	If status persists, give 20 mg/kg of phenobarbital by IV at 100 mg/min; when phenobarbital is given after a benzodiazepine, the risk of apnea or hypopnea is great and assisted ventilation is usually required
	If status persists, give anesthetic doses of drugs such as phenobarbital or pentobarbital; ventilatory assistance and vasopressors are virtually always necessary

From *JAMA* 270(7):857, 1993.
*Time starts at seizure onset. Note that a neurological consultation is indicated if the patient does not wake up, convulsions continue after the administration of a benzodiazepine and phenytoin, or confusion exists at any time during evaluation and treatment.
†*ECG*, Electrocardiogram; *IV*, intravenous line.

TABLE 11-15.—Methods of Giving Phenytoin

THERAPEUTIC RANGE* REACHED (AFTER INITIAL DOSE)	RATE OF ADMINISTRATION	ROUTE	COMMENT
20 minutes	1000 mg at 50 mg/min in adults (10-15 mg/kg at 25 mg/min in children)	IV	Always with pulse, BP, and respiration monitored; given by syringe; not mixed in bottle
4-6 hours	1000 mg stat in adults; then 300 mg/day (about 15 mg/kg stat in children; then 5 mg/kg/day)	PO	Local gastric upset is common; give with meals or milk
24-30 hours	300 mg every 8 hours for three doses; then 300 mg/day in adults (5 mg/kg every 8 hours for three doses; then 5 mg/kg in children)	PO	Mild ataxia is common initially
5-15 days	300 mg/day in adults (5 mg/kg/day in children)	PO	No unusual side effects

From Samuels MA: *Manual of neurologic therapeutics,* Boston, 1982, Little, Brown, p. 94.
*The therapeutic range is 5-20 μg/ml of serum.

STUPOR AND COMA

TABLE 11-16.—Harvard Criteria for Brain Death

Unresponsive: No vocal or motor response to intensely painful stimuli
Apneic: Room air breathing for 10 minutes; normal arterial CO_2 tension; turn off ventilator and observe; apnea for at least 3 minutes meets criteria
Areflexic: Pupils fixed and dilated; corneal and doll's eyes reflexes absent; no response to cold water calorics; flaccid extremities; no spontaneous blinking; no deep tendon reflexes
EEG: Flat EEG; repeated in 24 hours; patient must not be hypothermic or on barbiturates

Modified from Black P: *N Engl J Med* 299:7, 1978.

TABLE 11-17.—Stages of Rostrocaudal Deterioration With Central Herniation

LEVEL	CONSCIOUSNESS	PUPILS	EYE MOVEMENTS	OCULOVESTIBULAR RESPONSES	RESPIRATORY PATTERN	MOTOR FUNCTION
Diencephalic	Somnolence, stupor, or coma	Small, slightly reactive	Roving and conjugate	Abnormal calorics; doll's eyes response brisk	Sighing or Cheyne-Stokes	Generalized hypertonicity, bilateral pyramidal tract signs or decorticate posturing
Midbrain—upper pontine	Coma	Mid-size, fixed	Disconjugate	Difficult to elicit	Central neurogenic hyperventilation	Bilateral decerebrate posturing
Lower pontine—upper medullary	Coma	Mid-size, fixed	Absent	Absent	Tachypnea	Generalized flaccidity; bilateral extensor plantars, minimal flexion withdrawal
Medullary (terminal)	Coma	Dilated, fixed	Absent	Absent	Ataxic, gasping or apnea	Flaccidity

Modified from Mancall EL: *Alper's and Mancall's essentials of the neurologic examination,* ed 2, Philadelphia, 1981, FA Davis, p. 37.

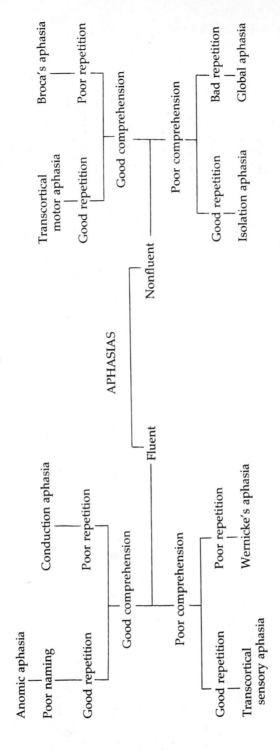

FIG 11-3.
Classification of aphasia. (From Rakel RE: *Textbook of family practice*, ed 3, Philadelphia, 1984, WB Saunders, p. 1174.)

TABLE 11-18.—COMPARISON OF MAJOR FORMS OF APHASIA

FORM	EXPRESSION	VERBAL COMPREHENSION	REPETITION	NAMING	READING COMPREHENSION	WRITING	LESION
Expressive (Broca's)	Nonfluent	Relatively intact	Impaired	Impaired	Variable	Impaired	Posteroinferior frontal (Broca's area)
Receptive (Wernicke's)	Fluent	Impaired	Impaired	Impaired	Impaired	Impaired	Posterosuperior temporal (Wernicke's area)
Global	Nonfluent	Impaired	Impaired	Impaired	Impaired	Impaired	Frontotemporal
Conduction	Fluent	Relatively intact	Impaired	Impaired	Variable	Impaired	Arcuate fasciculus; supramarginal gyrus
Nominal	Fluent	Relatively intact	Intact	Impaired	Variable	Variable	Angular gyrus; posterosuperior temporal
Transcortical motor	Nonfluent	Relatively intact	Intact	Impaired	Variable	Impaired	Anterior perisylvian
Transcortical sensory	Fluent	Impaired	Intact	Impaired	Impaired	Impaired	Posterior perisylvian

From Mancall EL: *Alper's and Mancall's essentials of the neurologic examination*, ed 2, Philadelphia, 1981, FA Davis, p. 113.

TUMORS

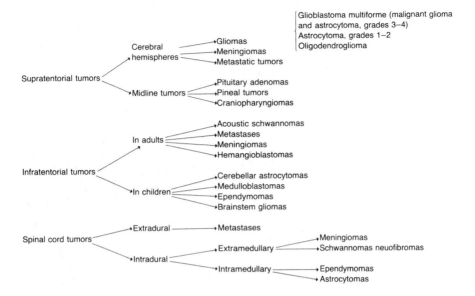

FIG 11-4.

Most frequent CNS tumors and their sites of predilection. (Modified from Samuels MA: *Manual of neurologic therapeutics,* Boston, 1982, Little, Brown & Co, p. 216.)

TABLE 11-19.—Drugs for the Treatment of a Migraine Headache

DRUG	DOSAGE (per event)	COMMENTS/SIDE EFFECTS
Sumatriptan (Imitrex)	6 mg subcutaneous injection per event; one 100-mg tablet orally per event; maximum dosage is three tablets or two injections	Serotonin (5-HT) antagonist. Expensive (about $35 per dose). Transient increase in blood pressure, may exacerbate angina Tingling, flushing, transient nausea are common
Ergotamine (Cafergot; DHE 45)	2-4 mg oral; 0.75-1 mg subcutaneous injection per event	Nausea, vomiting, abdominal pain, diarrhea
Nonsteroidal antiinflammatory drugs (Naproxen)	750-825 mg	Dyspepsia, GI hemorrhage. Any NSAID can be substituted
Metaclopramide (Reglan)	10 mg orally	Dopamine antagonist; rarely, may cause dystonia
Chlorpromazine (Thorazine)	0.1 mg/kg of body weight intravenously	Dopamine antagonist; tardive dyskinesia
Prochlorperazine	10 mg orally	Dopamine antagonist; tardive dyskinesia

From Welch KMA: Drug therapy of migraine, *N Engl J Med* 329(20):1477, 1993.

TABLE 11-20.—Drugs for the Prevention of a Migraine Headache

DRUG	DAILY DOSE	SIDE EFFECTS
Amitriptyline	10-150 mg	Weight gain, somnolence, dry mouth, cardiac arrhythmias, urinary retention
Methysergide	2-8 mg	Muscle cramps, insomnia, tissue fibrosis
Naproxen	1100 mg	Dyspepsia, gastritis, GI bleeding (may use other NSAID)
Nifedipine	30 mg	Headache, tachycardia, depression
Propranolol	40-320 mg 60-320 mg (long-acting)	Fatigue, bradycardia, bronchospasm
Verapamil	280-320 mg	Headache, bradycardia, weight gain, constipation, depression

PARKINSON'S DISEASE

TABLE 11-21.—Drugs Commonly Used for Parkinson's Disease

DRUG	AVAILABILITY	FREQUENCY AND ADMINISTRATION	COMMENTS
Amantadine	100-mg capsules	bid or tid (reduce with renal impairment)	Excreted unchanged in urine; initial effect reached 48 hours after administration; half-life, 2-4 hours; treat early disease or as adjunct to main therapy; initial dose 100 mg daily.
Trihexyphenidyl (Artane)	2.0- and 5.0-mg tablets; 0.4-mg/ml elixer; 5 mg sustained-release capsules	tid for tablets and elixer; qd or bid for sustained-release capsules	Additive to other agents; dry mouth, constipation, urinary retention, worsens glaucoma, impaired memory, and confusion.
Benztropine mesylate (Cogentin)	0.5-, 1.0-, and 2.0-mg tablets; injectable, 1 mg/ml	bid	Same as for trihexyphenidyl. May help control tremor only.
Levodopa with carbidopa (Sinemet)	10/100, 25/100, 25/250, and 50/200 (as Sinemet CR) mg tablets	tid (bid for CR)	Less effective as disease progresses; "on-off effect"; dose-related dyskinesias common; anorexia, nausea, hypotension, mental aberrations; taper gradually on discontinuance. Most effective of current drugs.

Continued.

TABLE 11-21.—Drugs Commonly Used for Parkinson's Disease—cont'd

DRUG	AVAILABILITY	FREQUENCY AND ADMINISTRATION	COMMENTS
Selegiline (Eldepryl)	5 mg	bid (breakfast and lunch)	Monoamine oxidase inhibitor. Side effects include nausea and orthostatic hypotension. Toxic interaction with Prozac and Demerol.
Bromocriptine (Parlodel)	1.25 mg	Everyday for 3 days, increase slowly up to 15 to 30 mg/day bid bid with meals	Dopamine antagonist; adjunctive rx with ʟ-dopa.
Pergolide (Permax)	0.05 mg	Everyday for 3 days, increase slowly from 1.5 to 3 mg/day tid	Same as for bromocriptine.

NOTE: Several surgical treatments have emerged for Parkinson's Disease. Currently only thalamotomy is well established for the treatment of unilateral tumor. Fetal transplants have resulted in improvement for some patients and appear to be relatively safe. The improvement is often minimal, however.

CARPAL TUNNEL SYNDROME

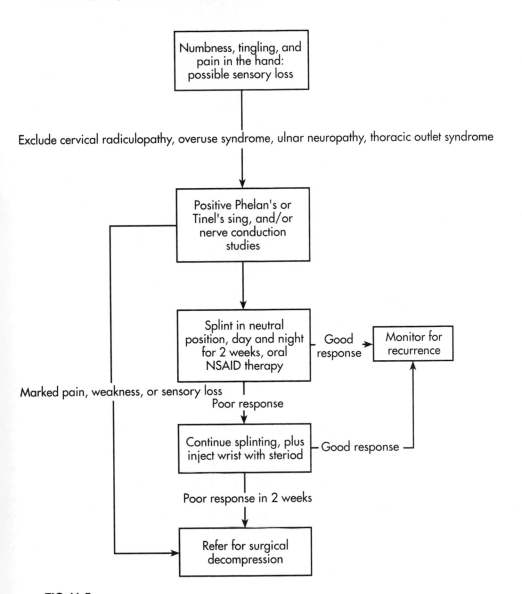

FIG 11-5.
Management strategies for carpal tunnel syndrome. (From Dawson DM: Entrapment neuropathies of the upper extremities, *NEJM* 329(27):2013, 1993.)

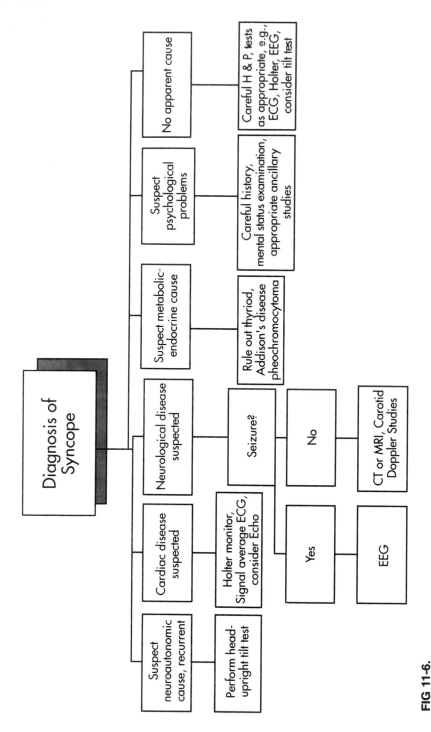

FIG 11-6.

Diagnosis of syncope. (Modified from Wolfe DA, Grubb BP, Kimmel SR: Head-upright tilt test: a new method of evaluating syncope, *Am Fam Physician* 47(1):151, 1993.)

12 *Mental Disorders and Mental Health*

Edward T. Bope

MOOD DISORDERS

Mood disorders represent a disturbance of mood with a manic or depressive syndrome. Mood is a prolonged emotion and is usually depression or elation (sad or happy). The mood disorders are subdivided into bipolar disorders and depressive disorders. To qualify as a bipolar disorder, there must have been one or more manic or hypomanic episodes. The DSM-IV, Diagnostic and Statistical Manual of Mental Disorders, Fourth Edition, is an excellent resource for the family physician.

Bipolar Disorders
Bipolar I Disorder (296.60)

There is a community prevalence of 0.5%. These patients have had one or more manic episodes and have often had previous major depressive episodes. The manic episode is not explained by schizoaffective disorder or is not superimposed on a psychotic disorder.

Bipolar II Disorder (296.89)

There is a community prevalence of 0.5%. These patients have recurrent major depressive episodes with one or more hypomanic episodes. Hypomanic episodes have the same characteristics as manic episodes but are not severe enough to impair the patient socially or occupationally or require hospitalization. If the hypomanic episode becomes manic, then the diagnosis becomes Bipolar I.

Cyclothymia (301.13)

This disorder must have occurred for 2 years for adults or 1 year for children and involves numerous hypomanic episodes (essentially like manic episodes except that they do not interfere with function) as well as recurrent periods of depressed mood (not severe or prolonged enough to be diagnosed as major depression). There is a prevalence of 0.4% to 1%.

Depressive Disorders

This is a very common disorder affecting the mood. There cannot be an organic factor as the etiology, nor is it a normal reaction to bereavement. Delusions or hallucinations may occur but not in the absence of mood symptoms. Naturally, there must be a depressive episode in which there is either a depressed mood or a loss of interest or pleasure in daily activities, or both. If both are present, then there must be at least three of the following findings (four if only one is present): (1) Increase or decrease in weight, (2) increase or decrease in sleep, (3) psychomotor agitation or retardation, and (4) fatigue, feelings of worthlessness or guilt, cognitive changes, and recurrent thoughts of death.

Major Depression (296.2)

The essentials of the diagnosis are a major depressive episode as described earlier without a history of a manic episode. Fifty percent of people who have major depression will have another episode. The range of incidence for females is 9% to 26%, and for males the incidence is 5% to 12%. The disorder is 1.5 to 3 times more common in first-degree relatives. Up to 15% of individuals with major depression die from suicide during this episode.

Dysthymia (Depressive Neurosis) (300.4)

Individuals with dysthymia have never had a manic episode. Symptoms of depressed mood have existed for 2 years (1 year for children) without evidence of a major depressive episode as defined before. While feeling depressed, these individuals must have at least two of the following three symptoms: (1) Increased or decreased appetite, (2) increase or decrease in sleep, (3) fatigue, low self-esteem, poor concentration or difficulty making decisions, and feeling of hopelessness.

Treatment of Mood Disorders
Bipolar Disorders

Psychotherapy is generally helpful in conjunction with medication but may be impossible in presenting episodes. Safety for individuals with bipolar disorder must be ensured since they could harm themselves in either the manic or depressive phase. Lithium carbonate is the most often prescribed drug, but other modalities and medications are also common.

Depressive Disorders

Assessing the risk of suicide is of immediate importance. When necessary or in doubt, force hospitalization. Rely on your judgment, not the patient's. Psychotherapy is certainly important, and drug therapy may be needed. Medication is generally selected, taking into account the side effect profile (some of which may be desirable). Table 12-2 lists these medications.

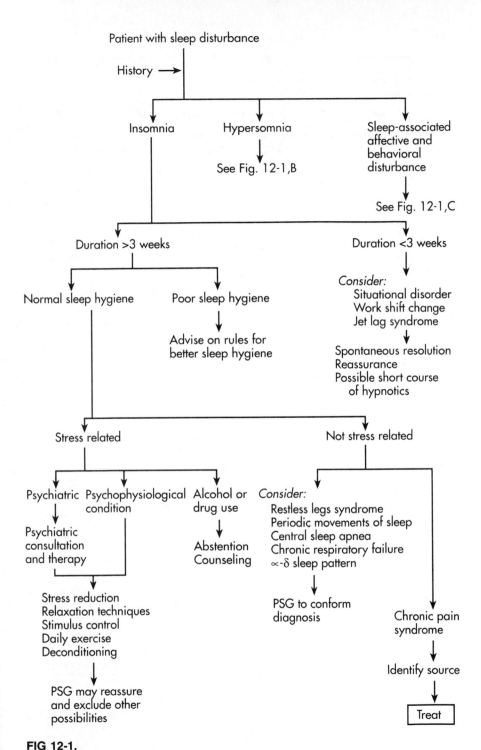

FIG 12-1.
Diagnosing sleep disorders. (From HL Greene, WP Johnson, MJ: Maricie *Decision making in medicine,* St. Louis, 1993, Mosby, pp. 351-353.)   *Continued.*

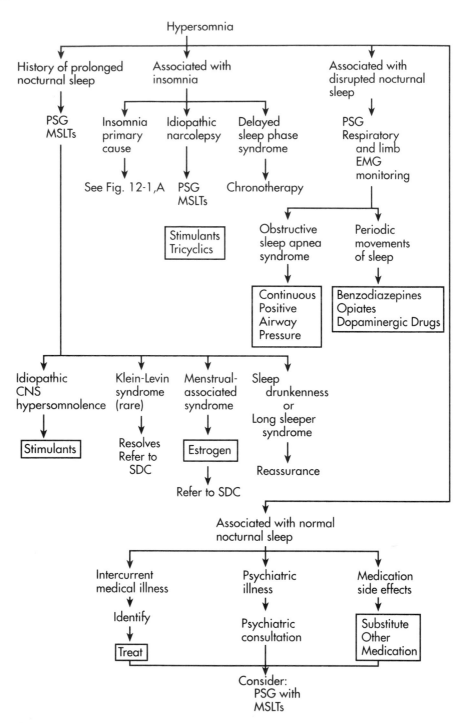

FIG 12-1, cont'd.
Diagnosing sleep disorders. (From HL Greene, WP Johnson, MJ: Maricie *Decision making in medicine,* St. Louis, 1993, Mosby, pp. 351-353.)

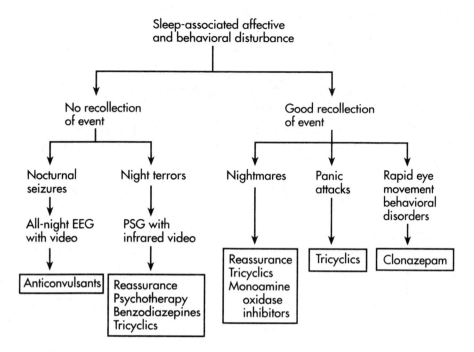

FIG 12-1, cont'd.
For legend see opposite page.

ANXIETY DISORDERS

TABLE 12-1.—ANXIETY DISORDERS

ICDA-9 CODE	DSM-IV CLASSIFICATION	DEFINITION: EXCESSIVE, IRRATIONAL WORRY PLUS:
300.22	Agoraphobia without panic disorder	Fear of being in a place where escape might be embarrassing
300.21	Panic disorder without agoraphobia	Fear of having a panic attack
309.21	Separation anxiety	Fear of separation from well-known people; onset before age 18
300.29	Specific phobia	Fear of an item
300.23	Social phobia	Fear of embarrassment or humiliation
300.3	Obsessive-compulsive disorder	Recurrent obsessions or compulsions
300.02	Generalized anxiety disorder	Nonstressor related, lasting ≥6 months
309.81	Posttraumatic stress disorder	Recurring thoughts of traumatic event
300.00	Anxiety disorder not otherwise specified	Do not meet other criteria
308.3	Acute stress disorder	Occurs within 4 weeks of a stressful event
293.89	Anxiety disorder resulting from a general medical condition	Physiologically linked to medical condition (e.g., thyrotoxicosis)
—	Substance induced anxiety	Related to chemical agent or withdrawal

TABLE 12-2.—ANTIDEPRESSANTS

CLASS	DRUG	DOSE*	NE	SER	ANTICHOLINERGIC	SEDATION	ORTHO
Tertiary Amines							
	Amitriptyline (Elavil and generic)	50-150 mg hs	++	++++	++++	++++	++
	Imipramine (Tofranil and generic)	50-150 mg hs	++	++++	++	++	+++
	Doxepin (Sinequan and generic)	50-150 mg hs	+	++	++	+++	++
	Clomipramine (Anafranil)†	25-250 mg hs	++	+++++	+++	+++	++
	Trimipramine (Surmontil)	50-150 mg hs	+	+	++	+++	++
Secondary Amines							
	Desipramine (Norpramin and generic)	50-150 mg hs	++++	++	+	+	+
	Nortriptyline (Aventyl and Pamelor)	25-100 mg hs	++	+++	++	++	+
	Protriptyline (Vivactil)	15-40 mg hs	++++	++	+++	+	+
Tetracyclic							
	Maprotiline (Ludiomil and generic)	50-150 mg hs	+++	+	++	++	+

NE, Norepinephrine; *SER*, serotonin; *Ortho*, orthostatic hypotension; *0*, none; *+*, slight; *++*, moderate; *+++*, high; *++++*, very high; *+++++*, extremely high.

*Doses listed are usual daily doses. Initiate the dosage at the low end of the range indicated and slowly titrate upwards over several days or weeks. The dosage in elderly patients or children should be reduced (see product labeling).

†Clomipramine is only indicated for obsessive-compulsive disorder.

‡Also inhibits dopamine uptake. To avoid seizures, dosage increases of bupropion must not exceed 100 mg in a 3-day period, and no single dose should exceed 150 mg. The maximum dose is 450 mg daily (150 mg tid).

Continued.

TABLE 12-2.—Antidepressants—cont'd

CLASS	DRUG	DOSE*	NE	SER	ANTICHOLINERGIC	SEDATION	ORTHO
Bicyclic	Fluoxetine (Prozac)	20-60 mg in the morning	+	+++++	0	0	+
Triazolopyridine	Trazodone (Desyrel and generic)	150-400 mg hs or twice daily	0	+++	+	+++	+++
Aminoketone	Bupropion‡ (Wellbutrin)	100 mg AM and PM for 3 days, then 100 mg tid	0/+	0/+	++	++	+
New Agents	Paroxetine (Paxil)	20-50 mg in the morning	0/+	+++++	0	0	0
	Sertraline (Zoloft)	50-200 mg in the morning	0/+	+++++	0	0	0
	Venlafaxine (Effexor)	75-150 mg in 2-3 daily doses	+++	+++	0	0	0

SCHIZOPHRENIA

TABLE 12-3.—SCHIZOPHRENIA: SYMPTOMS AND TREATMENT

DISORDER	MAJOR SYMPTOMS	TREATMENT PLAN
Schizophrenia	Delusions that may or may not have persecutory or jealousy content; auditory hallucinations; incoherence; decrease in level of functioning; symptoms present for 6 months at some time in life	See individual types
Catatonic	Mutism; negativism; rigid posture in inappropriate positions; may have motor excitement	Major tranquilizer*; hospitalization; structured protective environment
Disorganized	Incoherent; delusions in fragments only; affect blunted, inappropriate, or silly	Major tranquilizer; structured environment
Paranoid	Delusions that are persecutory, grandiose, or jealous; hallucinations of same three types	Major tranquilizer; supportive but not overly friendly environment
Undifferentiated	Prominent delusions; incoherence; tangential thinking; hallucinations; grossly disorganized; other types excluded	Major tranquilizer; structured environment; routine medical follow-up; socialization groups
Residual	Emotional blunting; social withdrawal; eccentric behavior; illogical behavior; loose associations; past history of one of the above types	Major tranquilizer; routine medical care

*See Table 12-5.

COGNITION OR MEMORY CHANGES

TABLE 12-4.—Cognition or Memory Changes

DISEASE	MAJOR SYMPTOMS	ETIOLOGY
Delirium	Clouded state of consciousness; disorientation; memory deficit; misinterpretations; illusions or hallucinations; incoherent; increased or decreased psychomotor activity. Symptoms develop over a short period	Systemic infections; metabolic disorders, including hypoxia; postoperative state; substance abuse
Dementia	Decrease intellectual ability leading to decrease in level of function; memory deficit; deficit in abstract thinking; impaired judgment aphasia; agnosia; state of consciousness clear	Primary degenerative dementia (Alzheimer's disease); CNS infection (HIV); brain trauma; toxic metabolic disturbances; vascular diseases; normal pressure hydrocephalus; neurological diseases
Amnestic syndrome	Long- and short-term memory deficit; clear state of consciousness; intellectual function intact	Head trauma; hypoxia; infarction; encephalitis; thiamine deficiency; alcohol abuse; substance abuse
Cognitive disorder not otherwise specified	Cognitive dysfunction often mild, presumed caused by general medical condition other than above	Mild neurocognitive disorder, postconcussion

TABLE 12-5.—PROPERTIES OF COMMON ANTIPSYCHOTIC AGENTS

CLASS	DRUG	DOSE*	EPS	SEDATION	ANTICHOLINERGIC	ORTHO
Aliphatic						
	Chlorpromazine (Thorazine and generic)	50-1000 mg daily in three doses	++	+++	++	+++
	Promazine (Sparine and generic)	50-1000 in four doses	++	++	+++	++
	Triflupromazine (Vesprin)	60-150 mg IM daily	++	+++	+++	++
Piperidine						
	Mesoridazine (Serentil)	50-400 mg in three doses	+	+++	+++	++
	Thioridazine (Mellaril and generic)	150-800 mg in three doses	+	+++	+++	+++
Piperazine						
	Acetophenazine (Tindal)	40-80 mg daily in three doses	+++	++	+	+
	Fluphenazine (Prolixin and generic)	0.5-10 mg once or twice daily	+++	+	+	+
	Perphenazine (Trilafon and generic)	12-24 mg in three doses	+++	+	+	+
	Prochlorperazine (Compazine and generic)	25-150 mg in three doses	+++	++	+	+
	Trifluoperazine (Stelazine and generic)	4-30 mg in two doses	+++	+	+	+

EPS, Extrapyramidal side effects; *O*, none; +, slight; ++, moderate; +++, high; ++++, very high.

*Doses listed are usual daily doses. Initiate the dosage at or below the low end of the range indicated and slowly titrate upwards over several days or weeks. The dosage in elderly patients or children should be reduced (see product labeling).

†Initial dose should be 25 mg once or twice daily and should be titrated to the target range by 14 days. The use of clozapine must be accompanied by weekly blood tests to detect agranulocytosis.

Continued.

TABLE 12-5.—PROPERTIES OF COMMON ANTIPSYCHOTIC AGENTS—cont'd

CLASS	DRUG	DOSE*	EPS	SEDATION	ANTICHOLINERGIC	ORTHO
Butyrophenone						
	Haloperidol (Haldol and generic)	1-15 mg in two or three doses	+++	+	+	+
Thioxanthene						
	Chlorprothixene (Taractan)	75-600 mg in three doses	++	+++	++	++
	Thiothixene (Navane and generic)	6-30 mg in three doses	+++	+	+	+
Dibenzodiazepine						
	Clozapine (Clozaril)	300-900 mg daily in one or two daily doses†	+	+++	+++	+++
Benzisoxazole						
	Risperidone (Risperdal)	4-16 mg in two daily doses	0	+	+	+
Diphenylbutylpiperidine						
	Pimozide (Orap)	1-10 mg in two or three doses	+++	++	++	+

BORDERLINE PERSONALITY DISORDER

TABLE 12-6.—BORDERLINE PERSONALITY DISORDER

According to the criteria set forth by the American Psychiatric Association in the DSM-IV, the patient begins in early adulthood to show five of the following nine features as characteristics of her or his current and/or long-term functioning:

Impulsivity or unpredictability in at least two areas that are potentially self-damaging: spending money, sex, gambling, substance abuse, overeating, inflicting self-harm

A pattern of unstable and intense interpersonal relationships

Inappropriate, intense anger or lack of control of anger (temper)

Identity disturbance described many times by metaphors ("I feel like a robot") and that may involve poor self-image or gender identity confusion

Marked shifts of mood lasting only a few hours and rarely a few days

Self-destructive acts like self-mutilation, frequent fights, or suicide gestures

Chronic feelings of boredom, loneliness, and emptiness

Concerned about real or imagined abandonment

Transient stress related paranoid ideation or dissociative symptoms

Treatment must be individualized, but the cornerstone is surely patience, support, and limits. Psychotherapy must be weekly for about 2 years. Medications, though not useful for the long-term, may be needed to control temporary crises.

State	Drug or Class
Emotional lability	Lithium carbonate
Anxiety states	Benzodiazepines
Psychotic episodes	Phenothiazines

ALCOHOLISM AND DETOXIFICATIONS

TABLE 12-7.—Alcoholism

Scope of Problem

Alcoholism is one of the leading causes of death and disability. It is certainly the nation's number one drug problem. Early recognition and treatment are important.

Features That May Indicate an Alcohol Problem

HISTORICAL FEATURES	SYMPTOMS	SIGNS
GI bleeding	Abdominal pain	Decreased levels of
Recent auto accident	Anxiety	consciousness
or arrest record	Depression	Tremors
Unusual trauma or frac-	Hallucinations	Spider nevus
ture	Insomnia	Abdominal tenderness
Blackouts with drinking	Headache	Hepatomegaly
Hypertension	Impotence	Splenomegaly
Heart disease		Testicular atrophy
Sexual dysfunction		Cigarette burns
Amenorrhea		Parotid gland enlarge-
Seizures		ment
Marital discord		Elevated BP
Legal or job problems		Gynecomastia
		Unexplained bruises

TABLE 12-8.—ALCOHOLISM SCREENING TESTS

Short Michigan Alcoholism Screening Test (SMAST)

	Yes	No
1. Do you feel you are a normal drinker? (By normal we mean do you drink less than or as much as most other people.)	(0 point)	(1 point)
2. Do others who are important to you ever worry or complain about your drinking?	(1 point)	(0 point)
3. Do you ever feel bad about your drinking?	(1 point)	(0 point)
4. Do friends or relatives think you are a normal drinker?	(0 point)	(1 point)
5. Are you always able to stop drinking when you want to?	(0 point)	(1 point)
6. Have you ever attended a meeting of Alcoholics Anonymous (AA) for yourself?	(3 points)	(0 point)
7. Has your drinking ever created problems between you and others who are important to you?	(1 point)	(0 point)
8. Have you ever gotten into trouble at work because of your drinking?	(1 point)	(0 point)
9. Have you ever neglected your obligations, your family, or your work for two or more days in a row because you were drinking?	(1 point)	(0 point)
10. Have you ever gone to anyone for help about your drinking?	(3 points)	(0 point)
11. Have you ever been in a hospital because of your drinking?	(3 points)	(0 point)
12. Have you ever been arrested for drunken driving, driving while intoxicated, or driving while under the influence of alcoholic beverages?	(1 point)	(0 point)
13. Have you ever been arrested, even for a few hours, because of other drunken behavior?	(1 point)	(0 point)

Scoring System

0-1 point—Normal
2 points—Possibly alcoholic
3 or more points—Probably alcoholic

CAGE Survey

Are you . . .

C utting down or feel the need to?
A nnoyed when people criticize your drinking?
G uilty about your drinking?
E ye-opening with a drink in the morning?

If you answered yes to any question, there is high probability of alcoholism.

TABLE 12-9.—Alcohol Detoxification Orders

Obtain current drinking history with emphasis on prior withdrawal experience; inquire specifically about other drug use (tranquilizers, sedatives, cocaine, etc.) in addition to alcohol
  Regular diet; between meal feeding as needed
  Up ad lib, with help first 24 hours
  Take vital signs every 3 hours
  Pajamas or hospital gown first 72 hours
  MOM 30 ml PO PRN
  Liquid antacid, 30 ml PO PRN
  Encourage PO fluid intake
  Unless otherwise specified, the following medications:
    Multivitamin tablets, 1 PO bid
    Thiamine HCl, 100 mg IM
    ASA, 650 mg, or Tylenol, 650 mg
    $MgSO_4$, if serum magnesium is low
PPD and *Candida* control
On admission, order the following lab tests: CBC with platelets, SMA 6/60 and 12/60, SGPT, GGT, PT, PTT, serum magnesium, folic acid, RPR, urinalysis, blood alcohol, urine drug screen, consider HIV
PA and lateral chest x-ray examination and ECG
Detoxification regimen:
  Phenobarbitol 60-90 mg every 6 hours PO
  Alternate with Diazepam 10-20 mg every 6 hours PRN
  Decrease the regimen daily if vital signs remain stable
Alternate regimen: Choose one or more of the following to sedate patient, then wean over 2-3 days:
  Chlordiaepoxide (Librium)
  Diazepam (Valium)
  Lorazepam (Ativan)
  Phenobarbitol
Additional meds used as adjuncts:
  Clonidine: to relieve autonomic hyperactivity
  Beta-blockers: for persistent tachycardia
For imminent delirium tremens, which usually occurs 48-72 hours after blood pressure, pulse, and respiration increase, use additional phenobarbitol or diazepam

---

TABLE 12-10.—Psychiatric Diagnoses to Consider when Physical Symptoms
are Unexplained

Alcohol or drug dependence
Anxiety disorders
   Generalized anxiety disorder (300.02)
   Panic disorder without agoraphobia (300.01)
Factitious disorder with physical signs and symptoms (300.19)
Mood disorders
   Major depressive disorder (296.2)
   Dysthymic disorder (300.4)
Somatoform disorders
   Somatization disorder (300.81)
   Hypochondriasis (300.7)

HOSTILE PATIENT

Patients may become hostile for a variety of reasons, including a long wait, offensive office personnel, or failure to get better. Two hostile persons cannot solve a problem. You will need to be the calm peacemaker, despite your tendency to defend yourself, your practice, and your office staff. Confrontation can lead the patient to think in medicolegal terms and will leave everyone uneasy. Try to clarify the issues and then discuss alternative solutions.

If a patient is hostile and exhibiting psychotic symptoms you may need to request police help. Remember not to antagonize the patient. Offering a shot to help the patient relax and feel better may allow you the opportunity to administer a major tranquilizer (Table 12-11).

Generally, state law permits involuntary hospitalization when the patient is either dangerous to himself or to others (including you). The police are often well versed in this procedure.

TABLE 12-11.—The Hostile and Dangerous Patient

Rapid sedation may be achieved with one of the following drugs:

Drug	Dose	Time Interval	Total 24-hour Dose
Haloperidol (Haldol)	2.5-10 mg IM	Every 30-60 minutes	100 mg
Chlorpromazine (Thorazine)	25-50 mg IM	Every 60 minutes	75 mg (except for extremely unmanageable patients)

RELAXATION THERAPY

TABLE 12-12.—RELAXATION THERAPY

Relaxation therapy can be used to relieve stress and tension in some patients. It can be done in 5-10 minutes in the office and repeated by the patient several times a day. It is best introduced in a quiet, uninterrupted atmosphere with the patient in a comfortable position. The patient should understand that he or she is not being hypnotized and will remain in control of his or her body. You will need to speak in a soft soothing monotone and continue talking until the therapy ends. You can use your own script or this sample: "You are going to relax to the best of your ability. Please close your eyes. As you relax you will feel tension leave your body, to be replaced by a calm soothing sensation. I want you to think of a pleasant landscape scene and see yourself relaxing there. Already you can feel your tense muscles relax. You may feel sleepy as relaxation takes over your body. With each breath you become more relaxed. Breathe in relaxation and exhale tension. Breathe in relaxation and exhale tension. With each breath you relax. Breathe in relaxation and breathe out all tension. Feel your arms and legs relax as we count to ten. 1 . . .2 . . .3 . . .4 . . .5 . . .6 . . .7 . . .8 . . .9 . . .10. [You may ad lib here and discuss each area of the body.] Now feel how calm you are becoming and see yourself resting in that pleasant landscape scene. Every part of your body is relaxing now, your arms, your legs, your feet, your back, and your scalp. Breathe in relaxation and exhale tension. Now as we count backwards from 10 to 1 you will become more alert and more rested. 10 . . . 9 . . . 8 . . . 7 . . . 6 . . . 5 . . . . Breathe in relaxation and exhale tension. At zero you will be alert and well rested . . . 4 . . . 3 . . . 2 . . . 1 . . . 0 . . . . Open your eyes and feel how relaxed you are."

COUNSELING TECHNIQUES

TABLE 12-13.—Counseling the Family or Individual

Counseling Format
Outline of Counseling Session
Build a therapeutic relationship
Assess the problem:
    Let each member describe the problem
    Reflect the problem to make sure you understand it
    Ask each member how it affects him or her
    Allow ventilation and give support
Problem solve:
    How has it been dealt with in the past?
    What can be done to change the problem?
Form a treatment plan
Summarize the session: First the patient, then the counselor

Counseling Techniques
Engaging the Family
The process of beginning a trusting relationship is more difficult with the family
    than with an individual. Some guidelines are to talk to all family members,
    beginning the session by addressing each member with polite social ques-
    tions. It is usually best to not address the patient first, particularly if it is a
    child. Make an attempt to pull in the member who seems the most reserved.
    Recognize the member whose opinion is valued—there probably is one—and
    make a point to honor this authority. Adopt the family's style of conversation
    so that everyone is at ease.
Initiating Discussion of the Problem
Open the discussion by asking a family member (other than the patient) how it
    came about that you are meeting today. Another approach is to ask what it is
    like being in this family these days. You may want to address this question to
    the youngest member since he/she is likely to be totally honest. When deal-
    ing with a child problem, it is best to ask the parent what problems the family
    needs to work on. Even though one member may have already given you
    details of the problem, it is better to let someone repeat it in front of the
    whole group. In supportive counseling sessions, such as grief, you may be
    the one to summarize the situation.
Structuring the Session
The family or individual must perceive you as able to lead the session to feel
    secure enough to talk about painful material. There may be a struggle for
    control and leadership. You must win this struggle to be an effective coun-
    selor. Doherty and Baird suggest six core family counseling rules:
    Each person has the right to speak without being interrupted.
    When you have announced a procedure or plan of action, do not become
        sidetracked, e.g., if you say you want to hear everyone's opinion, do not
        let an argument interrupt that plan.

Continued.

TABLE 12-13.—Counseling the Family or Individual—cont'd

Steer the family back to the issues at hand when they stray.

Resist requests for solutions if requests seem premature or inappropriate, e.g., "I think the solution will come from you as a family. I will have ideas to help you."

Take charge of the physical arrangement of the session. Observe the seats they choose. Rearrange when needed. A circle is often good.

Take charge of who attends the session, make sure everyone knows who is expected to come to each meeting and insist that they be there.

Defining the Problem

You may wish to define the problem by asking each member how he/she would like to see this relationship change. "What changes would you like to see?" You should encourage these to be specific, concrete, and positive.

History Taking

This should occupy less than a third of the initial interview. The two most basic pieces of information are the onset of the problem, and how the family or person has attempted to cope with it.

Remaining Neutral

To avoid casting family members in roles, you must believe that there are no villains or victims. Your support must be seen as distributed equally among the group.

Encouraging a Collaborative Set

Encourage the family to work on the problem together. Explain that they got to the problem together and now must pull together to get out.

Facilitate Family Discussion

Encourage the family to talk directly to one another during the session. They may resist and say that they feel silly, etc. If you have asked them to speak directly to each other, insist on it and don't back down. There are three good opportunities for this direct communication:

When a joint decision is being reached.

When a positive comment about a member is made to you, respond with "Why don't you *ask/tell* her that now."

If a member says another member will not listen, ask him if he will listen.

Modified from Doherty WJ, Baird MA: *Family therapy and family medicine,* New York, 1983, Guilford Press.

TABLE 12-13.—Counseling the Family or Individual—cont'd

Generally, communications must be practiced in the session before being used by the family. Give support when dealing with stress, grief, or dislocation. To be an effective counselor you must provide support, and to do that you must genuinely want to support them. Here are five guidelines:
Listen, let people express their feelings.
Let them know that you are with them emotionally by reflecting the emotion you hear them expressing, e.g., "You still miss him a lot."
Do not move ahead of the family emotionally by promising that they will feel better soon or that it may not be as bad as they think.
Mobilize support systems for the family or individual.
Teach when you can clarify a situation. The art is to teach when information is needed and back out when the family processes that information.
Challenge the Family
It is often best to let a member challenge the group. When a challenge is made a treatment plan should be in place.
Dealing with Resistance
The two most common primary care counseling forms of resistance are tardiness or absenteeism and arguing with you. Schedule problems should be addressed to see if there is a hidden meaning in the tardiness. If not, you may want to confront them by saying "My time is important to me, and I would like you to respect it." If a member wants to argue with you, ask that he/she simply think about what you have said, or encourage him/her to describe how he/she sees the issues and how he/she would like to change things. You may gain valuable information by following their lead. Don't work hard to persuade the family that you are right, maybe you aren't.

Making Behavioral Contracts
You should encourage all members to identify clearly the specific, concrete changes they are willing to make. This must be done in a cooperative, non-hostile group mood. Members must be willing to make the changes in good faith so that the others will make their changes. The family should plan to evaluate the contract to see if it is working.

After-Session Assignments
It may be useful to follow through on some issues that arise during the session. For example, if sharing household tasks is an issue, you might help the family make specific assignments for the week. If the parents want to spend more time together, let them make specific plans for an event that week. Follow up on these assignments. Failure to follow through would be an important family dynamic to address.

13 *Surgical Care*
Charles W. Smith, Jr.

SUTURES AND LACERATIONS

TABLE 13-1.—GUIDELINES FOR SUTURE REMOVAL

SITE	NO. OF DAYS
Eyelid	3
Other head and neck	4-6
Extremities and trunk	7
Back and feet	10-14

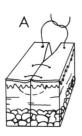
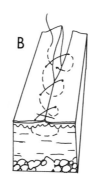
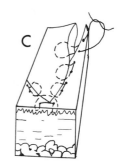
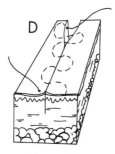
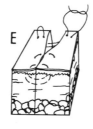
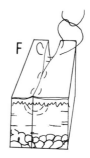

FIG 13-1.
Technique for suturing epidermis. Any of the techniques illustrated are acceptable. **A,** Simple interrupted suture, good for irregular wounds. **B,** Simple running suture, only for linear wounds (tends to invert), quick to do. **C,** Half-buried mattress suture, good for flaps. **D,** Subcuticular suture, good results (leaves no skin marks). **E,** Vertical mattress suture, good for thick and thin skin (e.g., scalp, eyelid), good eversion. **F,** Horizontal mattress suture, looks bad early but achieves good eversion later; must be applied loosely. (From Stuzin JM, Engrav LH, Buehler PK: *Postgrad Med* 71:81, 1982.)

TABLE 13-2.—Types of Suture Material

MATERIAL	COMPOSITION	INDICATIONS FOR USE	COMMENTS
Absorbable			
Plain "catgut"	Sheep intestine connective tissue	Small blood vessels and subcutaneous fat	Causes marked inflammatory reaction in 1 week
Chromic	Same, impregnated with chromic oxide	Same, especially if longer approximation is needed (e.g., bowel closure)	Causes less tissue reaction than catgut
Dexon	Polyglycolic acid	Has almost replaced catgut	Less tissue reaction, lasts about 6 weeks, stronger
Vicryl	Polyglactin	To close deep portions of a wound	Lasts 35 days, strong; little tissue reaction
Nonabsorbable			
Silk	Silk	Artery ligation; use in infected fields	Strong, easy to use, low tissue reactivity
Cotton	Cotton	Same as silk	Not as strong as silk; maintains itself better in tissue than silk
Synthetic	Nylon Dacron Polypropylene	Internal surgery, when ease of use not critical; skin closure	Strong, low tissue reaction, somewhat hard to tie
Wire	Stainless steel wire	Closing abdomen and chest	Least tissue reactivity, very strong; hard to tie

Modified from McCredie JA, Burns GP: Operating room management. In McCredie J, ed: *Basic surgery*, New York, 1977, Macmillan, pp. 236-237.

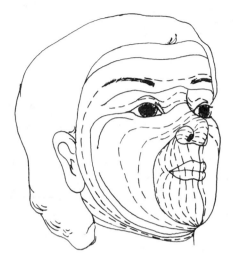

FIG 13-2.
Facial skin lines. (From Riley WB: Wound healing and problem scars. In Barrett BM, ed: *Manual of patient care in plastic surgery,* Boston, 1982, Little, Brown, p. 132.)

TABLE 13-3.—Immunization Schedule

Verify a history of tetanus immunization from medical records so that appropriate tetanus prophylaxis can be accomplished.

HISTORY OF ADSORBED TETANUS TOXOID (Doses)	TETANUS-PRONE WOUNDS		NONTETANUS-PRONE WOUNDS	
	Td*	TIG	Td*	TIG
Unknown or fewer than 3	Yes	Yes	Yes	No
3 or more†	No‡	No	No§	No

From *Advanced trauma life support course manual,* Chicago, 1989, American College of Surgeons.
Td, Tetanus and diphtheria toxoids adsorbed (for adult use); *TIG,* tetanus immune globulin (human).
*For children less than 7 years old: DTP (DT, if pertussis vaccine is contraindicated) is preferable to tetanus toxoid alone. For persons 7 years old and older, Td is preferable to tetanus toxoid alone.
†If only three doses of fluid toxoid have been received, a fourth dose of toxoid, preferably an adsorbed toxoid, should be given.
‡Yes, if more than 10 years since last dose.
§Yes, if more than 5 years since last dose. (More frequent boosters are not needed and can accentuate side effects.)

BURNS

TABLE 13-4.—DEPTH OF BURN INJURY

DEPTH OF CLASSIFICATION	STRUCTURAL DAMAGE	CAUSAL AGENT	CLINICAL APPEARANCE	SENSATION
First-degree	Only superficial layers of epidermis devitalized; dilation of intradermal vessels	Ultraviolet exposure Very short flash	Erythema; blanches with pressure	Present
Second-degree (partial thickness)	Destruction of epidermis to basal layer; deeper skin appendages preserved in dermal layer; clefting of epidermis with fluid collection	Spillage of scalding material Flash Some chemicals	Blister formation, erythema, weeping; superficial skin can be wiped away; erythematous areas should blanch with pressure	Present
Third-degree (full thickness)	Destruction of all skin elements, epidermal and dermal; coagulation of subdermal blood vessels	Flame Immersion Some chemicals	Dry, pale white, charred, leathery, inelastic, visible thrombosed vessels; sometimes red from fixed hemoglobin and will not blanch	Absent
Fourth-degree (involvement of muscle, bone, and other deep structures)	Destruction of all skin elements along with necrosis of deeper structures	Electricity Flame occasionally	Deeply charred, shrunken, often with exposed bones; explosive appearing	Absent

From Lewis ML: *Thermal injuries.* In Wilkins EW, ed: *MGH textbook of emergency medicine,* ed 3, Baltimore, 1988, Williams & Wilkins, p. 762.

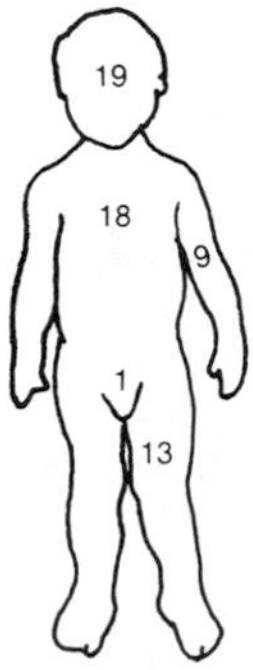

		Child	Adult
Rule of Nines	Head	19%	9%
	Arms	9%	9%
	Front Torso	18%	18%
	Back Torso	18%	18%
	Genitals	1%	1%
	Legs	13%	18%
		100%	**100%**

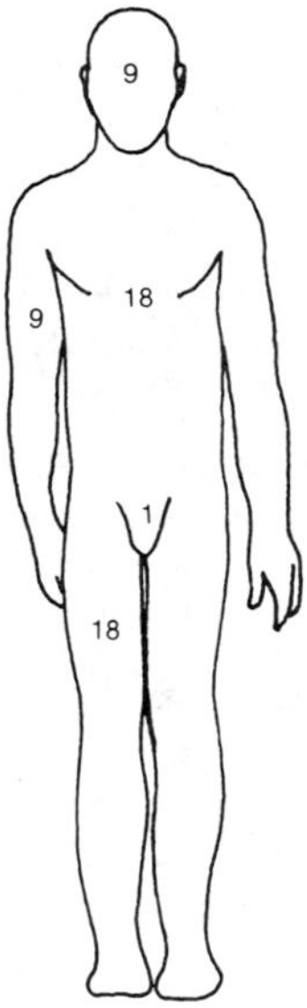

FIG 13-3.
The rule-of-nines estimation of burned body area. (From Bass CB: Burns. In Barrett BM, ed: *Manual of patient care in plastic surgery,* Boston, 1982, Little Brown, p, 292.)

TABLE 13-5.—BURN TREATMENT

Criteria for Hospitalizing Burn Patients
Second-degree burns of more than 30% of body surface area
Third-degree burn of face, hands, and feet
Third-degree burn of more than 10% of body surface area
Significant respiratory injury suspected
All electrical burns
Suspected child abuse

Fluid Replacement in Burn Patients*
First 24 Hours, Lactated Ringer's Solution
4 ml × weight (kg) × % burn (total body surface area)
Give ½ in first 8 hours; ¼ in second 8 hours; remaining ¼ in third 8 hours
24-48 Hours
Decrease total amount by half
Add colloid (Plasmanate or albumin, 7-8 ml/kg) to maintain plasma volume
48 Hours to 10 Days
Add oral liquids, advance as soon as possible to high-protein, high-calorie diet
Give additional colloid as needed
PRBCs to keep hematocrit >30%

Outpatient Burn Management†
Treat pain with appropriate dose of narcotic
Apply cool compresses to burn or place in cool water
Cleanse area with povidone-iodine solution
Give appropriate tetanus prophylaxis
Leave blisters intact (if large, evacuate aseptically and leave skin intact)
Cover burn with vaseline gauze, then a bulky dressing
Wrap area with Kerlix or Kling dressing
Change dressing every 3 days
Debride all devitalized tissue every dressing change
Continue until healing is complete

*Modified from Bass CB: Burns. In Barrett BM, ed: *Manual of patient care in plastic surgery,* Boston, 1982, Little, Brown, pp. 296-297.

†Modified from Bass CB: Burns. In Barrett BM, ed: *Manual of patient care in plastic surgery,* 1982, Boston, Little, Brown, p. 313.

ASSESSMENT OF SURGICAL RISK

TABLE 13-6.—AMERICAN BOARD OF ANESTHESIOLOGY CLASSIFICATION
OF PREOPERATIVE RISK

CLASS	DESCRIPTION
I	No known risk
II	Mild to moderate disease (e.g., well-controlled diabetes)
III	Severe disease present (e.g., complicated diabetic)
IV	Life-threatening disease (e.g., severe angina)
V	Patient moribund (e.g., ruptured aortic aneurysm)

Modified from Deutsch S: Anesthesia. In Papper S, Williams GR, eds: *Manual of medical care of the surgical patient,* ed 2, Boston, 1981, Little, Brown.

TABLE 13-7.—Weighting of Cardiac Risk Factors for Noncardiac Surgery[†]

CRITERIA	POINTS[*]
Historical	
Age over 70 years	5
Myocardial infarction in previous 6 months	10
Examination	
S_3 gallop/jugular venous distention	11
Significant aortic valvular stenosis	3
ECG	
Premature atrial contractions or rhythm other than sinus	7
More than five premature ventricular contractions/minute	7
General Status	
Abnormal blood gases	3
K^+/HCO_3 abnormalities	3
Abnormal renal function	3
Liver disease/bedridden	3
Operation	
Emergency	4
Intraperitoneal/intrathoracic/aortic	3
TOTAL POSSIBLE	62

Cardiac Morbidity and Mortality Caused by Anesthesia and Surgery[††]

Points	Cardiac Risk Class[**]	Cardiac Death Rate (%)	Serious Cardiac Complications (%)	Without Serious Complications (%)
0-5	I	0.2	0.7	99
6-12	II	2.0	5.0	93
13-25	III	2.0	11.0	86
≥26	IV	56.0	22.0	22

[*]Use point total to estimate risk of complications.

[**]I, Healthy patient; II, slightly compromised (e.g., dyspnea on moderate exertion); III, moderately compromised (e.g., dyspnea on mild exertion); IV, severly compromised (e.g., dyspnea at rest).

[†]Modified from Goldman L, et al: *N Engl J Med* 297:845, 1977.

[††]From Brunner EA, Eckenhoff JE: Anesthesia. In Sabiston DC, ed: *Davis-Christopher textbook of surgery,* ed 12, Philadelphia, 1981, WB Saunders, p. 213.

LOCAL ANESTHESIA

TABLE 13-8.—COMMONLY USED LOCAL ANESTHETIC AGENTS

TECHNIQUE	LOCAL ANESTHETIC	CONCENTRATION RANGE (%)	DURATION OF ACTION	MAXIMAL SAFE DOSE (mg)
Topical anesthesia (mucous membranes)	Lidocaine	2-4	15 minutes	100
	Cocaine	4-10	30 minutes	100-200
	Tetracaine	1-2	45 minutes	40
	Benzocaine	2-10	Several hours	—
Local infiltration	Procaine	0.5	¼-½ hours	1000
	Lidocaine	0.5-1	½-1 hour	500
	Mepivacaine	0.5-1	½-1 hour	500
	Tetracaine	0.025-0.1	2-3 hours	75
Major nerve block	Lidocaine	1-2	1-2 hours	500
	Mepivacaine	1-2	1-2¼ hours	500
	Tetracaine	0.1-0.25	2-3 hours	75
Epidural anesthesia	Procaine	1-2	½-1 hour	1000
	Lidocaine	1-2	¾-1½ hour	500
	Mepivacaine	1-2	1-2¼ hours	500
	Tetracaine	0.1-0.25	2-3 hours	75
	Bupivacaine	0.25-0.75	2-4 hours	150
Spinal anesthesia	Procaine	5	½-1 hour	—
	Lidocaine	5	¾-1½ hours	—
	Tetracaine	0.5	1-2 hours	—
Intravenous regional anesthesia	Lidocaine	0.25-0.5	Varies	100-150

From Brunner EA, Eckenhoff JE: Anesthesia. In Sabiston DC, ed: *Davis-Christopher textbook of surgery*, ed 12, Philadelphia, 1981, WB Saunders, p. 197.

TRAUMA

TABLE 13-9.—Evaluation and Treatment of the Trauma Patient

Airway
Use nasotracheal, endotracheal, tracheostomy, or oral airway as indicated
Assess arterial blood gases
Assess chest wall stability
Give O_2 at 2 L/min

Vital Signs
Monitor pulse, BP, and respirations every 10-15 minutes and record
Insert nasogastric tube and Foley catheter; record intake and output

Cardiovascular System
Start 16-gauge or larger IV line
Give Ringer's lactate to keep urine output $\geq$ 30 ml/hr
Apply MAST garment and inflate if BP <80 mm Hg systolic
Check all peripheral pulses
Place on cardiac monitor
Obtain chest x-ray radiograph

Neurological System
Assess level of consciousness and motor and sensory function
If unconscious, treat as if patient had cervical spine injury
If neck or head injury, obtain cervical spine x-ray radiograph

Abdomen
Assess for tenderness, guarding, or rebound
If patient is unconscious, peritoneal tap is indicated
If hematuria is present, obtain IVP and cystogram

Musculoskeletal
Splint fractures
Clean wounds with saline; apply pressure dressings

Other
Labs
Obtain CBC, coagulation profile, BUN, glucose, type and hold, and urinalysis
Arrange Transfer as Indicated
Send copies of all records
History must be "ample":
   A, *A*llergies noted
   M, *M*edications and therapy given
   P, *P*ast history
   L, *L*ast meal
   E, *E*vents leading to injury

Modified from *University of Iowa hospitals and clinics emergency treatment Protocols.*

TABLE 13-10.—Glasgow Coma Scale

Evaluate and plot periodically to follow comatose patient. An initial score of ≥7 points indicates a poor prognosis in the trauma patient.

Best Verbal Response

No response	1 point
Speech incomprehensible	2 points
Inappropriate speech	3 points
Confused speech	4 points
Oriented	5 points

Eye Opening

Not open	1 point
Opens in response to pain	2 points
Response to speech	3 points
Spontaneous	4 points

Best Motor Response

No response	1 point
Extensor response	2 points
Abnormal flexion	3 points
Withdrawal	4 points
Localizes	5 points
Obeys commands	6 points

BREAST MASSES AND BREAST CANCER

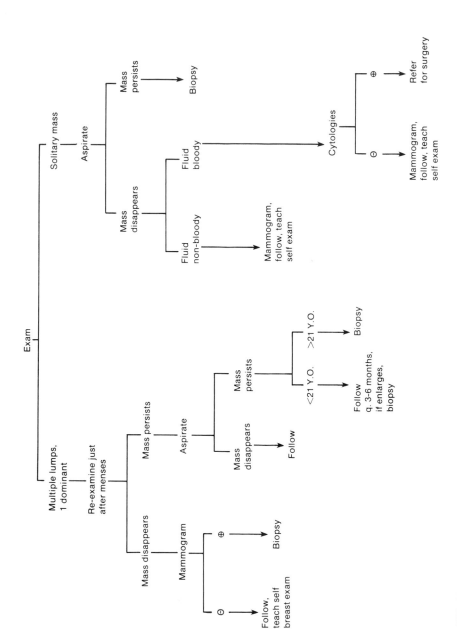

FIG 13-4.
Management of breast masses.

INTESTINAL OBSTRUCTION AND ABDOMINAL PAIN

TABLE 13-11.—Differentiating Paralytic Ileus from Intestinal Obstruction

ASPECT	PARALYTIC ILEUS	MECHANICAL OBSTRUCTION
Symptoms		
Pain	Diffuse, mild aching pain, bloating sensation	Cramping, often severe, mid- to low-abdominal pain
Vomiting	Occasional, mild vomiting episodes	Bilious or feculent vomiting
Physical Signs		
Distention	Early marked distention, persistent	Moderate distention, worsens over time
Bowel sounds	Decreased or absent bowel sounds	Increased bowel sounds with rushes
Tenderness	Mild, diffuse tenderness to palpation	Mild, diffuse tenderness to palpation
X-ray Signs		
Stomach gas	Usually increased	Sometimes present, normal amount
Bowel gas	Marked throughout small and large bowel	Only proximal to obstruction
Fluid in bowel	Minimal	Large amount
"Stepladder" pattern	Occasionally seen	Often seen
Air/fluid levels in loop of bowel (upright film)	Same level across mid-abdomen	Different levels; "J-loops" seen

Modified from Condon RE, Brient B: Intestinal obstruction. In Condon RE, Nyhus LM, eds: *Manual of surgical therapeutics,* ed 2, Boston, 1972, Little, Brown.

TABLE 13-12.—DIFFERENTIAL DIAGNOSIS OF BILIARY COLIC, ACUTE CHOLECYSTITIS, AND SUPPURATIVE COMPLICATIONS OF ACUTE CHOLECYSTITIS

SYMPTOM	BILIARY COLIC	ACUTE CHOLECYSTITIS	SUPPURATIVE COMPLICATED CHOLECYSTITIS
Pain	Crampy	Steady	Steady
Nausea	Usually present	Usually present	Usually present
Vomiting	Occasional	Often present	Often present
Onset	Usually meal-related	Occasionally meal-related	Occasionally meal-related
Fever	Absent	99° F-100° F	Usually 102° F or more
WBC count	<10,000	10,000-15,000	Usually >15,000
Bilirubin	Normal	1-4 mg/100 ml	Often >4 mg/100 ml
Course	Resolves in 1-4 hours	Resolves in 24-48 hours	Requires surgery acutely

Modified from Carey LC, Ellison EC: Acute cholecystitis. In Sabiston DC, ed: *Davis-Christopher textbook of surgery,* ed 12, Philadelphia, 1981, WB Saunders, p. 1265.

DECUBITUS ULCERS

TABLE 13-13.—TREATMENT OF DECUBITUS ULCERS

STAGE	DESCRIPTION	TREATMENT
I	Erythema, edema, punctate hemorrhages, superficial blisters or blebs	Remove pressure, eliminate shear forces, gentle cleaning every 6-8 hours; topical antibiotics and fine mesh gauze; Opsite or Duoderm is a good alternative
II	Full-thickness skin loss; erythematous halo; defects <3 cm	Consider excision and primary closure
III	Same as II, but defects >3 cm	Eliminate pressure, debride devitalized tissue; wet to dry dressings every 6 hours until wound is ready to graft, then use split-thickness skin graft
IV	Crater base with yellow-gray eschar; pus exudes from periphery surrounding red halo	Debride, in stages if needed; pack wound with damp gauze, covered with dry gauze at skin surface, every 6-8 hours; graft with full-thickness graft after 2-3 weeks
V	Cone-shaped defect; small skin opening with undermining and cavern formation	Extend wound and debride as above; treatment same as for stage IV
VI	Chronic ulcerative defect; often present months or years; bone often visible	Hospitalization; attention to nutrition, patient positioning; usually requires skin flap surgery

Modified from Agris J: Pressure ulcers. In Barrett BM, ed: *Manual of patient care in plastic surgery,* Boston, 1982, Little, Brown, pp. 347-363.

CLINICAL PRACTICE GUIDELINES: PRESSURE ULCERS IN ADULTS

An algorithm (Fig. 3-5) was developed as a visual display of the conceptual organization, procedural flow, decision points, and preferred management path discussed in the 1992 AHCPR pressure ulcer guideline. It begins at the point of admission to an acute care hospital, rehabilitation hospital, nursing home, home care program, or other health care facility or program. Numbers in the algorithm refer to the annotations in the legend of Fig. 13-5.

Pressure Ulcer Prediction and Prevention Algorithm

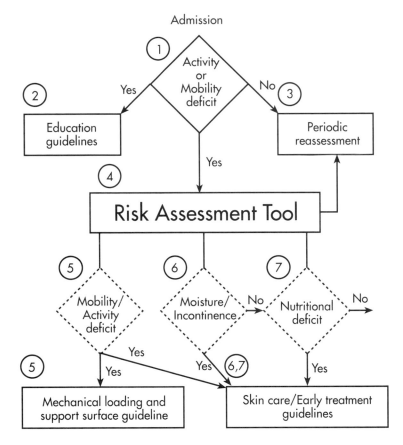

FIG 13-5.

1. *Activity or Mobility Deficit:* Bed- or chair-bound individuals or those whose ability to reposition is impaired should be considered at risk for pressure ulcers. Identification of additional risk factors (immobility, moisture/incontinence, and nutritional deficit) should be undertaken to direct specific preventive treatment regimes.

2. *Educational Program:* Educational programs for the prevention of pressure ulcers should be structured, organized, and comprehensive and directed at all levels of health care providers, patients, and family or caregivers.

3. *Reassessment:* Active, mobile individuals should be periodically reassessed for changes in activity and mobility status. The frequency of reassessment depends on patient status and institutional policy.

FIG 13-5—cont'd.

4. *Risk Assessment Tools:* Clinicians are encouraged to select and use a method of risk assessment that ensures systematic evaluation of individual risk factors. Many risk assessment tools exist, but only the Norton Scale (see Table 13-14) and Braden Scale have been tested extensively.

   Risk assessment tools include the following risk factors: mobility/ activity impairment, moisture/incontinence, and impaired nutrition. Altered level of consciousness (or altered sensory perception) is also identified as a risk factor in most assessment tools. Identification of individual risk factors Table 13-15 is helpful in directing care.

5. *Mobility/Activity Deficit:*
   For bed-bound individuals:

- Reposition at least every 2 hours.
- Use pillows or foam wedges to keep bony prominences from direct contact.
- Use devices that totally relieve pressure on the heels.
- Avoid positioning directly on the trochanter.
- Elevate the head of the bed as little and for as short a time as possible.
- Use lifting devices to move rather than drag individuals during transfers and position changes.
- Place at-risk individuals on a pressure-reducing mattress. *Do not use donut-type devices.*

For chair-bound individuals:
- Reposition at least every hour.
- Have patient shift weight every 15 minutes if possible.
- Use pressure-reducing devices for seating surfaces. *Do not use donut-type devices.*
- Consider postural alignment, distribution of weight, balance and stability, and pressure relief when positioning individuals in chairs or wheelchairs.
- Use a written plan.

For skin care
- Inspect skin at least once a day.
- Individualize bathing schedule. Avoid hot water. Use a mild cleansing agent.
- Minimize environmental factors such as low humidity and cold air. Use moisturizers for dry skin.
- Avoid massage over bony prominences.
- Use proper positioning, transferring, and turning techniques.
- Use lubricants to reduce friction injuries.
- Institute a rehabilitation program.
- Monitor and document interventions and outcomes.

Continued.

FIG 13-5—cont'd.

6. *Moisture/Incontinence:*

- Cleanse skin at time of soiling.
- Minimize skin exposure to moisture. Assess and treat urinary incontinence. When moisture cannot be controlled, use underpads or briefs that are absorbent and present a quick-drying surface to the skin.

7. *Nutritional Deficit:*

- Investigate factors that compromise an apparently well-nourished individual's dietary intake (especially protein or calories) and offer him or her support with eating.
- Plan and implement a nutritional support and/or supplementation program for nutritionally compromised individuals.

Risk should be periodically reassessed. Care should be modified according to the level of risk. Frequency of reassessment depends on patient status and institutional policy. (From U.S. Department of Health and Human Services, Rockville, Md, AHCPR Publication No. 92-0047, May 1992.)

TABLE 13-14.—Norton Scale: Pressure Ulcer Risk Assessment Tool

Name	Date	PHYSICAL CONDITION		MENTAL CONDITION		ACTIVITY		MOBILITY		INCONTINENT		TOTAL SCORE*
		Good	4	Alert	4	Ambulant	4	Full	4	Not	4	
		Fair	3	Apathetic	3	Walk/help	3	Slightly limited	3	Occasional	3	
		Poor	2	Confused	2	Chairbound	2	Very limited	2	Usually/urine	2	
		Very bad	1	Stupor	1	Stupor	1	Immobile	1	Doubly	1	

From Norton D, McLaren R, Exton-Smith AN: *An investigation of geriatric nursing problems in the hospital*, London 1962, National Corporation for the Care of Old People (now the Centre for Policy on Ageing).

*Low score (e.g., <12) indicates higher risk for pressure ulcer.

THYROID NODULES

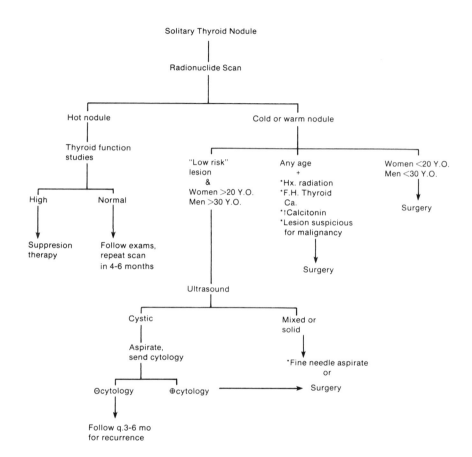

*Undertake if close follow up, good
 cytology lab, and experience in procedure

FIG 13-6.
Management of thyroid nodules.

NATURE OF OPERATION	LIKELY PATHOGENS	RECOMMENDED DRUGS	ADULT DOSAGE BEFORE SURGERY[a]
Clean			
Cardiac			
Prosthetic valve, coronary artery bypass, other open-heart surgery, pacemaker implant	*Staphylococcus epidermidis, S. aureus, Corynebacterium,* enteric gram-negative bacilli	Cefazolin or cefuroxime *or* vancomycin[c]	1-2 g IV[b] 1 g IV
Vascular			
Arterial surgery involving the abdominal aorta, a prosthesis, or a groin incision	*S. aureus, S. epidermidis,* enteric gram-negative bacilli	Cefazolin *or* vancomycin[c]	1-2 g IV 1 g IV
Lower extremity amputation for ischemia	*S. aureus, S. epidermidis,* enteric gram-negative bacilli, clostridia	Cefazolin *or* vancomycin[c]	1 g IV 1 g IV
Neurosurgery			
Craniotomy	*S. aureus, S. epidermidis*	Cefazolin *or* vancomycin[c]	1 g IV 1 g IV
Orthopedic			
Total joint replacement, internal fixation of fractures	*S. aureus, S. epidermidis*	Cefazolin *or* vancomycin[c]	1-2 g IV 1 g IV

From *Med Lett* 35(906):94, Oct. 1993.

[a]Parenteral prophylactic antimicrobials can be given as a single intravenous dose just before the operation. Cefazolin can also be given intramuscularly. For prolonged operations, additional intraoperative doses should be given every 4-8 hours for the duration of the procedure.

[b]Some consultants recommend an additional dose when patients are removed from bypass during open heart surgery.

[c]For hospitals in which methicillin-resistant *S. aureus* and *S. epidermidis* frequently cause wound infection, or for patients allergic to penicillins or cephalosporins. Rapid IV administration may cause hypotension, which could be especially dangerous during induction of anesthesia. Even if the drug is given over 60 minutes, hypotension may occur; treatment with diphenhydramine (Benadryl, and others) and further slowing of the infusion rate may be helpful (Maki DG et al, *J Thorac Cardiovasc Surg,* 104:1423, 1992). For procedures in which enteric gram-negative bacilli are likely pathogens, such as vascular surgery involving a groin incision, cefazolin should be included in the prophylaxis regimen.

[d]After appropriate diet and catharsis, one gram of each at 1 PM, 2 PM, and 11 PM the day before an 8 AM operation.

[e]Patients with previous pelvic inflammatory disease, previous gonorrhea, or multiple sex partners.

[f]Divided into 100 mg one hour before the abortion and 200 mg one half hour after.

[g]For "dirty" surgery, therapy should usually be continued for five to 10 days.

[h]For bite wounds, in which likely pathogens may also include oral anaerobes, *Eikenella corrodens* (human), and *Pasteurella multocida* (dog and cat), some *Medical Letter* consultants recommend use of amoxicillin-clavulanic acid (Augmentin) or ampicillin-sulbactam (Unasyn).

Continued.

NATURE OF OPERATION	LIKELY PATHOGENS	RECOMMENDED DRUGS	ADULT DOSAGE BEFORE SURGERY[a]
Ophthalmic	S. aureus, S. epidermidis, streptococci, enteric gram-negative bacilli, Pseudomonas	Gentamicin or tobramycin or neomycin-gramicidin-polymyxin B,	Multiple drops topically over 2 to 24 hours
		Cefazolin	100 mg subconjunctivally at end of procedure
Clean-Contaminated			
Head and Neck Entering oral cavity or pharynx	S. aureus, streptococci, oral anaerobes	Cefazolin or clindamycin	1-2 g IV 600-900 mg IV
Abdominal, Gastroduodenal	Enteric gram-negative bacilli, gram-positive cocci	High risk, gastric bypass, or percutaneous endoscopic gastrostomy only: cefazolin	1 g IV 1 g IV
Biliary Tract	Enteric gram-negative bacilli, enterococci, clostridia	High risk only: cefazolin	
Colorectal	Enteric gram-negative bacilli, anaerobes	Oral: neomycin plus erythromycin base[d] Parenteral: cefoxitin or cefotetan	1 g IV
Appendectomy	Enteric gram-negative bacilli, anaerobes	Cefoxitin or cefotetan	1 g IV
Gynecological, Vaginal, or Abdominal Hysterectomy	Enteric gram-negative bacilli, anaerobes, group B streptococci, enterococci	Cefazolin	1 g IV
Cesarean Section	Same as for hysterectomy	High risk only: cefazolin	1 g IV after cord clamping
Abortion	Same as for hysterectomy	First trimester high risk[e]: aqueous penicillin G or doxycycline	1 million U IV 300 mg PO[b]
		Second trimester: cefazolin	1 g IV
Dirty Surgery			
Ruptured viscus[g]	Enteric gram-negative bacilli, anaerobes, enterococci	Cefoxitin or cefotetan with or without gentamicin or clindamycin plus gentamicin	2 g IV every 6 hours 1-2 g IV every 12 hours 1.5 mg/kg IV every 8 hours 600 mg IV every 6 hours 1.5 mg/kg IV every 8 hours
Traumatic wound[g,h]	S. aureus, group A strepto-	Cefazolin	1-2 g IV every 8 hours

TABLE 13-16.—ABDOMINAL AORTIC ANEURYSM

Risk of Rupture
<4.0 cm, risk is about 2%
Between 4 and 5 cm, risk is between 3% and 12% within 5 years
>5.0 cm, risk is between 25% and 41% within 5 years

Diagnosis
Ultrasonography sensitivity almost 100%
Measurement by this technique is very accurate
CT sensitive and specific and provides additional information about shape
MRI may be best but is too expensive to be routinely used
Role of aortography preoperatively debatable, but many surgeons use

Surgery
If size >5 cm, most surgeons recommend resection
If 4-5 cm, obtain ultrasound every 6 months, and operate if expansion of 0.5 cm

From Desforges JF: Abdominal aortic aneurysm, *N Engl J Med* 328(16):1167, 1993.

TABLE 13-17.—LAPAROSCOPIC SURGERY

CURRENTLY ACCEPTED PROCEDURES	INDICATION	COMMENTS
Diagnostic laparoscopy	Evaluation of abdominal pain	Avoid unneeded appendectomy; overall accuracy 80-99 per cent
	Staging of malignant tumors	Tumors less than 1-2 cm often missed; accuracy in assessing liver disease 90%; good for second look ovarian tumors
Laparoscopic cholecystectomy	Evaluation of abdominal trauma	Accuracy over 90%; doesn't visualize retroperitoneum.
	Cholecystitis	Less pain, shorter hospital stay, faster recovery; death <1%; rate of bile duct injury only slightly greater (< or = 0.5%)

LAPAROSCOPIC PROCEDURES GAINING ACCEPTANCE	COMMENTS
Appendectomy	Limited trials show shorter hospital stay, less pain, fewer wound infections
Exporation of the common duct	90% of common duct stones extractable with a basket
Repair of inguinal hernia	Patch repair most common; requires general anesthetic
Laparoscopic colon resection	Combination of laparoscopic and extracorporeal techniques
GI reflux surgery	Procedure similar to Nissen fundoplication;
Peptic ulcer surgery	Rarely needed because of excellent drugs available; highly selective vagotomy; omental patch can be used for acute perforation

From Soper NJ, Brunt LM, Kerbl, K: Laparoscopic general surgery, *N Engl J Med* 330(6):409, 1994.

14 Care of Children

Edward T. Bope

IMMUNIZATIONS

TABLE 14-1.—IMMUNIZATIONS: GENERAL PRINCIPLES

It is more important that every child receive every immunization than that a rigid schedule is followed. Absolute contraindications to immunizations are as follows:
Immune deficiency in child or family member
γ-Globulin within 3 months
Relative contraindications to immunizations are as follows:
A febrile illness
Febrile convulsions or neurological disorders
If a scheduled dose of DTP or TOPV is missed, it is not necessary to repeat the series, no matter how long the interval is
Premature infants can be started on immunizations when they weigh >10 lb
Live virus vaccines, e.g., TOPV, MMR, and Varivax should be given 1 month apart.

SCREENING AND HEALTH MAINTENANCE

TABLE 14-2.—Recommended Schedule for Active Immunization of Infants and Children

AGE	IMMUNIZATION		APPROXIMATE COST* (WHOLESALE)	
Birth	HBV no. 1		$16.00	
2 months	HBV no. 2		$16.00	
	TOPV no. 1		$12.80	
	DTP no. 1	} *or* Tetramune no. 1+	$5.40	$27.50+
	HbCV no. 1		$15.70	
4 months	DTP no. 2	} *or* Tetramune no. 2+	$5.40	$27.50+
	HbCV no. 2		$15.70	
	TOPV no. 2		$12.80	
6 months	DTP no. 3	} *or* Tetramune no. 3+	$5.40	$27.50+
	HbCV no. 3		$15.70	
9 months	HBV no. 3		$12.80	
12-18 months	VV		$39.94	
15-18 months	MMR no. 1		$31.00	
	TOPV no. 3		$12.80	
	DTaP no. 1		$16.00	
	HbCV no. 4		$16.00	
5 years	MMR no. 2		$31.00	
	DTaP no. 2		$16.00	
	TOPV no. 4		$12.80	
Every 10 years after age 5	Td		$7.50 (pediatric) $6.80 (adult)	
10 years and older	HBV series if not given before age 10		$120.00/series	

HBV, Hepatitis B vaccine; *TOPV,* trivalent oral polio vaccine (suspension of live attenuated poliovirus types 1, 2 and 3); *DTP,* diptheria-tetanus-pertussis (inactivated *Corynebacterium diphtheriae, Clostridium tetani,* killed strains of *Bordetella pertussis); HbCV,* Haemophilus influenza type-B conjugate vaccine (conjugate of oligosaccharides of the capsular antigen); *MMR,* measles·mumps-rubella (live attenuated measles, mumps, and rubella viruses); *DTaP,* diphtheria-tetanus-acellular pertussis; *Td,* tetanus (full dose)—diphtheria (reduced dose); *VV,* Varivax.
*1994 prices.

TABLE 14-3.—IMMUNIZATION SCHEDULE FOR CHILDREN WHO DID NOT START
IMMUNIZATIONS BEFORE 12 MONTHS

TIME LINE	GENERAL SCHEDULE	USAGE GUIDELINES
For Ages 12 Months to 7 Years		
First visit	DTP no. 1, TOPV no. 1, MMR, PPD, Hib no. 1	
2 months	DTP no. 2, TOPV no. 2, Hib no. 2	Hib no. 2 and no. 3 not needed if starting >15 months
4 months	DTP no. 3, Hib no. 3	Hib no. 2 and no. 3 not needed if starting >15 months
10-16 months	TOPV no. 3, DTP no. 4, or DTaP	
12-18 months	VV	
At entry to school (age 4-6 years)	TOPV no. 4, MMR, DTP no. 5, or DtaP	DTP no. 5 and TOPV no. 4 are not needed if previous set was given after age 4
For Ages 7 or Older		
First visit	Td, TOPV no. 1, MMR, PPD, Hib no. 1, Hep. B	
1 month	Hep. B	
2 months	Td, TOPV no. 2, Hib no. 2	Hib no. 2 not needed if >12 years old
6 months	Hep. B	
8-14 months	Td, TOPV no. 3	Repeat Td at 10 years from this visit
11-12 years	MMR	

DTP, Diphtheria-tetanus-pertussis; *TOPV,* trivalent oral polio vaccine; *MMR,* measles-mumps-rubella; *PPD,* Purified protein derivative; *Hib,* Haemophilus influenzae B. vaccine; *Hep. B,* Hepatitis B vaccine; *VV,* Varivax.

TABLE 14-4.—IMMUNIZATION GUIDELINES

IMMUNIZATION	AGENT	SIDE EFFECTS	USAGE GUIDELINES
Diphtheria	Toxoid	Fever, pain, erythema, induration, nodule	Seizure disorder of previous CNT symptoms are contraindications to further pertussis doses; can be given during afebrile gastrointestinal or respiratory disease
Pertussis	Killed pertussis	"	"
Tetanus	Toxoid	"	"
DtaP	Toxoid	Fever, local reactions, and minor systemic symptoms in 10%-33%	May be used after first three doses of DTP. No reports of fever, febrile seizure, crying, hypotonic, hyporesponsive episodes
Polio	Three strains of live attenuated polio virus	None common	May be given to pregnant mother if exposed to polio; if parents have not been immunized, give adults 2-3 doses of IPV (inactivated polio virus) before immunizing children
Measles	Live attenuated mumps virus	None	MMR may be used prophylactically if exposed to disease, although not guaranteed to prevent disease. Live measles and mumps vaccine contraindicated only if patient has had anaphylactic or anaphylactoid reaction subsequent to egg ingestion
Rubella	Live attenuated rubella virus	Fever, rash, arthralgia, arthritis, neuropathy	All must be satisfied in postmenarchal female: Not pregnant Absence of rubella titer Prevent pregnancy for 3 months Give consequences of pregnancy Warn of side effects
Haemophilus	Purified capsular polysaccharide	Mild febrile and local reaction	May be used at 18 months for high risk of day care children
Varicella	Live attenuated varicella vaccine	Pain, redness, swelling, fever, and noninjection site varicella-like rash	Do not give to immunocompromised patients; do not use in patients less than 1 year of age; do not administer with other live viruses; may occasionally cause latent varicella zoster

DtaP, Diphtheria-tetanus-acellular pertussis; *DTP,* diphtheria-tetanus-pertussis.

EVALUATION OF THE NEWBORN

TABLE 14-5.—Evaluation of the Newborn

Apgar Score
The newborn is evaluated at 1 and 5 minutes after birth. Points are given to each of the five criteria and added for a total score. The 5-minute score is the one most useful in predicting neonatal and long-term prognosis.

Condition	Apgar Score
Best condition	8-10
Moderately depressed	5-7
Severely depressed	≤4

TABLE 14-6.—Determining the Apgar Score

ASPECT	POINTS		
	0	1	2
Heart rate	Absent	Slow (<100)	>100
Respiratory effort	Absent	Slow, irregular	Good, crying
Muscle tone	Limp	Some flexion of extremities	Active motion
Response to catheter in nostril (tested after oropharynx is clear)	No response	Grimace	Cough or sneeze
Color	Blue or pale	Body pink; extremities blue	Completely pink

Modified from Apgar V: *JAMA* 168:1985, 1958.

TABLE 14-7.—Conditions of High Risk for the Newborn

ANTENATAL	NATAL	POSTNATAL
Maternal age <16 or >35	Abnormal fetal heart rate	Birth asphyxia
Maternal diabetes	Abnormal presentation, such as breech or face	Fetal malformations
Maternal hypertension		HIV infection
Maternal hemorrhage		Hypothermia
Maternal hypoxia	Cesarean section	Macrosomia
Maternal infection	Chorioamnionitis	Meconium staining
Maternal drug therapy	Heavy sedation of mother	Preterm infant
Reserpine		Respiratory distress
Lithium carbonate	Maternal hypotension	Small-for-dates infant
Magnesium	Maternal infection, herpes, HIV, group B streptococcus.	
Alcohol		
Adrenergic blocking drugs	Meconium-stained fluid	
Maternal substance abuse	Mid- or high-forceps delivery	
Cocaine	Multiple births	
Heroin, alcohol	Polyhydramnios	
Methadone	Precipitus delivery	
Maternal anemia or isoimmunization	Premature delivery	
Smoking	Prolapsed cord	
	Prolonged labor	
	Prolonged rupture of membranes	
	Shoulder dystocia	

TABLE 14-8 A.—Drugs Used in Pediatric Advanced Life Support*

DRUG	DOSE	REMARKS
Adenosine	0.1 to 0.2 mg/kg Maximum single dose: 12 mg	Rapid IV bolus
Atropine sulfate	0.02 mg/kg per dose	Minimum dose: 0.1 mg Maximum single dose: 0.5 mg in child, 1.0 mg in adolescent
Bretylium	5 mg/kg: may be increased to 10 mg/kg	Rapid IV
Calcium chloride 10%	20 mg/kg per dose	Give slowly
Dopamine hydrochloride	2-20 µg/kg per minute	α-Adrenergic action dominates at ≥15-20 µg/kg per minute
Dobutamine hydrochloride	2-20 µg/kg per minute	Titrate to desired effect
Epinephrine For bradycardia	IV/IO: 0.01 mg/kg (1:10 000) ET: 0.1 mg/kg (1:1000)	Be aware of effective dose of preservatives administered (if preservatives are present in epinephrine preparation) when high doses are used
For asystolic or pulseless arrest	First dose: IV/IO: 0.01 mg/kg (1:10 000) ET: 0.1 mg/kg (1:1000) Doses as high as 0.2 mg/kg may be effective Subsequent doses: IV/IO/ET: 0.1 mg/kg (1:1000) Doses as high as 0.2 mg/kg may be effective	Be aware of effective dose of preservative administered (if preservatives present in epinephrine preparation) when high doses are used
Epinephrine infusion	Initial at 0.1 µg/kg per minute Higher infusion dose used if asystole present	Titrate to desired effect (0.1-1.0 µg/kg per minute)
Lidocaine	1 mg/kg per dose	
Lidocaine infusion	20-50 µg/kg per minute	
Sodium bicarbonate	1 mEq/kg per dose or 0.3 × kg × base deficit	Infuse slowly and only if ventilation is adequate

*IV, Intravenous route; IO, intraosseous route; ET, endotracheal route.
From Pediatric advanced life support: *JAMA* 268:2268, 1992, American Medical Association.

TABLE 14-8 B.—Preparation of Infusions

DRUG	PREPARATION*	DOSE
Epinephrine	0.6 × body weight (kg) equals mg added to diluent† to make 100 mL	Then 1 mL/h delivers 0.1 µg/kg/min; titrate to effect
Dopamine, dobutamine	6 × body weight (kg) equals milligrams added to diluent to make 100 mL	Then 1 mL/h delivers 1 µg/kg/min; titrate to effect
Lidocaine	120 mg of 40-mg/mL solution added to 97 mL of 5% dextrose in water, yielding 1200 µg/mL solution	Then 1 mL/kg per hour delivers 20 µg/kg per minute

*Standard concentration may be used to provide more dilute or more concentrated drug solution, but then individual dose must be calculated for each patient and each infusion rate:

$$\text{Infusion rate (mL/h)} = \frac{\text{weight (kg)} \times \text{dose (µg/kg/min)} \times 60 \text{ min/h}}{\text{concentration (µg/mL)}}$$

†Diluent may be 5% dextrose in water, 5% dextrose in half-normal saline, normal saline, or Ringer's lactate.
From Pediatric advanced life support: *JAMA* 268:2268, 1992, American Medical Association.

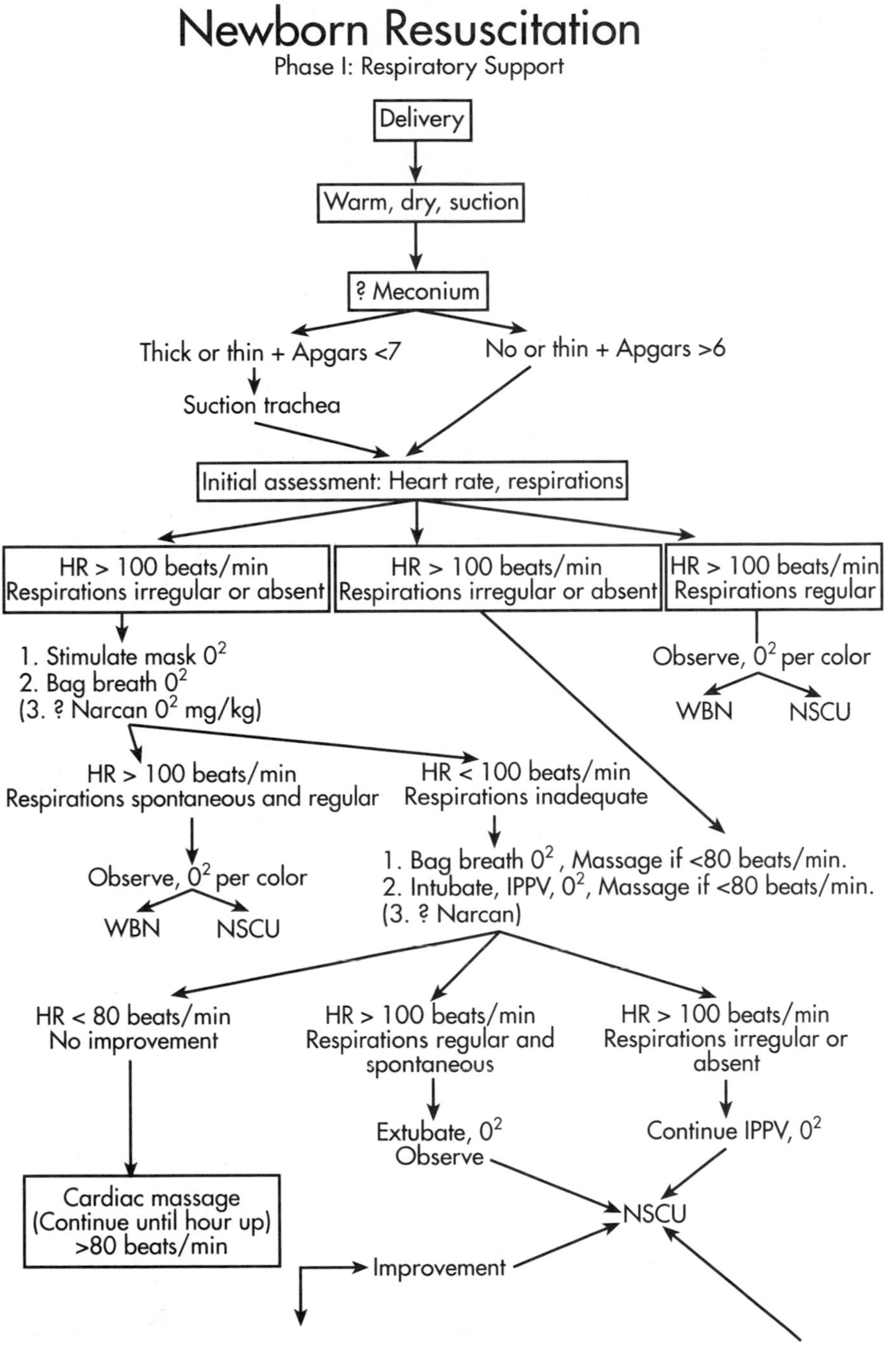

Newborn Resuscitation
Phase I: Respiratory Support

Delivery

↓

Warm, dry, suction

↓

? Meconium

Thick or thin + Apgars <7 ← → No or thin + Apgars >6

Suction trachea

Initial assessment: Heart rate, respirations

| HR > 100 beats/min | HR > 100 beats/min | HR > 100 beats/min |
| Respirations irregular or absent | Respirations irregular or absent | Respirations regular |

1. Stimulate mask 0^2
2. Bag breath 0^2
(3. ? Narcan 0^2 mg/kg)

Observe, 0^2 per color

WBN   NSCU

HR > 100 beats/min   HR < 100 beats/min
Respirations spontaneous and regular   Respirations inadequate

Observe, 0^2 per color

WBN   NSCU

1. Bag breath 0^2, Massage if <80 beats/min.
2. Intubate, IPPV, 0^2, Massage if <80 beats/min.
(3. ? Narcan)

HR < 80 beats/min   HR > 100 beats/min   HR > 100 beats/min
No improvement   Respirations regular and   Respirations irregular or
          spontaneous   absent

Extubate, 0^2 Continue IPPV, 0^2
Observe

Cardiac massage
(Continue until hour up)
>80 beats/min

NSCU

Improvement

FIG 14-1.
Newborn resuscitation phase I: respiratory support. (Courtesy Patrick Wall, MD, Riverside Methodist Hospitals, Columbus, Ohio.)

Newborn Resuscitation
Phase II: Drug Support

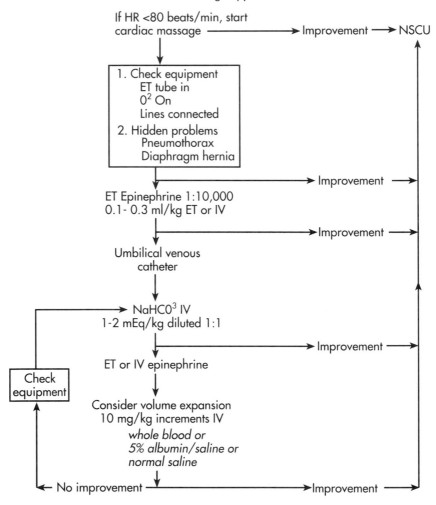

If HR <80 beats/min, start
cardiac massage ————————————→ Improvement ——→ NSCU

1. Check equipment
   ET tube in
   0^2 On
   Lines connected
2. Hidden problems
   Pneumothorax
   Diaphragm hernia

—————————————→ Improvement ——→

ET Epinephrine 1:10,000
0.1- 0.3 ml/kg ET or IV

—————————————→ Improvement ——→

Umbilical venous
catheter

$NaHCO^3$ IV
1-2 mEq/kg diluted 1:1

—————————————→ Improvement ——→

ET or IV epinephrine

Check
equipment

Consider volume expansion
10 mg/kg increments IV
*whole blood or
5% albumin/saline or
normal saline*

←— No improvement ——————————→ Improvement ——→

FIG 14-2.
Newborn resuscitation phase II: drug support. (Courtesy Patrick Wall, MD, Riverside Methodist Hospitals, Columbus, Ohio.)

GROWTH AND DEVELOPMENT

TABLE 14-9.—Developmental Assessment and Guidance

AGE	GROSS MOTOR	VISUAL MOTOR	LANGUAGE	SOCIAL	GUIDANCE
1 month	Raises head slightly from prone, makes crawling movements, lifts chin up	Has tight grasp, follows to midline	Alert to sound (e.g. by blinking, moving, startling)	Regards face, spontaneous smile	Car seats, fever control, thermometers, talking to baby, sleeping, stimulating mobiles
2 months	Holds chin in midline, lifts chest off table, head up 45 degrees	No longer clenches fist tightly, follows object past midline	Smiles after being stroked or talked to	Acts increasingly alert, recognizes parent, may smile spontaneously	
3 months	Supports self on forearms in prone, holds head up steadily	Holds hand open at rest, pulls at clothing, follows in circular fashion, puts hands together	Coos (produces long vowel sounds in musical fashion), squeals, laughs	Reaches for familiar people or objects; anticipates feeding, regards own hand	Car seats, diet, stimulating safe toys, babysitters
4-5 months	Rolls front to back, back to front, sits well when propped, supports on wrists, shifts weight, can bear weight on legs	Move arms in unison to grasp, touches cube placed on table, follows 180 degrees	4 months: orients to voice 5 months: orients to bell, says "ah goo," razzes	Enjoys looking around environment	
6 months	Sits well, puts feet in mouth in supine position	Reaches with either hand, transfers, uses raking grasp	Babbles (imitates speech sounds) 8 months: says "mama/dada" indiscriminately	Work for toy, feed self, recognize strangers	Car seats, stair gates, electric cord and outlet covers, crawling, stranger anxiety, peek-a-boo, banging toys

Modified from *The Harriet Lane handbook*, ed 13, Chicago, 1993, Mosby.

Continued.

TABLE 14-9.—Developmental Assessment and Guidance—cont'd

AGE	GROSS MOTOR	VISUAL MOTOR	LANGUAGE	SOCIAL	GUIDANCE
9 months	Creeps, crawls, cruises, pulls to feet, likes to stand, pivots when sitting	Uses overhand pincer grasp, probes with forefinger, holds bottle, finger-feeds	Imitates sounds 10 months: waves bye-bye	Starts to explore environment	Car seats, water bath safety, finger-foods, cup weaning, teeth care, first book, appropriate discipline, ipecac
11 months	Stands for 2 seconds		Follows one-step command with gesture, says "mama/dada" discriminately		
12 months	Walks alone or with hand held, pivots when sitting, cooperates with dressing	Uses mature pincer grasp, throws objects, lets go of toys, hand release	One word	Imitates actions, comes when called, cooperates with dressing, indicates wants, plays ball with examiner	Car seats, books, water safety, burns, scalds, diet, decreases appetite, riding toys, pull toys, temper tantrums, nightmares, toilet training
13 months	Stands alone				
14 months	Stoops and recovers, walks well		Two words		
15 months	Walks well, creeps upstairs, walks backwards	Scribbles in imitation of examiner	Follows one-step command without gesture, uses two words	Drinks from cup	
18 months	Runs, throws toy from standing without falling	Turns 2-3 pages at a time, fills spoon and feeds self	Uses three words, points to one body part when named, uses mature jargoning, includes intelligible words	Copies parent in tasks (e.g., sweeping, dusting), plays in company of other children, uses spoon, fork	

Age	Gross Motor	Fine Motor	Language	Personal-Social	Safety
21 months	Squats in play, goes up steps, kicks ball forward	Builds tower of two blocks, drinks well from cup	Points to three body parts, uses two-word combination	Asks to have food and to go to toilet	Car seats, books, playground safety, babysitter, giving up blanket etc., appropriate discipline, learning to play with others
24 months	Walks up and down steps without help, throws ball overhand	Turns pages one at a time, removes shoes, pants, etc., build tower of six cubes	Uses 50 words, two-word sentences, three pronouns; names objects in pictures		
30 months	Jumps with both feet off floor, throws ball overhand	Unbuttons, holds pencil in adult fashion, differentiates horizontal and vertical lines	Appropriate use of pronouns, understands concept of "1", repeats two digits	Tells first and last names when asked, gets drink without help	
3 years	Pedal tricycle, can alternate feet when going up steps	Dresses and undresses partially, dries hands if reminded, draws a circle	Tells story about experiences, knows his or her sex	Shares toys, takes turns, plays well with others	
4 years	Hops, skips, alternates feet going down stairs	Buttons clothing fully, catches ball	Knows all colors, says song or poem from memory	Tells "tall tales"; plays cooperatively with a group of children	Consideration should be given to discussing "private" areas and setting limits for those areas
5 years	Skips, alternating feet; jumps over low obstacles	Ties shoes, spreads with knife	Prints first name, asks meaning of words, prepares cereal	Plays competitive games, abides by rules, likes to help in household tasks	

Modified from *The Harriet Lane Handbook*, ed 13, Chicago, 1993, Mosby.

TABLE 14-10.—Time of Appearance of Sexual Characteristics: American Girls

ASPECT	DESCRIPTION	AGE
Pelvis	Female contour assumed and fat deposition begins	8-10 years
Breasts	First hypertrophy or budding	10.4-12.9 years
	Further enlargement and pigmentation of nipples	11.1-13.4 years
	Histological maturity	12-17 years
Vagina	Secretion begins and glycogen content of epithelium increases with change in cell type	11.1-13.4 years
Pubic hair	Initial appearance	10.4-12.9 years
	Abundant and curly	11.8-14.3 years
Axillary hair	Initial appearance	9-15 years
Acne	Varies considerably	9-17 years

TABLE 14-11.—Time of Appearance of Sexual Characteristics: American Boys

ASPECT	DESCRIPTION	AGE
Breasts	Some hypertrophy, often assuming a firm nodularity	11-15 years
	Disappearance of hypertrophy	12-16 years
Testes and penis	Increase in size begins	10.4-14.5 years
	Rapid growth	12-15 years
Pubic hair	Initial appearance	10.5-14.5 years
	Abundant and curly	12.8-15.4 years
Axillary hair	Initial appearance	11-15 years
Facial and body hair	Initial appearance	12-16 years
Acne	Varies considerably	11-18 years

TABLE 14-12.—DENTAL DEVELOPMENT

| | DECIDUOUS TEETH | | | | PERMANENT TEETH ERUPTION | |
| | ERUPTION | | SHEDDING | | | |
	MAXILLARY	MANDIBULAR	MAXILLARY	MANDIBULAR	MAXILLARY*	MANDIBULAR*
Central incisors	6-10 months	5-8 months	7-8 years	6-7 years	7-8 years (4)	6-7 years (3)
Lateral incisors	8-12 months	7-10 months	8-9 years	7-8 years	8-9 years (6)	7-8 years (5)
Cuspids	16-20 months	16-20 months	11-12 years	9-11 years	11-12 years (12)	9-11 years (7)
First premolar	—	—	—	—	10-11 years (8)	10-12 years (9)
Second premolar	—	—	—	—	10-12 years (10)	11-13 years (11)
First molars	10-18 months	10-18 months	9-11 years	9-12 years	6-7 years (1)	6-7 years (2)
Second molars	20-30 months	20-30 months	10-12 years	11-13 years	12-14 years (13)	12-13 years (14)
Third molars	—	—	—	—	17-30 years (15)	17-30 years (16)

NOTE: Sexes are combined, although girls tend to be slightly advanced over boys. Averages are approximate values derived from various studies.
*Numbers in parentheses give order of eruption.

HYPERBILIRUBINEMIA

TABLE 14-13.—COMMON CAUSES OF JAUNDICE IN THE FIRST WEEK OF LIFE

DIAGNOSIS	CLINICAL AND LABORATORY DATA
Physiological jaundice	Observed on day 2-4 after birth. Transient. Elevated indirect serum bilirubin. Peak <12.9 mg/dl on day 3-4 term, or >15 mg/dl day 5-7 preterm.
Hemolytic disease, Rh incompatibility	Onset usually within 24 hours. Hepatosplenomegaly. Petechiae. Rh-negative mother; Rh-positive infant. Anemia with reticulocytosis. Positive Coombs' test. Elevated indirect serum bilirubin. Nucleated red cells in peripheral blood smear. Worsens with subsequent pregnancy.
ABO incompatibility	Jaundice appears within 24 hours. Mild anemia and hepatosplenomegaly may be present with reticulocytosis. Mother, O blood group; infant, either A or B group. Peripheral blood smear reveals microcytosis and nucleated red cells.
Congenital spherocytosis	Anemia and splenomegaly. Spherocytes on peripheral blood smear. Elevated indirect serum bilirubin. Coombs' test negative.
Jaundice associated with breast-feeding	Jaundice appears between fourth and fourteenth day of life. May reach very high levels (12-20 mg/dl) during second or third week. Disappears rapidly when formula is substituted; however, this is usually unnecessary.

TSB Level, mg/dl (μmol/L)				
Age, hours	Consider phototherapy†	Phototherapy	Exchange transfusion if intensive phototherapy fails‡	Exchange transfusion and intensive phototherapy
≤24	...	...	...	...
25-48	≥12(170)	≥15(260)	≥20(340)	≥25(430)
49-72	≥15(260)	≥18(310)	≥25(430)	≥30(510)
>72	≥17(290)	≥20(340)	≥25(430)	≥30(510)

TSB LEVEL (mg/dl)*

*	TSB, Total serum bilirubin.
†	Phototherapy at these TSB levels is a clinical option, meaning that the intervention is available and may be used *on the basis of individual clinical judgment.*
‡	Intensive phototherapy should produce a decline of TSB of 1-2 mg/dl within 4 to 6 hours, and the TSB level should continue to fall and remain below the threshold level for exchange transfusion. If this does not occur, it is considered a failure of phototherapy.
§	Term infants who are clinically jaundiced at ≤24 hours old are not considered healthy and require further evaluation.

FIG 14-3.
Management of hyperbilirubinemia in the healthy term neonate. (From Practice Parameter: Management of Hyperbilirubinemia in the Healthy Term Newborn, *Pediatrics* 94(4):565, 1994.)

TABLE 14-14.—Ruling Out Physiological Jaundice

Criteria that Rule Out the Diagnosis of Physical Jaundice*
1. Clinical jaundice the first 24 hours of life.
2. Total serum bilirubin concentrations increasing by more than 5 mg/dl (85 μmol/L) per day.
3. Total serum bilirubin concentration exceeding 12.9 mg/dl (221 μmol/L) in a full-term infant on days 3-4, or 15 mg/dl (257 μmol/L) in a premature infant on days 5-7.
4. Direct serum bilirubin concentration exceeding 2 mg/dl (34 μmol/L).
5. Clinical jaundice persisting for >1 week in a full-term infant or 2 weeks in a premature infant.

*The absence of these criteria does not imply that the jaundice *is* physiological. In the presence of any of these criteria, the jaundice must be investigated.

SPECIFIC FORMULAS FOR SPECIFIC PROBLEMS

TABLE 14-15.—Specific Formulas for Specific Problems

PROBLEM	FORMULA
Lactose intolerance	ProSobee, Isomil, Nursoy (lactose-free formulas)
Malabsorption of fat	Portagen, Osmolite (contains medium-chain triglycerides)
Protein intolerance	Nutramigen (hydrolyzed protein, Portagen, Alimentum, Pregestimil (hydrolyzed protein and medium-chain triglycerides)
Prematurity	Premature Enfamil, Premie SMA
Inborn errors:	
Amino acid	Lofenalac (low phenylalanine content)
Galactosemia	Nutramigen (galactose free), Soy formulas (galactose free)
Fructose	Similac, Enfamil, SMA (fructose free)

COMMON INFECTIOUS DISEASES

TABLE 14-16.—COMMON INFECTIOUS DISEASES

DISEASE	INCUBATION	PRODROME	SIGNS AND SYMPTOMS	ISOLATION	TREATMENT
Chickenpox (varicella)	10-21 days	Minimal	Mixture of macules, papules, vesicles; spreads from trunk to extremities for 5-20 days	Until all lesions are crusted; infectious 2 days before appearance	Symptomatic, bed rest, antipyretics, topical antipruritics such as Calamine lotion
Diphtheria	2-6 days	Rapid onset of signs and symptoms	Moderate fever, malaise, sore throat; gray, tenacious membrane in throat; respiratory distress	Until two negative nose and throat cultures 24 hours apart	Antitoxin, erythromycin or penicillin G
Fifth disease (erythema infectiosum)	6-14 days	None	Maculopapular rash on face with circumoral pallor (slapped cheek) and spreading to extremities; rash lasts a few days to a few weeks and is brought out by warmth	Not needed	None
Hepatitis A	15-20 days	Rapid onset	Fever, anorexia, headache, abdominal pain, liver enzyme elevation, jaundice	Stool, urine, and blood for 1 month	Bed rest, fluids, immune serum γ-globulin to contacts

Continued.

TABLE 14-16.—COMMON INFECTIOUS DISEASES—cont'd

DISEASE	INCUBATION	PRODROME	SIGNS AND SYMPTOMS	ISOLATION	TREATMENT
Hepatitis B	6 weeks to 6 months	Insidious onset	Slight fever and mild gastrointestinal upset, jaundice, hepatomegaly, elevated liver enzymes	Body excretions until surface antigen negative	Bed rest, fluids, hepatitis B immune globulin to intimate contacts, ISG to others
Herpangina (coxsackie virus group A)	?	None	High fever, vomiting, ulcers of oral mucosa for 5-6 days	2-6 days	Symptomatic
Meningococcal meningitis	1-7 days	URI, fever, headache, diarrhea	Meningitis, purpuric or petechial rash; septic arthritis	Until 24 hours after first antibiotic	Penicillin or ampicillin chloramphenicol, cefotaxime, ceftriaxone, or cefuroxime
Mononucleosis	2-8 weeks	None	Fatigue, anorexia, exudative tonsillitis, lymphadenopathy, splenomegaly; maculopapular rash not unusual	Avoid saliva contact for 3 months	Symptomatic
Mumps	14-21 days	None	Asymptomatic in 30%-40% of patients; swelling and pain of the salivary glands; fever	Communicable from 7 days before to 9 days after occurrence of swelling	Symptomatic, bed rest, isolation, until salivary swelling is gone, analgesics

Disease	Incubation	Prodrome	Characteristics	Communicability	Treatment
Poliomyelitis	7-14 days usual; 5-35 days maximum	Fever, lassitude, GI upset	Paralysis heralded by nuchal rigidity and stiffness of back; pain and tenderness in affected muscles	Secretions 1 week, stool 6 weeks	Supportive, bed rest, active physiotherapy when pain subsides
Roseola (exanthem subitum)	1-15 days	3-4 Days of sustained high fever	Fine pink rash begins at defervescense and lasts 2 days; seen from 6 months to 3 years of age	Unknown	Fever control
Rubella, German measles, 3-day measles	14-21 days	Lymphadeno-pathy, fever, headache, malaise	Maculopapular discrete rash appears on face and rapidly spreads to trunk and proximal extremities, lasting 1-3 days; postauricular and suboccipital lymphadenopathy	Communicable from 7 days before until 5 days after rash appears	None
Rubeola (measles)	10-12 days	High fever, cough, coryza, and conjunctivitis for 3 days	Koplik's spots appear 1-2 days before maculopapular rash; rash is confluent and spreads from hairline to face, then body; lasts 4-5 days	From fifth day of incubation to fifth day after rash appears	Symptomatic care of cough, coryza, conjunctivitis
Whooping cough (pertussis)	5-10 days, 21 days maximum	1-3 weeks of cough, coryza, and occasional emesis	Short paroxysmal cough ending with inspiratory "whoop"	5-10 Days on treatment	Erythromycin Corticosteroids and albuterol may reduce coughing paroxysms

TABLE 14-17.—RESPIRATORY DISORDERS

BRONCHIOLITIS/RESPIRATORY SYNCYTIAL VIRUS	ASTHMA	PNEUMONIA	EPIGLOTTITIS	LARYNGOTRACHEOBRONCHITIS
Onset: 3 months-3 years	Onset: infancy to adulthood	Onset: all ages	2-7 years	<3 yr
Previous history negative	Previous history often positive	Previous history often negative	Previous history often negative	Previous history of rhinorrhea and cough
Frequent in winter	Frequent all seasons	Frequent in winter	Any season	Late fall and winter
Afebrile or mildly febrile	Usually afebrile	Febrile	39.4° C (103° F)	39° C-40° C (102° F-104° F)
Prolonged expiration	Prolonged expiration	No prolonged expiration	Normal expiration	Normal expiration
Inspiratory and expiratory obstruction	Expiratory obstruction	Obstructive respiratory usually lacking	Inspiratory stridor	Inspiratory obstruction, barking cough
Respiratory distress marked	Respiratory distress mild to marked	Respiratory distress mild to marked	Respiratory distress marked	Respiratory distress mild to marked
Usually hyperresonant	Usually hyperresonant	Usually hyperresonant	No wheezing	Wheezing may be present
Wheezing, rales, or rhonchi	Wheezing	Rales		Bilateral
Chest findings bilateral	Chest findings bilateral	Chest findings either unilateral or bilateral	Bilateral	
Lymphocytosis	Eosinophilia	Lymphocytosis or "viral" or "bacterial" white count and differential, polymorphonuclear leukocytosis	Elevated WBC count (>18,000/mm³)	Normal WBC count
Hyperaeration	Hyperaeration	Pneumonic infiltrate or consolidation	Normal chest x-ray findings; abnormal neck x-ray findings	Normal neck and chest x-ray findings
Antibiotic in severe cases	Bronchodilation, epinephrine	Appropriate antibiotic if bacterial	Ampicillin and chloramphenicol	Cool mist, observe

OTITIS MEDIA

TABLE 14-18.—OTITIS MEDIA

Diagnosis
Hyperemic tympanic membrane
Opacity of tympanic membrane
Bulging and poor mobility of tympanic membrane
Fever not always present, and when present, should remind you to look for con-
comitant disease, e.g., pneumonia, URI
Earache (variable)

Etiology
Newborns
Gram-negative bacilli
Infants
Streptococcus pneumoniae 40%
Haemophilus influenzae 20%
Group A β-hemolytic streptococci

Treatment
See Table 14-19.

TABLE 14-19.—TREATMENT OF OTITIS MEDIA*

ANTIBIOTIC	DOSE (mg/kg/day)	DOSES/ DAY	DURATION (Days)
Ampicillin	50-200	qid	10
Amoxicillin	30-50	tid	10
Amoxicillin/clavulanate K	40	tid	10
Cefaclor	40-50	bid	10
Erythromycin/sulfisoxazole	50/150	qid	10
Trimethoprim/sulfamethoxazole	10/50	bid	10

*Other treatment modalities include analgesia, heat, and antipyretics.

PARASITIC INFECTIONS

TABLE 14-20.—PARASITIC INFECTIONS IN CHILDREN

PARASITE	DIAGNOSIS	DRUG		DOSAGE
Pinworm (*Enterobius vermicularis*)	Demonstration under microscope, ova on tape applied and removed from anus, or visualization of pinworm (white and looks like an eyelash)	*Drug of choice:*	Pyrantel pamoate (Antiminth)	11 mg/kg once (maximum 1 g); repeat after 2 weeks
		Alternative:	Mebendazole (Vermox)	100 mg single dose; repeat in 2 weeks
Giardiasis (*Giardia lamblia*)	Multiple stool examinations	*Drug of choice:*	Metronidazole (Flagyl)	15 mg/kg/day in 3 doses for 5 days
		Alternatives:	Quinacrine (Atabrine)	6 mg/kg/day in 3 doses after meals for 5 days (maximum dose 300 mg/day)
			Furazolidone (Furoxone)	6 mg/kg/day in 4 doses for 7-10 days

Disease (organism)	Diagnosis		Drug	Dose
Roundworm (*Ascaris lumbricoides*)	Adult worm vomited or passed in stool	*Drug of choice:*	Mebendazole (Vermox)	100 mg twice daily for 3 days
		Alternative:	Pyrantel pamoate (Antiminth)	11 mg/kg once (maximum 1 g)
Visceral larva migrans (*Toxocara canis, T. cati*)	Generally by history of exposure to cats and dogs; may be anemic; signs include fever, hepatomegaly	*Drug of choice:*	Diethylcarbamazine (Hetrazan)	6 mg/kg/day in 3 doses for 7-10 days
		Alternative:	Thiabendazole (Mintezole)	44 mg/kg/day in 2 doses for 7 days
Tapeworm (*Taenia saginata, T. solium*)	Demonstration of worm segments or eggs in stool	*Drug of choice:*	Praziquantel (Biltricide)	5-10 mg/kg in a single dose
			Niclosamide (Niclocide)	11-34 kg: A single dose of 1 g (2 tablets), then 1 tablet (500 mg) daily for 6 days >34 kg: A single dose of 1.5 g (3 tablets), then 2 tablets (1 g) daily for 6 days

FEBRILE SEIZURES

TABLE 14-21.—FEBRILE SEIZURES

Definition
Tonic-clonic seizure <15 minutes
Occur in children aged 3 months to 5 years
Fever present
No evidence of intracranial infection by sign or symptom; spinal tap should be
  done if there is any suspicion of infection of the CNS

Risk Factors
Family history
Abnormal neurodevelopmental status
Atypical seizures
Past history of febrile seizures—about one third who have one seizure will have
  more episodes

Treatment
Temperature control is needed with each subsequent illness
Anticonvulsant therapy is not routinely instituted

MENINGITIS

Fever, headache, nuchal rigidity, irritability, nausea, vomiting, and altered mental status are all symptoms of meningitis. The two most common types are aseptic and bacterial (Table 14-22). The spinal fluid should be cultured for TB, fungus, and viruses as well.

TABLE 14-22.—MENINGITIS

CSF	ASEPTIC MENINGITIS	BACTERIAL MENINGITIS
Gram stain	Negative	May be positive
Opening pressure	Elevated	Elevated
WBC count	50-4000/mm^3	100-60,000/mm^3 mostly PMN
Protein	NL or increased	Elevated
Glucose	NL or increased	Decreased

TABLE 14-23.—GRAM STAIN: DIRECTED THERAPY FOR MENINGITIS

STAIN MORPHOLOGY	LIKELY ORGANISM	FIRST CHOICE	ALTERNATE
Gram-negative cocci in chains or pairs	*Streptococcus pneumoniae* Group B streptococci	Penicillin G plus gentamicin for 24 hours	Cefotaxime or chloramphenicol, vancomycin as third line
Gram-positive cocci in clusters	*Staphyloccus*	Nafcillin (β-lactamase $-$) Vancomycin (β-lactamase $+$)	Vancomycin, trimethoprim-sulfamethoxazole
Gram-negative cocci	*Neisseria meningitidis*	Penicillin G	Ceftriaxone, chloramphenicol, cefotaxime
Gram-negative coccobacilli	*Haemophilus influenzae*	Ceftriazone or cefotaxime	Chloroamphenicol plus ampicillin, trimethoprim-sulfamethoxazole
Gram-negative enteric rods	*E. coli* *Klebsiella* *Salmonella* *Serratia* *Pseudomonas*	Cefotaxime, ceftriaxone, or ceftazidime plus aminoglycoside	Trimethoprim-sulfamethoxazole
Gram-positive rods	*Listeria monocytogenes*	Ampicillin plus aminoglycoside	Trimethoprim-sulfamethoxazole

TABLE 14-24.—Presumptive Therapy for Bacterial Meningitis

AGE GROUP	PATHOGENS	THERAPY
<1 month	Group B streptococci Gram-negative enteric bacilli *Listeria monocytogenes* *Haemophilus influenzae* *Streptococcus pneumoniae* *Neisseria meningitidis* *Staphylococcus aureus* (predominantly in premature infants)	Ampicillin plus amino-glycoside or ampicillin plus cefotaxime; 20% of *H. influenzae* is ampicillin resistant
1-3 months	*H. influenzae* *N. meningitidis* *S. pneumoniae* Group B streptococci	Ampicillin plus cefotaxime; 20% of *H. influenzae* is ampicillin resistant
3 months-9 years	*H. influenzae* *S. pneumoniae* *N. meningitidis*	Cefotaxime or ceftriaxone or ampicillin plus chloramphenicol; 20% of *H. influenzae* is ampicillin resistant
>9 years and adults	*N. meningitidis* *S. pneumoniae* *H. influenzae*	Penicillin G, ceftriaxone, cefotaxime

Modified from Rakel RE: *Conn's current therapy,* Philadelphia, 1994, WB Saunders.

TABLE 14-25.—CSF Characteristics in the Normal Child and Some Neurological Disorders

CONDITION	INITIAL PRESSURE (MM H₂O)	APPEARANCE	CELLS/ML	PROTEIN (MG/DL)	GLUCOSE (MG/DL)	OTHER TESTS	COMMENTS
Normal	<180	Clear	0-5 lymphocytes. First 3 months, 1-3 PMNs. Neonates, up to 30 lymphocytes, 20-50 RBCs	15-35 (lumbar). 5-15 (ventricular). Up to 150 (lumbar) for short time after birth; to 6 months, up to 65	50-80 (two thirds of blood glucose). May be increased after seizure	CSF IgG index; <0.7 U = CSF IgG/ Serum IgG CSF albumin/ Serum albumin Lactate dehydrogenase (LDH), 2-27 IU/L	CSF protein in first month may be up to 170 mg/dl in small-for-dates or premature infants. No increase in WBCs due to seizure
Bloody tap	Normal or low	Bloody (sometimes with clot)	One additional WBC/700 RBCs.* RBCs not crenated	One additional mg/800 RBCs*	Normal	RBC number should fall between first and third tube; wait 5 minutes between tubes	Spin down fluid; supernatant will be clear and colorless
Bacterial meningitis, acute	200-750+	Opalescent to purulent	Up to 1000s, mostly PMNs. Early, few cells	Up to 100s	Decreased; may be none	Smear and culture mandatory. LDH > 24 IU/L. Bacterial antigen tests.	Very early, glucose may be normal. Immunofluorescence tests

Continued.

From Hay WW et al: *Current pediatric diagnosis and treatment,* ed 12, East Norwalk, Conn., 1995, Appleton & Lange.
*Many studies document pitfalls in using these ratios because of WBC lysis. Clinical judgment and repeat taps may be necessary to rule out meningitis in this situation.

TABLE 14-25.—CSF Characteristics in the Normal Child and Some Neurological Disorders—cont'd

CONDITION	INITIAL PRESSURE (MM H₂O)	APPEARANCE	CELLS/ML	PROTEIN (MG/DL)	GLUCOSE (MG/DL)	OTHER TESTS	COMMENTS
Bacterial meningitis, partially treated	Usually increased	Clear or opalescent	Usually increased. PMNs usually predominate	Elevated	Normal or decreased	LDH usually >24 IU/L	Smear and culture often negative
Tuberculous meningitis	150-750+	Opalescent; fibrin web or pellicle	250-500, mostly lymphocytes. Early, more PMNs	45-500; parallels cell count	Decreased; may be none	Smear for acid-fast organism; CSF culture and inoculation	NOTE: Bacterial meningitis may be superimposed
Fungal meningitis	Increased	Variable; often clear	10-500. Early, more PMNs; then mostly lymphocytes	Elevated and increasing	Decreased	India ink preparations, cryptococcal antigen, culture, inoculations, immunofluorescence tests	Often superimposed in patients who are debilitated or on immunosuppressive or tumor therapy
Aseptic meningoencephalitides (poliomyelitis)	Normal or slightly increased	Clear unless cell count >300	0 to few hundred, mostly lymphocytes; PMNs predominate early	20-125	Normal; may be low in mumps	CSF, stool, throat wash for viral cultures. LDH < 28 IU/L (90% < 24 IU/L)	Acute and convalescent antibody titers. In mumps, up to 1000 lymphocytes; serum amylase often elevated. Rarely, several thousand cells present in enteroviral infection

Neurosyphilis	Normal to 400	Clear unless protein is very high	10-100, mostly lymphocytes	25-150; higher in meningitis	Normal	Positive CSF serology. CSF IgG index increased	Blood serology positive in untreated cases; *Treponema pallidum* immobilization test positive
Parainfectious encephalomyelitis	80-450, usually increased	Usually clear	0-50, mostly lymphocytes	15-75	Normal	CSF IgG index may be increased. Oligoclonal bands variable	No organisms. Fulminant cases resemble bacterial meningitis.
Polyneuritis Early Late	Normal and occasionally increased	Normal Xanthochromic if protein high	Normal; occasionally slight increase	Normal 45-1500	Normal	Bacterial cultures negative; globulin may be elevated	Try to find cause (viral infections, toxins, lupus, infectious mononucleosis, diabetes)
Meningeal carcinomatosis	Often elevated	Clear to opalescent	Cytologic identification of tumor cells	Often mildly to moderately elevated	Often depressed	Cytology	Seen with leukemia, medulloblastoma, meningeal melanosis, histiocytosis X. NOTE: May mimic meningitis
Brain abscess	Normal or increased	Usually clear	5-500 in 80%; mostly PMNs	Usually slightly increased	Normal; occasionally decreased		Cell count related to proximity to meninges; findings as in purulent meningitis if abscess perforates

STOOLING DISORDERS

TABLE 14-26.—STOOLING DISORDERS WITH DIARRHEA

CONDITION	FIRST-STAGE SCREENING	SECOND-STAGE SCREENING	SPECIFIC DIAGNOSTIC STUDIES
Hirschsprung's disease (1)*	Abdominal radiograph	Barium enema	Rectal biopsy
Stenosis of the bowel (1)	Abdominal radiograph	Gastrointestinal series	Exploratory laparotomy
Milk protein sensitivity (1)	Cow's milk elimination	Rechallenge with cow's milk	Consistent response to cow's milk protein
Agammaglobulinemia (Swiss type) (1)	Peripheral blood smear (lymphocytes)	Serum protein electrophoresis	Biopsy of lymph nodes
Disaccharide intolerance (1,2)	Stool pH—test for reducing substances	Tolerance test for sugars	Trial carbohydrate elimination; may use fructose
Cystic fibrosis (1,2)	Sweat test	—	Repeat sweat test
Celiac disease (2,3)	History	Trial of gluten-free diet	Intestinal biopsy
Ulcerative colitis (3)	Stool guaiac	Sigmoidoscopy, barium enema	
Ova and parasites	Stool cultures	Repeat stool cultures	
Antibiotic associated toxin (1,2,3)	Culture for *C. difficile*	Sigmoidoscopy	Culture

*Age at onset: (1), Infant; (2), toddler; (3), toddler or older child.

TABLE 14-27.—Stooling Disorders with Constipation

CLINICAL	HIRSCHSPRUNG'S DISEASE	ENCOPRESIS
Age	Birth or soon after; male > female	After age 4
Toilet training	Usually successful	Usually successful initially
Constipation	Yes	Yes
Toilet use	Usually	Infrequent
Soiling	Rarely	Constant
Rectum	Usually empty	Stool present
Stool	Pellet or ribbonlike; offensive odor	Very large. Some retain and others deposit in inappropriate places
Evaluation	Plain x-ray examination and barium enema; rectal biopsy	Psychiatric since many will have retardation or serious psychopathology
Resolution	Surgery	Psychotherapy, behavior modification

RABIES

TABLE 14-28.—GUIDELINES FOR POSTEXPOSURE RABIES PROPHYLAXIS*

ANIMAL SPECIES	CONDITION OF ANIMAL AT TIME OF ATTACK	TREATMENT
Domestic dog or cat	Healthy and available for 10 days of observation	None, unless animal develops rabies
	Suspicious	HRIG and HDCV or RVA; discontinue after 5 days if animal is healthy
	Rabid	HRIG and HDCV or RVA
	Unknown	Consult public health officials; if treatment is indicated, give HRIG and HDCV or RVA
Wild animals; skunk, bat, fox, coyote, raccoon, bobcat, and other carnivores	Regard as rabid unless proven negative by laboratory test	HRIG and HDCV or RVA
Other animals; livestock, rodents, rabbits, and hares	Consider individually. Bites of provoked squirrels, hamsters, guinea pigs, gerbils, chipmunks, rats, mice, other rodents, rabbits, and hares almost never call for antirabies prophylaxis.	Local or state public health officials should be consulted concerning questions that arise about the need for rabies prophylaxis.

*HRIG, Human rabies immune globulin; HDCV, human diploid cell vaccine; RVA, rabies vaccine adsorbed. Regimen is: Day 0 HRIG + HDCV or RVA, day 3, 7, 14, and 28 HDCV or RVA alone. HRIG dosage is 20 IV/kg half dose IM and half dose in wound edge. HDCV and RVA dose is 1.0 ml IM (deltoid).

ATTENTION DEFICIT

TABLE 14-29.—Attention-Deficit Hyperactivity Disorder (ADHD)

ADHD is a syndrome of behavior, not a psychiatric disease. It affects 5%-15% of school-aged children. The diagnosis is made by observing the child and eliciting a history of the following behaviors from the child's parents and teachers:

Increased motion activity	Impulsiveness
Distractibility	Antisocial behavior
Short attention span	Learning disabilities
Restlessness	Poor academic performance

Treatment may involve only reassurance of teachers and parents and manipulation of the environment such as a definite home routine and structured rather than open classroom with frequent breaks. When this behavior interferes with academic and social performance, drug therapy should be considered.
Workup includes a physical, lab if indicated, and psychological and IQ tests.

TABLE 14-30.—Drug Therapy for Attention-Deficit Hyperactivity Disorder (ADHD)

DRUG	AGE (YEARS)	INITIAL DOSE	SUBSEQUENT DOSE
Methylphenidate (Ritalin)	6-8 9-12	5 mg in AM 10 mg in AM	Increase daily dose by 5 mg each week to a maximum of 60 mg/day. Ritalin SR 20 mg available
Pemoline (Cylert)	6	37.5 mg in AM	Increase daily dose by 18.75 each week to a maximum of 112.5 mg/24 hr
Dextroamphetamine (Dexedrine)	3-5 6-7	2.5 mg qd 5 mg qd	Raise daily dose 5 mg each week until desired response (maximum 40 mg/day)
Imipramine (Tofranil)	6 7-8	10 mg in AM 25 mg in AM	Divide dose, and each week increase by 10 mg daily until desired response (maximum 75 mg/day)

RHEUMATIC FEVER

There is a high probability of acute rheumatic fever if two major criteria or one major and two minor criteria are present, supported by evidence of recent Group A streptococcal infection such as scarlet fever, increased ASO titer, or positive throat culture (Table 14-31).

TABLE 14-31.—THE DIAGNOSIS OF RHEUMATIC FEVER: JONES CRITERIA REVISED

MAJOR CRITERIA	MINOR CRITERIA
Carditis	Arthralgia
Chorea	Fever
Erythema marginatum	Previous rheumatic fever or rheumatic heart disease
Polyarthritis	Prolonged PR interval
Subcutaneous nodules	Elevated sedimentation rate, C-reactive protein, or leukocytosis

TABLE 14-32.—DIFFERENTIAL DIAGNOSIS OF RHEUMATIC FEVER, RHEUMATOID ARTHRITIS, AND SYSTEMIC LUPUS ERYTHEMATOSUS

ASPECT	RHEUMATIC FEVER	JUVENILE RHEUMATOID ARTHRITIS	SYSTEMIC LUPUS ERYTHEMATOSUS
Age trend	5-15 years	5 yr	9-15 years
Sex ratio	Equal	Girls 1.5:1	Girls 8:1
Joint findings			
Pain	Severe	Moderate	—
Swelling	Nonspecific	Nonspecific	Nonspecific
Tenderness	Severe	Moderate	—
Bone x-ray	None	Frequent	Occasional
Morning stiffness	Yes	Yes	Yes
Rash	Erythema marginatum	Rheumatoid arthritis rash	Malar flush
Chorea	Yes	No	Rarely
Clinical carditis	Possible	Rare	Late
Laboratory tests			
WBC	Normal to high	Normal to high	Decreased to normal
Latex	Negative	+ (15%)	+ Occasionally
Sheep cell agglutination	Negative	+ (10%)	—
LE cell prep	Negative	+ (5%)	+ Always
Biopsy			
Skin rash	Nonspecific	Nonspecific	Diagnostic
Nodules	Nonspecific	Nonspecific	Nonspecific
Response to salicylates	Rapid	Slow, usually	Slow or none
Fever	Low grade	Low grade	Possible

PEDIATRIC SEDATION

TABLE 14-33.—PEDIATRIC SEDATION

MEDICATION	DOSE (mg/kg/dose)			
	PO	IV	IM	PR
Diazepam	0.15-0.3	0.5-0.1	Painful	—
Lorazepam	—	0.05	0.05	—
Midazolam	0.05-0.08	0.05-0.08	—	0.05-0.08
Pentobarbitol	2.0-6.0	0.5-1.0	2.0-6.0	2.0-6.0
Promethazine	—	—	0.5-1.0	—
Chlorpromazine	—	0.5-1.0	0.5-1.0	—
Chloral hydrate	25-100	—	—	25-100
Hydroxyzine	—	—	25-100	—

ANEMIA

TABLE 14-34.—DISTINGUISHING COMMON CAUSES OF ANEMIA

	IRON DEFICIENCY	β-THALASSEMIA TRAIT	CHRONIC INFLAMMATION	LEAD POISONING
Reticulocyte count	Low	Low	Normal	Low
RDW	↑	↓	Normal	↓
Ferritin	↓	Normal to↑	Normal	↓to normal
FEP	↑	Normal	↑	↑
Iron	↓	Normal	↓	↓to normal
TIBC	↑	Normal	↓	
Electrophoresis	Normal	↑HbA$_2$ or F	Normal	Normal
ESR	Normal	Normal	↑	Normal
Smear	Hypochromic, target cells	Normochromic, microcytic	Varies	Basophilic stippling

From Johnson K: *The Harriet Lane handbook,* ed 13, St. Louis, 1993, Mosby.

AGE-SPECIFIC HEMATOLOGY VALUES

TABLE 14-35.—AGE-SPECIFIC HEMATOLOGY VALUES

AGE	HGB (g%), MEAN (−2 SD)	HCT (%), MEAN (−2 SD)	MCV (fl), MEAN (−2 SD)	MCHC (g% RBC), MEAN (−2 SD)	RETIC (%)	WBC/mm³ × 1000, MEAN (+2 SD)	PLATELETS (10³/mm³), MEAN (+2 SD)
26-30 weeks gestation*	13.4 (11)	41.5 (34.9)	118.2 (106.7)	37.9 (30.6)	—	4.4 (2.7)	254 (180-327)
28 weeks	14.5	45	120	31.0	(5-10)	—	275
32 weeks	15.0	47	118	32.0	(3-10)	—	290
Term† (cord)	16.5 (13.5)	51 (42)	108 (98)	33.0 (30.0)	(3-7)	18.1 (9-30)‡	290
1-3 days	18.5 (14.5)	56 (45)	108 (95)	33.0 (29.0)	(1.8-4.6)	18.9 (9.4-34)	192
2 weeks	16.6 (13.4)	53 (41)	105 (88)	31.4 (28.1)		11.4 (5-20)	252
1 months	13.9 (10.7)	44 (33)	101 (91)	31.8 (28.1)	(0.1-1.7)	10.8 (4-19.5)	
2 months	11.2 (9.4)	35 (28)	95 (84)	31.8 (28.3)			
6 months	12.6 (11.1)	36 (31)	76 (68)	35.0 (32.7)	(0.7-2.3)	11.9 (6-17.5)	
6 month-2 years	12.0 (10.5)	36 (33)	78 (70)	33.0 (30.0)		10.6 (6-17)	(150-350)
2-6 years	12.5 (11.5)	37 (34)	81 (75)	34.0 (31.0)	(0.5-1.0)	8.5 (5-15.5)	"
6-12 years	13.5 (11.5)	40 (35)	86 (77)	34.0 (31.0)	(0.5-1.0)	8.1 (4.5-13.5)	"
12-18 years							
Male	14.5 (13)	43 (36)	88 (78)	34.0 (31.0)	(0.5-1.0)	7.8 (4.5-13.5)	"
Female	14.0 (12)	41 (37)	90 (78)	34.0 (31.0)	(0.5-1.0)	7.8 (4.5-13.5)	"
Adult							
Male	15.5 (13.5)	47 (41)	90 (80)	34.0 (31.0)	(0.8-2.5)	7.4 (4.5-11)	"
Female	14.0 (12)	41 (36)	90 (80)	34.0 (31.0)	(0.8-4.1)	7.4 (4.5-11)	"

From Johnson K: *The Harriet Lane handbook* ed 13, St. Louis, 1993, Mosby.

*Values are from fetal samplings.

†Under 1 m/o, capillary Hgb exceeds venous: 1 hour-3.6 g difference; 5 days-2.2 g difference; 3 weeks-1.1 g difference.

‡Mean (95% confidence limits).

15 *The Musculoskeletal System*

Edward T. Bope

ARTHROCENTESIS

TABLE 15-1.—ARTHROCENTESIS

Indications
Analysis of joint fluid
Relief of pain by drainage of an effusion
Installation of medication (Table 15-2)
Drainage of hemarthrosis

Contraindications
Infection in skin or soft tissue
Coagulation disorder

General Technique
Identify landmarks and mark site with indelible ink
Use aseptic technique
Inject local anesthesia in the overlying skin and subcutaneous tissues
Choose syringe appropriate for effusion size: 3-50 ml
Advance needle with negative pressure
Remove effusion
Apply sterile bandage

Technique (Site Approach)
Shoulder (Anterior Approach)
Seat patient with hand in lap
Palpate the glenohumeral joint (between the coracoid process and humeral
head)
Internally rotate shoulder and feel the joint groove lateral to the coracoid
Direct the needle (20-22 gauge) dorsally and medially into the joint space
A slight superior direction will avoid the neurovascular bundle

Continued.

541

TABLE 15-1.—ARTHROCENTESIS—cont'd

Shoulder (Posterior Approach)
Rotate the patient's arm internally by having the patient place the hand on the
    opposite shoulder
Palpate the acromion process
Insert the needle 1 cm below the posterior tip of the acromion
Direct it anteriorly and medially to the humeral head
    Wrist (Dorsal Approach)
Patient should be sitting with pronated palm flexed slightly over a rolled towel
Mark the bony process of the distal radius and ulna
Direct the needle into the groove between the two bony processes just lateral to
    the extensor pollicis longus tendon
    Elbow
Place patient's relaxed arm on pillow in lap 45 degrees from full extension
Turn palm toward abdomen or pillow
Palpate the lateral epicondyle
The shallow depression distal to it represents the joint
Enter perpendicular to the joint with a 22-gauge needle
    Ankle (Medial Approach)
Place foot at 45 degrees plantar flexion with heel on table
Palpate medial malleolus
Insert needle 1.2 cm proximal and volar to the distal end of medial malleolus
Direct the needle 45 degrees posteriorly, slightly upward and medial
    Knee (Medial Approach)
Patient should be supine with a relaxed knee (patella freely moveable)
Mark the inferior plane of the patella (the underside)
Direct the needle (18 gauge) parallel to the inferior plane of the patella
Compression of the suprapatellar pouch may help aspiration

INTRAARTICULAR INJECTION

TABLE 15-2.—INTRAARTICULAR STEROID INJECTIONS

Mix 1% lidocaine and steroid:
    For elbow or ankle, 10-40 mg of methylprednisolone acetate in 0.5 ml of 1%
        lidocaine
    For knee or shoulder, 40-80 mg of methylprednisolone acetate in 1 ml of 1%
        lidocaine
Use the approaches listed in Table 15-1 to enter the joint
Aspirate to be sure you are not in a vessel
Inject and apply a sterile bandage
Advise patient that there may be an initial irritation from the steroid lasting less
    than 24 hours
This may need to be repeated for severe inflammation
Bursae overlie these joints and can be injected with the same preparation

---

TABLE 15-3.—Assessment of Synovial Fluid

PRESUMPTIVE DIAGNOSIS	APPEARANCE	MUCIN CLOT/ VISCOSITY	CELL COUNT (WBCs/mm³)	PERCENT POLYS (PMNs)	PROTEIN (g/dl)	ALBUMIN (g/dl)	GLUCOSE PERCENT OF SERUM	CRYSTALS	CULTURE/ SMEAR	COMMENTS
Normal	Clear, straw colored	Good/high	<200	<20	1.0-4.0	1.0-2.0	Same	None	0	—
Noninflammatory										
Trauma	Clear, turbid red or xanthochromic	Good/high	<2000	<30	1.3-5.0	2.5	Same	None	0	Many RBCs, few cartilage fragments
Osteoarthritis	Clear, straw colored	Fair to good/high	<2000	20-60	2.9-5.5	2.5	Same	None	0	Many cartilage fragments
Systemic lupus erythematosus	Clear or turbid	Good/high	0-9000	<20	1.5-4.0	2.5	Same	None	0	LE cells
Inflammatory										
Rheumatoid arthritis	Turbid, greenish yellow	Poor/low	3000-50,000	60-95	3.0-6.0	2.5-3.7	75-100	None	0	Latex positive, ragocytes, low complement
Gout	Turbid, white	Poor/low	100-160,000	50-95	2.5-5.0	1.5-3.5	Same	Sodium urate	0	Strongly negative birefringence

Continued.

TABLE 15-3.—Assessment of Synovial Fluid—cont'd

PRESUMPTIVE DIAGNOSIS	APPEARANCE	MUCIN CLOT/ VISCOSITY	CELL COUNT (WBCs/mm³)	PERCENT POLYS (PMNs)	PROTEIN (g/dl)	ALBUMIN (g/dl)	GLUCOSE PERCENT OF SERUM	CRYSTALS	CULTURE/ SMEAR	COMMENTS
Pseudo-gout	Clear turbid	Fair/low	50-75,000	30-95	—	—	Same	Calcium pyro-phos-phate	0	Weakly positive birefrin-gence many RBCs
Rheumatic fever	Slightly tur-bid	Good/low	0-60,000	60-90	1.5-5.0	2.5	Same	None	0	—
Reiter's disease	Turbid	Fair/low	700-45,000	>60	2.5-6.0	2.0-3.6	—	None	—	PMNs in macro-phages
Infectious Bacterial	Turbid, gray or yellow	Poor/low	50,000-300,000	>90	2.8-6.8	1.5-3.8	<50	None	+	Bacteria on Gram stain, often negative in gono-coccal arthritis
Tubercu-lous	Turbid, gray or yellow	Poor/low	2500-100,000	50	4.0-6.0	2.8-4.2	50-75	None	+	Acid-fast on smear 20%; cul-ture 80%; biopsy 90%

ORTHOPEDIC MANEUVERS

TABLE 15-4.—ORTHOPEDIC MANEUVERS/TESTS

Knee Valgus Stress Test	To test medial collateral ligament
Patient:	Supine, leg extended and supported by examiner
Examiner:	Beside extremity tested with one hand on distal lateral femur and other on medial tibia below the joint line
Technique:	Apply medial pressure on femur while distracting tibia laterally. Note amount of opening of medial knee. It should be minimal. Compare with other leg
Knee Varus Stress Test	To test lateral collateral ligament
Patient:	Supine, leg extended and supported by examiner
Examiner:	Beside extremity tested with one hand on distal medial femur and other on the lateral tibia below the joint line
Technique:	Apply lateral pressure on the femur while distracting the tibia medially. Note amount of opening of lateral knee. It should be minimal. Compare to other leg
Straight Leg Raise	To test for protrusion of disk causing radicular pain
Patient:	Supine
Examiner:	Gently hold leg at knee and ankle
Technique:	Slowly raise the leg through 60 degrees of motion. Pain will be felt if positive between 30 degrees and 60 degrees in back, hip, and leg
Spurling Test	To test for cervical restriction or foramen restriction
Patient:	Seated on stool
Examiner:	Standing with hands on patient's head
Technique:	Apply downward pressure with neck straight, left, left posterior, right, right posterior. Elicited pain or neurological symptom is positive test
McMurray Sign	To test for tears in medial and lateral menisci
Patient:	Supine and relaxed with knee completely bent
Examiner:	Standing at the side of the injured limb
Technique:	Grasp the heel and rotate the foot externally while abducting the leg and extending the knee. A click or pain is significant for lateral tear. Opposite maneuver can be positive for medial tear and is done by rotating the foot internally and abducting the leg while extending the knee

Continued.

TABLE 15-4.—Orthopedic Maneuvers/Tests—cont'd

Apprehension Test	To test for patella subluxation.
Patient:	Seated
Examiner:	Hand on affected patella
Technique:	Gently push the patella laterally. A start of apprehension is positive. If negative, examiner can extend the knee and then passively flex the knee while gently pushing the patella laterally
Anterior Drawer Sign	To test the anterior cruciate
Patient:	Supine, hip flexed 45°, knee flexed 90 degrees
Examiner:	Sitting on patient's ipsilateral foot
Technique:	Place hands around the tibia just below the joint line Apply anterior force and note the amount of anterior motion. Always compare with other knee
Lachman Test	When the knee cannot be flexed
Patient:	Supine, hip and knee extended
Examiner:	Standing beside patient
Technique:	Grasp the femur with one hand and the tibia below the joint line. Apply a distracting force to the tibia and note the excursion
Posterior Drawer Sign	To test the posterior cruciate
Patient:	Supine, hip flexed, 45 degrees, knee flexed 90 degrees
Examiner:	Sitting on patient's ipsilateral foot
Technique:	Same as anterior drawer sign, except apply posterior force on tibia

TABLE 15-5.—Volume of Steroid for Injection*

AREA	VOLUME (ML)
Large joints	0.5-2.0
Small joints	0.2-1.0
Bursae	0.5-1.5
Tendon sheaths	0.1-0.5
Ganglia	0.2-1.0

*Volume is steroid only. Most often the volume is doubled by adding 1% lidocaine as vehicle.

AVERAGE RANGES OF JOINT MOTION

TABLE 15-6.—Average Ranges of Joint Motion

JOINT	DEGREES
Shoulder	
Horizontal flexion	135
Horizontal extension	—
Neutral abduction	170
Forward flexion	158
Backward extension	53
Inward rotation	70
Outward rotation	90
Elbow	
Flexion	146
Extension	0
Forearm	
Pronation	71
Supination	84
Wrist	
Flexion	73
Extension	71
Radial deviation	19
Ulnar deviation	33
Hip	
Beginning position flexion	—
Flexion	113
Extension	28
Abduction	48
Adduction	31
Inward rotation	45
Outward rotation	45
Knee	
Beginning position flexion	—
Flexion	134
Ankle	
Flexion (plantar)	48
Extension (dorsiflexion)	18
Fore Part of the Foot	
Inversion	33
Eversion	18

From *Manual of orthopaedic surgery,* Chicago, 1966, American Orthopedic Association.

SCOLIOSIS SCREENING

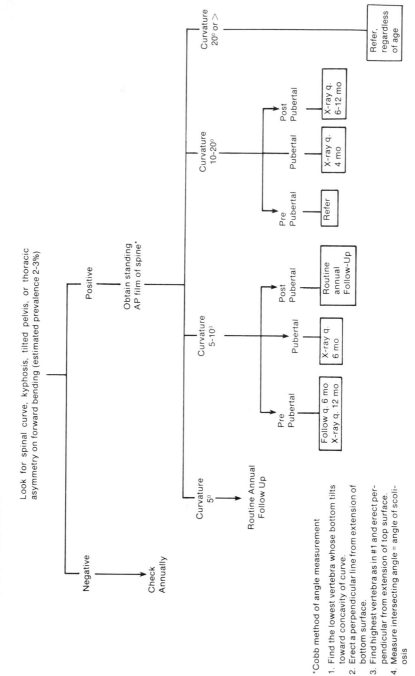

Look for spinal curve, kyphosis, tilted pelvis, or thoracic asymmetry on forward bending (estimated prevalence 2-3%)

Negative → Check Annually

Positive → Obtain standing AP film of spine*

Curvature 5° → Routine Annual Follow Up

Curvature 5-10°
- Pre Pubertal → Follow q. 6 mo X-ray q. 12 mo
- Pubertal → X-ray q. 6 mo
- Post Pubertal → Routine annual Follow-Up

Curvature 10-20°
- Pre Pubertal → Refer
- Pubertal → X-ray q. 4 mo
- Post Pubertal → X-ray q. 6-12 mo

Curvature 20° or > → Refer, regardless of age

*Cobb method of angle measurement

1. Find the lowest vertebra whose bottom tilts toward concavity of curve.
2. Erect a perpendicular line from extension of bottom surface.
3. Find highest vertebra as in #1 and erect perpendicular from extension of top surface.
4. Measure intersecting angle = angle of scoliosis

FIG 15-1.
Scoliosis screening and follow-up.

DISEASES WITH POLYARTHRITIS

TABLE 15-7.—DIFFERENTIAL DIAGNOSIS OF DISEASES WITH POLYARTHRITIS

ASPECT	RHEUMATOID ARTHRITIS	GONOCOCCAL ARTHRITIS	RHEUMATIC FEVER	JOINT MANIFESTATIONS OF INFECTIOUS DISEASES	OSTEOARTHRITIS	GOUT
Age	Adults under 40	Young adults	Children and young adults	Children, mainly	Middle age	Middle age
Etiology	Nonspecific or infectious	Gonococcus	Probably allergic from hemolytic streptococcus	Allergic or specific infectious	Metabolic disturbance; senescence	Disturbance of purine metabolism
Mode of onset	Usually insidious; occasionally acute	Acute	Acute	Acute	Insidious	Acute
Involvement	Periarticular and synovial; no effusion	Periarticular and synovial; moderate effusion	Periarticular and synovial; very little effusion	Periarticular and synovial; rarely, purulent effusion	Spurring and lipping of bones at joints	Accumulation of sodium monourate in joint spaces and ends of bones
Joints affected	Many, large and small	Often multiple, sometimes monarticular; knees, ankles, wrists, elbows, feet	Multiple and migratory; mainly large joints	Usually multiple	Mainly weight-bearing joints and distal phalangeal joints of fingers	Frequently multiple; sometimes monarticular; toes and fingers often
Result	General debility; joint ankylosis and deformity	Little general effect; may go on to ankylosis	No residual joint trouble; residual cardiac involvement	Usually no residual joint involvement; occasionally suppurative arthritis	General health good; no ankylosis; mainly pain	Swellings due to deposits of urates (tophi); urates may be discharged through skin

Continued.

TABLE 15-7.—Differential Diagnosis of Diseases With Polyarthritis—cont'd

ASPECT	RHEUMATOID ARTHRITIS	GONOCOCCAL ARTHRITIS	RHEUMATIC FEVER	JOINT MANIFESTATIONS OF INFECTIOUS DISEASES	OSTEOARTHRITIS	GOUT
Diagnostic aids	Increased sedimentation rate of RBC; presence of streptococcus agglutinins in blood	Presence of genitourinary gonorrhea; positive complement fixation test; gonococci in joint fluid; therapeutic test	Severe acute infectious manifestations; cardiac involvement; relief of pain by salicylates	Manifestations of the disease of which the arthritis is a complication	Absence of evidence of infection	High blood uric acid; increased urate content of urine; presence of urate crystals in discharging crystals
X-ray findings	Rarefaction of ends of bones; thinning of joint space	Soft tissue swelling when acute; "moth-eaten" bone ends when chronic	Negative	Negative	Spurring and lipping of bones	Punched-out areas at ends of bones after years of disease
Course	Chronic with acute exacerbations	Acute or chronic	Acute with recurrences	Acute	Chronic	Chronic with acute exacerbations

From Yater, WM: *Fundamentals of internal medicine*, ed 4, New York, 1954, Appleton-Century-Crofts.

RHEUMATOID ARTHRITIS

TABLE 15-8.—Diagnostic Criteria for Rheumatoid Arthritis

Classic Rheumatoid Arthritis
Requires 7 of the following criteria. Criteria 1-5 must be continuously present for at least 6 weeks

Definite Rheumatoid Arthritis
Requires 5 of the following criteria. Criteria 1-5 must be continuously present for at least 6 weeks

Probable Rheumatoid Arthritis
Requires 3 of the following criteria. One of criteria 1-5 must be continuously present for at least 6 weeks
Criteria
1. Morning stiffness
2. Pain on motion or tenderness in at least one joint*
3. Soft tissue swelling in at least one joint*
4. Swelling of at least one other joint within past 3 months*
5. Symmetric joint swelling*—same joint both sides of body; distal phalangeal joint does not count
6. Subcutaneous nodules*
7. X-ray changes: decalcification adjacent to affected joint
8. Positive rheumatoid factor
9. Poor mucin precipitate from synovial fluid
10. Histologic changes in synovium
11. Histologic changes in nodules

Possible Rheumatoid Arthritis
Requires 2 of the following criteria and joint symptoms continuously present for at least 6 weeks
1. Morning stiffness
2. Pain on motion or tenderness recurring or persisting for 3 weeks*
3. History or observation of joint swelling
4. Subcutaneous nodules*
5. Elevated sedimentation rate or C-reactive protein
6. Iritis

Modified from Schumacher HR, ed: *Primer on the rheumatic diseases,* ed 9, Atlanta, 1988, Arthritis Foundation, p. 316.
*Observed by physician.

TABLE 15-9.—Rheumatoid Factor

Rheumatoid factor is an antibody found in many disease states but in high titer in rheumatoid arthritis. It can occur in 5% of normal patients less than 60 years old and in 30% of normal patients over 80 years old.

The following are other diseases associated with elevated levels of rheumatoid factor:

Ankylosing spondylitis
Chronic active hepatitis
Cirrhosis
Dermatomyositis
Enteropathic arthritis
Idiopathic pulmonary fibrosis
Juvenile chronic arthritis
Leprosy
Psoriatic arthritis
Sarcoidosis
Sjögren's syndrome
Subacute bacterial endocarditis
Systemic lupus erythematosus

TABLE 15-10.—Juvenile Rheumatoid Arthritis (JRA)

SYNDROMES	PERCENT OF CASES OF JRA	SIGNS AND SYMPTOMS	PROGNOSIS
Systemic onset disease Male > female; median age at onset, 5 years	25	Fever, rash, arthritis, myalgia and distinctive extra-articular manifestations such as lymphadenopathy, splenomegaly, hepatomegaly, pericarditis, pneumonitis, pleuritis; ANA and RF are negative	One third become disabled; chronic, progressive
Polyarticular disease Seronegative: Female > male; median age at onset, 2 years	25	Insidious onset, initially involves small joints of hands and feet; RF negative, 25% are ANA positive	One sixth become disabled
Seropositive: female > male; median age at onset, 12 years	10	Insidious onset, initially involves hands and feet; RF positive, ANA negative, nodules, tendonitis, HLA-B27 present in 75%	Rapidly progressive
Pauciarticular Female > male; median age at onset, 2-4 years	30	Involves one or a few joints, most commonly knees and ankles; 50% have chronic iridocyclitis; RF negative, ANA positive in 50%	Good prognosis, mild disability

OSTEOARTHRITIS AND OTHER JOINT DISORDERS

TABLE 15-11.—JOINT DISORDERS

Osteoarthritis (Degenerative Joint Disease)
Loss of joint cartilage and bone hypertrophy
Present in 85% of people >70 years old
Symptoms begin in fifth and sixth decades
Joint pain with use of weight-bearing
Heberden's nodes found on dorsolateral aspect of base of distal phalanx
Sedimentation rate is normal
Rheumatoid factor negative

Systemic Lupus Erythematosus (SLE)
Diagnosis
Patient must have four of the following manifestations, not necessarily at the
  same time:
  Malar rash
  Discoid rash
  Photosensitivity
  Oral or nasopharyngeal ulcers
  Arthritis (2 or more joints)
  Pleuritis or pericarditis
  Urine casts or proteinuria >0.5 g/24 hr
  Seizures or psychosis
  Hematological disorder:
    Hemolytic anemia
    or leukopenia <4000/mm^3 on two occasions
    or lymphopenia <1500/mm^3 on two occasions
    or thrombocytopenia <100,000/mm^3
  Immune Disorder
    LE cells
    or anti-DNA
    or antismooth muscle
    or false positive serological test for syphilis for 6 months
  Antinuclear antibody

TABLE 15-11.—Joint Disorders—cont'd

Acute Gouty Arthritis
Arthritis Foundation Classification Criteria
One or more of the following:
    Urate crystals in joint fluid
    Tophus containing urate crystals
    Six of the following:
        More than one attack
        Maximum inflammation in one day
        Attack of monoarticular arthritis
        Observed joint erythema
        First metatarsophalangeal joint painful or swollen
        Unilateral attack at first metatarsophalangeal joint
        Unilateral attack at tarsal joint
        Suspected tophus
        Hyperuricemia
        X-ray evidence of asymmetric swelling within a joint
        X-ray evidence of subcortical cysts without erosions
        Negative joint fluid culture during attack

Raynaud's Phenomenon
A common disorder with female predominance (5:1) manifested as episodic transient pallor of the fingers when exposed to cold. The pallor is followed by cyanosis and finally by rubor and pain. Episodes may last from minutes to hours. In 50%-90% of cases there is no associated systemic disease.

Pseudogout (Calcium Pyrophosphate Deposition Disease)
Three forms
1. Acute arthritis
2. Chondrocalcinosis
3. Progressive oligoarticular disease
10% of patients also have hyperparathyroidism or hemochromatosis
Synovial fluid (see Table 15-3)
X-ray films may reveal calcifications in menisci or hyaline cartilage
There is a hereditary form (autosomal dominant)
Treatment: Antiinflammatory agents

SHOULDER PAIN

TABLE 15-12.—SHOULDER PAIN: DIAGNOSIS, EVALUATION, AND TREATMENT

ENTITY	CHARACTER OF PAIN, HISTORY	PHYSICAL FINDINGS	X-RAY FINDINGS	TREATMENT
Glenohumeral osteoarthritis	Dull, aching, not severe	Crepitus, decreased ROM	Degenerative changes of joint	Conservative*
Rotator cuff injury	Chronic pain, history of weakness in arm elevation	Pain in active abduction between 70-100 degrees; positive "drop arm" sign	Normal or degenerative changes of greater tuberosity	Surgery if total, otherwise conservative*
Bicipital tendonitis	Pain, anterior shoulder; radiates to biceps and forearm; limited abduction	Tender to palpatation in bicipital groove; pain on resisted elbow flexion or wrist supination	Irregularity of bicipital groove (requires special views); X-ray findings are usually normal	Conservative* plus steroid injection over bicipital groove
Adhesive capsulitis (frozen shoulder)	Pain and stiffness often follows prior shoulder condition, i.e., prolonged immobility	Restricted active and passive ROM, all planes	Localized osteopenia; otherwise normal	Prevention: Early mobilization of shoulder injuries; steroid injection plus conservative*; active and passive ROM
Calcific tendonitis/subacromial bursitis	Sudden, severe, diffuse pain, radiates to deltoid; cannot sleep on side; greater prevalence in diabetics	Severe pain on active abduction; tender over upper deltoid and teres major	Fluffy calcific deposit in supraspinatus tendon or other rotator cuff tendons	Conservative*; treat pain; intrabursal steroid inection; rest, but mobilize as soon as possible

	Symptoms	Examination	X-ray	Treatment
Thoracic outlet syndrome	Pain in shoulder and/or arm, plus fullness or numbness	Decreased sensation, muscle weakness, decreased radial pulse; positive Adson's maneuver (decreased pulse plus reproduces symptoms)	Cervical rib on chest x-ray film	Postural training; surgery if recurrent
Referred shoulder pain	Many types, usually diffuse and vague; consider neck, arm, hand pain	Examination of shoulder should be normal; increased by neck motion	Normal	Diagnose underlying cause, (e.g., nerve root compression, lung/plueral disease, MI, subphrenic abscess)
Inpingement syndrome	Pain has gradual onset; increased pain with activity	Pain with elevation, loss of forward flexion and internal rotation	Normal	Rest from offending activity; NSAID; subacromial steroid injection
Fibrositis	Aching pain in muscles between shoulder and neck; aggravated by stress or cold	Diffuse tenderness, some trigger points of pain		Reassurance, warm modalities, NSAID

*Conservative treatment: sling, ASA, or NSAID; cold packs for acute; hot packs for chronic pendulum qid.

LOW BACK PAIN

TABLE 15-13.—LOW BACK PAIN

Differential Diagnosis
Mechanical low back pain:
   Ligament sprain
   Acute or chronic muscle pain
Herniated nucleus pulposis
Degenerative joint disease
"Facet syndrome"
Congenital spinal anomalies
Rheumatic disease (RA, anklyosing spondylitis)
Referred pain (GI, GU, GYN)
Metastatic bone lesions

Symptoms
Stiffness (muscular component)
Ache in AM (inflammation)
Numbness, weakness, paresthesia, ↑ with Valsalva's maneuver, radiation (neurological component, radiculopathy)
Bladder, bowel, or sexual dysfunction (sacral radiculopathy, cord tumor)

Examination
Observe lordosis: Loss of lordosis represents body's attempt to remain rigid and protect a sore back
Palpate for trigger points
With the patient supine, flex the hip by lifting the extended leg. If pain is produced, note the position. This indicates pain with nerve stretching
Check reflexes

Test	Nerve Root	Nerve
Knee jerk	L2, L3, L4	Femoral
Ankle jerk	L5, S1, S2	Posterior tibial

Check motor strength

Test	Nerve	Muscle
Squat	L2, L3, L4	Quadriceps
Toe walk	L4, L5	Anterior tibialis
Great toe extension	L5	Extensor hallucis longus

TABLE 15-13.—Low Back Pain—cont'd

Further testing when needed

Test	Implication
EMG	Confirms, localizes and quantifies neurological defect
MRI or CT scan with myelogram	Evaluates for herniated disk, spinal stenosis, or extradural masses
Lumbrosacral x-rays	Evaluates for disk space narrowing, DJD facet joints, tumor, anomalies
Sedimentation rate	Screens for rheumatic diseases
Urinalysis	Infection, proteinuria

Acute Treatment
Strict bed rest for severe pain of any cause
Antiinflammatory medications for DJD or acute injury
Consider oral steroids for radicular pain if unresponsive to NSAID
Analgesics
Heat for mild to moderate stiffness
Point specific ice massage in severe pain
Muscle relaxants
Corset for short-term immobilization in selected cases

Chronic Treatment
Weight loss
Physical therapy for stretching and long-term muscle conditioning program
Encourage program of aerobic conditioning
Surgical consult if documented neurological defect and failure to respond to conservative therapy

*Courtesy Paul Dusseau, MD, Riverside Family Practice Center, Columbus, Ohio.

COMMON MONORADICULAR SYMPTOMS

TABLE 15-14.—Common Monoradicular Symptoms and their Cause

AFFECTED NERVE ROOT	PAIN	TENDERNESS	PARESTHESIAS AND SENSORY DEFECT	WEAKNESS, FASCICULATION, AND ATROPHY	REFLEX CHANGES
Fifth cervical	Numbness and localized shoulder pain	Shoulder	Shoulder	Deltoid	Biceps reflex is inconsistently affected
Sixth cervical	Radiation from neck into lateral arm and forearm; interscapular pain	Lower cervical spine, brachial plexus	Dorsal and lateral aspect of thumb	Biceps	Diminished biceps reflex
Seventh cervical	Across back of shoulder and down posterolateral forearm to middle finger	Lower cervical spine, brachial plexus	Index finger and usually middle finger	Triceps	Depressed or absent triceps reflex
Eighth cervical	Radiation from neck into medial arm and forearm; interscapular pain	Lower cervical spine, brachial plexus, ulnar nerve	5th and ulnar half of 4th finger ulnar side of hand below wrist	Intrinsic hand muscles	None

Fourth lumbar	Posterolateral aspect of thigh, across patella to anteromedial lower leg	Midlumbar spine, femoral nerve	Anterior thigh just above knee	Quadriceps	Depressed or absent knee reflex
Fifth lumbar	Back pain radiating into buttocks and posterior aspect of thigh, anterolateral leg and medial foot and great toe	Low lumbar spine, sciatic and occasionally superficial peroneal nerves	Dorsum of foot and great toe	Dorsiflexors of foot and great toe	None
First sacral	Posterior aspect of thigh and leg; posterolateral foot and lateral toes	Lumbrosacral junction, sciatic nerve	Lateral aspect of foot and small toe	Plantar flexors of foot (calf) and toes	Depressed or absent ankle reflex

SPORTS INJURIES

TABLE 15-15.—COMMON SPORTS INJURIES

INJURY/CONDITION	HISTORY	SPECIAL TESTING/HISTORY	TREATMENT	RESUMPTION OF SPORTS
Ligamentous injuries of the knee	Twisting injuries with pain and swelling	Testing is specific for ligament injured	Treatment is dependent on grade of injury	When knee is minimally painful, stable, range of motion is good, and patient can run in place, hop on affected leg, run figure-of-8 in both directions, start and stop quickly
Medial collateral	Lateral force	Valgus stress test	Grade I (pain, swelling, stable): ice, compression dressing; grade II (pain, swelling, moderate unstable): cylinder cast 4-6 weeks; grade III (marked instability): usually surgical but may improve with immobilization	
Lateral collateral	Medial force	Varus stress test		
Anterior cruciate	"Pop" or "snap" heard in 50%	Anterior drawer sign		
Posterior cruciate		Posterior drawer sign		
Meniscus tear	Twisting injury followed by swelling, locking, pain and negative ligament stress test	Arthroscopy; knee locking or "giving way" is typical	Surgical resection, often through arthroscope	Minimal pain, good range of motion
Patella subluxation	Generally bilateral knee pain, squatting, climbing stairs	Clicking on squatting and pain on climbing stairs	Quadriceps strengthening; patellar cut-out brace	When comfortable
Corns, calluses, blisters	Painful hypertrophic skin changes	May need x-ray examination to see if there is underlying structural deformity	Padding, reduction of source of friction	When comfortable

Subungual hematoma	Traumatic hematoma with pain	Trauma	Evacuation of hematoma with perforation of nail by hot paper clip or needle	When comfortable
Stress fractures	Repetitive stress like running; sudden or gradual onset of pain and swelling	Most common in shafts of first, second, third metatarsals	Short leg cast for 3-4 weeks then weight-bearing but protected	Gradually when asymptomatic
Plantar fasciitis	Burning ache along fascia, worse with activity	X-ray examination may show calcaneal spurs	Ice, Achilles tendon stretch, antiinflammatory drug	With good warm-up after improving
Achilles tendinitis	Repeated stress to the Achilles tendon, pain and swelling	None	Limit running while acute; antiinflammatory drug	When asymptomatic with aggressive Achilles tendon stretch program
Shin splints	Aching pain in posteromedial aspect of lower leg after running	None	Ice and rest; tendon stretching	When asymptomatic, tendon stretch program; avoid hard surfaces
Hamstring pull	Pain in back of thigh or at hamstring origin in pelvis	X-ray examination may show avulsion injury	Ice, rest, stretch program	When asymptomatic, good warm-up needed to avoid reinjury
Brachial plexus injury	Hyperextension of neck with counter traction of arm	Numbness in arm and fingers lasting ≤5 minutes	Protect shoulder	If lasting <5 min, may resume

TABLE 15-16.—Sports Medicine Head Injuries

Mild Concussion (Grade I)
No loss of consciousness
Brief headache
Dazed behavior, mental confusion
Lack of coordination
Ringing in ears
Return to play: 20 minutes after symptoms clear if first concussion. If second concussion, then 1 week after symptoms clear. After third mild concussion, terminate contact sports for season and obtain neurological consultation

Moderate Concussion (Grade II)
Loss of consciousness <2 minutes
Headache
Change in behavior
Numbness
Weakness
Return to play: After 24 hours of observation and 1 week after symptoms clear if first concussion. If second moderate concussion, terminate season or return after 1 asymptomatic month. Terminate sport after third concussion

Severe Concussion (Grade III)
Loss of consciousness >2 minutes
Headache
Change in behavior
Lack of coordination
Weakness
Return to play: Consider only after emergency treatment, hospitalization, neurosurgical evaluation and recommendation, and asymptomatic 1 month. If second concussion, terminate sport for season. May return following year if asymptomatic. Terminate sport after third concussion

TABLE 15-17.—Heat Illness

Heat injuries include syncope, cramps, exhaustion, and stroke. These are all preventable, and an unlimited water supply must be readily available for the athletes. Sling psychrometer and wetbulb reading are useful guides for practice precautions.
<66° F: No precautions necessary
67° F-77° F: Unlimited water available, and all athletes must be encouraged to drink whether thirsty or not
78° F-94° F: Alter practice schedule to a lighter routine and lighter clothing, withhold heat illness susceptible athletes
>95° F: No practice
Weight loss of individual athletes after practice during conditioning will identify susceptible or "at risk" athletes

General Guidelines for Practice Weight Loss
3% Loss, safe
5% Loss, susceptible to heat illness
7% Loss, dangerous because subsequent sweating capability is severely limited, and heat stroke is likely

PHYSICAL THERAPY MODALITIES

TABLE 15-18.—Physical Therapy Modalities

MODALITY	ACTION	INDICATIONS	CONTRAINDICATIONS	HOW TO ORDER
Moist Heat				
Hot packs	Circulation Muscle relaxation	Muscle spasm Joint contracture	Sensory loss Malignant tumor Open lesions	20 minutes
Whirlpool	Cleansing Muscle relaxation	Open lesions Muscle spasm	Poor heat tolerance Cortisone withdrawal	20 minutes
Therapeutic pool	Decrease gravity to aid in exercise	To aid exercise and ambulation training	Cardiovascular disease	Temperature 94°-96°; progress from shallow to deep water; continue exercise after leaving water
Dry Heat				
Diathermy	Circulation Muscle relaxation	Muscle spasm Chronic pain Adhesive capsulitis	Metallic implants Coagulation defects Sensory loss Open lesions Malignancy	20 minutes, 3 times/week, for 1-2 weeks
Infrared		Muscle spasm Relief of pain Promotes healing of open lesions	Sensory loss Excessive scar tissue	Buy infrared bulb, keep 20 inches from skin; direct it perpendicular to skin for 30 minutes; may repeat after cooling skin 1 hour

Continued.

TABLE 15-18.—Physical Therapy Modalities—cont'd

MODALITY	ACTION	INDICATIONS	CONTRAINDICATIONS	HOW TO ORDER
Deep Heat Ultrasound	Muscle relaxation	Joint pain Contractures	Application to eyes Pregnancy, malignancy Caution S/P laminectomy	10-15 minutes
Cold packs, ice massage		Acute trauma	Raynaud phenomena Cryoglobulinemia	Freeze water in paper cups; peel away paper at open end; massage affected area with circular movement
Intermittent traction	Spine distraction	Cervical DJD Lumbar DJD Herniated disk	Unstable vertebrae Malignancy Pregnancy Spinal cord disease	50-60 lb (maximum of 10 for neck); intermittently; need PT instruction
Paraffin baths	Minimizes pain Heats joint capsule	Arthritis	Sensory loss which could lead to burns	5-10 min per treatment; home units and MITS are available with PT instruction

CASTING TECHNIQUES

TABLE 15-19.—Casting Techniques

General Principles
Fiberglass
Lightweight and can endure moisture
Wear gloves
Use specially designed nylon stockinette and padding, which is designed to dry
  quickly if it gets wet
Use small width such as 4 inch for leg, 2 inch for hand, and 3 inch for wrist;
  wrap around forearm, so that "tucks" are not needed as with plaster
Wet the roll; there will be a thermal reaction during curing, which is not a haz-
  ard
Apply fiberglass spirally with a little more tension than plaster
Trimming is difficult but can be done with Bohler's scissors before the fiberglass
  sets
Be sure to evert all edges
The cast can be trimmed or cut after it has set with a cast removal saw
Plaster
The hotter the water, the faster the plaster will set
Stockinette should be the first layer applied
Next, line the extremity with padding (e.g., Webril)
Extra padding or felt should be applied to bony prominences
Wear gloves (protection and smoothing of plaster)
Soak plaster until bubbling stops, squeeze gently, then apply
Start plaster at either end
Advance plaster about one third to one half width of roll per turn
Six or seven layers are the usual thickness needed
Turn stockinette onto plaster and incorporate into cast to form smooth soft edge
Sculpt plaster with both hands while applying
Do not pull plaster tight as you roll it
Check capillary filling and for paresthesias every 1-2 hours for first 24 hours
  while awake; office follow-up in 24-48 hours
Short Arm Cast
For nondisplaced fractures of the forearm and wrist
Have an assistant hold patient's arm in 90 degree flexion with arm partially ex-
  tended while applying case
Extend cast to, not beyond, MCP joints
Include thumb, if for navicular fracture
Hold wrist in 15-20 degree extension
If thumb spica, hold thumb in "neutral" position
Use 4" plaster (2" may be used for hand and thumb)
Short Leg Cast
For nondisplaced fractures of the lower leg and ankle
Apply with patient on end of table, knee at 90 degree flexion
Keep ankle in neutral position avoiding plantar flexion
Use 6-inch plaster (4-inch may be used around ankle)
After applying one or two layers, fold four 4-inch splints longitudinally and place
  one on each side and front and back of ankle
Apply one additional layer and trim as needed
If walking cast is desired, fill arch of foot with splints to make a flat surface; ap-
  ply rubber "walker" and secure with a plaster bandage

16 Poisoning and Overdose

Barry L. Carter

TABLE 16-1.—General Management for Systemic Poisoning Before Patient is Seen by the Emergency Department

Emesis
Recent evidence suggests gastric lavage is more effective than emesis, which is no longer used in the emergency department. However, syrup of ipecac (not the fluid extract) is still useful for administration in the home, private office, or in transport from remote locations. Vomiting occurs in 90% of patients within 20-30 minutes of poisoning, and it may remove 30%-50% of the stomach contents.
Timing
If there is no ipecac in the home or setting, and the emergency department is near, the patient should be transported immediately. However, if the emergency department is more than a 30-minute drive, and there is a pharmacy within 10-15 minutes, the patient should be transported to the pharmacy to obtain syrup of ipecac before being transported to the emergency department.
Contraindications
Decreased level of consciousness or active seizures
Caustic ingestions
Ingested material that leads to rapid, significant neurological symptoms
Ingestion of petroleum distillates or hydrocarbons
Relative Contraindications
Severe hypertension or respiratory disease
Patient with high risk of hemorrhagic disorder
Age <6 months
Late-stage pregnancy
Dose for Syrup of Ipecac
6-12 months, 5-10 ml (not recommended for nonhealth care facility use in this age group)
1-12 years, 15 ml
>12 years, 30 ml
Follow dose with 4-8 oz of water or clear liquid. If emesis does not occur within 20 minutes, the dose of ipecac and 4-8 oz of fluids should be repeated.
General Procedures:
Patient should be transported to the emergency department with containers of the ingested poison for inspection of all remaining uningested substances. A large container should be sent with patient for vomitus. Vomitus should be saved and inspected for tablets, capsules, or other particles to determine the success of the emesis (Table 16-2).

Modified from Olson KR: *Poisoning and drug overdose,* Norwalk, Conn., 1994, Appleton & Lange, p. 345; Tenenbein M, et al: *Ann Emerg Med* 16:838, 1987.

TABLE 16-2.—GENERAL MANAGEMENT FOR SYSTEMIC POISONING IN THE EMERGENCY
DEPARTMENT OR HOSPITAL

There is controversy concerning the use of gastric lavage, activated charcoal,
and cathartics. Part of this relates to studies that show that charcoal is just as
effective when used alone as when it is used following gut emptying (e.g.,
lavage or emesis). Emesis is no longer recommended once the patient pre-
sents to the emergency department and recent data suggest that charcoal
should be the primary treatment for poisoning and overdose.

Gastric Lavage
Lavage is generally not very effective when delayed more than 60 minutes after
poison is ingested. However, it is still routinely performed up to 1-2 hours
postingestion. For some drugs that delay gastric emptying (e.g., anticholin-
ergics, salicylates, or tricyclics), gastric lavage may be effective even after
more prolonged delays. Lavage is generally not indicated for small or moder-
ate overdoses when activated charcoal can be given immediately.
Indications
Removal of large overdoses of liquids, solid drugs, or poisons
Method to administer activated charcoal or cathartics in patients who cannot
take them orally
To dilute and remove corrosives and/or to empty the stomach before endoscopy
Contraindications
Active seizures, coma, or obtunded patient
Large sustained-release dosage forms may not be returned, and whole bowel
irrigation may be preferable to removing tablets or capsules intact
Methods
1. If the patient is unconscious, insert and inflate a cuffed endotracheal tube
before performing gastric lavage to prevent aspiration.
2. Place patient in the left lateral decubitus position.
3. Use the largest diameter tube possible, 36-40 F in adults or 32-36 F in children.
4. Immediately withdraw as much of the stomach contents as possible, and
perform toxicology analysis.
5. Administer 60-100 g (1 g/kg) of activated charcoal down the tube before initiating lavage to begin adsorption of the substance.
6. Lavage with tepid water or normal saline at 15 ml/kg/cycle in children and up
to 200-400 ml/cycle in adults. Repeat lavage until a total of 2 L is administered or until passes are clear and free of tablets, capsules, or toxic material.

Activated Charcoal
Activated charcoal is effective for adsorption of most toxins *except* boric acid,
acids, alkali, alcohols, iron, or lithium.

Modified from Olson KR: *Poisoning and drug overdose,* Norwalk, Conn., 1994, Appleton &
Lange, pp. 44-49; Tenenbein M, et al: *Ann Emerg Med* 16:838, 1987; Watson WA: *Drug
Intell Clin Pharm* 21:160, 1987; Rodgers GC, Matyunas NJ: *Pediatr Clin North Am* 33:261,
1986; Albertson TE, et al: *Ann Emerg Med* 18:56, 1989; Tenenbein M, et al: *Arch Intern
Med* 147:905, 1987.

Continued.

TABLE 16-2.—GENERAL MANAGEMENT FOR SYSTEMIC POISONING IN THE EMERGENCY
DEPARTMENT OR HOSPITAL—cont'd

Availability
Powder or liquid suspensions in sorbitol in bottles containing 12.5, 25, 30, or 50
    g (Charcoaid, Liqui-Char, Superchar)
Indications
Can be used with essentially any toxic ingestion to limit toxin absorption from
    the gut
Multiple doses of charcoal can serve as intestinal dialysis and enhance elimina-
    tion of some drugs from the systemic circulation even after the drug has been
    absorbed
Charcoal is given even if the toxin is not known
It was previously thought that administration of charcoal before the use of ace-
    tylcysteine would inactivate the acetylcysteine, but it is now known that this is
    insignificant
Dosage
1 g/kg (for adults the dose is 60-100 g) orally or via gastric tube
One or two doses may be repeated at 1-2 hour intervals following large inges-
    tions
Repeat Doses of Charcoal (Intestinal Dialysis)
When a constant amount of charcoal is available in the gut, the intestine can
    serve as a site to attract drug from the systemic circulation and has been
    shown to enhance the systemic elimination of the following:

Barbiturates	Carbamazepine
Cyclosporine	Dapsone
Digoxin	Digitoxin
Nadolol	Phenylbutazone
Phenytoin	Salicylate
Theophylline	Tricyclic antidepressants

The dosage is 20-30 g (0.5-1 g/kg) every 2-3 hours given orally or through the
    gastric tube. This dose is generally given for 24-48 hours. The sorbitol may
    cause large-volume diarrhea, which can lead to fluid and electrolyte distur-
    bances. Repeat charcoal dose is contraindicated in ileus or GI obstruction.

TABLE 16-2.—General Management for Systemic Poisoning in the Emergency Department or Hospital—cont'd

Cathartics
There are few data that support the efficacy of cathartics.
Indications
Particularly useful with charcoal to help move the contents through the GI tract
Used to speed the passage of drugs not adsorbed to charcoal (e.g., iron)
Contraindications
Ileus or obstruction (absence of bowel sounds)
Caustic ingestions
CHF (sodium-containing agents)
Renal impairment (magnesium-containing agents)
Recent bowel surgery
Dosage
Give sorbitol 70% (1-2 ml/kg) or magnesium citrate 10% (3-4 ml/kg) along with activated charcoal or mixed as a slurry
Repeat one-half the original dose if there is no charcoal stool within 6-8 hours

Whole Bowel Irrigation
Has become an accepted procedure for eliminating some toxins; the principle is that large volumes are used to force the intestinal contents through the GI tract
Indications
Large ingestions of iron, lithium, or other drugs that are not adsorbed well to charcoal
May be effective for large ingestions of sustained-release or enteric-coated products that are not removed by gastric lavage
Contraindications
1. Ileus or intestinal obstruction
2. Seizures, coma, or obtunded patient
Method
Bowel preparation solution, polyethylene glycol-electrolyte solution (CoLyte, GoLYTELY, OCL) is administered by nasogastric tube at a rate of 500 ml/hr in children or 2 L/hr in teenagers and adults. Irrigation is continued until rectal effluent is the same as the infusate. Be prepared for a large volume stool in 1-2 hours. Pass a rectal tube, or have the patient sit on a commode.

Hemodialysis and Hemoperfusion
In most instances these methods are unnecessary and should be initiated by an individual knowledgeable in clinical toxicology. An understanding of the physical-chemical characteristics of the toxin are necessary. In many cases, these methods are not effective or may be dangerous.

TABLE 16-3.—ACETAMINOPHEN INGESTION

Products
Tylenol, Liquiprin, Tempra, Anacin-3, Tylenol with codeine, Darvocet, Comtrex, Excedrin ES, Sominex 2, many others.

Symptoms and Toxicity
In toxic overdoses, acetaminophen overwhelms the ability of glutathione to detoxify one of the hepatotoxic metabolites of the drug.
Early Symptoms
Within a few minutes to a few hours after ingestion, the only symptoms are anorexia, nausea, and vomiting.
Late Symptoms
Symptoms often improve over 24-48 hours, but bilirubin, hepatic enzymes, and PT levels rise. After 72-96 hours following a large ingestion, jaundice, coagulation defects, and encephalopathy secondary to hepatic necrosis may occur. Renal failure and death may occur.

Estimating Risk of Hepatotoxicity

HOURS AFTER ACUTE INGESTION	NO RISK (μg/ml)	POSSIBLE RISK (μg/ml)	PROBABLE RISK (μg/ml)
4	<150	150-200	>200
6	<100	100-150	>150
8	<75	75-100	>100
10	<50	50-75	>75
12	<40	40-50	>50
14	<22	22-40	>40
16	<18	18-22	>22
18	<12	12-18	>18
20	<8	8-12	>12
22	<5	5-8	>8
24	<4	4-5	>5

To use the table: An acetaminophen serum level should be drawn 4 hours following ingestion. Levels can also be drawn after 4 hours with patients who present late or to obtain serial levels. Levels drawn before 4 hours are not reliable when estimating risk.

Note that salicylates may falsely elevate acetaminophen levels by 10%. Based on the time the serum level is drawn, estimate the probability that hepatotoxicity will occur. Serum levels in the possible or probable categories should receive acetylcysteine (e.g., 4-hour serum level over 150 μg/ml).

Modified from Rumack BH, Matthews H: *Pediatrics* 55:871, 1975; Rumack BH: *Pediatr Clin North Am* 33:691, 1986; Lewis RK, Paloucek FP: *Clin Pharm* 10:765, 1991; Brent J: *Ann Emerg Med* 22:1860, 1993.

TABLE 16-3.—ACETAMINOPHEN INGESTION—cont'd

Treatment
Prehospital
Ipecac-induced emesis may be effective if given within 60 minutes of ingestion. Give activated charcoal if available.
In the Emergency Department
Activated charcoal and a cathartic should be given within 1-2 hours after ingestion. Consider multidose charcoal for polydrug poisoning. It was once thought that charcoal inactivated acetylcysteine, but this is now known to be insignificant.
It is recommended that acetylcysteine be withheld until the results of the 4-hour serum level are known.
If the serum level is in the possible or probable risk category, initiate acetylcysteine.
Acetylcysteine should be given as soon after the 4-hour window as possible. However, it is very effective when started within 8 hours of ingestion. While it may be less effective after 10-36 hours, the drug is still beneficial and should be given late in the course of overdose. *Free consultations can be obtained from the Rocky Mountain Poison Center at 1-800-525-6115, 24 hours daily.*
Oral acetylcysteine (Mucomyst) 20% should be mixed to prepare a 5% solution in carbonated beverage or fruit drink.
Loading dose: 140 mg/kg PO or NG
Maintenance: 70 mg/kg every 4 hours for 17 doses
If vomiting occurs within 1 hour of a dose, repeat that dose. Cold solutions and a straw may increase palatability.
Intravenous acetylcysteine is used in Canada and Europe. The sterile injectable form is not available in the United States except through an investigational protocol with the National Capital Poison Center or the Rocky Mountain Poison Center: 150 mg/kg IV over 15 minutes, then 50 mg/kg IV over the next 4 hours and 100 mg/kg IV over the last 16 hours (300 mg/kg over 20 hours).
Monitor liver function tests, electrolytes, CBC, glucose, BUN, creatinine, and prothrombin time in all patients.

TABLE 16-4.—Poisoning by Aspirin and Other Salicylates

Products
Bayer aspirin, Anacin, Bufferin, Ecotrin, Ascriptin, Alka-Seltzer, Magan, Trilisate, Pepto-Bismol, oil of wintergreen

Signs and Symptoms
Acute Ingestion
Nausea, vomiting, tinnitus, lethargy, hyperpnea, mixed respiratory alkalosis, and metabolic acidosis. With severe ingestions, coma, seizures, hypoglycemia, hyperthermia, and death
Chronic Ingestion
Confusion, dehydration, metabolic acidosis, cerebral edema, and pulmonary edema

Severity
Ingestions of >150 mg/kg are expected to cause toxicity; ingestions of 300-500 mg/kg are serious; and ingestions of >500 mg/kg are potentially lethal. Chronic ingestion of much lower doses may be toxic.

Estimating Risk
Measure serum levels 6 hours or later after acute ingestion. Levels measured before 6 hours may indicate toxicity but may not reflect severity. Levels can continue to rise because of sustained-release products or large tablet mass. Compare the level with the following estimation of severity. Make serial determinations to examine serum level characteristics and elimination.

HOURS AFTER ACUTE INGESTION	POTENTIALLY MILD (mg/dl)	POTENTIALLY MODERATE (mg/dl)	POTENTIALLY SEVERE (mg/dl)
6	45-65	65-90	>90
12	35-52	52-72	>72
24	22-35	35-50	>50
30	20-30	30-40	>40
36	15-25	25-32	>32
42	12-20	20-28	>28
48	10-15	15-20	>20
60	—	10-13	>13

Modified from Snodgrass WR: *Pediatr Clin North Am* 33:381, 1986; Olson KR: *Poisoning and drug overdose,* Norwalk, Conn., 1994, Appleton & Lange, pp. 277-280.

TABLE 16-4.—Poisoning by Aspirin and Other Salicylates—cont'd

Therapy (Begin before serum level is known)
Prehospital
Ipecac-induced emesis may be effective if given within 60 minutes of ingestion. Give activated charcoal if available.
In the Emergency Department
Maintain airway; assist ventilation; administer oxygen; and obtain blood gases and chest x-ray radiograph.
Activated charcoal and a cathartic should be given within 1-2 hours after ingestion. With very large ingestions (>30 g), doses of 300-600 g of charcoal may be necessary and 25-50 g doses can be given at 3-5 hour intervals.
Treat metabolic acidosis with intravenous sodium bicarbonate, and do *not* allow serum pH to fall below 7.4.
Fluid management: Initially give Ringer's lactate in D_5W at 10-15 ml/kg/hr for 1-2 hours to achieve a urine flow of 3-6 ml/kg/hr. Then continue D_5W containing bicarbonate (about 20-35 mEq/L depending on the degree of acidosis), potassium (about 20-40 mEq/L unless renal failure is present), sodium (40-50 mEq/L), and chloride (50 mEq/L) at a rate of 4-6 ml/kg/hr until salicylate level is below the mild values noted above. Attempt to maintain urinary pH > 7.0-8.0. Maintenance fluids can then be administered at 2-3 ml/kg/hr.
Monitoring: Fluid therapy may contribute to pulmonary edema, and this must be monitored. Also monitor blood gases, blood glucose, electrolytes, anion gap, BUN, creatinine, prothrombin time, chest x-ray examination, urine pH, urine specific gravity, I/O, and salicylate levels.
Hemodialysis corrects acid-base and fluid abnormalities and very effectively removes salicylate. Hemodialysis is indicated for patients with acute ingestion and serum levels greater than 120 mg/dl, or severe acidosis and other symptoms of intoxication; patients with chronic intoxication with serum levels greater than 60 mg/dl accompanied by acidosis, confusion, or lethargy; or any patient with severe manifestations of intoxication.

Modified from Snodgrass WR: *Pediatr Clin North Am* 33:381, 1986; Olson KR: *Poisoning and drug overdose,* Norwalk, Conn., 1994, Appleton & Lange, pp. 277-280.

TABLE 16-5.—OVERDOSE WITH ANTICHOLINERGIC DRUGS (ATROPINE, BELLADONNA, ANTIHISTAMINES)

Products
Hyoscyamine (Anaspaz, Levsin), atropine, scopolamine, belladonna tincture, methscopolamine (Pamine), clidinium (Quarzan), glycopyrrolate (Robinul), mepenzolate (Cantil), methantheline (Banthine), propantheline (Pro-Banthine), dicyclomine (Bentyl), diphenhydramine (Benadryl), many others, including combination products and generic drugs

Signs and Symptoms
Dry mouth, mydriasis, flushing, urinary retention, decreased bowel sounds, fever, tachycardia, hypertension, AV dissociation, restlessness, irritability, delirium, hallucinations, hyperthermia, coma. Drowsiness and ataxia with antihistamines

Therapy
Prehospital
Ipecac-induced emesis may be effective if given within 60 minutes of poison ingestion. Give activated charcoal if available.
In the Emergency Department
Maintain airway; assist ventilation; administer oxygen; obtain blood gases, glucose, and electrolytes; and perform ECG monitoring.
Activated charcoal and a cathartic should be given. Repeat dose charcoal (gastrointestinal dialysis) is not effective.
Lavage may not be necessary if charcoal can be given immediately. However, it may be effective long after ingestion, since these drugs slow GI motility.
Tachycardia may respond to propranolol.
Physostigmine
Indications:
   1. To establish the diagnosis of anticholinergic poisoning—most non-CNS signs and symptoms will disappear in minutes if the diagnosis is correct
   2. To treat severe symptoms that cannot be managed supportively such as delirium, urinary retention, severe sinus tachycardia, and hyperthermia
Contraindications:
   Tricyclic antidepressant overdose, gangrene, asthma, GI or GU obstruction, cardiovascular disease, or in patients receiving depolarizing neuromuscular blocking agents
Dosage: Adults, 1-2 mg (children 0.02 mg/kg) IV at a rate of 1 mg/min with cardiac monitoring; may repeat every 20-30 minutes
Dialysis is not effective for enhancing elimination.

Modified from Olson KR. *Poisoning and drug overdose,* Norwalk, Conn., 1994, Appleton & Lange, pp. 75-76 and 370-378.

TABLE 16-6.—INGESTION OF CAUSTIC SUBSTANCES

Signs and Symptoms
Oral pain, vomiting, drooling, refusal to drink, chest or abdominal pain, edema
or ulceration of the palate and pharynx

Treatment
Do not attempt to chemically neutralize (e.g., vinegar or bicarbonate). *Do not*
induce emesis or give charcoal (charcoal interferes with endoscopy).
Immediately dilute with water or milk.
Gastric lavage may be beneficial, and a soft flexible tube should be used. Re-
peated passes of water or saline should be given, and the pH should be
checked with each pass.
Endoscopy
Attempting to predict which patients require endoscopy has been controversial.
Some asymptomatic patients will still have significant burns. However, recent
data suggest that endoscopy is not necessary in totally asymptomatic patients. Patients with symptoms of dysphagia, pain, drooling, vomiting, or oral
burns should receive endoscopy.
Steroids
Steroid use remains controversial but may reduce stricture formation for
second- or third-degree burns. Use IV methylprednisolone, 2 mg/kg/day, or
the equivalent, and continue for 2-3 weeks (e.g., prednisone 1 mg/kg/day) or
until reepithelialization has occurred. Corticosteroids increase the risk of infection and prophylactic antibiotics are often given.

Follow-up
Close follow-up will be necessary to detect stricture formation and to perform
dilation or surgery as necessary.
These patients may be at high risk for the development of esophageal carcinoma (as early as 13 years and a mean of 40 years later), and they should
be followed for this disease.

Modified from Rothstein FC: *Pediatr Clin North Am* 33:665, 1986; Olson KR: *Poisoning and drug overdose,* Norwalk, Conn., 1994, Appleton & Lange, pp. 126-128; Howell JM, et al: *Am J Emerg Med* 10:421, 1992; Gorman RL, et al: *Am J Emerg Med* 10:189, 1992.

TABLE 16-7.—DIGITALIS GLYCOSIDE POISONING (DIGOXIN, DIGITOXIN)

Products
Crystodigin, Lanoxin, Lanoxicaps, several plants such as oleander, foxglove, lily
of the valley, and rhododendron

Signs and Symptoms
Acute Ingestion
Nausea, vomiting, hyperkalemia (with large ingestions), bradycardia, supraven-
tricular arrhythmias, first- or second-degree heart block; with large ingestions
PAT with block, ventricular ectopy with block, third-degree block, ventricular
tachycardia
Chronic Ingestion
Nausea, vomiting, CNS disturbances, arrhythmias (see acute ingestion), and
abnormal vision, usually hypokalemia

Assessment
Potential toxicity is increased by hypokalemia, hypomagnesemia, or hypercalcemia.
Digoxin levels drawn within 6 hours are still in the distributive phase, may not
reliably represent the degree of toxicity, and should be repeated later.
Serum digoxin level does not predict toxicity. Therefore treatment should be
based on clinical assessment. Healthy children often tolerate high digoxin levels with little toxicity (e.g., levels < 10 ng/ml).

Therapy
Prehospital
Induce emesis within 1 hour of poison ingestion. Give activated charcoal if
available.
In Emergency Department
Begin continuous ECG monitoring and serial electrolytes, digoxin levels, and
magnesium and calcium levels. Monitor for at least 24 hours, since distribu-
tion into the tissues can be delayed.
Multiple-dose charcoal (see Table 16-2) can markedly increase digoxin elimina-
tion long after ingestion or even with chronic toxicity. Administer with a cathar-
tic.
Do not give potassium until electrolyte status is known.
Symptomatic Bradycardia or Heart Block
Atropine 0.5-1 mg (0.01 mg/kg in children) IV; may repeat every 5 minutes for
2-4 doses
Temporary pacemaker may be needed for persistent symptomatic bradycardia.
Ventricular Arrhythmias

Modified from Lalonde RL, et al: *Clin Pharmacol Ther* 37:367, 1985; Lake KD, et al: *Pharmacotherapy,* 4:161, 1984; Cole PL, Smith TW: *Drug Intell Clin Pharm* 20:267, 1986; Le-
wander WJ, et al: *Am J Dis Child* 140:770, 1986; Olin BR: *Facts and Comparisons,* St. Louis,
1994, Facts and Comparisons, pp. 712b-712d.
*Each vial contains 40 mg. Dosages for children are expressed as mg; dosages for adults
are expressed as number of vials needed.

TABLE 16-7.—DIGITALIS GLYCOSIDE POISONING (DIGOXIN, DIGITOXIN)—cont'd

Lidocaine 1-1.5 mg/kg IV load, then 1-4 mg/min IV infusion. Can repeat bolus of 0.5-1 mg/kg every 8-10 minutes for a total of 2-4 bolus doses. For patients with CHF, who are elderly, or who have hepatic dysfunction, use half of these bolus doses and infusion rates.

Or

Phenytoin 1-2 mg/kg IV (*do not* give faster than 50 mg/min); repeat every 5 minutes up to 10 doses or 1 g maximum dose. Maintenance dose is 4-8 mg/kg/day.

Do not give quinidine, procainamide, or bretylium.

Antidote: Digibind

Digibind can begin to reverse signs of toxicity in 30-60 minutes.

Indications:

Life-threatening arrhythmias

Severe hyperkalemia (>5 mEq/L)

Ingestion of >10 mg in adult

Ingestion of >4 mg in a child

Steady state serum concentrations >10 ng/ml

Dosage Estimate for Digibind Following a Single Ingestion

NUMBER OF TABLETS OR CAPSULES INGESTED	DOSE (mg)	DOSE IN NUMBER OF VIALS
25	340	8.5
50	680	17
75	1000	25
100	1360	34
150	2000	50
200	2680	67

Estimate of Digibind Dose Based on Serum Digoxin Concentrations: (for Exact Dosage Calculations, See Package Insert)

WEIGHT (kg)	SERUM DIGOXIN CONCENTRATION (ng/ml)*						
	1	2	4	8	12	16	20
5	2 mg	4 mg	8 mg	15 mg	22 mg	30 mg	40 mg
10	4 mg	8 mg	15 mg	30 mg	40 mg	60 mg	80 mg
20	8 mg	15 mg	30 mg	60 mg	80 mg	120 mg	160 mg
60	0.5 vial	1 vial	2 vials	3 vials	5 vials	6 vials	8 vials
70	1 vial	2 vials	3 vials	5 vials	8 vials	11 vials	13 vials
80	1 vial	2 vials	3 vials	6 vials	9 vials	12 vials	15 vials
100	1 vial	2 vials	4 vials	8 vials	11 vials	15 vials	19 vials

TABLE 16-8.—HYDROCARBON INGESTIONS

Signs and Symptoms

Most morbidity and mortality are from aspiration pneumonitis, but ingestion can lead to systemic toxicity. Symptoms include choking, coughing, tachypnea, respiratory effort, nausea, vomiting, fever, irritability, drowsiness, lethargy, seizures, and coma. Toxicity is highly variable and dependent on the type of hydrocarbon.

Treatment

Prehospital

Do not induce emesis, which may increase the risk of aspiration. Give activated charcoal if it is available.

In Emergency Department

Most accidental ingestions are less than 5-10 ml, and toxicity is rare. However, if the ingestion was large and recent, consider gastric lavage. Administer activated charcoal and a cathartic.

For suspected large ingestions: Monitor BP, heart rate and rhythm, respiratory rate, electrolytes, glucose, BUN, creatinine, liver function studies, and ECG.

For suspected pneumonitis: Examine and observe for at least 6-8 hours, monitoring chest x-ray findings and blood gases. If symptoms of aspiration pneumonitis (coughing, choking, wheezing) are not present by 4-6 hours, then pneumonitis will probably not occur.

All patients who become symptomatic should be admitted.

Do not use steroids.

Avoid epinephrine or other catecholamines, which may induce arrhythmias.

Do not use prophylactic antibiotics unless the patient is debilitated or has preexisting respiratory disease. Infectious pneumonia can be difficult to distinguish because of fever or other signs of aspiration, and Gram stains and cultures should be performed.

Modified from Simon JE: *Pediatr Clin North Am* 33:411, 1986; Truemper E, et al: *Pediatr Emerg Care* 3:187, 1987; Olson KR: *Poisoning and drug overdose,* Norwalk, Conn., 1994, Appleton & Lange, pp. 178-180.

TABLE 16-9.—INSECTICIDES (CARBAMATES AND ORGANOPHOSPHATES)

Signs and Symptoms

Rapidly absorbed through skin and mucous membranes. Symptoms progress rapidly and occur within minutes and almost always before 12 hours of exposure.

Salivation, lacrimation, urination, defecation (SLUD), vomiting, bronchospasm, bronchorrhea, miosis, sweating, diaphoresis, fasciculations, tremors, convulsions, coma, and respiratory arrest. Pneumonitis may occur with petroleum-based liquid insecticides.

Therapy

Prehospital

Patient should remove all contaminated clothing and wash with soap and water including hair and under nails. Eyes should be irrigated with copious water or saline.

Administer activated charcoal for ingestions, if available. Emesis should be avoided because of the potential for the rapid development of symptoms.

In Emergency Department

All individuals assisting with decontamination must wear protective clothing and gloves following large exposures.

Administer activated charcoal and cathartics. Gastric lavage may be helpful for recent ingestions.

Maintain airway, assist ventilation, and give oxygen.

Observe patients for at least 6-8 hours.

Obtain RBC acetylcholinesterase if possible (this must be obtained before the use of 2-PAM). RBC acetylcholinesterase levels that are 20%-50% of normal indicate mild poisoning; levels 10%-20% of normal are considered moderate poisoning; levels <10% of normal are considered severe poisoning.

Atropine will not treat muscle weakness because of nicotinic receptor stimulation, and patients can still develop respiratory depression.

   Adult dose: 1-2 mg every 10-30 minutes

   Children: 0.05 mg/kg every 10-30 minutes

   Very large doses may be necessary (40-50 mg daily are common, and much higher doses may be needed). Do not underdose. The endpoint should be drying of secretions, elimination of wheezing, and elevation of heart rate (if the patient had bradycardia). It will be necessary to continue atropine for 24 hours (up to 5-10 days for lypophilic poisons) and then taper slowly.

Pralidoxime (2-PAM) is the specific antidote for organophosphates. It may be effective for carbamates, but some authors consider it ineffective for carbamates. It should be used as soon as possible and when unknown insecticides are involved. The drug will reverse muscular weakness and fasciculations.

   Dose: 1-2 g (25-50 mg/kg in children) in 100-200 ml D_5W infused over 10-15 minutes. The dose can be repeated if muscle weakness or fasciculations are not relieved.

Do not give morphine, theophylline, physostigmine, phenothiazines, ethacrynic acid, or furosemide. These are contraindicated.

Modified from Mortensen ML: *Pediatr Clin North Am* 33:421, 1986; Tafuri J, Roberts J: *Ann Emerg Med* 16:193, 1987; Olson KR: *Poisoning and drug overdose,* Norwalk, Conn., 1994, Appleton & Lange, pp. 118-119, 240-242.

TABLE 16-10.—IRON INGESTION

Products

Ferrous sulfate (20% elemental iron), ferrous gluconate (12% elemental iron), ferrous fumarate (33% elemental iron), Feosol, Fer-in-Sol, Mol-Iron, Niferex, and multiple vitamins with iron

Signs and Symptoms

Toxicity occurs as a result of the direct corrosive effects of iron in the GI tract. Iron also causes vasodilation and vascular damage, hepatic damage, and coagulopathy. Following are the four phases that have been described:

Phase I (within 6 Hours of Ingestion)

Abdominal pain, vomiting, diarrhea (often bloody), hemorrhagic gastritis. Most patients do not progress beyond Phase I but uncommonly, shock, renal failure, and death may result from massive fluid and blood loss

Phase II (Stability—6-24 Hours)

Improvement of symptoms except lethargy. Most patients continue to improve, but severe cases progress to Phase III. Some patients progress to Phase III rapidly without a noticeable Phase II

Phase III (within 12-48 Hours of Ingestion)

Shock, cardiovascular collapse, GI hemorrhage, hepatic necrosis, coma, hypoglycemia, metabolic acidosis, bleeding abnormalities, and seizures

Phase IV (2-8 Weeks After Ingestion)

Occurs following severe GI effects and includes pyloric or antral stenosis or stricture leading to obstruction

Evaluation and Therapy

Prehospital

Induce emesis with syrup of ipecac, unless contraindicated. Charcoal does not adsorb iron.

Observe for severe symptoms if dose is <40 mg/kg.

In Emergency Department

Support airway, breathing, and circulation. Correct shock, electrolyte imbalance, or hypoglycemia. Large IV volumes may be necessary, and urine output should be maintained at least 1-2 ml/kg/hr.

Modified from Tenenbein M: *J Pediatr* 111:142, 1987; Mann KV, et al: *Clin Pharm* 8:428, 1989; Klein-Schwartz W, et al: *Clin Pediatr* 29:316, 1990; Olson KR: *Poisoning and drug overdose,* Norwalk, Conn., 1994, Appleton & Lange, pp. 189-191.

TABLE 16-10.—IRON INGESTION—cont'd

Obtain serum iron within 2-4 hours after ingestion, since this provides the best correlation with severity of poisoning. Serum iron >350 μg/dl should be considered potentially toxic. In the past, serum iron >TIBC was used to estimate toxicity, but this is now known to be unreliable.

Lavage with normal saline. *Do not* use phosphate solutions or deferoxamine lavage.

Obtain abdominal x-ray film after lavage to identify remaining iron and to determine need for whole bowel irrigation.

If tablets are seen on x-ray film following emesis and/or lavage, perform whole bowel irrigation by administering bowel preparation solution (e.g., CoLyte or GoLYTELY), 500 ml/hr in children (2 L/hr in adults) by gastric tube until rectal effluent is the color of the irrigation solution. Be prepared for large volume stool.

Deferoxamine challenge can be given while awaiting laboratory results. First obtain a baseline urine sample. Then the challenge dose is 15 mg/kg/hr IV for 2 hours. Then obtain a posttreatment urine sample; a pink-orange (vin rosé) color indicates iron complex and a significant ingestion, but urine color change may not be a reliable guide to toxicity.

Patients with serum iron >350 μg/dl, severe symptoms, or ingestion >40 mg/kg should receive chelation therapy with deferoxamine.

Deferoxamine dosage is 15 mg/kg/hr IV by a constant infusion not to exceed a daily dose of 6 g. (Higher rates have been given for massive ingestions, but these may result in greater hypotension or anaphylactic-like reactions). The duration of therapy is controversial. For patients who display a vin rosé color change in the urine, it is recommended that deferoxamine be continued for 24 hours after the disappearance of the vin rosé color. Other authors recommend that deferoxamine be continued until the serum iron concentration is less than 100 μg/dl.

TABLE 16-11.   Lead Poisoning and Screening

Signs and Symptoms
Acute Ingestion
Acute ingestion of several grams can result in abdominal pain, hemolytic anemia, and hepatitis.
Chronic Poisoning
Anorexia, weight loss, irritability, fatigue, headache, insomnia, myalgias, hypertension, and anemia. Low-level exposure in children may result in impaired behavioral development and decreased intelligence. Severe cases may signal impending encephalopathy and include ataxia, persistent vomiting, irritability, weakness, paralysis, severe anemia or frank papilledema, seizures, and coma.

Screening and Diagnosis
The new CDC guidelines recommend that all children between the ages of 6 months and 6 years be screened for lead. Ideally, screening should occur between 6 and 72 months of age for all children. Low-risk patients should be screened at 12 months and again at 24 months. High-risk patients or those with possible exposure should be screened immediately. Children 6-16 years of age with a history suggestive of lead exposure or with learning disabilities should be screened.
To Determine High Risk Ask the Following Questions:
1. Does the child live in or regularly visit a house with peeling or chipping paint built before 1978, including day care or relatives' home?
2. Does the child live in or regularly visit a house built before 1978 with planned or ongoing renovation or remodeling?
3. Does the child have a sibling, housemate, or playmate with confirmed lead poisoning?
4. Does the child live with an adult whose job or hobby involves exposure to lead?
5. Does the child live near an active lead smelter, battery recycling plant, or other industry likely to release lead?

Modified from: Centers for Disease Control: *Preventing lead poisoning in young children;* 1991. DHHS publication no. 5:37-304; Illinois Department of Public Health: *Guidelines for the detection and management of lead poisoning for physicians and health care providers,* April 1992.

TABLE 16-11.—LEAD POISONING AND SCREENING—cont'd

If Blood Lead (Venous Sample) Is:

<9 μg/dl—child is Class I, monitor at well child visits.

10-14 μg/dl—child is Class IIA, rescreen in 6 months and then periodically as indicated. If level has not increased, then monitor at well child visits. Many children in this range should trigger community-wide lead poisoning prevention activities.

15-19 μg/dl—child is Class IIB and should receive nutritional and educational interventions and be rescreened every 3 months until lead is below 15 μg/dl.

20-44 μg/dl—child is Class III and requires medical evaluation and may need pharmacological intervention. Environmental evaluation and remediation should take place.

45-69 μg/dl—child is Class IV and requires medical evaluation, including chelation therapy and environmental interventions.

≥70 μg/dl—child is Class V, which is a medical emergency. Medical and environmental management must begin immediately.

Lead poisoning is a reportable disease, and cases should be reported to the local department of public health.

Erythrocyte protoporphyrin (EP) was previously used for diagnostic purposes, but it is insensitive for lead levels below 30 μg/dl, and it lags behind rising lead levels. However, EP levels and concurrent blood lead determinations are useful for monitoring postchelation therapy.

Other Diagnostic Tests

If blood lead is 25-44 μg/dl, the CaEDTA provocation test will determine whether there will be a response to chelation therapy (do not use if blood lead is >44 μg/dl).

1. Administer 10 ml/kg of $D_5$1/4NS bolus over 20 minutes.
2. Collect all urine or use adhesive urine bag.
3. Give CaEDTA 25 mg/kg IV infusion in 150 ml $D_5$1/4NS over 30-45 minutes.
4. Continue infusion of $D_5$1/4NS at 1.5 times hourly maintenance rate after EDTA infusion is complete.

Continued.

TABLE 16-11.—LEAD POISONING AND SCREENING—cont'd

5. Collect all urine when EDTA is started for 8 hours in lead-free container.
6. Test result is the ratio of lead excretion (μg) divided by EDTA dose (in mg). A ratio of $\geq$0.6 is positive and suggests benefits from further doses of EDTA (see below).
7. If ratio is <0.6, consider repeat provocation test after iron supplementation (if iron is deficient). If ratio is <0.6 in the face of adequate iron stores, consider alternative therapies.

Iron deficiency test: Iron deficiency can exacerbate lead poisoning. Patients with blood lead values over 20 μg/dl should also be evaluated for iron deficiency. Ferritin is the most sensitive indicator of iron status, but serum iron and TIBC can be used with discretion. Hgb, HCT, and reticulocyte count are not sensitive, and EP is not specific enough to diagnose iron deficiency.

Other tests: Flat plate of abdomen, long bone x-ray examination, RBC microscopic examination for basophilic stippling are not sensitive for diagnosis or management and should not be used for routine workup. Abdominal x-ray film can be helpful when there is evidence of acute ingestion.

Therapy

Blood Lead 25-44 μg/dl (Class III)

Monitor blood lead levels and screen for iron deficiency.

Perform CaEDTA provocation test (above); if ratio is $\geq$0.6, give CaEDTA 1000 mg/m^2/day for 5 days IV over 1 hour or IM mixed with procaine.

If provocation ratio is <0.6, give no treatment but monitor blood lead, and perform CaEDTA provocation test periodically.

Blood Lead 45-69 μg/dl (Class IV)

Monitor blood lead levels and screen for iron deficiency.

Give succimer 10 mg/kg or 350 mg/m^2 orally every 8 hours for 5 days, then reduce dose to every 12 hours for 14 days. Monitor liver function studies. Succimer is preferred unless there is a problem with compliance (emits a rotten egg, sulfur odor, and patient may not comply). If compliance is a problem, give CaEDTA.

TABLE 16-11.—LEAD POISONING AND SCREENING—cont'd

Or

CaEDTA 1000 mg/m^2/day for 5 days, preferably by continuous infusion or divided doses through a heparin lock. Additional cycles may be needed, depending on lead levels, but there should be 2 weeks between cycles, unless more prompt treatment is indicated.

Blood Lead >70 μg/dl (Class IV) or Symptoms Other than Encephalopathy at Lower Blood Levels

Monitor blood lead levels, and screen for iron deficiency.

Give BAL (British antilewisite, or dimercaprol) 300 mg/m^2/day (start with 50 mg/m^2 IM every 4 hours); then after 4 hours, do the following:

Start CaEDTA 1000 mg/m^2/day for 5 days preferably by continuous infusion or divided doses through a heparin lock.

BAL may be discontinued after 3 days if blood lead is <50 μg/dl.

Interrupt therapy for 2 days.

Treat for 5 additional days with BAL and CaEDTA if blood lead remains high.

Other cycles may be necessary, depending on blood lead rebound from bone stores or other sources.

Blood Lead >70 μg/dl (Class IV) with Acute Encephalopathy

Monitor blood lead levels, and screen for iron deficiency.

Give BAL (British antilewisite, or dimercaprol) 450 mg/m^2/day (start with 75 mg/m^2 IM every 4 hours); then after 4 hours do the following:

Start CaEDTA 1500 mg/m^2/day for 5 days preferably by continuous infusion or divided doses through a heparin lock.

Interrupt therapy for 2 days.

Treat for 5 additional days with BAL and CaEDTA if blood lead remains high.

Other cycles may be necessary, depending on blood lead rebound from bone stores or other sources.

TABLE 16-12.—POISONING WITH OPIATES (NARCOTICS) AND THEIR ANALOGUES

Signs and Symptoms
Lethargy, respiratory depression, apnea, constricted pupils (dilated with anoxia), flaccid musculature, slow respirations, cyanosis, hypotension, shock, and seizures

Therapy
Prehospital

If ipecac can be administered at the scene within a few minutes of exposure, it should be given. However, use caution since progressive lethargy and coma can develop.

Give activated charcoal if available.

In Emergency Department

Maintain airway and intubate and ventilate if necessary. Treat coma, seizures, hypotension, or pulmonary edema if they occur.

Immediately give naloxone (Narcan) to any patient with depressed mental status of unknown cause. Narcan dose is 0.4-2 mg IV. Repeat dose every 2-3 minutes if no response to a total dose of 10-20 mg if opiate overdose is strongly suspected. Narcan has a short duration so once improvement has occurred, the dose may need to be administered every 30-60 minutes for opiates with long durations of action.

For large ingestions or long-acting opiates, consider a Narcan infusion. Mix Narcan in normal saline or D_5W and infuse at 0.4-0.8 mg/hr titrated to effect. Continue infusion for 24-48 hours, but attempt to wean the dose every 12 hours while monitoring the patient's vital signs and respiratory rate.

Give activated charcoal and cathartics every 3-4 hours until charcoal appears in the stool. Lavage is not necessary if charcoal can be given promptly.

Modified from Olson KR: *Poisoning and drug overdose,* Norwalk, Conn., 1994, Appleton & Lange, pp. 238-240.

TABLE 16-13.—Poisoning with Tricyclic Antidepressants (TCAs)

Products
Amitriptyline (Elavil), nortriptyline (Pamelor), imipramine (Tofranil), doxepin (Sinequan), trimipramine (Surmontil), amoxapine (Asendin), desipramine (Norpramin), protriptyline (Vivactil), clomipramine (Anafranil), maprotiline (Ludiomil)

Signs and Symptoms
Lethal dose is generally considered to be 1000 mg in an adult and doses of 10-20 mg/kg are considered life-threatening. Serum levels are not reliable in predicting severity.

Hypotension, shock, arrhythmias, tachycardia, AV block, mydriasis, sedation, coma, seizures, irritability, restlessness, delirium, urinary retention, decreased bowel sounds, and fever

QRS prolongation to 0.1 seconds or longer suggests serious toxicity (except with amoxapine, which causes seizures and coma without changing the QRS). Hypotension is independent of QRS prolongation, and hypotension may predict arrhythmias and pulmonary edema.

Therapy
Prehospital
Do not induce emesis because of the potential for rapid development of seizures.
Administer activated charcoal if available.
In Emergency Department
Do not induce emesis because of the potential for rapid development of seizures.
Maintain airway and assist ventilation; be prepared for rapid development of respiratory arrest.
If patient has CNS depression, give Narcan, dextrose, and thiamine.
Lavage with large-bore tube (36-40 F). Give repeated doses of charcoal for intestinal dialysis (see Table 16-2) and cathartics.
Monitor electrolytes, glucose, BUN, creatinine, CPK, ABGs, ECG, and chest x-ray films.
Acidosis increases the toxicity of TCAs. Alkalinization with either hypertonic sodium bicarbonate (1-2 mEq/kg IV) and/or hyperventilation should be given to reverse hypotension, ventricular arrhythmias, widened QRS (>0.1 seconds), ventricular arrhythmias or acidosis. The pH should be kept between 7.45 and 7.55.
Hypotension should be treated with hypertonic sodium bicarbonate, fluids, and, if necessary, vasopressors such as norepinephrine or phenylephrine. If inotrope is needed, dobutamine is preferred.
Seizures must be treated aggressively because they can increase free TCA concentrations and increase toxicity. Treat acute seizures with IV diazepam 0.1 mg/kg per dose, and switch to IV phenytoin (15 mg/kg IV over 30 minutes) for long-term control.

Modified from: Frommer DA, et al: *JAMA* 257:521, 1987; Hoffman JR, et al: *Am J Emerg Med* 11:336, 1993; Crome P: *Med Toxicol* 1:261, 1986.

Continued.

TABLE 16-13.—POISONING WITH TRICYCLIC ANTIDEPRESSANTS (TCAs)—cont'd

Cardiotoxicity should be treated with hypertonic sodium bicarbonate and/or hyperventilation, which can reverse widened QRS, hypotension, and arrhythmias. Arrhythmias should initially be treated with bicarbonate and lidocaine, and the patient can be switched to phenytoin (15 mg/kg IV over 30 minutes) for long-term control. β-blockers can cause cardiodepression and should be used with caution.

Avoid the use of physostigmine, which may lead to bradycardia, seizures, and asystole. It should only be used cautiously for frank and severe anticholinergic psychosis.

If the patient is asymptomatic, monitor at least 6-12 hours because of possible delayed absorption and toxicity. The patient can then be discharged for psychiatric evaluation.

If isolated tachycardia resolves with time or volume repletion and no further toxic signs manifest, the patient can be discharged for psychiatric evaluation.

If tachycardia does not resolve, or other symptoms develop, the patient should be admitted to the ICU. Do not discharge the patient unless she or he is asymptomatic and without arrhythmias for at least 24 hours.

TABLE 16-14.—CARBON MONOXIDE POISONING

Signs, Symptoms, and Laboratory Tests

Carboxyhemoglobin (COHb)

Symptoms	*Signs*
Loss of consciousness	Neurological deficits
Headache	Note: "cherry red" coloration is rare
Lethargy	*Lab tests*
Seizures	Elevated blood COHb level
Nausea/vomiting	Metabolic acidosis
Dizziness	Abnormal drug screen if suicide attempt
Confusion	Ischemic changes or dysrhythmia on EKG
Visual disturbance	
Weakness	
Dyspnea	
Chest pain	

Complications

Arrhythmias, pulmonary edema, myoglobinuria and renal failure, seizures, cerebral edema, visual defects, or temporary blindness

Late Complications

Personality changes, decreased mentation, visual impairment, agnosia, and movement disorders

Therapy

Immediately remove the patient from the source of carbon monoxide.

Maintain airway and assist ventilation.

Administer 100% oxygen until COHb levels are <5%-10%. (CO half-life at room air is 5 hours, and this drops to 90 minutes with 100% oxygen, and with hyperbaric oxygen it is <30 minutes).

Consider transfer for hyperbaric oxygen therapy in cases of severe carbon monoxide poisoning, as manifest by:

1. Blood carboxyhemoglobin (COHb) level ≥ 25%, or
2. Anginal pain or ischemia on electrocardiogram, or
3. Loss of consciousness (including transient), or
4. Neurological impairment

    Note: These criteria are independent. Consider hyperbaric oxygen treatment if any one is present. Age or pregnancy is not a contraindication to hyperbaric treatment.

Modified from Norkool DM, Kirkpatrick JN: *Ann Emerg Med* 14:1168, 1985; Zimmerman SS, Truxal B: *Pediatrics* 68:215, 1981.

TABLE 16-15.—THEOPHYLLINE AND AMINOPHYLLINE TOXICITY AND POISONING

Products
Aerolate, Slo-bid, Slo-Phyllin, Theolair, Quibron, Elixophyllin, and Theo-Dur

Signs and Symptoms
Chronic Toxicity
Levels > 20-25 mg/L: Nausea, vomiting, diarrhea, insomnia, tremor, tachycardia, irritability, headache (seizures and death rarely occur at 20-25 mg/L)
Levels > 30-35 mg/L: Tachycardia, arrhythmias, seizures, hypotension, cardiac arrest
Acute Toxicity
Acute single dose of 16-20 mg/kg can produce serum levels of 30-40 mg/L and 50 mg/kg can produce serum levels over 100 mg/L.

Therapy
Prehospital
If the patient is not already vomiting, administer syrup of ipecac if it can be given within 30 minutes of poison ingestion. Administer activated charcoal if it is available.
In Emergency Department
Support cardiac and respiratory status, establish airway, start IV, and administer oxygen.
Obtain serial theophylline levels but begin therapy before the results are known.
Insert large gastric tube (36-40 F) and lavage. Give repeat doses of charcoal for intestinal dialysis for any patient with serum levels <100 mg/L (see Table 16-2). This method should be performed even in the absence of symptoms.
Give cathartics to allow evacuation of the charcoal.
Administer whole bowel irrigation (see Table 16-2).
If seizures occur, treat initially with IV diazepam. For long-term treatment, phenobarbital should be used. Avoid phenytoin.
If serious ventricular arrhythmias occur, treat with lidocaine or procainamide.
For tachycardia, treat with low-dose propranolol or esmolol. For patients with asthma, verapamil may slow the ventricular rate for atrial arrhythmias.
For serious, life-threatening toxicity, charcoal hemoperfusion will rapidly remove theophylline. Hemoperfusion is indicated if the patient has cardiorespiratory failure, hepatic dysfunction, recurrent seizures or serum level > 100 mg/L (some clinicians use if serum levels > 60 mg/L). Hemodialysis is not as effective as hemoperfusion, but it can be used.

Modified from Olson KR: *Poisoning and drug overdose,* Norwalk, Conn., 1994, Appleton & Lange, pp. 295-297; Park GD, et al: *Arch Intern Med* 146:969, 1986; Albert S: *Pediatr Clin North Am* 34:61, 1987; Shannon M: *Ann Intern Med* 119:1161, 1993.

TABLE 16-16.—Poisoning with Ethylene Glycol

Sources
Auto radiator antifreeze or coolant and brake fluid

Lethal Dose
The lethal oral dose of 100% (e.g., antifreeze) is approximately 1.5 mL/kg or 100 ml for an adult.

Signs and Symptoms
Early (4-5 Hours):
Nausea, vomiting, ataxia, nystagmus, hypothermia, and fever
Late (4-12 Hours):
Calcium oxalate crystals in urine, renal failure, anion gap acidosis, hyperventilation, seizures, coma, cardiac conduction disturbances and arrhythmias, pulmonary edema, and cerebral edema.

Therapy
Prehospital:
Treat with syrup of ipecac if it can be given within a few minutes of the ingestion.
In the Emergency Department:
Maintain airway; provide cardiopulmonary support.
Perform gastric lavage quickly. Do not give activated charcoal unless other poisons are suspected, since it does not adsorb ethylene glycol.
Administer ethanol (which has a higher affinity for alcohol dehydrogenase). Give IV or PO loading dose of 7.5-10 ml/kg of a 10% ethanol in D_5W (or 1 ml/kg of 95% ethanol in fruit juice), then a maintenance dose of 1-2 ml/kg/hr IV of a 10% ethanol in D_5W or 0.15 ml/kg/hr of 95% ethanol in fruit juice PO. During hemodialysis, the infusion rate should be increased to 2-3.5 ml/kg/hr IV of a 10% ethanol solution.
Continuously monitor blood ethanol levels. The desired serum concentration is 100 mg/dl (20 mmol/L).
Administer pyridoxine 100 mg IV or IM, folate 50 mg IV or IM, and thiamine 100 mg IM, which may increase the rate of metabolism of ethylene glycol.
Hemodialysis is indicated along with ethanol therapy for serum ethylene glycol > 50 mg/dl, with renal failure or with suspected ethylene glycol poisoning with an osmolar gap > 10 mOsm/L.

Modified from Olson KR: *Poisoning and drug overdose,* Norwalk, Conn., 1994, Appleton & Lange, pp. 162-163; Litovitz T: *Pediatr Clin North Am* 33:311, 1986.

TABLE 16-17.—POISONING WITH METHANOL

Sources
Carburetor fluid, gas antifreeze, model engine fuel, windshield washer fluid, and bootleg whiskey.

Lethal Dose
The fatal dose is as low as 30 ml of 100% methanol but death has occurred with 15 ml of 40%. Serum methanol levels > 20 mg/dl are toxic and levels > 40 mg/dl are very serious.

Signs and Symptoms
Early
Intoxication as with ethanol, nausea, vomiting, slurred speech, and CNS depression
Late (Up to 30 Hours)
Anion gap, metabolic acidosis, blurred or cloudy vision, yellow spots, central scotoma, reversible or irreversible blindness, seizures, coma, and death

Therapy
Prehospital
Treat with syrup of ipecac if it can be given within a few minutes of the ingestion.
In the Emergency Department
Maintain airway; provide cardiopulmonary support.
Perform gastric lavage quickly. Do not give activated charcoal unless other poisons are suspected, since it does not adsorb methanol.
Metabolic acidosis should be treated with IV sodium bicarbonate.
Administer ethanol (which has a higher affinity for alcohol dehydrogenase). Give IV or PO loading dose of 7.5-10 ml/kg of a 10% ethanol in D_5W (or 1 ml/kg of 95% ethanol in fruit juice), then a maintenance dose of 1-2 ml/kg/hr IV of a 10% ethanol in D_5W or 0.15 ml/kg/hr of 95% ethanol in fruit juice PO. During hemodialysis, the infusion rate should be increased to 2-3.5 ml/kg/hr IV of a 10% ethanol solution.
Continuously monitor blood ethanol levels. The desired serum concentration is 100 mg/dl (20 mmol/L).
Administer folate 50 mg IV or IM, which may increase the rate of metabolism of methanol.
Hemodialysis is indicated along with ethanol therapy for serum methanol > 40 mg/dl, metabolic acidosis, or with suspected methanol poisoning with an osmolar gap > 10 mOsm/L.

Modified from Olson KR: *Poisoning and drug overdose,* Norwalk, Conn., 1994, Appleton & Lange, pp. 215-217; Litovitz T: *Pediatr Clin North Am* 33:311, 1986.

17 *Blood Disorders and Cancer*

Charles E. Driscoll

HEMOSTASIS

TABLE 17-1.—Pathological Bleeding

Pathological bleeding may be classified as a disorder of primary hemostasis (vascular fragility or platelet function [cellular]) or secondary hemostasis (plasma coagulation factors).
Localize the defect by history and physical examination as follows:

History	Vascular	Cellular	Plasma
Bleeding from multiple sites		+	+
Hemarthrosis; large ecchymoses			+
Petechiae, purpura, mucosal bleeding	+	+	
Bleeding after trauma		Immediate	Delayed
Congenital disorders; prior bleeding episodes			+

Order selective screening tests to complete the diagnosis.
    Primary hemostasis assessment
        Platelet count, bleeding time, bone marrow examination, von Willebrand's factor antigen
    Secondary hemostasis assessment
        Prothrombin time (PT), partial thromboplastin time (PTT), fibrinogen, coagulation factor assays

595

TABLE 17-2.—PRESUMPTIVE DIAGNOSIS OF COMMON BLEEDING DISORDERS BASED ON ROUTINE SCREENING TESTS

PRESUMPTIVE PROBLEM	PLATELET COUNT	BLEEDING TIME	PROTHROMBIN TIME (PT)	PARTIAL THROMBOPLASTIN TIME (PTT)	THROMBIN TIME (TT)	MISCELLANEOUS
Thrombocytopenia	↓	N,↑	N	N	N	
Platelet function defect or vascular defect	N	↑	N	N	N	
Von Willebrand's disease	N	↑	N	↑	N	$\downarrow VIII_{cr}$, $\downarrow VIII_{ag}$, $\downarrow VIII_{vWF}$
Extrinsic pathway defect (VII)	N	N	↑	N	N	
Intrinsic pathway defect (VIII, IX, XI, XII, prekallikrein, high-molecular-weight kininogen, inhibitor)	N	N	N	↑	N	
Common pathway or multiple pathway defects, excluding fibrinogen	N	N	↑	↑	N	
Fibrinogen deficiency or dysfunction, vitamin K deficiency, liver disease, primary fibrinolysis	N	N	↑	↑	↑	High levels of fibrin(ogen) degradation products (FDP)
Disseminated intravascular coagulation	↓	N,↑	↑	↑	↑	High levels of FDP
Factor XIII deficiency	N	N	N	N	N	Positive clot solubility

Modified from Blacklow RS, ed: *MacBryde's signs and symptoms: applied pathologic physiology and clinical interpretation*, ed 6, Philadelphia, 1983, JB Lippincott, p. 551.
N, Normal; ↓, decreased; ↑, increased.

TABLE 17-3.—HYPERCOAGULABLE STATES

Suspect when unusual, recurrent thromboses or thromboembolism in a young person with no predisposing factors (e.g., surgery).

Hereditary Disorders
 Protein C Deficiency (Vitamin K-Dependent Clot Inhibitor)
Heterozygous autosomal dominant transmission
Prevalence of 1 in 300 individuals
Dx by functional and immunoassay of Protein C
Causes disease in newborns, skin necrosis, purpura
Responsible for up to 10% of thromboses in <45 years of age
 Protein S Deficiency (Vitamin K-Dependent Clot Inhibitor)
Codominant autosomal transmission
Prevalence of 1 in 15,000 individuals
Dx by functional and immunoassay of Protein S
Responsible for 5%-8% of thromboses in patients <45 years of age
Often starts in the early teen years
 Antithrombin III (Inhibits Final Coagulation Cascade)
Autosomal dominant transmission
Measure antithrombin III levels, Dx if <60% of normal
Responsible for 2%-4% of thromboses in patients <45 years of age
Often starts in early childhood
 Dysfibrinogenemia
Can be inherited or spontaneous mutation
A prolonged thrombin time suggests this disorder

Acquired Disorders
 IgG Antiphospholipid Antibodies
Responsible for spontaneous abortion, arterial and venous thrombi
Lupus anticoagulant present
A PTT that is prolonged and does not correct with a 1:1 mix suggests the dx
 Malignancy
Increased platelet adhesion
Procoagulant factors involved
 Other Conditions
Surgery, trauma, estrogens, pregnancy, renal disease, sepsis, varicose veins, CHF, myeloproliferative disorder

---

TABLE 17-4.—CHARACTERISTICS OF COAGULATION FACTORS

FACTOR	DESCRIPTIVE NAME	SOURCE	APPROXIMATE HALF-LIFE (hr)	FUNCTION
I	Fibrinogen	Liver	120	Substrate for fibrin clot (CP)
II	Prothrombin	Liver VKD	60	Serine protease (CP)
V	Proaccelerin, labile factor	Liver	12-36	Cofactor (CP)
VII	Serum prothrombin conversion accelerator, proconvertin	Liver VKD	6	? Serine protease (EP)
VIII	Antihemophilic factor or globin	Endothelial cells and ? elsewhere	12	Cofactor (IP)
IX	Plasma thromboplastin component, Christmas factor	Liver VKD	24	Serine protease (IP)
X	Stuart-Prower factor	Liver VKD	36	Serine protease (CP)
XI	Plasma thromboplastin antecedent	? Liver	40-84	Serine protease (IP)
XII	Hageman factor	? Liver	50	Serine protease, contact activation (IP)
XIII	Fibrin stabilizing factor	? Liver	96-180	Transglutaminase (CP)
Prekallikrein	Fletcher factor	? Liver	?	Serine protease, contact activation (IP)
High-molecular-weight kininogen	Fitzgerald factor Flaujeac or Williams factor	? Liver	?	Cofactor, contact activation (IP)

From Blacklow RS, ed: *MacBryde's signs and symptoms: applied pathologic physiology and clinical interpretation*, ed 6, Philadelphia, 1983, JB Lippincott, p. 539.
VKD, Vitamin K-dependent; *CP*, common pathway; *EP*, extrinsic pathway; *IP*, intrinsic pathway.

DISSEMINATED INTRAVASCULAR COAGULOPATHY

Disseminated intravascular coagulation (DIC), or consumption coagulopathy, may need to be differentiated from other coagulation disorders (Table 17-5). Causes of DIC include septic shock, severe RDS, malignancies, rickettsial diseases, head trauma, obstetrical hemorrhage, and postoperative state (especially after lung or prostate surgery).

TABLE 17-5.—COMPARISON OF DIC AND ENTITIES CONFUSED WITH DIC

ASPECT	DIC	LIVER DISEASE	VITAMIN K LOW	DILUTIONAL	LUPUS ANTICOAGULANT	SEPSIS WITHOUT SHOCK
PTT	P	P	P	P	P	P
PT	P	P	P	P	N	P
FIB	R	R	N	R	N	E
II	R	R	R	R	N	R
V	R	R	N	R	N	E
VIII	R	N-E	N	R	N	E
PLT	R	N-R	N	R	N	N-R
FSPs	+	+/−	0	0	0	0
SOL FIB	+	0	0	0	0	0
TT	P	Only if chronic	N		P	N	P
Test to confirm	FSPs	II, VII IX, X	II, VII IX, X		PTT Will not correct with protamine	Blood culture

PTT, Partial thromboplastin time; *PT*, prothrombin time; *II, V, VII, VIII, IX, X*, clotting factors; *PLT*, platelets; *FSPs*, fibrinolytic split products; *SOL FIB*, soluble fibrin; *TT*, thrombin time; *P*, prolonged; *R*, reduced; *N*, normal; +, present; *0*, absent; *E*, elevated.

RED AND WHITE BLOOD CELLS

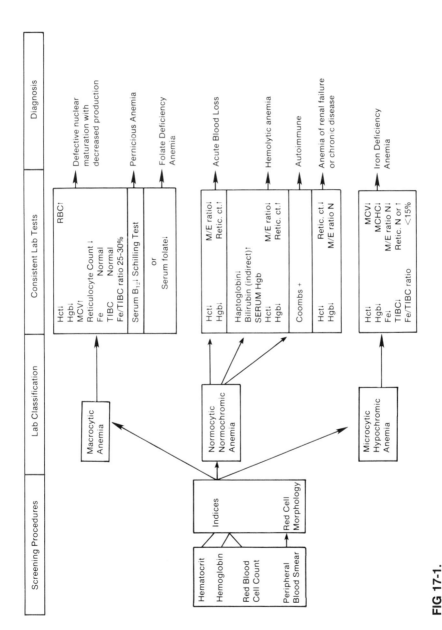

FIG 17-1.

Laboratory diagnosis of anemia. (From Bolinger AM, Korman NR: Anemias. In Young LY, Koda-Kimble MA, eds: *Applied therapeutics: the clinical use of drugs*, ed. 4, Vancouver, Wash, 1988, Applied Therapeutics, p. 1053.)

Reticulocyte Response

TABLE 17-6.—Diagnostic Considerations Based on Erythrokinetic Measurements, RBC Size, and RBC Heterogeneity in Anemia

MCV fl	RDW (%)	HYPOPROLIFERATIVE Reticulocyte Response RPI less than 2, or Absolute Reticulocytes* less than 100,000	INEFFECTIVE Reticulocyte Response	PROLIFERATIVE Reticulocyte Response RPI greater than 2, or Absolute Reticulocytes* greater than 100,000
<85	<15.5	Chronic disease		Nonanemic thalassemia
	>13.5	Iron deficiency	Sideroblastic anemia	Anemic thalassemia Hb H disease Hb S-thalassemia
75 to 105	<15.5	Acute blood loss Aplastic anemia Chronic disease Hypothyroidism		Hereditary RBC membrane disorder Nonanemic hemoglobinopathy or enzymopathy Hemolytic anemia (especially non-immune) Acute blood loss
	>13.5	Myelodysplasia Myeloproliferative disorder	Early or mixed nutritional deficiency Myelodysplasia Sideroblastic anemia	Anemic hemoglobinopathy or enzymopathy Hemolytic anemia (especially immune)
>95	<15.5	Aplastic anemia Hypothyroidism Myelodysplasia	Myelodysplasia Cobalamin or folate deficiency Myelodysplasia	Hb SS
	>13.5	Myeloproliferative disorder	Myeloproliferative disorder Sideroblastic anemia	Hemolytic anemia (especially immune)

From Maksem JA: The Nature of Anemias, *Mercy Medicine and Surgery* 3:6, 1992.

RPI, Reticulocyte production index $= \dfrac{\text{corrected reticulocyte count}}{\text{reticulocyte maturation index}}$

(Corrected reticulocyte count $= \dfrac{\text{Patient's hematocrit}}{\text{Normal hematocrit}} \times$ Reticulocyte count)

*Absolute reticulocyte count = Raw reticulocyte %/100 × RBC

TABLE 17-7.—Differential Diagnosis of the Hypochromic-Microcytic States

BLOOD PARAMETER	DEFICIENCY	TRANSFERRIN DEFECT	DEFECT IN IRON UTILIZATION	DEFECT IN IRON REUTILIZATION
Peripheral Blood				
Microcytosis *(M)* versus hypochromia *(H)*	M > H	M > H	M > H	M < H
Polychromatophilic targeted cells	Absent	Absent	Present	Absent
Stippled red cells	Absent	Absent	Present	Absent
RDW	Increased	Increased	Increased	Normal
Serum Iron				
Iron-binding capacity	↓:↑	↓:↓	↑:Normal	↓:↓
Percent saturation of transferrin	<10%	0	>50%	>10%
Serum Ferritin (normal 30-300 ng/ml)	<12	(No data available)	>400	30-400
Bone Marrow				
Erythrocyte-granulocyte ratio (normal 1:3 to 1:5)	1:1-1:2	1:1-1:2	1:1-5:1	1:1-1:2
Marrow iron	Absent	Present	Increased	Present
Ringed sideroblasts	Absent	Absent	Present	Absent

From Berkow R, Fletcher AJ, eds: Hematology and oncology. In *The Merck manual of diagnosis and therapy,* ed 16, Rahway, NJ, 1992, Merck & Co., p. 1149; modified from Frenkel EP: *Houston Med* June, vol 11, 1976.
RDW, Red blood cell volume distribution width expressing the degree of anisocytosis (i.e., variation in cell size).

TABLE 17-8.—Characteristics of the Thalassemias

CATEGORY	ANEMIA	MCV	PERCENT Hb A$_2$	PERCENT Hb F
β Thalassemia				
Heterozygous	Mild	↓	↑	Variable
Homozygous	Severe	↓	Variable	↑ up to 90%
βδ Thalassemia				
Heterozygous	Mild	↓	N or ↓	>5%
Homozygous	Moderate-severe	↓	Absent	100%
α Thalassemia				
Single gene defect	None	N-↓	N	N
Double gene defect	Mild	↓	N-↓	<5%
Triple gene defect	Moderate	↓	N-↓ (Hb H or Bart's Hb present)	Variable

From Berkow R, Fletcher AJ, eds: Hematology and oncology. In *The Merck manual,* ed 15, Rahway, NJ, 1987, Merck & Co, p. 1123.

TABLE 17-9.—Normal Microhematocrit Values

AGE	AVERAGE NORMAL	MINIMAL NORMAL
Children of Both Sexes		
At birth	56.6	51.0
First day	56.1	50.5
End of first week	52.7	47.5
End of second week	49.6	44.7
End of third week	46.6	42.0
End of fourth week	44.6	40.0
End of second month	38.9	35.1
End of fourth month	36.5	32.9
End of sixth month	36.2	32.6
End of eighth month	35.8	32.3
End of tenth month	35.5	32.0
End of first year	35.2	31.7
End of second year	35.5	32.0
End of fourth year	37.1	33.4
End of sixth year	37.9	34.2
End of eighth year	38.9	35.1
End of twelfth year	39.6	35.7
Men		
End of fourteenth year	44	39.6
End of eighteenth year	47	42.3
18-50 years	47	42.3
50-60 years	45	40.5
60-70 years	43	38.7
70-80 years	40	36.0
Nonpregnant Women		
14-50 years	42	36
50-80 years	40	36
Pregnant Women		
End of fourth month	42	30
End of fifth month	40	30
End of sixth month	37	30
End of seventh month	37	30
End of eighth month	39	30
End of ninth month	40	30

Courtesy Dr. M. Strumia.

TABLE 17-10.—Normal Leukocyte Count in Peripheral Blood

	LEUKOCYTE COUNT (CELLS/mm³)	
AGE	AVERAGE	95% RANGE*
Birth	18,100	9000-30,000
12 hours	22,800	13,000-38,000
24 hours	18,900	9400-34,000
1 week	12,200	5000-21,000
2 weeks	11,400	5000-20,000
4 weeks	10,800	5000-19,500
2 months	11,000	5500-18,000
4 months	11,500	6000-17,500
6 months	11,900	6000-17,500
8 months	12,200	6000-17,500
10 months	12,000	6000-17,500
12 months	11,400	6000-17,500
2 years	10,600	6000-17,000
4 years	9100	5500-15,500
6 years	8500	5000-14,500
8 years	8300	4500-13,500
10 years	8100	4500-13,500
12 years	8000	4500-13,500
14 years	7900	4500-13,000
16 years	7800	4500-13,000
18 years	7700	4500-12,500
20 years	7500	4500-11,500
21 years	7400	4500-11,000

Modified from Albritton EC: *Standard values in blood,* Philadelphia, 1952, WB Saunders, pp. 50-51.
*Average value ± 2 SD.

TABLE 17-11.—NORMAL LEUKOCYTE DIFFERENTIAL COUNT IN PERIPHERAL BLOOD*

AGE	SEGMENTED NEUTROPHILS		BAND NEUTROPHILS		EOSINOPHILS		BASOPHILS		LYMPHOCYTES		MONOCYTES	
	%	No./mm³	%	No./mm³	%	No./mm³	%	No./mm³	%	No./mm³	%	No./mm³
At birth	52	9400	9.1	1,650	2.2	400	0.6	100	31 ± 5	5500	5.8	1050
12 hours	58	13,200	10.2	2,330	2.0	450	0.4	100	24	5500	5.3	1200
24 hours	52	9800	9.2	1,750	2.4	450	0.5	100	31	5800	5.8	1100
1 week	39	4700	6.8	830	4.1	500	0.4	50	41	5000	9.1	1100
2 weeks	34	3900	5.5	630	3.1	350	0.4	50	48	5500	8.8	1000
4 weeks	30	3300	4.5	490	2.8	300	0.5	50	56 + 15	6000	6.5	700
2 months	30	3300	4.4	490	2.7	300	0.5	50	57	6300	5.9	650
4 months	29	3300	3.9	450	2.6	300	0.4	50	59	6800	5.2	600
6 months	28	3300	3.8	450	2.5	300	0.4	50	61	7300	4.8	580
8 months	27	3300	3.3	410	2.5	300	0.4	50	62	7600	4.7	580
10 months	27	3200	3.3	400	2.5	300	0.4	50	63	7500	4.6	550
12 months	28	3200	3.1	350	2.6	300	0.4	50	61	7000	4.8	550
2 years	30	3200	3.0	320	2.6	280	0.5	50	59	6300	5.0	530
4 years	39	3500	3.0	270	2.8	250	0.6	50	50 ± 15	4500	5.0	450
6 years	48	4000	3.0	250	2.7	230	0.6	50	42	3500	4.7	400
8 years	50	4100	3.0	250	2.4	200	0.6	50	39	3300	4.2	350
10 years	51	4200	3.0	240	2.4	200	0.5	40	38 ± 10	3100	4.3	350
12 years	52	4200	3.0	240	2.5	200	0.5	40	38	3000	4.4	350
14 years	53	4200	3.0	240	2.5	200	0.5	40	37	2900	4.7	380
16 years	54	4200	3.0	230	2.6	200	0.5	40	35 ± 10	2800	5.1	400
18 years	54	4200	3.0	230	2.6	200	0.5	40	35	2700	5.2	400
20 years	56	4200	3.0	230	2.7	200	0.5	40	33	2500	5.0	380
21 years	56	4200	3.0	220	2.7	200	0.5	40	34 ± 10	2500	4.0	300

Modified from Albritton EC: *Standard values in blood*, Philadelphia, 1952, WB Saunders, pp. 50-51.
*Average values based on the average normal leukocyte counts in Table 17-10.

IMMUNE FACTORS

T cells (thymus-dependent) and B cells (lymphocytes from bursa of Fabricius) cannot be separated morphologically, but a functional assessment is possible. T cells are screened by a white cell count with differential; B cells are evaluated by means of immunoglobulin assay.

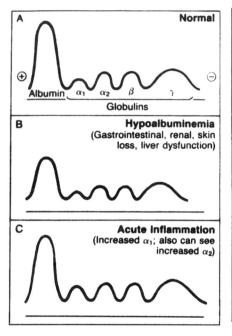
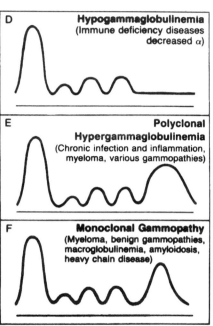

FIG 17-2.

Serum immunoelectrophoretic patterns. (From Goodwin JS: Clinical assessment of the immune system: Which tests? When? In Goodwin JS, ed: *Mediguide to inflammatory diseases,* New York, 1983, Dellacorte, vol. 1, no. 2, p. 2.)

HIV INFECTION

TABLE 17-12.—TESTING AND COUNSELING FOR HIV INFECTION

Acute Retroviral Syndrome
 3 days-3 weeks after exposure
 Mononucleosis-like syndrome
 Fever, skin rash, myalgias, arthralgias, lymphadenopathy, malaise, sore
  throat, headache, photophobia, GI symptoms
 (Neurological symptoms, weight loss, elevated SGOT level in some patients)

Chronic HIV Infection
 PGL* = nodes ≥ 1 cm at ≥ 2 extrainguinal sites persisting > 3 months
 Patients with clinical disease may also have fever, fatigue, diarrhea, weight
  loss (10% of ideal), night sweats
 Declining T-lymphocyte count
 Oral hairy leukoplakia
 Herpes infections
 Enlarged liver and spleen
 Chronic vaginitis
 Dermatological disorders

History Questions
 Prior blood transfusions
 IV drug use
 Sex with men, women, or both
 Number of sexual partners
 Known HIV+ sex partner or partner of high risk
 Oral, anal, or vaginal sex
 Exchanged money or drugs for sex, sex with prostitute

Early Physical Findings
 Severe seborrheic dermatitis
 Candidiasis
 Oral hairy leukoplakia
 Herpes zoster
 Kaposi's sarcoma
 CMV retinitis
 PID
 Cervical dysplasia/cancer
 Lymphadenopathy
 Pneumocystis or TB
 Encephalopathy/neuropathy

Pretest Counseling
 Informed consent obtained; benefits and risks of testing explained
  Benefits
   Reduce risky behaviors
   Diminish anxiety
   Reduce further transmission
   Conception counseling
   Immunomodulation therapy/antiretroviral prophylaxis

Continued.

TABLE 17-12.—Testing and Counseling for HIV Infection—cont'd

Risks
    Psychological trauma
    Social ostracism and discrimination
    Insurance problems
    Preoccupation with and exaggeration of symptoms
Ask why patient wants test
Give estimate of how likely he or she is to be positive based on type of exposure and type of fluid or tissue
Ask how he or she will feel and what will be done if positive
Explain limits of HIV antibody test; false-positives/negatives
Educate regarding safe sex
Testing
    HIV antibodies develop within 3 months of infection for most patients but can remain seronegative for up to 36 months
    Lab abnormalities supporting need for HIV testing
        Low serum cholesterol level, lymphopenia, anemia, thrombocytopenia; high ESR, low LDH, low serum globulin levels, or positive VDRL result
    Two-step testing
        ELISA: Enzyme-linked immunosorbent assay
            Repeat if positive, and if positive second time, then do next step
        Western blot test (WBT): Identification of specific antibody bands

	Negative	False-Positive	True-Positive	False-Negative
ELISA	–	+/ + or –	+/++/+	– Within 3 months of exposure
WBT	Not run	–	+	Not run

Posttest Counseling
    Done in person, never over the phone.
    Assurance of confidentiality
    Educate concerning prognosis, medical and social resources, how to prevent transmission of infection, sexual contact notification, danger signals of infection
    Evaluate and manage emotional response
    Need for clinical monitoring
    Refer to support group
    Minimal laboratory assessment of asymptomatic patients CBC, UA, VDRL, Pap, PPD, hepatitis serology, T-cell subsets (number and percent of CD4 cells; CD4:8 ratio)

*PGL, Persistent generalized lymphadenopathy.

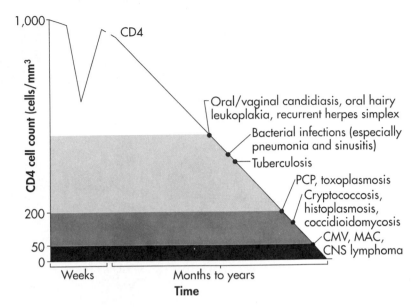

FIG 17-3.
Relationship between CD_4 cell count and HIV-associated diseases. The CD_4 cell count is widely used to reflect the state of the immune system. As the count declines from an average of 1000 cells/mm³ in the asymptomatic stage toward zero in advanced AIDS, the patient becomes vulnerable to certain diseases that afflict only severely immunocompromised hosts. (From Worth LA: Preventing opportunistic infections in patients with AIDS, *Hosp Med* 30:26, 1994.)

TABLE 17-13.—COMMON ANTIRETROVIRAL THERAPY USED FOR PATIENTS INFECTED WITH HIV

DRUG AND HOW SUPPLIED	INDICATIONS	DOSAGE ADULTS/TANNER IV AND V*	DOSAGE INFANTS AND CHILDREN TANNER I AND II*	SELECTED ADVERSE REACTIONS†	PATIENT INSTRUCTIONS
Zidovudine (Retrovir, AZT, ZDV) 100 mg capsules, 50 mg/5ml, 10 mg/ml injection	First-line agent when CD$_4$ count <500 alone or with ddC	100 mg orally every 4 hours (5 doses/day) daily When given with ddC, the dosage is 200 mg every 8 hours daily	180 mg/m^2 orally every 6 hours daily	Anemia, granulocytopenia, nausea, headache, confusion, myositis, anorexia, hepatitis, seizures, nail discoloration	Not a cure. Headache may disappear, watch for signs of anemia (dizziness, weakness)
Didanosine (Videx, ddI) 25-, 50-, 100-, 150-mg tablets, 100, 167, 250, 375 mg powder for oral solution, 2, 4 g pediatric oral solution	Intolerance to ZDV, disease progression on ZDV, or taking ZDV > 8 weeks	<45 kg: 100 mg orally every 12 hours daily >45 kg: 200 mg orally every 12 hours daily	100 mg/m^2 orally every 12 hours daily	Pancreatitis (potentially fatal), peripheral neuropathy, peripheral retinal atrophy (children only), nausea, diarrhea, confusion, seizures	Not a cure. Take on empty stomach. Always chew 2 tablets (one is an antacid buffer) thoroughly and swallow. May be dispersed in water or

					apple juice. Advise patients of signs of pancreatitis or peripheral neuropathy
Zalcitabine (Hivid, ddC) 0.375-0.75-mg tablets, 0.1 mg/ml syrup	Approved only for combination with ZDV	<45 kg: 0.375 mg orally every 8 hours daily >45 kg: 0.75 mg orally every 8 hours daily	0.005-0.01 mg/kg orally every 8 hours daily	Pancreatitis, peripheral neuropathy, aphthous ulcers, esophageal ulcers, stomatitis, cutaneous eruptions, thrombocytopenia	Not a cure. Take each dose with 200 mg ZDV three times daily. Advise patients of signs of pancreatitis or peripheral neuropathy

Modified from *Clinical practice guideline: evaluation and management of early HIV infection:* AHCPR Publication No. 94-0572, 1994. For copy of the guidelines, call 800-342-AIDS.

*Adolescents in Tanner stage I or II should receive the pediatric dosage. Adolescents in Tanner stage IV or V should receive adult doses. Those in Tanner stage III should have dosages individualized based on their rapid growth.

†Only includes a selected list of adverse reactions; consult product labeling for a complete list.

TABLE 17-14.—Common Therapy for Prevention of Pneumocystis Carinii Pneumonia

DRUG AND HOW SUPPLIED	INDICATIONS	DOSAGE ADULTS/TANNER IV AND V*	DOSAGE INFANTS AND CHILDREN TANNER I & II*	SELECTED ADVERSE REACTIONS†	PATIENT INSTRUCTIONS AND COMMENTS
Trimethoprim-Sulfamethoxazole (Bactrim or Septra DS tablet) contains 160 mg TMP and 800 mg SMX, pediatric suspension contains 40 mg TMP and 200 mg SMX per 5 ml	Most commonly used drug for primary (CD$_4$ <200) and secondary prophylaxis; also treatment of acute PCP or other bacterial infections	1 DS tablet orally 3 times per week on alternate days *Or* 1 DS tablet every day	150 mg/m^2 TMP with 750 mg/m^2 SMX; total oral daily dose given 3 times/week; or divided in 2 doses and given on 3 alternate days each week; *Or* divided in 2 doses given 7 days per week	Skin rash, Stevens-Johnson syndrome, fever, drug allergy, arthralgia, toxic epidermal necrolysis, hematological (anemia, neutropenia, thrombocytopenia), nausea, vomiting hepatitis	Take with full glass of water. Adverse reactions are more common than in non-HIV patients. Additive marrow suppression with ZDV
Pentamidine (Nebupent) 300 mg aerosol (vial must be dissolved in 6 ml sterile water and used with Respirgard II nebulizer	Prophylaxis of PCP (injectable form is indicated for acute treatment)	300 mg every 4 weeks; nebulized dose over 30-45 minutes at a flow of 5-9 L/min from 40-50 lb per sq inch air or oxygen source	>5 years—same inhalation dose as for adults	Bronchospasm with cough, metallic taste, pneumothorax, extrapulmonary *P. carinii* infection, increased risk of transmission of *Mycobacterium tuberculosis*	Refrain from smoking before use. Patients with bronchoconstriction may require inhaled dilator. Use only Respirgard II nebulizer. Not to be used in

Drug	Indication	Pediatric dose	Adult dose	Adverse reactions	Comments
Dapsone (DDS) 25-, 100-mg tablets	Alone for PCP prophylaxis. (Used with trimethoprim for treatment)	50–100 mg total daily oral dose divided into two daily doses or administered as single daily dose given 2–7 times per week	1 mg/kg orally as a single daily dose given 7 days per week	Agranulocytosis, aplastic anemia, hemolytic anemia in G6PD deficiency, methemoglobinemia, bullous and exfoliative dermatitis, erythema nodosum, erythema multiforme, peripheral neuropathy; nausea, vomiting, hepatitis	patients with active TB or who are suspected to have TB Take 2 hours before antacid, H$_2$-blocker or ddl. Anemia is dose related and may be aggravated by coadministration of ZDV. Requires an acidic gastric pH for optimal absorption

Modified from *Clinical practice guideline: evaluation and management of early HIV infection:* AHCPR Publication No. 94-0572, 1994. For copy of the guidelines, call 800-342-AIDS.

*Adolescents in Tanner stage I or II should receive the pediatric dosage. Adolescents in Tanner stage IV or V should receive adult doses. Those in Tanner stage III should have dosages individualized based upon their rapid growth.

†Only includes a selected list of adverse reactions. Consult product labeling for a complete list.

TABLE 17-15.—OTHER COMMON THERAPIES USED FOR PATIENTS INFECTED WITH HIV

DRUG AND HOW SUPPLIED	INDICATIONS	DOSAGE	SELECTED ADVERSE REACTIONS	PATIENT INSTRUCTIONS	COMMENTS
Atovaquoné (Mepron) 250-mg tablets	Treatment of mild to moderate PCP in patients intolerant to TMP-SMX	750 mg with food 3 times daily for 21 days	Rash, nausea, vomiting, diarrhea, headache, fever	Take all tablets with food to increase absorption	Absorption reduced with diarrhea and increased with fatty meals (>23 g)
Clotrimazole (Mycelex) 10-mg troches	Treatment of oral candidiasis	1 troche 5 times daily for 14 days	Loss of taste, nausea, vomiting	Allow troches to slowly dissolve in mouth	Not effective for esophageal candidiasis
Ketoconazole (Nizoral) 200-mg tablets	Treatment of oral or esophageal candidiasis or other mucocutaneous fungal infections	200-400 mg once daily for 7-14 days. Children >3 years of age take 3.3-6.6 mg/kg/day as single daily dose	Hepatotoxicity, adrenal insufficiency, impotence, gynecomastia	Take 2 hours before antacid, H$_2$-blockers or ddl. *Do not take* with Seldane or Hismanal	Requires acidic gastric pH for absorption; higher doses may be needed in HIV patients. Drug interaction with Seldane or Hismanal has led to ventricular arrythmias and torsades de pointes. Other drug interactions occur

Drug	Indication	Dose	Side effects	Patient instructions	Comments
Itraconazole (Sporanox) 100-mg capsules	Treatment of histoplasmosis or oral candidiasis	200 mg once daily up to 200 mg twice daily taken with food	Nausea, vomiting, hepatotoxicity	Take 2 hours before antacid, H₂-blockers or ddl. *Do not take* with Seldane or Hismanal	Requires acidic gastric pH for absorption; higher doses may be needed in HIV patients. Drug interaction with Seldane or Hismanal has led to ventricular arrythmias and torsades de pointes. Other drug interactions occur
Fluconazole (Diflucan) 50-, 100-, 200-mg tablets 200 mg/100 ml injection, 400 mg/200 ml injection	Treatment of oral or esophageal candidiasis, Treatment or suppression of *Cryptococcus neoformans* meningitis	Oral candidiasis: 200 mg first day, then 100 mg daily for 14 days. *C. neoformans* meningitis: 400 mg first day, then 200-400 mg daily	Nausea, vomiting, headache, hepatotoxicity	Inform doctor if symptoms not improving	Absorption not affected by gastric pH or food. Resistant strains of Candida have been reported. Meningitis should be treated for 10-12 weeks after negative CSF.

Continued.

TABLE 17-15.—OTHER COMMON THERAPIES USED FOR PATIENTS INFECTED WITH HIV—cont'd

DRUG AND HOW SUPPLIED	INDICATIONS	DOSAGE	SELECTED ADVERSE REACTIONS	PATIENT INSTRUCTIONS	COMMENTS
Nystatin (Mycostatin) 100,000 U/ml oral suspension 200,000 U troches	Treatment of oral candidiasis	Suspension: 2-3 ml each side of mouth, 4 times daily for 7-14 days Troche: 1 or 2 troches 4-5 times daily for 7-14 days	Anorexia, vomiting, diarrhea, loss of taste	Swish around mouth for 1 minute and swallow. Do not eat or drink for 30-60 minutes	Minimal systemic absorption. Not effective for esophageal candidiasis.
Pyrimethamine (Daraprim) 25-mg tablets	Treatment and suppression of toxoplasmosis in combination with sulfadiazine or clindamycin	50-75 mg daily with sulfadiazine for 1-3 weeks, dosage may then be reduced 50% and given for another 4-5 weeks	Anorexia, vomiting, bone marrow suppression		Concomitant use of leucovorin may reduce bone marrow suppression.
Sulfadiazine 500-mg tablets	Treatment and suppression of toxoplasmosis in combination with pyrimethamine	4-8 g daily in 4 divided doses along with pyrimethamine (see above) or clindamycin	Hypersensitivity reactions (can be severe), bone marrow suppression	Report rash, sore throat or fever immediately. Take with a full glass of water.	Contraindicated in patients with sulfa allergy
Clindamycin (Cleocin) 75-, 150-, 300-mg capsules	Second line for treatment and suppression of toxoplasmosis when used in combination with pyrimethamine	Adults: 300-600 mg 4 times daily Children: 8-16 mg/kg/day divided into 3 or 4 equal doses	Diarrhea, including *Clostridium difficile* colitis or pseudomembranous colitis, rash	Report diarrhea or rash to your doctor immediately	Has also been used as second-line therapy in combination with primaquine for the treatment of PCP

Acyclovir (Zovirax) 800-mg tablets 200-mg capsules 200 mg/5 ml suspension	Treatment of herpes simplex and herpes zoster, and for suppression of recurrent infections	Herpes simplex: 200 mg every 4 hours (5 times daily) for 10 days Herpes zoster: 800 mg every 4 hours (5 times daily) for 7-10 days Chronic suppression of herpes simplex: 400 mg twice daily for up to 12 months	Nausea, vomiting, CNS toxicity with high doses and/or renal impairment	Not a cure. Inform doctor if infection fails to heal	Dosage must be reduced with reduced renal function. Resistant herpes simplex has been reported in AIDS patients
Ganciclovir (Cytovene) powder for injection 500 mg/vial	Treatment and maintenance therapy for CMV retinitis	Induction: 5 mg/kg IV (over 1 hour) every 12 hours for 14-21 days Maintenance: 5 mg/kg IV (over 1 hour) once daily, given indefinitely. Reduce dose in renal impairment.	Neutropenia, anemia, thrombocytopenia, thrombophlebitis	Use sterile technique in drug administration; report any signs of fever or line-related infection (redness, warmth, and tenderness)	Need long-term central line placement; additive bone marrow suppression when used with AZT, TMP-SMX, pyrimethamine

Continued.

TABLE 17-15.—OTHER COMMON THERAPIES USED FOR PATIENTS INFECTED WITH HIV—cont'd

DRUG AND HOW SUPPLIED	INDICATIONS	DOSAGE	SELECTED ADVERSE REACTIONS	PATIENT INSTRUCTIONS	COMMENTS
Foscarnet (Foscavir) 24 mg/ml injection	Treatment and maintenance therapy for CMV retinitis and for herpes simplex resistant to acyclovir	Induction: 60 mg/kg (over 1 hour) every 8 hours for 14-21 days Maintenance: 90-120 mg/kg/day (over 2 hours), given indefinitely. Reduce dose in renal impairment	Renal failure, electrolyte abnormalities (hypercalcemia or hypocalcemia, hyperphosphatemia or hypophosphatemia), nausea, vomiting, thrombophlebitis, seizure	Regular ophthalmological examinations are necessary. Drink plenty of fluids. Report severe nausea, vomiting, diarrhea, fever, or line-related infections	Solution needs to be diluted (1:1) if foscarnet is to be given via a peripheral line
Rifabutin (Mycobutin) 150-mg capsules	Prophylaxis against *Mycobacterium avium* complex (MAC), patients with $CD_4 <$ 100 without active MAC or TB infection	300 mg once daily. May use 150 mg 2 times daily if nausea or vomiting is a problem	Rash, nausea, vomiting, rarely neutropenia	Advise patients that the drug causes an orange-red discoloration of body fluids	Not effective for TB prophylaxis. Should use with INH in PPD-positive patients. Rule out active TB and MAC before using. Enzyme inducer that may have many drug interactions

Drug	Use	Dose	Adverse effects	Administration notes	Comments
Clarithromycin (Biaxin) 250-, 500-mg tablets	Used in combination treatment for MAC infections	500 mg every 12 hours	Nausea, vomiting, abdominal pain	May be taken without regard to food	Should not be used alone for MAC, development of resistance may occur. May increase theophylline and carbamazepine serum levels
Clofazimine (Lamprene) 50-, 100-mg capsules	Used in combination treatment for MAC infections	100 mg daily	Rash, skin discoloration (common), red-brown discoloration of cornea, lacrimal fluid, abdominal pain, nausea, vomiting, diarrhea	Inform patients of potential change in skin and eye color, and it may discolor tears, sweat, sputum, urine, and feces	Drug is a bright-red dye and, drug crystals may deposit and accumulate in tissues. Most side effects are dose related and reversible
Ciprofloxacin (Cipro) 250-, 500-, 750-mg tablets	Used in combination treatment for TB or MAC infections	750 mg every 12 hours. Reduce dose in renal impairment	Nausea, vomiting, diarrhea, headache, dizziness, rash, crystalluria	Take at least 2 hours before antacid. Drink plenty of fluids	Drug interactions may increase serum levels of theophylline, warfarin, cyclosporine, digoxin, and phenytoin

Modified from *Clinical practice guideline: evaluation and management of early HIV infection:* AHCPR Publication No. 94-0572, 1994. For copy of the guidelines, call 800-342-AIDS.

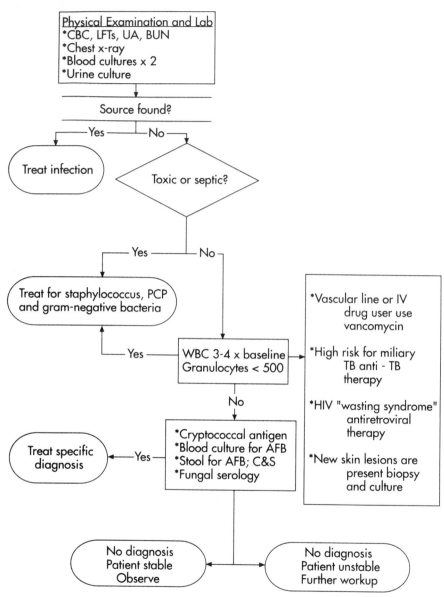

FIG 17-4.
Fever in HIV Patients with CD_4 counts < 200.

CANCER DETECTION

TABLE 17-16.—CLINICAL AND LABORATORY FEATURES OF VARIOUS FORMS OF CHRONIC LEUKEMIA COMMONLY SEEN AT DIAGNOSIS

SYMPTOMS	PHYSICAL FINDINGS	LABORATORY FINDINGS
Chronic Myelocytic Leukemia (CML)		
Abdominal discomfort, fullness	Slight hepatomegaly	Blood
Fatigue	Mild to moderate splenomegaly	Philadelphia chromosome (Ph[1])
Malaise		Granulocytic leukocytosis
Night sweats		Mild normochromic normocytic anemia
Weight loss		Thrombocytosis (platelet count >450,000/ mm^3)
		Increase in vitamin B_{12} serum level and binding activity
		Decrease in leukocyte alkaline phosphatase (LAP) activity
		Bone marrow
		Basophilia
		Eosinophilia
		Hypercellularity with elevated myeloid-erythroid ratio
Chronic Lymphocytic Leukemia (CLL)		
Same as in CML	Anemia	Blood
	Lymphadenopathy	Lymphocytosis
	Hepatomegaly	Positive Coombs' test
	Splenomegaly	Hypogammaglobulinemia
	Thrombocytopenia (degree of all depending on disease stage)	Neutropenia
		Bone marrow
		Lymphocytosis

From Hurd DD: *Postgrad Med* 73(5):217, 1983.

Continued.

TABLE 17-16.—Clinical and Laboratory Features of Various Forms of Chronic Leukemia Commonly Seen at Diagnosis—cont'd

SYMPTOMS	PHYSICAL FINDINGS	LABORATORY FINDINGS
Hairy-cell Leukemia (HCL)		
Same as in CML	Moderate to massive splenomegaly Mild hepatomegaly Minimal lymphadenopathy	Blood Pancytopenia Mononuclear cells with cytoplasmic extensions (hairy cells) Leukocyte count $<3000/mm^3$ Granulocytopenia Moderate thrombocytopenia Normochromic normocytic anemia
Prolymphocytic Leukemia (PLL)		
Same as in CML	Massive splenomegaly Moderate hepatomegaly No significant lymphadenopathy	Blood Extreme leukocytosis (leukocyte count $>100,000/mm^3$) Mild anemia Thrombocytopenia

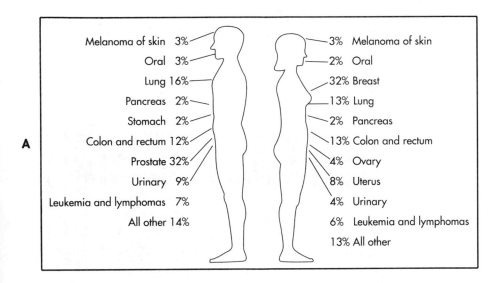

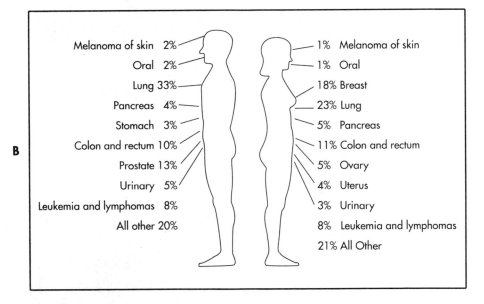

FIG 17-5.
A, 1994 Estimated cancer incidence by site and gender (excluding basal and squamous cell skin cancers and carcinoma in situ). **B,** 1994 estimated cancer deaths by site and gender. (From Silverberg E, Boring CC, Squires TS: *Cancer J Clin* 44:7, 1994.)

TABLE 17-17.—Risk Assessment for Cancer

FACTOR	INCREASED RISK FOR CANCER
Carcinogenic Factor	
Alcohol	Head and neck, esophagus
Alkylating agents	Leukemia, bladder
Aromatic amines	Bladder
Asbestos	Lung, mesothelioma
Estrogen	Uterus
Other chemicals	
Radiation (especially thyroid, spine, skin, breast)	Leukemia, sarcoma thyroid
Tobacco products	Lung, head and neck, larynx
Cigarettes	
Cigars	
Pipe	
Chew	
Note: Some combinations are very dangerous	
Alcohol and tobacco	Head and neck, esophagus
Asbestos and tobacco	Very high incidence of lung cancer
Genetic Predisposition	
Dysplastic nevus syndrome	Melanoma
Familial cancers of breast, ovary, uterus, colon	Breast, ovary, uterus, colon
Multiple endocrine neoplastic syndrome	Neuroendocrine
Polyposis coli	Colon
von Recklinghausen's neurofibromatosis	CNS
Personal History of Cancer	
Breast	Breast, colon, uterus, ovary
Cervix	Rectum
Colon	Colon, prostate, ovary
Lung	Lung, larynx, oral cavity, bladder

Modified from Costanza ME, et al: Cancer prevention and detection: strategy for the office practice. In American Cancer Society: *Cancer: a manual for practitioners,* ed 6, Boston, 1982, American Cancer Society, Massachusetts Division, pp. 6-7.

TABLE 17-17.—Risk Assessment for Cancer—cont'd

FACTOR	INCREASED RISK FOR CANCER
Lymphoma	Leukemia (especially if heavily treated with chemotherapy or radiotherapy)
Oral cavity	Oral cavity (particularly if patient continues to smoke), lung, larynx, bladder
Ovary	Leukemia (if treated with alkylating chemotherapy)
Uterus	Rectum
Family History of Cancer	
Breast, colon, lung, melanoma, prostate, stomach	Breast, colon, lung, melanoma prostate, stomach
Certain Associated Diseases	
Cirrhosis of liver	Liver
Colonic polyps, ulcerative colitis	Colon
Dermatomyositis	Viscera
Molar pregnancy	Choriocarcinoma
Paget's disease	Osteogenic sarcoma
Pernicious anemia, achlorhydria	Stomach
Scleroderma	Bronchiolar carcinoma
Sjögren's syndrome	Lymphoma
Undescended testes	Testes
Other	
Early or multiple coital partners	Cervix
Nulliparity, late parity	Breast
Obesity, nulliparity	Uterus

TABLE 17-18.—American Cancer Society Guidelines for Early Detection of Cancer in Asymptomatic Patients

TEST OR PROCEDURE	POPULATION		
	SEX	AGE (years)	FREQUENCY
Sigmoidoscopy, flexible	M/F	50 and over	Every 3 to 5 years
Stool occult blood test	M/F	50 and over	Every year
Digital rectal examination	M/F	40 and over	Every year
DRE and PSA	M	50 and over	Every year
Pap test and pelvic examination	F	All women who are, or who have been, sexually active, or who have reached age 18, should have an annual Pap test and pelvic examination. After a woman has had three or more consecutive satisfactory normal annual examinations, the Pap test may be performed less frequently at the discretion of her physician.	
Endometrial Tissue sample	F	At menopause, if women at high risk*	
Breast self-examination	F	20 and over	Every month
Physician breast examination	F	20-40	Every 3 years
		Over 40	Every year
Mammography	F	40-49	Every 1-2 years
		50 and over	Every year
Chest x-ray			Not recommended
Sputum cytology			Not recommended
Health counseling and cancer checkup†	M/F	Over 20	Every 3 years
	M/F	Over 40	Every year

From Summary of The American Cancer Society, *Recommendations for the early detection of cancer in asymptomatic persons,* 88-30M, revised Jan. 1994, No. 3409-PE.
*History of infertility, obesity, failure to ovulate, abnormal uterine bleeding, tamoxifen, or unopposed estrogen therapy.
†To include examination for cancers of the thyroid, testicles, prostate, ovaries, lymph nodes, oral region, and skin.

TABLE 17-19.—COMMON CONCERNS OF CANCER PATIENTS AND THEIR FAMILIES

Questions
What will happen next?
What treatments will I need (drugs, surgery, radiation)?
How do I tell my friends, family, and employer?
Is this cancer curable, or will it kill me?
How much time do I have?
Will there be pain?
How will I pay for all the treatment?
How do people die from this cancer?
Will the cancer affect my sex life?
Is cancer contagious?
How do I get what I want and need?

Strategies
Read or consult with someone about the particular cancer before breaking the news.
Know where to go for more facts (e.g., American Cancer Society).
Teach appropriate coping skills for relaxation, stress reduction, and pain relief.
Encourage open communication and questions.
Facilitate expression of emotions.
Provide for spiritual and psychosocial supportive care.
Stay involved as an active patient/family advocate.
Involve others in helping the patient and family (e.g., visiting nurse and hospice team).

TABLE 17-20.—EVALUATION OF PATIENTS WITH CARCINOMA OF AN UNKNOWN PRIMARY SITE TO IDENTIFY THOSE WHOSE TUMORS MAY BE TREATABLE

CARCINOMA	CLINICAL EVALUATION	PATHOLOGICAL STUDIES	SPECIAL SUBGROUPS	THERAPY	PROGNOSIS
Adenocarcinoma (well differentiated or moderately well differentiated)	Abdominal CT; serum PSA in men, mammography in women	PSA stain in men; status of ERs and PRs in women	Women with axillary-node involvement	Treat as primary breast cancer	Poor for entire group (median survival 4 months); better for subgroups
			Women with peritoneal carcinomatosis	Surgical cytoreduction + chemotherapy effective in ovarian cancer	
			Men with blastic bone metastases, high serum PSA, or PSA tumor staining	Hormonal therapy for prostate cancer	
			Patient with single peripheral nodal site of involvement	Lymph-node dissection ± radiotherapy	

Squamous carcinoma	Panendoscopy for cervical-node presentation; pelvic + rectal examination, anoscopy for inguinal presentation	None	Cervical adenopathy	Radiotherapy ± neck dissection	5-year survival, 25%-50%
			Inguinal adenopathy	Inguinal-node dissection ± radiotherapy	Potential long-term survival
Poorly differentiated carcinoma or adenocarcinoma	Chest, abdominal CT; serum hCG, AFP	Immunoperoxidase staining, electron microscopy, chromosomal analysis	Atypical germ-cell tumors (identified by chromosomal abnormalities only)	Treatment for germ-cell tumor	Treatment results similar to those for extragonadal germ-cell tumor
			Neuroendocrine tumors	Cisplatin-based therapy	10%-20% cured with therapy; high overall response rate
			Predominant tumor location in retroperitoneum, peripheral nodes	Cisplatin, etoposide, and bleomycin	

From Hainsworth JD, Grew FA: Treatment of patients with cancer of an unknown primary site, *N Engl J Med* 329:257, 1993.

CT, Computed tomography; *PSA*, prostate-specific antigen; *ER*, estrogen receptor; *PR*, progesterone receptor; *hCG*, human chorionic gonadotropin; *AFP*, α-fetoprotein.

TABLE 17-21.—UNDIAGNOSED CANCERS PRESENTING AS AN EMERGENCY

EMERGENCY	SIGNS AND SYMPTOMS	PROBABLE SITE	CANCER TYPE
Superior vena cava syndrome	Dyspnea, face swelling, cyanosis	Right upper chest	Small cell lung, lymphoma, ovary, breast, testicle
Malignant pericardial effusion	Dyspnea, cough, chest pain, orthopnea, tamponade	Heart	Metastatic lesion, lymphoma, leukemia
Severe back or neck pain	Radicular pain, spasticity, weakness	Spinal cord compression	Breast, lung, prostate, lymphoma, melanoma, GI
Altered mental status	Confusion, coma, lethargy, $\uparrow Ca^{++}$	Brain	Lung, breast, prostate, brain

TABLE 17-22.—Symptomatic Metastases in Patients With Cancer

GENERAL AREA OF METASTASES	COMMON SYMPTOMS	POSSIBLE PHYSICAL FINDINGS	INITIAL DIAGNOSTIC TESTS	POSSIBLE SPECIFIC FINDINGS
Lung and mediastinum	Hemoptysis,* dyspnea, dry cough, pleuritic pain, hoarseness	Bronchospasm, stridor, rhonchi, distended neck veins, pulsus paradoxus, Horner's syndrome, cord paralysis	Chest radiography	Intrapulmonary metastases, tracheal or caval compression by tumor masses,† pleural effusion,* pericardial effusion,* rib fracture
CNS	Headaches, mental confusion, extremity weakness,† visual difficulty, leg pain, bowel or bladder control loss†	Papilledema, deficits of cranial nerves, muscle strength, tendon reflexes, sensation, cranial function, sphincter tone	*Not* lumbar puncture; brain scan, spine radiographs, serum calcium, ? bone scan, ? myelogram, ? CT scan	Intracranial metastases,* spinal cord compression (either epidural or vertebral body metastases)†
Bone metastases	Pain with weight-bearing, radiating pain, pleuritic pain, nighttime pain, obtundation	Point tenderness to percussion, decreased tendon reflexes	Radiography, bone scan, serum calcium	Large lytic metastases* with impending vertebral body collapse or pathological fracture, diffuse metastases with hypercalcemia*
Abdomen and pelvis	Pain, vomiting, GI bleeding, obstipation, fatigue	Tenderness, distention, abnormal or absent bowel sounds, ascites, hepatomegaly, palpable masses, blood in stool	Radiography, hematocrit, leukocyte count, blood urea nitrogen	Bowel obstruction,† bowel perforation,† diffuse metastases, liver metastases, urinary obstruction*

From Osteen RT, McDonouh EF, Harris JR: The history and physical examination for cancer detection. In American Cancer Society: *cancer: a manual for practitioners*, ed 6, Boston, 1982, American Cancer Society, Massachusetts Division, p. 27.
*Urgent treatment sometimes indicated.
†Emergency treatment usually necessary for good palliation.

TABLE 17-23.—THE PARANEOPLASTIC SYNDROMES

CONDITION OR SUBSTANCE	DIAGNOSIS	TUMOR
Inappropriate ADH	Low serum osmolality and Na$^+$, high urinary sodium	Oat cell lung, thymoma, pancreas, lymphoma
ACTH	Excess adrenocortical hormones, abnormal GII	Oat cell, bronchial carcinoid, islet cell of pancreas, pheochromocytoma, ovary
Parathormone	Hypercalcemia, low serum phosphorus, high urinary calcium, no bony metastases, metabolic alkalosis	Lung squamous cell, head and neck, kidney, ovary, cervix, hepatoma, pancreas
Insulin	Hypoglycemia	Pancreatic insulinoma, hepatoma, mesothelioma, fibrosarcoma
hCG	Elevated serum hCG	Hepatoblastoma, stomach, lung, melanoma, ovary, carcinoid
Erythropoietin	Hematocrit >54% in men, 47% in women; normal leukocyte alkaline phosphatase	Renal cell, Wilms', sarcoma, hepatoma, cerebellum, uterus, ovary, pheochromocytoma
Thyroid-stimulating substance	Elevated serum T$_3$ and T$_4$; thyroid scan diffusely active	Trophoblastic tumors of testes, choriocarcinoma, moles
Gastrin	High serum gastrin, diarrhea, steatorrhea, GI ulcerations (Zollinger-Ellison syndrome)	Pancreatic islet cell, pheochromocytoma, lung cancer
Vasoactive intestinal peptide	Hypokalemia, hypochlorhydria, hypercalcemia, severe watery diarrhea (Verner-Morrison syndrome)	
Serotonin, kinins, histamine, prostaglandins	Elevated serum 5-HIAA	Carcinoid with hepatic metastases
Prolactin	Hyperprolactinemia	Renal
Placental alkaline phosphatase	Elevated serum alkaline phosphatase	Lung, breast, colon, ovary, pancreas, stomach, cervix, lymphoma
Growth hormone	Elevated serum GH	Lung, endometrium
Encephalomyelitis	Mental changes, nystagmus, ataxia, sensory deficit	Lung
Anti–Purkinje cell antibodies	Cerebellar atrophy, gait abnormality, nystagmus	Breast, ovary
Lambert-Eaton syndrome	Proximal lower extremity muscle weakness	Lung (small cell)

TABLE 17-24.—Skin and Connective Tissue and Other Changes

CONDITION	DIAGNOSIS	TUMOR
Acanthosis nigricans	Pigmented hyperkeratosis in skin flexures of axillae and perineum; pruritus	Stomach and other visceral adenocarcinomas
Icthyosis	Generalized drying and scaling	Lung, Hodgkin's disease
Dermatomyositis	Violaceous malar and extremity skin rash; proximal muscle weakness and pain; elevated serum CPK, aldolases, and transaminases	Stomach, breast, lung
Hypertrophic pulmonary osteoarthropathy	Clubbing of fingers and toes, polyarticular arthritis, periosteal proliferation	Lung
Reverse myasthenia gravis	Lambert-Eaton syndrome: males over 40 with proximal muscle weakness, facilitation after repeated stimuli	Oat cell lung (true myasthenia-thymoma)
Carcinomatous neuropathy	Symmetric motor, sensory, or mixed peripheral neuropathy	All types of malignancy
Proteinuria	Bence Jones proteinuria and renal amyloidosis	Multiple myeloma
	Extensive proteinuria with nephrotic syndrome	Breast, colon, lung, Hodgkin's disease

TABLE 17-25.—COMMON ONCOLOGICAL EMERGENCIES

EMERGENCY	IMPLICATION	TREATMENT OPTIONS
Ascites	Portal hypertension	Spironolactone, paracentesis
	Tumor extension	Tumor control
Bilateral ureteral obstruction	Tumor extension	Ureteral catheters, or percutaneous nephrostomies, hemodialysis
Bowel obstruction	Primary tumor or peritoneal metastases	Decompression by tube, surgery, or radiation
Bowel perforation	Rupture secondary to chemotherapy, radiation, or unattended obstruction	Fluids, antibiotics, surgical exploration
Disseminated infections: viral, fungal, parasitic	Immunocompromise	Organism specific, supportive
Disseminated intravascular coagulation	Seen in initial therapy of AML and prostate cancer	Fresh frozen plasma, heparin
Esophageal obstruction and perforation	Esophageal or gastric tumor extension	Nutritional support, tumor reduction
Hypercalcemia	Bone metastases, ectopic parathormone	Vigorous hydration, furosemide, mithramycin
Hypoglycemia	Insulinoma	50% glucose, tumor reduction
Hyperuricemia	Result of treatment of leukemias and lymphomas	Diuresis, alkalinization of urine, dialysis, allopurinol
Increased intracranial pressure	CNS tumor	Corticosteroids, surgery, radiation, chemotherapy

From Bope ET: Follow-up of the cancer patient: surveillance for metastases. In Driscoll CE, ed: *Primary care: the management of the cancer patient,* Philadelphia, 1987, WB Saunders, pp. 391-401; modified from Rubin P, Arsenlau JC: *Clinical oncology: a multidisciplinary approach,* ed 6, New York, 1983, American Cancer Society, pp. 516-525.

TABLE 17-25.—COMMON ONCOLOGICAL EMERGENCIES—cont'd

EMERGENCY	IMPLICATION	TREATMENT OPTIONS
Lactic acidosis	Rapidly growing tumors, (e.g., lymphoma)	Sodium bicarbonate
Leukostasis	Leukemia (blastic crisis)	Chemotherapy (hydroxyurea 5000-6000 mg as single dose)
Pathological fractures	Lytic bone metastases	Orthopedic surgery, radiation
Pericardial tamponade	Metastatic tumor to pericardium, radiation pericarditis	Pericardiocentesis, surgery
Pleural effusion	Pleural metastases, ascites, CHF, tumor obstructing lymph system	Treat cause, thoracentesis
Pneumothorax and tension pneumothorax	Misadventure, tumor extension	Chest tube
Sepsis	Leukopenia	Antibiotics, cultures, supportive care
Spinal cord compression	Tumor extension	Corticosteroids, radiation, surgery, chemotherapy
Superior vena cava syndrome	Tumor extension	Radiation, chemotherapy
Thrombocytopenic hemorrhage	Myelosuppression	Platelets
Tumor lysis syndrome	Rapid necrosis of tumor secondary to chemotherapy	Diuresis, electrolyte management, dialysis
Upper airway obstruction	Tumor extension	Radiation, tracheostomy, chemotherapy
Visual changes	Ocular primary or metastasis	Radiation, chemotherapy

CANCER THERAPIES

TABLE 17-26.—Common Combination Chemotherapy Regimens

CANCER	REGIMEN (type of cancer)	DRUGS AND DOSAGES
Breast	1. ACe (Breast cancer, metastatic or recurrent)	Cyclophosphamide 200 mg/m^2/day, PO, days 3-6 Doxorubicin (Adriamycin) 40 mg/m^2, IV, day 1 Repeat every 21-28 days
	2. CAF (Breast cancer, metastatic disease)	Cyclophosphamide 100 mg/m^2/day, PO, days 1-14 Doxorubicin 30 mg/m^2/day, IV days 1 and 8 Fluorouracil 500 mg/m^2/days, IV, days 1 and 8 Repeat every 4 weeks until a total cumulative dose of 450 mg/m^2 of doxorubicin is given, then discontinue doxorubicin and substitute methotrexate 40 mg/m^2, IV, and increase fluorouracil to 600 mg/m^2, IV
	3. CMF (Breast cancer, metastatic or recurrent disease and various adjuvant regimens)	Cyclophosphamide 100 mg/m^2/day, PO, days 1-14 Methotrexate 40-60 mg/m^2/day, IV, days 1 and 8 Fluorouracil 600 mg/m^2/day, IV, days 1 and 8 Repeat every 28 days
	4. CMFP (Breast cancer, metastatic disease)	Same as CMF but fluorouracil is 700 mg/m^2/day days 1 and 8 plus Prednisone 40 mg/m^2/day, PO, days 1-14 Repeat every 28 days
	5. FAC	Fluorouracil 500 mg/m^2/day, IV, days 1 and 8 Doxorubicin 50 mg/m^2, IV, day 1 Cyclophosphamide 500 mg/m^2, IV, day 1 Repeat every 3 weeks

Modified from Carter BL: Common chemotherapeutic agents. In Driscoll CE, ed: *Primary care: management of the cancer patient,* Philadelphia, 1987, WB Saunders, pp. 293-315; Olin BR, ed: Antineoplastics.

TABLE 17-26.—Common Combination Chemotherapy Regimens—cont'd

CANCER	REGIMEN (type of cancer)	DRUGS AND DOSAGES
Hodgkin's Lymphoma	1. ABVD (Hodgkin's induction resistant to MOPP)	Doxorubicin 25 mg/m^2/day, IV, days 1 and 14 Bleomycin 10 units/m^2/day, IV, days 1 and 14 Vinblastine 6 mg/m^2/day, IV, days 1 and 14 Dacarbazine 375 mg/m^2/day, IV, days 1 and 14 Repeat every 38 days for 6 cycles
	2. A-COPP (Hodgkin's induction, children only)	Doxorubicin 60 mg/m^2, IV, day 1 Cyclophosphamide 300 mg/m^2/day, IV, days 14 and 20 Vincristine 1.5 mg/m^2/day, IV, days 14 and 20 (max 2 mg) Procarbazine 100 mg/m^2/day, PO, days 14-28 Prednisone 40 mg/m^2/day, PO, days 1-27 (first and fourth cycles; then days 14-27 during second, third, fifth, and sixth cycles) Repeat every 42 days for 6 cycles
	3. MOPP	Mechlorethamine 6 mg/m^2/day, IV, days 1 and 8 Vincristine 2 mg/m^2/day, IV, days 1 and 8 (max 2 mg) Procarbazine 100 mg/m^2/day, PO days 1-14 Prednisone 40 mg/m^2/day, PO, days 1-14 Repeat every 28 days for 6 cycles
Non-Hodgkin's Lymphoma	1. CHOP (Non-Hodgkin's lymphoma with unfavorable histology)	Cyclophosphamide 750 mg/m^2, IV, day 1 Doxorubicin 50 mg/m^2, IV, day 1 Vincristine 1.4 mg/m^2, IV, day 1 (max 2 mg) Prednisone 60 mg/day, PO, days 1-5 Repeat every 21-28 days for 6 cycles
	2. COP (Non-Hodgkin's lymphoma with unfavorable histology)	Cyclophosphamide 800-1000 mg/m^2, IV, day 1 Vincristine 1.4 mg/m^2, IV, day 1 (max 2 mg) Prednisone 60 mg/m^2/day, PO, days 1-5 Repeat every 21 days for 6 cycles

Continued.

TABLE 17-26.—Common Combination Chemotherapy Regimens—cont'd

CANCER	REGIMEN (type of cancer)	DRUGS AND DOSAGES
	3. C-MOPP (or COPP) (Hodgkin's or non-Hodgkin's lymphoma with unfavorable histology)	Cyclophosphamide 650 mg/m^2/day, IV, days 1 and 8 Vincristine 1.4 mg/m^2/day, IV, days 1 and 8 (max 2 mg) Procarbazine 100 mg/m^2/day, PO, days 1-14 Prednisone 40 mg/m^2/day, PO, days 1-14 Repeat every 28 days for 6 cycles
Leukemia (ALL)	1. MTX + MP + CTX	Methotrexate 20 mg/m^2/week, IV Mercaptopurine 50 mg/m^2/day, PO Cyclophosphamide 200 mg/m^2/week, IV Continue until relapse or after 3 years of remission
	2. VP	Vincristine 2 mg/m^2/week, IV, for 4-6 weeks (max dose 2 mg) Prednisone 60 mg/m^2/day, PO, in divided doses for 4 weeks Taper weeks 5-7
Leukemia (AML)	1. ArA-C ADR	Cytarabine 100 mg/m^2/day, continuous 24-hour infusion, for 7-10 days Doxorubicin 30 mg/m^2/day, IV, for 3 days
	2. ArA-C + DNR + Pred + MP	Daunorubicin 25 mg/m^2, IV, for 1 day Cytarabine 80 mg/m^2/day, IV, for 3 days Prednisolone 40 mg/m^2/, PO, daily Mercaptopurine 100 mg/m^2, PO, daily Repeat weekly until remission, then repeat every month
Leukemia (CLL)	1. CHL + Pred	Chlorambucil 0.4 mg/kg/day, PO, for 1 day every other week Prednisone 100 mg/day, PO, for 2 days every other week Adjust CHL according to blood counts and increase every 2 weeks by 0.1 mg/kg until toxicity or disease control
	2. M-2 (also used for multiple myeloma)	Vincristine 0.03 mg/kg, IV, day 1 (max 2 mg) Carmustine 0.5 mg/kg, IV, day 1 Cyclophosphamide 10 mg/kg, IV, day 1 Melphalan 0.25 mg/kg/day, PO, days 1-4 Prednisone 1.0 mg/kg/day, PO, days 1-7, then taper to day 21 Continue treatment cycle throughout remission period until progression of disease
Lung	1. CAMP (nonoat cell)	Cyclophosphamide 300 mg/m^2/day, IV, days 1 and 8 Doxorubicin 20 mg/m^2/day, IV, days 1 and 8 Methotrexate 15 mg/m^2/day, IV, days 1 and 8

TABLE 17-26.—Common Combination Chemotherapy Regimens—cont'd

CANCER	REGIMEN (type of cancer)	DRUGS AND DOSAGES
		Procarbazine 100 mg/m^2/day, PO, days 1-10 Repeat every 28 days
	2. CAV (small cell)	Cyclophosphamide 750 mg/m^2, IV, every 3 weeks Doxorubicin 50 mg/m^2, IV, every 3 weeks Vincristine 2 mg, IV, every 3 weeks
	3. CHOR (small cell)	Cyclophosphamide and doxorubicin doses same as CAV but give both drugs on days 1 and 22 Vincristine 1 mg, IV, days 1, 8, 15, 22 Radiation total dose, 3000 rad, 10 daily fractions over a 2-week period beginning with day 36
	4. FAM (nonoat cell, also used for gastric and pancreatic but daily schedule differs)	Fluorouracil 600 mg/m^2/day, IV, days 1, 8, 28, 36 Doxorubicin 30 mg/m^2/day, IV, days 1 and 28 Mitomycin 10 mg/m^2, IV, day 1 Repeat every 8 weeks
	5. MACC (nonoat cell)	Methotrexate 40 mg/m^2, IV, day 1 Doxorubicin 40 mg/m^2, IV, day 1 Cyclophosphamide 400 mg/m^2, IV, day 1 Lomustine 30 mg/m^2, PO, day 1 Repeat every 21 days
Soft Tissue Sarcomas	1. CYVADIC	Cyclophosphamide 500 mg/m, IV, day 1 Vincristine 1.4 mg/m^2, IV, days 1 and 5 (max 2 mg) Doxorubicin 50 mg/m^2, IV, day 1 Dacarbazine 250 mg/m^2/day, IV, days 1-5 Repeat every 21 days
	2. VAC standard	Vincristine 2 mg/m^2/week, IV, weeks 1-12 (max 2 mg) Dactinomycin 0.015 mg/kg/day, IV, for 5 days, every 3 months for 5-6 courses (max 0.5 mg/day) Cyclophosphamide 2.5 mg/kg/day, PO, continue for 2 years
Testicular (Disseminated)	1. VBP	Vinblastine 0.2 mg/kg/day, IV, days 1 and 2 (every 3 weeks for 5 courses) Cisplatin 20 mg/m^2/day, IV infusion over 15 minutes, 6 hours after vinblastine, days 1-5; repeat every 3 weeks for 3 courses Bleomycin 30 U/week, IV, 6 hours after vinblastine on the second day of each week for 12 weeks to a total cumulative dose of 360 U

TABLE 17-27.—IMMEDIATE TOXICITIES OF COMMONLY USED CHEMOTHERAPEUTIC AGENTS

AGENT	TRADE NAME	LOCAL IRRITANT	ANAPHYLAXIS	FACIAL FLUSHING	FEVER	NAUSEA AND VOMITING	MUCOSITIS	ALOPECIA	SKIN REACTIONS	MISCELLANEOUS
Alkylating Agents										
Chlorambucil	Leukeran									
Cyclophosphamide	Cytoxan		+	+	+	++	+	++	Rash, dermatitis ↑PIG*	Hemorrhage, cystitis, SIADH
Melphalan	Alkeran		+			+			Dermatitis PIG, dermatitis	
Mechlorethamine	Mustargen	+++	+		+	+++				
Antimetabolites										
Cytarabine (ARA-C)	Cytosar-U	+			+	+	+			
5-Fluorouracil (5-FU)	Adrucil				+	++	++	+	↑PIG, rash, photo sensitivity	Ataxia, cerebellar syndrome
Mercaptopurine (6-MP)	Purinethol	+			+	+/−	++	+++	↑PIG, dermatitis	Headache, weakness
Methotrexate	Methotrexate		+		+†	+/−	++‡	+	Dermatitis	Renal toxicity
Thioguanine (6-TG)	Tabloid					+/−			Rash	
Vinca Alkaloids										
Vinblastine	Velban	++			+	+	+	+	Dermatitis, rash, pruritus	Constipation, SIADH
Vincristine	Oncovin	++			+	+	+	+	Dermatitis, pruritus, rash	Constipation, SIADH
Antibiotics										
Actinomycin D	Cosmegen	++	+			+++	+++	+/−	↑PIG, folliculitis	Acneiform lesions

Drug	Trade name							Dermatologic	Other
Bleomycin	Blenoxane	+	+++	+	++		++	↑PIG, urticaria, dermatitis	Pneumonitis
Daunorubicin	Cerubidine	+	++	++	++	++	+++	Rash, urticaria	Cardiotoxicity
Doxorubicin	Adriamycin	+++	+	++	+++	+++	+++	↑PIG, rash, urticaria	Drowsiness, cardiotoxicity
Mitomycin	Mutamycin	++	+	+	+	+	+	Dermatitis	Lethargy, weakness
Nitrosoureas									
BiCNU Carmustine (BCNU)									
CeeNU Lomustine (CCNU)									
Miscellaneous Agents									
L-Asparaginase	Elspar	++	++	+	++		++	Urticaria	Pancreatis, lethargy
5-Azacytidine				++				Rash	
Busulfan	Myleran			+				↑PIG, rare urticaria	Pulmonary toxicity
Cisplatin	Platinol	+	+	+++			+++		Renal toxicity
Imidazole carboxamide (dacarbazine)	DTIC-Dome	+	+	+++			+++		Flulike syndrome
Prednisone	Prednisone	+	+	+				↑PIG, photosensitivity	
Procarbazine	Matulane	+§	+/-	;				Rash (10%), dermatitis	Constipation

Modified from Spiegel RJ: *Cancer Treat Rev* 8:197, 1981.
*PIG indicates increased pigmentation.
†A 10% incidence after intrathecal administration.
‡Increased incidence with high-dose infusions.
§Increased with concomitant alcohol use.

TABI F 17-28. CURAIIVE DOSES OF RADIATION FOR SPECIFIC TUMORS

2000-3000 rad
Acute lymphocytic leukemia
Central nervous system

3000-4000 rad
Neuroblastoma
Seminoma
Wilms' tumor

4000-4500 rad
Hodgkin's disease
Non-Hodgkin's lymphoma

5000-6000 rad
Ewing's tumor
Embryonal cancer
Lymph nodes, metastatic
Ovarian cancer
Medulloblastoma
Retinoblastoma
Postop RT in head and neck and GI
  cancer
Squamous cell and basal cell skin
  cancers

6000-6500 rad
Larynx (<1 cm)
Breast cancer (lumpectomy)
Pancreas

7000-7500 rad
Bladder cancers
Cervical cancer
Lung cancer (<3 cm)
Lymph nodes, metastatic (1-3 cm)
Oral cavity (2-4 cm)
Oro-naso-laryngo-pharyngeal cancer
Endometrial cancer
Breast cancer (>5 cm)
Glioblastoma
Head and neck cancer (>4 cm)
Lymph nodes, metastatic (>6 cm)
Melanomas
Soft tissue sarcoma (>5 cm)
Thyroid cancer

Courtesy Hamed Tewfik, M.D., Director of the Iowa City Cancer Center, 1994.

TABLE 17-29.—Reporting Results of Cancer Therapy: Recommendations for Grading of Acute and Subacute Toxicity

	GRADE 0	GRADE 1	GRADE 2	GRADE 3	GRADE 4
Hematological (Adults)					
Hemoglobin (g/dl)	≥11.0	9.5-10.9	8.0-9.4	6.5-7.9	<6.5
Leukocytes (1000/mm^3)	≥4.0	3.0-3.9	2.0-2.9	1.0-1.9	<1.0
Granulocytes (1000/mm^3)	≥2.0	1.5-1.9	1.0-1.4	0.5-0.9	<0.5
Platelets (1000/mm^3)	≥100	75-99	50-74	25-49	<25
Hemorrhage	None	Petechiae	Mild blood loss	Gross blood loss	Debilitating blood loss
Gastrointestinal					
Bilirubin	≤1.25 × N*	1.26-2.5 × N	2.6-5 × N	5.1-10 × N	>10 × N
SGOT/SGPT	≤1.25 × N	1.26-2.5 × N	2.6-5 × N	5.1-10 × N	>10 × N
Alkaline phosphatase	≤1.25 × N	1.26-2.5 × N	2.6-5 × N	5.1-10 × N	>10 × N
Oral	None	Soreness/erythema	Erythema, ulcers, can eat solids	Ulcers, requires liquid diet only	Alimentation not possible
Nausea/vomiting	None	Nausea	Transient vomiting	Vomiting requiring therapy	Intractable vomiting
Diarrhea	None	Transient, <2 days	Tolerable but >2 days	Intolerable, requiring therapy	Hemorrhagic dehydration

From Miller AB, et al: *Cancer* 47:207, 1981.

*N, Upper limit of normal.

†Constipation does not include constipation resulting from narcotics.

‡Pain—only treatment-related pain is considered, not disease-related pain. The use of narcotics may be helpful in grading pain, depending on the tolerance of the patient.

NOTE: The World Health Organization recommends standardized recording of data related to patient therapies for malignancy. Family physicians, often engaged in follow-up care of patients with malignancy, are encouraged to use this observation system.

Continued.

TABLE 17-29.—REPORTING RESULTS OF CANCER THERAPY: RECOMMENDATIONS FOR GRADING OF ACUTE AND SUBACUTE TOXICITY—cont'd

	GRADE 0	GRADE 1	GRADE 2	GRADE 3	GRADE 4
Renal, Bladder					
BUN or blood urea	≤1.25 × N	1.26-2.5 × N	2.6-5 × N	5-10 × N	>10 × N
Creatinine	≤1.25 × N	1.26-2.5 × N	2.6-5 × N	5-10 × N	>10 × N
Proteinuria	None	1+; <0.3 g/dl	2 to 3+; 0.3-1.0 g/dl	4+; >1.0 g/dl	Nephrotic syndrome
Hematuria	None	Microscopic	Gross	Gross with clots	Obstructive uropathy
Pulmonary	None	Mild symptoms	Exertional dyspnea	Dyspnea at rest	Complete bed rest required
Fever-Drug	None	Fever <38° C	Fever 38° C-40° C	Fever >40° C	Fever with hypotension
Allergic	None	Edema	Bronchospasm, no parenteral therapy needed	Bronchospasm, parenteral therapy required	Anaphylaxis
Cutaneous	None	Erythema	Dry desquamation, vesiculation, pruritus	Moist desquamation, ulceration	Exfoliative dermatitis, necrosis requiring surgical intervention
Hair	None	Minimal hair loss	Moderate, patchy alopecia	Complete alopecia but reversible	Nonreversible alopecia
Infection (Specify site)	None	Minor infection	Moderate infection	Major infection	Major infection with hypotension

Cardiac					
Rhythm	None	Sinus tachycardia	Unifocal PVC, atrial arrhythmia	Multifocal PVC	Ventricular tachycardia
Function	None	Asymptomatic, but abnormal cardiac sign	Transient symptomatic dysfunction, no therapy required	Symptomatic dysfunction responsive to therapy	Symptomatic dysfunction nonresponsive to therapy
Pericarditis	None	Asymptomatic effusion	Symptomatic, no tap required	Tamponade, tap required	Tamponade, surgery required
Neurotoxicity					
State of consciousness	Alert	Transient lethargy	Somnolent <50% of waking hours	Somnolent >50% of waking hours	Coma
Peripheral	None	Paresthesias and/or decreased tendon reflexes	Severe paresthesias and/or mild weakness	Intolerable paresthesias and/or marked motor loss	Paralysis
Constipation†	None	Mild	Moderate	Abdominal distention	Distention and vomiting
Pain‡	None	Mild	Moderate	Severe	Intractable

GENERAL CARE OF THE CANCER PATIENT

TABLE 17-30.—Steps to Successful Control of Cancer Pain

1. Evaluate *physical* (visceral), *psychological* (anxiety, grief, and depression), and *social* (isolation, anger, and withdrawal) aspects.
2. Identify specific sources of pain (direct tumor involvement, pain of cancer therapy, or pain unrelated to tumor or therapy).
3. Assess intensity of pain. Use a simple 1 to 5 scale (1 = minimal, 5 = maximal) or define by using McGill-Melzack Pain Questionnaire.*
4. Use oral medications when possible, given every 4 hours regularly rather than PRN.
5. Always start concomitant bowel program with bulk laxative or wetting agent to alleviate constipation.
6. Administer medications in a stepwise fashion according to degree of need.

Patient's Rating	Intensity	Medication
1-2	Mild	Nonnarcotic: ASA, acetaminophen NSAID (especially for peripheral pain or bony metastases) ± adjunct†
2-3	Moderate	Weak narcotic: oxycodone, codeine ± adjunct
4-5	Severe	Narcotic: morphine, hydromorphone ± adjunct

7. Antiemetic measures may be required during first 1 to 2 weeks of initiating narcotic therapy.

*Melzack R: *Pain* 1:277, 1975.
†Adjunct, Benzodiazapine, tricyclic, and haloperidol.

TABLE 17-31.—THE NARCOTIC AND NONNARCOTIC ANALGESIC DRUGS WITH ORAL/RECTAL FORMULATIONS FOR CANCER PAIN*

CLASS	DRUG NAME	DOSE EQUIVALENTS (mg)		DURATION OF ACTION (HR)	PEAK EFFECT (HR)	USUAL ORAL DOSE (mg)	AVAILABLE FORMULATIONS	COMMENTS
Nonnarcotic								
	Aspirin	650		4-6	1/2-11/2	650-975 every 4 hours	Tablet, liquid, suppository	Antiinflammatory effect GI side-effects limit use
	Acetamino-phen	650		4-6	1/2-11/2	650-975 every 4 hours	Tablet, liquid, suppository	Lacks antiinflammatory effect, better tolerated than aspirin
Narcotic Agonists		(Dose equivalent to morphine 10 mg IM)						
		Oral	Intramuscular					
Mild-moderate pain	Codeine	200	130	4-6	1-11/2	60 every 4 hours	Tablet, liquid, injection	Most patients will not tolerate oral doses 90 mg every 4 hours, antitussive
	Oxycodone	30	15	3-5	1-11/2	30 every 4 hours	Tablet, liquid, injection	Antitussive, tolerated better than codeine by some patients

Continued.

TABLE 17-31.—THE NARCOTIC AND NONNARCOTIC ANALGESIC DRUGS WITH ORAL/RECTAL FORMULATIONS FOR CANCER PAIN—cont'd

CLASS	DRUG NAME	DOSE EQUIVALENTS (mg)	DURATION OF ACTION (HR)	PEAK EFFECT (HR)	USUAL ORAL DOSE (mg)	AVAILABLE FORMULATIONS	COMMENTS
	Propoxyphene	50	2-4	1-1½	50 every 4-6 hours	Tablet	Usually in combination with nonopioid may accumulate if renal failure
Moderate-severe pain	Morphine	30	3-4	½-1½	30 every 4 hours	Tablet, liquid sustained release, suppository, injection	The "standard." First-pass ratio oral: IM is 6:1, all doses thereafter at 2:1. Also available in liquid concentrate.
	Methadone (Dolophine)	20	4-8	1-2	20 every 4 hours	Tablet, injection	Can accumulate rapidly, somewhat more expensive than morphine
	Meperidine (Demerol)	300	2-4	½-1	75-150 every 3 hours	Tablet, injection	Most patients will not tolerate oral doses >150 mg; not recommended for cancer patients

Drug						Forms available	Comments
Hydromorphone (Dilaudid)	8		4-6	½-1½	4-8 every 4 hours	Tablet, liquid, suppository, injection	Good potency, large dose concentrated in small volume
Levorphanol (Levo-Dromoran)	4		4-8	½-1	2-4 every 6 hours	Tablet, injection	Slightly longer acting than morphine, lipophilic
Oxymorphone (Numorphan)	—		4-6	½-1½	10 rectally every 4 hours	Suppository and injection	No oral form available
Fentanyl transdermal patch (Duragesic)	(100 µg/hr = morphine 2 mg/hr)		48-72	—	—	Patch	Patches deliver 25, 50, 75 and 100 µg/hr
Mixed Agonist/ Antagonist							
Pentazocine (Talwin)	180	60	3-4	½-1	280 every 4 hours	Tablet, injection	Only oral form available in combination with naloxone, aspirin, or acetaminophen. Hallucinations in elderly, decreases narcotic effectiveness.

TABLE 17-32.—HELP FOR SPECIFIC PAIN SYNDROMES

CAUSES	INTERVENTIONS
Nerve root compression	Surgical decompression; dexamethasone 4-8 mg PO bid; nerve block
Headache from intracranial mass	Dexamethasone 4-8 mg PO bid (dosing up to 20 mg qid may be required); palliative radiation; doxepin or amitriptyline (tertiary amines) to raise CNS serotonin levels
Intestinal colic	Lomotil, 1-2 tablets PO every 4-6 hours *or* loperamide 2 mg PO every 6 hours; stool softener; nasogastric decompression
Bladder/rectal spasm pain	Belladonna 15 mg with opium (30 or 60 mg) in rectal suppository every 4-6 hours; chlorpromazine 10-25 mg q4-6h
Postherpetic neuralgia	Amitriptyline 25-150 mg PO qd; Sinemet 2 tabs tid; clonazepam 0.5 mg PO tid; other anticonvulsants such as carbamazepine, phenytoin, and valproic acid
Phantom limb pain	Narcotics, steroids, and TENS unit; carbamazepine
Oropharyngeal pain	Swish and swallow 15 ml 2% viscous lidocaine every 2 hours; artificial saliva; antimonilial agent if fungal
Muscle spasm pain	Amitriptyline 75 qhs if fibromyositis; massage, heat and narcotic; inject trigger points; baclofen 5-20 mg PO tid; dantrolene sodium 24-100 mg tid, cyclobenzaprine HCl 10 mg tid or diazepam 2-10 mg qid

TABLE 17-33.—MANAGEMENT OF COMMON SYMPTOMS

CONDITION	TREATMENTS
Anorexia	Frequent small feedings, high caloric supplements; sherry or wine, ½ hr ac; prednisone, 10-20 mg bid-tid, or fluoxymesterone, 5 mg tid; Periactin, 4 mg tid
Dry or painful mouth	Mouthwash of equal parts H_2O_2, glycerine, saline, and mouthwash; carboxymethylcellulose, 5 ml PRN; lidocaine, 2% viscous, 5-15 ml swish every 4 hours
Dysphagia	Antacids; metoclopramide, 5-10 mg qid; antifungal for candidiasis
Hiccoughs	Pharyngeal irritation with dry swallow of granulated sugar, simethicone; chlorpromazine, 25-50 mg every 4-6 hours; dexamethasone, phenytoin, or carbamazepine
Nausea/vomiting	Metoclopramide, 5-10 mg qid for gastroparesis associated with intraabdominal tumors; prochlorperazine, 10 mg qid, or haloperidol, 0.5 mg tid are first-line agents; second-line agents added to these are pyridoxine, 50 mg qid, or cyclizine, 25 mg qid
Colic or intestinal obstruction	Loperamide, 2-4 mg qid; dexamethasone, 8-10 mg tid
Dyspnea/cough	O_2, bronchodilators, opiates, hyoscine 0.4-0.6 mg sub Q, glucocorticoids
Fungating ulcers	Povidine-iodine 4% in liquid paraffin (1:1 to 1:4)—cleanse wound and apply gauze soaked in this preparation; gauze soaked in epinephrine 1:1000 will control capillary bleeding; judicious use of collagenase or dextranomer; 1% metronidazole solution applied
Pruritus	Biliary itch may be relieved by Questran, 4 g qid; antihistamines; steroids; crotamiton cream; tranquilizers
Decubitus	Frequent turning; egg-crate mattress, water bed or sheepskin; wet lesions dried with hair dryer; magnesium and aluminum hydroxide (Maalox) topically; Opsite, Tegaderm, or Stomahesive
Urinary retention	Bethanechol, 10-30 mg tid, Foley catheter
Urinary frequency	Evaluate for hypercalcemia and infection; flavoxate, 100 mg tid

TABLE 17-34.—Management of Chemotherapy-Induced Nausea and Vomiting

AGENTS	DOSE	ROUTE	SCHEDULE
Regimen 1: Combine the Following Drugs			
Metoclopramide	2 mg/kg	IV	20 minutes prechemo and every 2 hours for 2 doses
Dexamethasone	20 mg	IV	30 minutes prechemo
Diphenhydramine*	50 mg	IV	30 minutes prechemo
Regimen 2: Combine the Following Drugs			
Metoclopramide	3 mg/kg	IV	30 minutes prechemo and 1.5 hours after
Dexamethasone	20 mg	IV	30 minutes prechemo
Diphenhydramine*	50 mg	IV	Prechemo and 1.5 hours postchemo-therapy
Lorazepam	1.25 mg/m^2	IV	30 minutes prechemo and every 2 hours after PRN
Regimen 3: Combine the Following Drugs			
Dexamethasone	12 mg	PO	Night before and every 4 hours on treatment day
	20 mg	IV	Prechemo and 1.5 hours postchemo-therapy
Prochlorperazine	5-10 mg	PO	Night before and every 2-4 hours on treatment day
Diazepam	5 mg	PO	Night before and on treatment day
Metoclopramide	1 mg/kg	IV	Prechemo and 1.5 hours postchemo-therapy
Diphenhydramine*	50 mg	IV	Prechemo and 1.5 hours postchemo-therapy
Regimen 4: Combine the Following Drugs			
Diphenhydramine*	50 mg	IV	Prechemo, then every 6 hours PRN
Droperidol	1 mg	IV	Prechemo, then every 6 hours PRN
Metoclopramide	2 mg	IV	Prechemo and every 2 hours postchemo-therapy for 3 doses, then PRN
Dexamethasone	10 mg	IV	Prechemo
Regimen 5: Combine the Following Drugs†			
Methylprednisolone	125-250 mg	IV	Prechemo
Ondansetron	8 mg	IV	Prechemo, repeat at 4 and 8 hours

Modified from Tortorice PV, O'Connell MB: Management of chemotherapy-induced nausea and vomiting, *Pharmacotherapy* 10:129, 1990; Finley RS: Nausea and vomiting. In Young LY, et al, *Handbook of applied therapeutics,* Vancouver, 1989, Applied Therapeutics, pp. 85-99.

*Diphenydramine is used to prevent extrapyramidal side effects from metoclopramide and/or the antipsychotic drugs.

†Regimen 5 is the least sedating. The other regimens can be very sedating.

FOLLOW-UP RECOMMENDATIONS FOR COMMON CANCERS

TABLE 17-35.—Breast Cancer Follow-Up

	MONTHS												THEN EVERY 12 MONTHS
	3	6	9	12	15	18	21	24	30	36	42	48	
History													
Complete	●	●	●	●				●		●		●	●
Self-examination	●	●	●		●	●	●		●		●		
Lumps	●	●	●		●	●	●		●		●		
Pain	●	●	●		●	●	●		●		●		
Cough, dyspnea	●	●	●		●	●	●		●		●		
Weight loss, anorexia	●	●	●		●	●	●		●		●		
Physical													
Complete	●	●	●	●				●		●		●	●
Chest wall, axillae	●	●	●		●	●	●		●		●		
Remaining breast tissue	●	●	●		●	●	●		●		●		
Lymph nodes	●	●	●		●	●	●		●		●		
Abdomen, liver	●	●	●		●	●	●		●		●		
Skin, eyes (jaundice)	●	●	●		●	●	●		●		●		
Chest	●	●	●		●	●	●		●		●		
Bones	●	●	●		●	●	●		●		●		
Pelvis				●				●		●		●	

From Fischer DS, Ungaro PC, Wilhelm MC: Cancer follow-up: How much is enough? *Patient Care* 26(11):201-224, 1992.

ALT, Serum alanine aminotransferase; *AST*, serum aspartate aminotransferase; *CEA*, carcinoembryonic antigen; *LDH*, lactate dehydrogenase.

KEY: ● Recommended by all consultants
○ Not recommended by all consultants
□ If patient was treated with lumpectomy and radiotherapy

NOTE: With regard to frequency of follow-up visits, this table shows the minimum recommendation. Some of the consultants recommend shorter intervals between follow-up visits or tests.

Continued.

TABLE 17-35.—Breast Cancer Follow-Up—cont'd

	MONTHS												THEN EVERY 12 MONTHS
	3	6	9	12	15	18	21	24	30	36	42	48	
Other													
Mammography		□		●		□		●		●		●	●
CBC				○				○		○		○	○
Serum calcium				○				○		○		○	○
Serum LDH				○				○		○		○	○
Serum alkaline phosphatase				○				○		○		○	○
Serum CEA				○				○		○		○	○
Serum phosphorus				○				○		○		○	○
Serum AST and ALT				○				○		○		○	○
Chest x-ray examination				○				○				○	Every other year
Bone scan		○		○									
Liver scan/ultrasonography				○									

TABLE 17-36.—Colon and Rectal Cancer Follow-Up

	FIRST YEAR MONTHS				SECOND-FIFTH YEAR MONTHS		THEN EVERY 12 MONTHS
	3	6	9	12	6	12	
History							
Complete				●		●	●
Weight loss, anorexia	●	●	●		●		
Bowel function (pain, change, blood)	●	●	●		●		
Abdominal pain	●	●	●		●		
Pruritus	●	●	●		●		
Dark urine	●	●	●		●		
Physical							
Complete				●		●	●
Abdomen, liver	●	●	●		●		
Stoma	●	●	●		●		
Rectum	●	●	●		●		
Lymph nodes	●	●	●		●		
Skin (jaundice)	●	●	●		●		
Other							
CBC	●	●	●	●	●	●	●
Fecal occult blood	○	●	○	○	●	●	●
Liver function		○		●	○	●	●
Serum CEA		●		●	In 2nd yr only	●	●
Endoscopy: Sigmoidoscopy and barium enema		●		●	In 2nd yr only	●	●
Or							
Colonoscopy				●	Every other yr after 3rd yr		
Liver scan/ ultrasonography				○		○	○
Chest x-ray examination				○		○	○

From Fischer DS, Ungaro PC, Wilhelm MC: Cancer follow-up: How much is enough? *Patient Care* 26(11):201, 1992.

CEA, Carcinoembryonic antigen.

KEY: ● Recommended by all consultants
○ Not recommended by all consultants

NOTE: With regard to frequency of follow-up visits, this table shows the minimum recommendation. Some of the consultants recommend shorter intervals between follow-up visits or tests.

TABLE 17-37.—PROSTATE CANCER FOLLOW-UP

| | MONTHS | | | | | | | THEN EVERY 12 MONTHS |
	3	6	9	12	16	20	24	
History								
Complete				●			●	●
Urinary symptoms	●	●	●		●	●		
Bone pain	●	●	●		●	●		
Cardiac symptoms	●	●	●		●	●		
Sexual problems	●	●	●		●	●		
Depression	●	●	●		●	●		
Radiation-induced problems	●	●	●		●	●		
Physical								
Complete				●			●	●
Prostatic bed, surgical field, meatus	●	●	●		●	●		
Rectum	●	●	●		●	●		
Lymph nodes	●	●	●		●	●		
Bladder	●	●	●		●	●		
Other								
Urinalysis	●	●	●	●	●	●	●	●
Prostate-specific antigen	○	●	○	●	○	○	●	●*
CBC		○		○			○	○
Chest x-ray examination		○		●			●	●
Pelvic x-ray examination/ ultrasound		○		●			●	●
Bone scan				○				
BUN		○		○			○	○
Serum creatinine		○		○			○	○

From Fischer DS, Ungaro PC, Wilhelm MC: Cancer follow-up: How much is enough? *Patient Care* 26(11):201, 1992.
KEY: ● Recommended by all consultants
○ Not recommended by all consultants
NOTE: With regard to frequency of follow-up visits, this table shows the minimum recommendation. Some of the consultants recommend shorter intervals between follow-up visits or tests.
*Many experts recommend follow-up at 6-month intervals.

TABLE 17-38.—CERVICAL CANCER FOLLOW-UP

	FIRST YEAR				SECOND-FIFTH YEAR		THEN EVERY 12 MONTHS
	MONTHS				MONTHS		
	3	6	9	12	6	12	
History							
Complete				●		●	●
Vaginal bleeding, spotting, discharge	●	●	●		●		
Bone pain	●	●	●		●		
Leg edema	●	●	●		●		
Weight loss, anorexia	●	●	●		●		
Abdominal distension	●	●	●		●		
Bowel function	●	●	●		●		
Bladder function	●	●	●		●		
Physical							
Complete				●		●	●
Pelvis	●	●	●		●		
Rectum	●	●	●		●		
Abdomen	●	●	●		●		
Breasts	●	●	●		●		
Lymph nodes	●	●	●		●		
Colposcopy*	○	○	○		○	○	○
Other							
Urinalysis	●	●		●	●	●	●
Fecal occult blood	●	●		●	●	●	●
Pap smear		●	●	●	●	●	●
CBC				○	○	○	○
Serum CEA and CA 125					○		○
Chest x-ray examination				●		●	●
IVP				●		○	

From Fischer DS, Ungaro PC, Wilhelm MC: Cancer follow-up: How much is enough? *Patient Care* 26(11):201, 1992.

CEA, Carcinoembryonic antigen; *IVP,* intravenous pyelogram.

KEY: ● Recommended by all consultants
○ Not recommended by all consultants

NOTE: With regard to frequency of follow-up visits, this table shows the minimum recommendation. Some of the consultants recommend shorter intervals between follow-up visits or tests.

*If cervix was not removed.

TABLE 17-39.—Endometrial Cancer Follow-Up

	FIRST YEAR MONTHS				SECOND-FIFTH YEAR MONTHS		THEN EVERY 12 MONTHS
	3	6	9	12	6	12	
History							
Complete				●		●	●
Vaginal bleeding, spotting, discharge	●	●	●		●		
Pelvic pain	●	●	●		●		
Leg edema	●	●	●		●		
Weight loss, anorexia	●	●	●		●		
Abdominal distension, enlargement	●	●	●		●		
Estrogen supplementation	●	●	●		●		
Physical							
Complete				●		●	●
Pelvis	●	●	●		●		
Rectum	●	●	●		●		
Abdomen	●	●	●		●		
Breasts	●	●	●		●		
Lymph nodes	●	●	●		●		
Other							
Urinalysis	●			○	○	○	○
Fecal occult blood	●	●		●	●	●	●
Pap smear		●	●	●	●	●	●
CBC		○		○	○	○	○
Serum CEA and CA 125				○		○	○
Liver function studies				○	○	○	
Chest x-ray examination				●		●	●
IVP				○		○	

From Fischer DS, Ungaro PC, Wilhelm MC: Cancer follow-up: How much is enough? *Patient Care* 26(11):201, 1992.

CEA, Carcinoembryonic antigen; *IVP*, intravenous pyelogram.

KEY: ● Recommended by all consultants
○ Not recommended by all consultants

NOTE: With regard to frequency of follow-up visits, this table shows the minimum recommendation. Some of the consultants recommend shorter intervals between follow-up visits or tests.

TABLE 17-40.—HODGKIN'S DISEASE FOLLOW-UP

	FIRST YEAR			SECOND-FIFTH YEAR		THEN EVERY 12 MONTHS
	MONTHS			MONTHS		
	1	3, 6, 9	12	4, 8	12	
History						
Complete			●		●	●
Weight loss, anorexia	●	●		●		
Fever	●	●		●		
Pruritus	●	●		●		
Pain (alcohol induced)	●	●		●		
Lumps	●	●		●		
Night sweats	●	●		●		
Respiratory symptoms	●	●		●		
Physical						
Complete			●		●	●
Lymph nodes	●	●		●		
Abdomen, liver, spleen	●	●		●		
Skin	●	●		●		
Oropharynx	●	●		●		
Chest	●	●		●		
Other						
CBC	●	●	●	●	●	●
Chest x-ray examination	●	●	●	●	●	●
Serum alkaline phosphatase	●		●		●	●
Serum LDH	●		●		●	●
Serum bilirubin	●		●		●	●
Serum AST	●		●		●	●
Urinalysis	●		●		●	●
ESR	○		○		○	○
Thyroid function		□	□			
Gallium scan			○			
Abdominal x-ray examination or CT scan		◇	◇		◇	◇

From Fischer DS, Ungaro PC, Wilhelm MC: Cancer follow-up: How much is enough? *Patient Care* 26(11):201, 1992.

AST, Serum aspartate aminotransferase; CT, computed tomography; LDH, lactate dehydrogenase.

KEY: ● Recommended by all consultants
○ Not recommended by all consultants
□ At 6 months in first year, if patient received radiation therapy near thyroid gland
◇ At 6 months in first year, if patient had intraabdominal Hodgkin's disease
NOTE: With regard to frequency of follow-up visits, this table shows the minimum recommendation. Some of the consultants recommend shorter intervals between follow-up visits or tests.

TABLE 17-41.—Non-hodgkin's Lymphoma Follow-Up

	FIRST YEAR			SECOND-FIFTH YEAR		THEN EVERY 12 MONTHS
	MONTHS			MONTHS		
	1	3, 6, 9	12	4, 8	12	
History						
Complete			●		●	●
Weight loss, anorexia	●	●		●		
Fever	●	●		●		
Pain	●	●		●		
Lumps	●	●		●		
Night sweats	●	●		●		
Respiratory symptoms	●	●		●		
GI symptoms	●	●		●		
CNS symptoms	●	●		●		
Physical						
Complete			●		●	●
Lymph nodes	●	●		●		
Abdomen, liver, spleen	●	●		●		
Skin	●	●		●		
Oropharynx	●	●		●		
Chest	●	●		●		
Neurological examination	●	●		●		
Other						
CBC		●	●	●	●	●
Chest x-ray examination		●	●	●	●	●
Serum alkaline phosphatase	●		●		●	●
Serum LDH	●		●		●	●
Serum bilirubin	●		●		●	●
Serum AST	●		●		●	●
Urinalysis	●		●		●	●
Gallium scan			○			
Abdominal x-ray examination or CT scan	□		●		□	□

From Fischer DS, Ungaro PC, Wilhelm MC: Cancer follow-up: How much is enough? *Patient Care* 26(11):201, 1992.

AST, Serum aspartate aminotransferase; *CT,* computed tomography; *LDH,* lactate dehydrogenase.

KEY: ● Recommended by all consultants
○ Not recommended by all consultants
□ At 6 mo in first yr, if patient had diffuse large cell lymphoma

NOTE: With regard to frequency of follow-up visits, this table shows the minimum recommendation. Some of the consultants recommend shorter intervals between follow-up visits or tests.

18 *Nutrition*

Charles W. Smith, Jr.

NUTRITIONAL ASSESSMENT

TABLE 18-1.—Nutritional Assessment

A nutritional assessment includes the following parameters:

Diet History
A diet history includes obtaining a typical day's intake of food plus information about weight change, patterns of eating, changes in appetite, taste, food intolerance, and digestive disorders. Educational needs and potential drug-nutrient interactions are also evaluated.

Nutrient Intakes
When a nutritional assessment is ordered, a 3-day nutrient intake is automatically performed. This includes calculation of calories, protein, fat, and carbohydrate from all food, formula, and IV solutions. Nutrient intakes may also be ordered separately for 3-day periods for patients suspected of having a poor dietary intake.

Nutritional Needs
To determine a patient's caloric and protein needs, the following four factors are calculated:
1. BEE (Basal Energy Expenditure)
A factor calculated from the patient's weight, height, and age
The following Harris-Benedict equations are used:

$$\text{Male} = 66 + [13.7 \times \text{Wt (kg)}] + [5 \times \text{Ht (cm)}] - [6.8 \times \text{Age (yrs)}]$$
$$\text{Female} = 655 + [9.6 \times \text{Wt (kg)}] + [1.7 \times \text{Ht (cm)}] - [4.7 \times \text{Age (yrs)}]$$

From Clinical Staff, Dietary Department, University of Iowa Hospitals and Clinics: Recent advances in thereapeutic diets, ed 4, Ames, Iowa, 1989, Iowa State University Press.
*Optimal parameters.
†Optional for preoperative patients.
‡Detailed instructions and feeding protocols can be found in the Enteral Nutrition Handbook (1989), available for purchase from the Dietary Department, University of Iowa Hospitals and Clinics.

Continued.

TABLE 18-1.—Nᴜᴛʀɪᴛɪᴏɴᴀʟ Assᴇssᴍᴇɴᴛ—cont'd

2. Activity Needs
A factor added to the BEE based on the patient's physical activity level

Percentage Above Basal	Classification	Groups of Individuals
20	Limited activity	Bed rest, anorexia nervosa
30	Minimum activity	Up and about, but inactive, women > 50 years old
40	Average activity	Most women, men > 50 years old
50	Average activity	Most men
60	Exercisers	Those who engage in physical exercise daily (20-30 minutes or more)
70	Heavy Work	Physical laborers

3. Metabolic Needs
A factor added to the BEE based on the patient's clinical status

Percentage Above Basal	Condition
13	Fever (increase 13% for each 1° C above normal)
20	Minor operation
35	Skeletal trauma (long bones)
40-60	Major sepsis
20-40	Moderate infection
20	Mild infection
5-25	Peritonitis
30	Soft tissue trauma
25	Cancer
10	Need for weight gain

4. Protein Needs
A factor calculated from the patient's weight (g pro/kg) and based on the patient's metabolic state

Metabolic State	Protein Needs (g/kg/day)
Nonstress	0.8-1.0
Elective surgery	1.5
Polytrauma	1.5-1.75
Sepsis	2.0
Burn	1.5-2.0

Laboratory Data

The following laboratory tests should be ordered to obtain biochemical data on nutritional status:

Serum albumin

Serum transferrin

Hemoglobin

Hematocrit

Total lymphocyte count

Serum glucose

Anthropometric Measurements

To determine the extent of depletion, specific physical parameters may also be evaluated. The following three parameters are measured:

1. Height/weight—compared with ideal weight
2. Midarm muscle circumference—a measure of the patient's lean body mass or the degree of protein depletion*
3. Triceps skinfold—an indirect measure of body fat*

Delayed Hypersensitivity Skin Testing*

Four skin tests for cell-mediated immunity are sometimes utilized for evaluating nutritional status. Lack of response to the antigen indicates anergy, or failure of the body's defense system to recognize foreign protein and to fight infection. The four antigens are:

1. PPD
2. Mumps
3. *Candida albicans*
4. Streptokinase/streptodornase

Prognostic Nutrition Index (PNI)†

PNI is a formula developed to preoperatively predict the risk of postoperative complications. If time permits, this may allow a patient's nutritional status to be improved before surgery. The formula is a percentage based on the following indicators:

Albumin (Alb)—g/dl

Triceps skinfold (TSF)—mm

Serum transferrin (TFN)—mg/dl

Delayed hypersensitivity skin testing (DH)

$$PNI(\%) = 158 - [16.6 \times Alb] - [.78 \times TSF] - [.20 \times TFN] - [5.8 \times DH]$$

Risk of postoperative morbidity and mortality:

<30% PNI = low risk

30-59% PNI = intermediate risk

>59% PNI = high risk

Summary Recommendations

After completion of the assessment,‡ the dietitian will summarize the parameters measured and make recommendations to improve the patient's nutritional status.

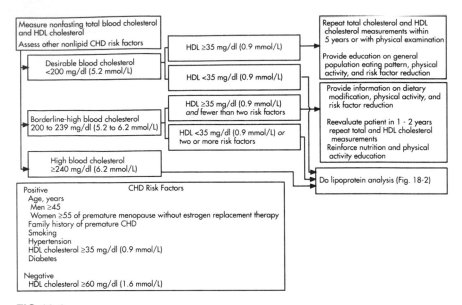

FIG 18-1.

Primary prevention in adults without evidence of coronary heart disease (CHD). Initial classification is based on total cholesterol and high-density lipoprotein (HDL) cholesterol levels. From Summary of the NCEP Adult Treatment Panel II Report: *JAMA* 269(23):3018, 1993.

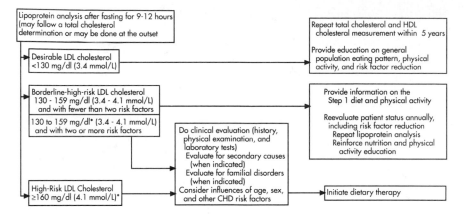

FIG 18-2.

Primary prevention in adults without evidence of coronary heart disease (CHD). Subsequent classification is based on low-density lipoprotein (LDL) cholesterol level. From Summary of the NCEP Adult Treatment Panel II Report: *JAMA* 269(23):3019, 1993.

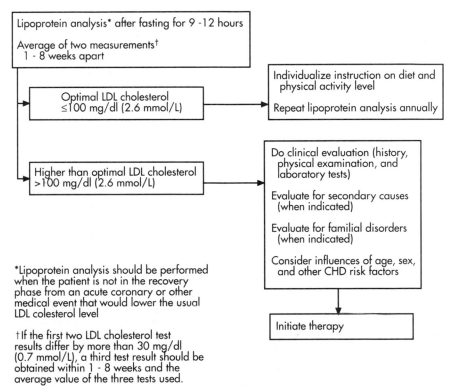

FIG 18-3.

Secondary prevention in adults with evidence of coronary heart disease (CHD). Classification is based on low-density lipoprotein (LDL) cholesterol level. From Summary of the NCEP Adult Treatment Panel II Report: *JAMA* 269(23):3020, 1993.

TABLE 18-2. –1983 METROPOLITAN LIFE INSURANCE HEIGHT-WEIGHT TABLES*

MEN

HEIGHT		WEIGHT (lb)		
FEET	INCHES	SMALL FRAME	MEDIUM FRAME	LARGE FRAME
5	2	128-134	131-141	138-150
5	3	130-136	133-143	140-153
5	4	132-138	135-145	142-156
5	5	134-140	137-148	144-160
5	6	136-142	139-151	146-164
5	7	138-145	142-154	149-168
5	8	140-148	145-157	152-172
5	9	142-151	148-160	155-176
5	10	144-154	151-163	158-180
5	11	146-157	154-166	161-184
6	0	149-160	157-170	164-188
6	1	152-164	160-174	168-192
6	2	155-168	164-178	172-197
6	3	158-172	167-182	176-202
6	4	162-176	171-187	181-207

WOMEN

HEIGHT		WEIGHT (lb)		
FEET	INCHES	SMALL FRAME	MEDIUM FRAME	LARGE FRAME
4	10	102-111	109-121	118-131
4	11	103-113	111-123	120-134
5	0	104-115	113-126	122-137
5	1	106-118	115-129	125-140
5	2	108-121	118-132	128-143
5	3	111-124	121-135	131-147
5	4	114-127	124-138	134-151
5	5	117-130	127-141	137-155
5	6	120-133	130-144	140-159
5	7	123-136	133-147	143-163
5	8	126-139	136-150	146-167
5	9	129-140	139-153	149-170
5	10	132-145	142-156	152-173
5	11	135-148	145-159	155-176
6	0	138-151	148-162	158-179

From the Metropolitan Life Insurance Company, New York, NY. Based on the Build study, 1979, Chicago, 1980, Society of Actuaries and Association of Life Insurance Medical Directors of America.

*Weight according to frame (ages 25 to 59) for men wearing indoor clothing weighing 5 lb and shoes with 1-inch heels; for women wearing indoor clothing weighing 3 lb and shoes with 1-inch heels.

TABLE 18-3.—CLINICAL SIGNS USED IN THE PHYSICAL EXAMINATION FOR NUTRITIONAL ASSESSMENT

ORGAN	NUTRIENT	CLINICAL SIGNS
Hair	Protein/Calories	Dry, brittle, fine, easily plucked, rough
Eyes	Vitamin A	Dry conjunctiva, Corneal softening, Bitot's spots (white or yellow sub-conjunctival)
	Riboflavin-Vitamin B_2	Circumcorneal injection
	Iron, folate, vitamin B_{12}	Conjunctival pallor
	Vitamin B_{12}	Optic neuritis
Skin	Vitamin A	Roughened, follicular hyperkeratosis, "crazy pavement" dermatitis
	Vitamin C	Petechiae, ecchymoses, curled hair follicles
	Vitamin K	Skin hemorrhages
	Niacin	Thickened pressure points, scaling, dry, hyperpigmented in sun-exposed areas
	Riboflavin-Vitamin B_2, Niacin	Nasolabial seborrhea
	Riboflavin-Vitamin B_2	Scrotal dermatitis
Nails	Iron	Spoon-shaped, brittle, ridged
Teeth	Fluoride	Gray or black spots (fluorosis)
Lips	Riboflavin-Vitamin B_2 Niacin	Cheilosis, scars and lesions, angular stomatitis
Tongue	Riboflavin-Vitamin B_2, Niacin, Vitamin B_6	Red, painful, atrophic, denuded, edema, fissured with atrophy of papillae
	Folate	Glossitis
Gums	Vitamin C, vitamin A	Gingivitis, periodontal disease, hypertrophy
Neck	Iodine	Goiter
Face	Protein/Calories	Enlargement of parotid gland
Skeleton	Calcium	Osteoporosis
	Vitamin C, vitamin D	Costochondral beading
	Vitamin D	Epiphyseal enlargement, cranial bossing, bowed legs, craniotabes, osteomalacia
Muscles/Fat	Thiamine-Vitamin B_1, Protein/Calories	Muscle tenderness and weakness, muscle wasting, loss of fat
	Vitamin D	Hypotonia
Heart	Thiamine-Vitamin B_1	Cardiomegaly, CHF, edema
Liver	Protein/Calories	Hepatomegaly
Neurological	Thiamine-Vitamin B_1	Hyporeflexia, hypesthesia, loss of vibratory sense, decreased DTRs, delirium
	Pyridoxine-Vitamin B_6	Peripheral neuropathy, dementia
	Vitamin B_{12}	Hyporeflexia, ataxia, loss of proprioception and vibration senses
	Niacin	Dementia
Gastrointestinal	Protein/Calories, niacin	Diarrhea

From MS Canu: *Handbook of clinical dietetics,* New Haven, 1981, Yale University Press. In Dwyer JT, Gallo JJ, Riechel W: Assessing nutritional status in elderly patients, *Am Fam Physician* 47(3):613, 1993.

DIETS

In 1992, a new educational food guide replaced the familiar "basic four" food groups. The pyramid gives a range for the number of servings in each of five food groups shown in the pyramid. When age, gender, and activity are taken into consideration, more specific advice about calories and number of servings is taken from Table 18-4.

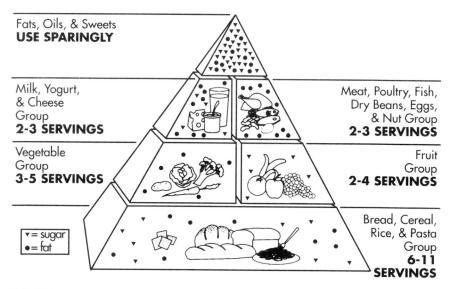

FIG 18-4.
Food Guide Pyramid, a guide to daily food choices.

TABLE 18-4.—ADVICE ABOUT CALORIES AND NUMBER OF SERVINGS

FOOD GROUP	WOMEN, SOME ELDERLY	CHILDREN, TEENAGE GIRLS, MOST MEN, ACTIVE WOMEN	TEENAGE BOYS, ACTIVE MEN
Bread	6	9	11
Vegetable	3	4	5
Fruit	2	3	4
Milk	2-3*	2-3*	2-3*
Meat	2 (5 oz total)	2 (6 oz total)	3 (7 oz total)
Fats	Use sparingly	Use sparingly	Use sparingly
Calories	~1600	~2200	~2800

*Women who are pregnant or breast-feeding, teenagers, and young adults to age 24 need three servings (see Table 18-5 for a definition of servings).

TABLE 18-5.—DEFINITION OF SERVINGS

BREAD	VEGETABLE	FRUIT	MILK	MEAT
1 slice of bread	1 cup of green leafy vegetable	1 medium apple or orange	1 cup of milk or yogurt	2-3 oz of cooked lean meat
1 oz of cereal	½ cup of other vegetable	½ cup of canned fruit	1½ oz of natural cheese	½ cup cooked dry beans
½ cup of pasta or rice	¾ cup of vegetable juice	¾ cup of fruit juice	2 oz of processed cheese	1 egg; 2 tbsp of peanut butter

TABLE 18-6.—DIETS

Pregnancy
Should contain recommended daily caloric allowance (1800-2400), plus 300 calories (see Table 18-9) and the following:
   3-4 servings of milk and cheese
   2-3 servings of meat, poultry, fish, or eggs
   ≥4 servings of vegetables or fruit
   ≥4 servings of bread and grain

Lactation
Recommended caloric requirement (1800-2400), plus 500 calories (same distribution as in pregnancy, plus 12 cups of fluid per day) (see Table 18-9).

Infant and Pediatric

Age	Fluids	Calories	Protein
0-6 months	140-160 ml/kg	kg × 117	kg × 2.2 g
6-12 months	125-135 ml/kg	kg × 108	kg × 2.0 g

Geriatric
Calories: 65-75-year-olds: reduce by 10%
          >75-year-olds: reduce by 25%
Protein: Should be ≥12% of calories. Protein requirements do not decline with age
Fat: Should be ≥30% of calories
Vitamins/minerals: Supplementation usually indicated. Consider calcium (800-1200 mg/day) in thin caucasian women

Soft (Mechanical Soft or Pureed)
For patients unable to chew, or as progression from liquid to regular diet. Is generally nutritionally adequate

Liquid
For postoperative or acute gastrointestinal conditions. Clear = little or no residue; "full" includes milk, strained soups, ice cream, and custard. Not nutritionally adequate.

Low Fiber (Low Residue)
Used for postoperative bowel surgery or acute exacerbations of inflammatory bowel disease. Contains minimal undigestible carbohydrate (e.g., cellulose and lignin), usually found in fruits, vegetables, and cereals.

Chronic Renal Failure
Restricted protein, sodium, potassium, and fluids, depending on type and severity of CRF. Protein restriction used when creatinine clearance is 25 ml/minute or less; potassium restriction if patient is oliguric or hyperkalemic. If clearance is ≤20 ml/min, use phosphate binder (e.g., Basalgel) to control hyperphosphatemia. A patient with end-stage renal disease not on dialysis should have approximately 0.6 mg/kg body wt/day of protein.

Continued.

TABLE 18 6.—Diets—cont'd

Hyperlipidemias
Hypertriglyceridemia (type IV, ↑ VLDL)
Decrease body weight and triglyceride levels by doing the following:
    Limiting CHO to 40% of caloric intake
    Using polyunsaturated fats when possible
    Restricting cholesterol and saturated fat intake
    Limiting alcohol intake
Hypercholesterolemia (type IIa, ↑ LDL) (see Table 18-17)
Reduce saturated fatty acids and cholesterol by doing the following:
    Decreasing ingested cholesterol to 300 mg/day
    Decreasing dairy and animal fats and substituting polyunsaturated fats
Mixed (↑ LDL and VLDL, type IIb)
Same as for type IIa + carbohydrate and alcohol restriction

Sodium-Restricted Diets
4-6 g: "No added salt"
4 g: Cook all foods without salt
2 g: Eliminate foods cooked or preserved in salt or with visible salt (e.g., saltine crackers)
1 g: Above, plus restriction of foods high in natural sodium

Diets for Weight Loss*

When diets are prescribed for weight loss, calories are reduced below the level necessary for maintenance of present body weight. At the same time, the intake of protein, vitamins, and minerals remains at or above the levels recommended by the National Research Council. The aim is to provide a diet tailored to the needs of the individual that will promote the use of stored body fat for energy without causing excessive loss of lean body mass.

An estimated 26% of the adult population in the United States is overweight or obese. Obesity is defined as *a body fat content of 25% or more in the male and greater than 30% in the female.* Overweight signifies a body weight above an arbitrary standard, usually defined in relation to height.

Obesity and overweight are associated with increased risk of hypertension, hyperlipidemia, cardiovascular disease, gout, diabetes, arthritis, and surgical complications. Many undesirable social and psychological consequences occur as well.

*From Clinical Staff, Dietary Department, University of Iowa Hospitals and Clinics: Recent advances in therapeutic diets, ed 4, Ames, Iowa, 1989, Iowa State University Press.

TABLE 18-7.—IDEAL BODY WEIGHT

The concept of ideal body weight is derived from data in which relative weight has been correlated with mortality. The Metropolitan Life Insurance Company tables are commonly used to determine desirable weight for height (see Table 18-2). The body mass index (weight in kilograms divided by height in meters squared) is also a convenient determination of desirable weight for height and can be calculated without the use of tables. The National Health and Nutrition Examination Survey II uses the following definitions for desirable body weight, overweight, and severe overweight:

Correlation of Body Mass Index with Weight Levels

$$\text{Body Mass Index (BMI)} = \frac{\text{weight in kg}}{\text{height in m}^2}$$

	Desirable Body Weight	20% Excess Weight	40% Excess Weight
Men	22.7	27.8	31.1
Women	21.1	27.3	32.3

The following is another method often used for estimating desirable body weight:

Women	Men
100 lb for the first 5 feet of height, plus 5 lb for each additional inch	106 lb for the first 5 feet of height, plus 6 lb for each additional inch

Determining Caloric Need

Determination of caloric need is used to anticipate the rate of loss and to assist in planning long-term goals. A calorie deficit of 500 to 1000 calories per day, which allows for a weight loss of 1 to 2 lb per week, is recommended.

The best methods for determining caloric needs consider weight (usually ideal weight if it can be decided), height, age, sex, and activity. Another influential factor is individual metabolic rate. The following formula can be used to quickly determine caloric need for adults:

Basal requirement + activity requirement = caloric need

Daily basal requirement = 1 cal × _____ kg ideal body weight × 24 hours

Activity requirement: 20% of basal if very sedentary
30% of basal if sedentary
40% of basal if moderately active
50% of basal if very active

The estimated caloric need for maintenance is then compared with the caloric intake calculated from a thorough diet history.

TABLE 18-0.—DIETS FOR WEIGHT LOSS

Selecting a Diet Plan

Several approaches can be used at University of Iowa Hospitals and Clinics to attain a hypocaloric diet. In all instances, assessments are made to determine advisability of vitamin and mineral supplementation, particularly at levels of less than 1200 kcal/day.

Exchange System. A balanced exchange system meal plan is designed based on individual preferences for a predetermined number of calories. An advantage of this method is the presumed development of good eating habits. A disadvantage is the time necessary to learn the system.

Calorie Counting. This method works well for the patient who has established good eating habits. He or she can then keep a diet diary and calculate calories on a daily basis.

Semistarvation. A very low calorie diet (200 to 600 kcal/day) results in significant physiological and biochemical changes. It should be carried out only with proper management and careful medical supervision. This approach to weight reduction may be desirable initially to enhance motivation, or when extensive weight loss is critical for patients with serious medical problems.

Protein-Sparing-Modified Fast (solid food version). The rationale for this diet is that high-quality protein will minimize the loss of lean muscle mass. Close medical supervision is required. The diet prescription is 1.0 to 1.5 g protein per kilogram ideal body weight, very low fat, and minimal carbohydrate. The only fat present in the diet is that found in fish, poultry, or other low-fat protein foods. Carbohydrate is obtained from three or more servings of low-calorie vegetables, included to promote compliance.

Specific Changes in Eating Habits. In some cases a significant number of calories can be eliminated by making changes in eating habits, without a "diet" per se. For example, a person drinking four cans of regular soda pop per day could eliminate 600 calories by altering that one behavior alone. Specific changes of this type can become well-defined attainable goals for the motivated individual.

TABLE 18-8.—Diets for Weight Loss—cont'd

Exercise and Behavior Modification

Successful weight management programs are those that include exercise and behavior modification techniques as well as a hypocaloric diet. The incorporation of exercise must be individualized according to motivational level and physical health. Assistance in determining physical activities that will be satisfying can be helpful, since enjoyable exercise routines tend to promote compliance. Obviously, exercise is a more significant variable in the younger person with only mild to moderate obesity than it is in the older individual who has other physical ailments. In any case, exercise is an important variable that should be included in weight management programs.

Behavior modification is based on the premise that behavior is controlled by environmental events that act as cues or stimuli and reinforcement. In weight management the emphasis is on changing behavior to decrease caloric consumption and to increase physical activity. Generally, the use of behavior modification involves the following four steps:

1. Identifying the behavior to be changed
2. Setting realistic goals for behavior change
3. Modifying the social and physical environment to support the behavior change
4. Reinforcing or rewarding the behavior change

In weight control programs, behaviors are identified by asking the patient to keep a diary. Information included in the diary varies from program to program but usually includes the following:

- Time of initiation of eating
- Time of termination of eating
- Place of eating
- Perceived mood
- Food selected
- Amount of food consumed by volume and often by calories

The information obtained is used to identify specific behaviors requiring change, as well as the stimuli and consequences controlling these behaviors. Self-monitoring does reveal patterns of behavior that the patient may not have previously recognized and that frequently can produce behavior change in and of itself. For effectiveness, the recording should occur immediately after the behavior.

Continued.

TABLE 18 8.—Diets for Weight Loss—cont'd

Appropriate goal setting involves the following principles:
- Goals should be established with patient involvement.
- Goals should be set at a moderate level of difficulty.
- Goals should be achievable and short term.
- Goals should be written and/or publicly stated.

Behavior modification programs attempt to help people reduce environmental cues associated with inappropriate behavior. The following are examples related to weight loss:
- Prepare small quantities of food and serve them on a small plate.
- Remove the refrigerator light.
- Rearrange cupboards to make problem foods difficult to see and reach.
- Establish one place in the house that is the only place to eat.
- Remove serving dishes from the table.

A goal of intervention programs is to develop immediate, tangible rewards for new appropriate behaviors, since those that are positively reinforced will be repeated.

TABLE 18-8.—DIETS FOR WEIGHT LOSS—cont'd

Evaluating Commercial Weight Loss Programs

The increasing prevalence of obesity in our country has made weight control a prime business venture. Many commercial weight loss promotions are based on unsound theories, which can be detrimental to health if followed for long periods.

Satisfactory weight loss programs are those that do the following:

1. Avoid promises of rapid weight loss (should not be substantially more than 1% of total body weight per week).
2. Provide all nutrients in adequate amounts using a balanced diet containing approximately 15% protein, 30% fat, and 55% carbohydrate.
3. Teach how to make wise choices from the conventional food supply, rather than creating dependency on special products or supplements.
4. Do not promote diets that are extremely low in calories, unless under the supervision of competent medical experts.
5. Encourage permanent, realistic life-style changes that include regular exercise and avoid the use of food as a coping device.
6. Avoid misrepresenting salespeople as "counselors" qualified to make nutrition recommendations.
7. Do not promote unproven or spurious weight loss aids such as starch blockers, diuretics, sauna belts, body wraps, ear stapling, passive exercise, or amino acid supplements.

TABLE 18-9.—Food and Nutrition Board, National Academy of Sciences—National Research Council Recommended Dietary Allowances,[a] Revised 1989 (Designed for the maintenance of good nutrition of practically all healthy people in the United States)

CATEGORY	AGE (YR) CONDITION	WEIGHT[b] (KG)	WEIGHT[b] (LB)	WEIGHT[b] (CM)	WEIGHT[b] (IN)	PROTEIN (g)	VITAMIN A (μg RE)[c]	VITAMIN D (μg)[d]	VITAMIN E (mg α-TE)[e]	VITAMIN K (μg)
Infants	0.0-0.5	6	13	60	24	13	375	7.5	3	5
	0.5-1.0	9	20	71	28	14	375	10	4	10
Children	1-3	13	29	90	35	16	400	10	6	15
	4-6	20	44	112	44	24	500	10	7	20
	7-10	28	62	132	52	28	700	10	7	30
Males	11-14	45	99	157	62	45	1000	10	10	45
	15-18	66	145	176	69	59	1000	10	10	65
	19-24	72	160	177	70	58	1000	10	10	70
	25-50	79	174	176	70	63	1000	5	10	80
	51+	77	170	173	68	63	1000	5	10	80
Females	11-14	46	101	157	62	46	800	10	8	45
	15-18	55	120	163	64	44	800	10	8	55
	19-24	58	128	164	65	46	800	10	8	60
	25-50	63	138	163	64	50	800	5	8	65
	51+	65	143	160	63	50	800	5	8	65
Pregnant,						60	800	10	10	65
lactating	First 6 months					65	1300	10	12	65
	Second 6 months					62	1200	10	11	65

From National Academy of Sciences: Recommended dietary allowances, ed 10, Washington, DC, 1989, National Academy Press.

[a]The allowances, expressed as average daily intakes over time, are intended to provide for individual variations among most normal persons as they live in the United States under usual environmental stresses. Diets should be based on a variety of common foods to provide other nutrients for which human requirements have been less well defined.

[b]Weights and heights of Reference Adults are actual medians for the U.S. population of the designated age, as reported by NHANES II. The median weights and heights of those under 19 years of age were taken from Hamill et al. (1979) The use of these figures does not imply that the height-to-weight ratios are ideal.

[c]Retinol equivalents. 1 retinol equivalent = 1 μg retinol or 6 μg β-carotene.

[d]As cholecalciferol. 10 μg cholecalciferol = 400 IU of vitamin D.

[e]α-Tocopherol equivalents. 1 mg d-α tocopherol = 1 α-TE.

[f]1 NE (niacin equivalent) is equal to 1 mg of niacin or 60 mg of dietary tryptophan.

	WATER SOLUBLE VITAMINS						MINERALS						
‑AMIN C (mg)	THIAMIN (mg)	RIBO-FLAVIN (mg)	NIACIN (mg NE)^f	VITAMIN B_6 (mg)	FOLATE (µg)	VITAMIN B_{12} (µg)	CALCIUM (mg)	PHOS-PHORUS (mg)	MAG-NESIUM (mg)	IRON (mg)	ZINC (mg)	IODINE (µg)	SELE-NIUM (µg)
30	0.3	0.4	5	0.3	25	0.3	400	300	40	6	5	40	10
35	0.4	0.5	6	0.6	35	0.5	600	500	60	10	5	50	15
40	0.7	0.8	9	1.0	50	0.7	800	800	80	10	10	70	20
45	0.9	1.1	12	1.1	75	1.0	800	800	120	10	10	90	20
45	1.0	1.2	13	1.4	100	1.4	800	800	170	10	10	120	30
50	1.3	1.5	17	1.7	150	2.0	1200	1200	270	12	15	150	40
60	1.5	1.8	20	2.0	200	2.0	1200	1200	400	12	15	150	50
60	1.5	1.7	19	2.0	200	2.0	1200	1200	350	10	15	150	70
60	1.5	1.7	19	2.0	200	2.0	800	800	350	10	15	150	70
60	1.2	1.4	15	2.0	200	2.0	800	800	350	10	15	150	70
50	1.1	1.3	15	1.4	150	2.0	1200	1200	280	15	12	150	45
60	1.1	1.3	15	1.5	180	2.0	1200	1200	300	15	12	150	50
60	1.1	1.3	15	1.6	180	2.0	1200	1200	280	15	12	150	55
60	1.1	1.3	15	1.6	180	2.0	800	800	280	15	12	150	55
60	1.0	1.2	13	1.6	180	2.0	800	800	280	10	12	150	55
70	1.5	1.6	17	2.2	400	2.2	1200	1200	320	30	15	175	65
95	1.6	1.8	20	2.1	280	2.6	1200	1200	355	15	19	200	75
90	1.6	1.7	20	2.1	260	2.6	1200	1200	340	15	16	200	75

TABLE 18-10.—Selected Drug-Induced Nutritional and Metabolic Effects

DRUG-INDUCED EFFECT	CLINICAL OBSERVATION
Electrolyte Imbalances	
Amphotericin B	Decreased serum K, Mg
Aluminum-containing antacids	Decreased serum PO_2
Magnesium-containing antacids	Increased serum Mg (severe renal failure)
Antibiotics (synthetic penicillins)	Decreased serum K
Antineoplastics (various)	Varies based on agent; decreased K, Mg, Na: Increased K
Cisplatin	Decreased serum Mg, other electrolytes
Corticosteroids	Decreased serum Ca, K, PO_1; increased serum Na
Glucose, insulin	Decreased serum K, Mg, PO_1 (anabolism)
Altered Acid-Base Balance	
Corticosteroids	Function of amount of acid lost in daily fluids as well as electrolytes
Diuretics (furosemide, ethacrynic acid)	Metabolic alkalosis
H_2-receptor antagonists	Metabolic alkalosis
	Blunts tendency to metabolic alkalosis in patients on nasogastric suction
Constipation	
Aluminum-containing antacids	Aluminum content changes intestinal motility
Anticholinergics	Reduced peristalsis
Antihistamines	Reduced peristalsis
Antipsychotics (phenothiazines)	Reduced peristalsis
Iron salts	Reduced peristalsis
Narcotic analgesics	Increased gastrointestinal tone, decreased gastrointestinal secretions, delayed gastric emptying, increased reabsorption of intestinal water
Tricyclic antidepressants	Reduced peristalsis
Diarrhea	
Alkylating agents	Chemical irritant effect
Antibiotics	Alteration of bowel flora, local gastrointestinal irritation
Antimetabolites	Chemical irritant effect
Colchicine	Inhibits intestinal epithelial cell mitosis and disaccharidase activity
Electrolyte solutions (potassium salts, sodium salts)	Hypertonicity causes osmotic diarrhea
Guanethidine	Increased gastrointestinal motility
Lactulose	Fermentation of unabsorbed sugar by intestinal bacteria with gastrointestinal irritation and increased lactic acid production

Laxatives	Stimulate hormone release, which increases gastrointestinal tract secretory activity
Magnesium salts (antacids, cathartics, electrolyte replacements)	Poor absorption from small intestine with osmotic diarrhea, hypertonicity
Potassium salts	Hypertonicity causes osmotic diarrhea
Quinidine	Increased gastrointestinal motility
Nausea and Vomiting	
Antibiotics	Direct gastrointestinal irritant effect
Antineoplastics	Rapid turnover time of intestinal cells
Digoxin	Drug toxicity
Iron salts	Direct gastrointestinal irritant effect with stimulation of vomiting center
Narcotic analgesics	Stimulation of medullary chemoreceptor trigger zone
Nonsteroidal antiinflammatory agents	Direct gastrointestinal irritant effect
Potassium salts	Direct gastrointestinal irritant effect with stimulation of vomiting center
Altered Glucose Metabolism	
Corticosteroids	Altered cellular uptake, altered insulin effectiveness
Diuretics	Hyperglycemia, glucosuria
Oral contraceptives	Hyperglycemia
	Hyperglycemia
Altered Protein Metabolism	
Chloramphenicol	Antianabolic effects
Corticosteroids	Amino acid transfer inhibited during protein synthesis
Indomethacin	Increased gluconeogenesis, increased BUN, UUN: negative nitrogen balance
Neomycin	Decreased amino acid absorption
Oral contraceptives	Decreased amino acid absorption
Tetracycline	Impaired vitamin B_6 status leading to amino acid plasma level alterations
Thyroid hormones	Increased BUN, UUN
Salicylates	Increased UUN
	Produce amino aciduria

Modified from Smith CH, Bidlack WR: Dietary concerns associated with the use of medications, *J Am Diet Assoc* 84(8):901, 1984.
BUN, Blood urea nitrogen; *UUN*, urinary urea nitrogen; *Ca*, calcium; *K*, potassium; *Na*, sodium; *PO₄*, phosphate.

TABLE 18-11.—Nutrient Analysis of Enteral

| | MILK BASED | | |
	INSTANT BREAKFAST	ENSURE	ISOCAL
Calories/ml	1	1.06	1.06
Carbohydrate source	Sucrose, corn syrup, lactose	Hydrolyzed corn starch, sucrose	Glucose oligosaccharides
Protein source	Milk, sodium casinate, soybean protein isolate	Soy protein isolate, sodium and calcium caseinates	Soy protein isolate, sodium and calcium caseinates
Fat source	Whole milk	Corn oil	MCT, soy oil
Protein g/L (%)	60 (22%)	37 (14%)	34 (13%)
Fat g/L (%)	32 (26%)	37 (31%)	44 (37%)
Carbohydrate g/L (%)	144 (50%)	145 (54%)	132 (50%)
Nonprotein calories: gN	88:1	153:1	167:1
mOsm/kg water	710	450	300
Na/K mEq/L	41/70	37/40	23/34
Ca/Phos mg/L	1600/1120	549/549	634/528
Vitamins, ml to meet 100% U.S. RDA	1400	1887	1890
Flavors	Chocolate, vanilla, strawberry	Chocolate, vanilla	Unflavored
Form	Powder	Liquid	Liquid
Uses/Features	Oral supplement, high protein	Oral supplement	Tube feeding
Manufacturer	Delmark Carnation	Ross	Mead-Johnson

| | ELEMENTAL | | HIGH |
	TOLEREX	VIVONEX T.E.N.	SUSTACAL HC
Calories/ml	1	1	1.5
Carbohydrate source	Glucose oligosaccharides	Maltodextrin and modified starch	Corn syrup solids, sugar
Protein source	Free amino acids	Crystalline amino acids	Sodium and calcium caseinates
Fat source	Safflower oil	Safflower oil	Corn oil
Protein g/L (%)	21 (8%)	38 (15%)	61 (16%)
Fat g/L (%)	1.5 (1%)	3 (2%)	58 (34%)
Carbohydrate g/L (%)	231 (92%)	206 (82%)	190 (50%)
Nonprotein calories: gN	281:1	139:1	134:1
mOsm/kg water	550	630	650
Na/K mEq/L	20/30	20/20	37/38
Ca/Phos mg/L	556/556	500/500	845/845
Vitamins, ml to meet 100% U.S. RDA	1800	2000	1180
Flavors	Unflavored	Unflavored	Vanilla
Form	Powder	Powder	Liquid
Uses/features	Tube feeding, lactose free, low fat	Jejunostomy tube feeding, high in glutamine	Oral supplement
Manufacturer	Norwich Eaton	Norwich Eaton	Mead-Johnson

Modified from Clinical Staff, Dietary Department, University of Iowa Hospitals and Clinics: *Recent*

Formulas and Supplements

	LACTOSE FREE	
OSMOLITE HN	PROFIBER	PRECISION ISOTONIC
1.06	1	1
Hydrolyzed corn starch	Hydrolyzed corn starch, soy fiber	Glucose oligosaccharides sucrose
Soy protein isolate, sodium and calcium caseinates	Sodium and calcium caseinates	Egg albumin
MCT, corn oil, soy oil	Corn oil	Partially hydrogenated soy oil
44 (17%)	40 (16%)	30
37 (30%)	40 (36%)	31
141 (53%)	132 (48%)	144
125:1	131:1	183:1
310	300	300
40/40	32/32	20/25
761/761	667/667	680/680
1321	1500	1560
Unflavored	Unflavored	Vanilla, orange
Liquid	Liquid	Powder
Tube feeding	High fiber tube feeding (14 g fiber/L)	Tube feeding isotonic lactose free
Ross	Sherwood Medical	Sandoz

CALORIC DENSITY	COMPONENTS	
TWO CAL HN	MICROLIPID	POLYCOSE LIQUID
2	4.5	2
Hydrolyzed corn starch, sucrose	—	Hydrolyzed corn starch
Soy protein isolate, sodium and calcium caseinates	—	—
Corn oil, MCT	Safflower oil	—
84 (17%)	—	—
91 (40%)	500	—
217 (43%)	—	500
125:1	—	—
690	80	850
46/59	—	30/2
1053/1053	—	200/30
950	—	—
Vanilla	Unflavored	Unflavored
Liquid	Liquid	Liquid
Tube feeding	Fat emulsion supplement	Carbohydrate supplement
Ross	Biosearch	Ross

advances in therapeutic diets, ed 4, Ames, Iowa, 1989, Iowa State University Press.

Continued.

TABLE 18-11.—NUTRIENT ANALYSIS OF ENTERAL

SUSTACAL	SUSTACAL WITH FIBER	VITANEED	CITROTEN
1	1.06	1	0.66
Sucrose, corn syrup solids	Maltodextrin, sugar, soy fiber	Maltodextrin, fruit and vegetables, soy fiber	Sucrose, maltodextrin
Soy protein isolate, sodium and calcium caseinates	Calcium and sodium caseinates, soy protein isolate	Beef puree, calcium and sodium caseinates	Egg albumin
Partially hydrogenated soy oil	Corn oil	Corn oil	Partially hydrogenated soy oil
61 (24%)	46 (17%)	40 (16%)	41 (25%)
23 (21%)	35 (30%)	40 (36%)	1.6 (21%)
140 (55%)	141 (53%)	128 (48%)	122 (55%)
79:1	120:1	131:1	76:1
620	450	300	495
41/54	31/36	30/32	31/18
1014/930	845/704	667/667	1048/1048
1080	1500	1500	1350
Strawberry, Vanilla	Vanilla	Unflavored	Fruit punch
Liquid	Liquid	Liquid	Powder
Oral supplement, high protein	High fiber tube feeding or supplement (6 g fiber/L)	Blenderized tube feeding	Oral supplement, low fat, low residue
Mead-Johnson	Mead-Johnson	Sherwood Medical	Sandoz

PRO-MIX PROTEIN	SUMACAL	GLUCEMIA
14.4 kcal/g	19 cal T	1
—	Maltodextrin	Hydrolyzed cornstarch, fructose
Whey protein	—	Sodium and calcium caseinates
—	—	Hi-oleic Safflower oil, soy oil
4 g/T	—	42 (17%)
0.2 g/T	—	56 (33%)
0.2 g/T	5 gm/T	94 (50%)
—	—	120:1
30	680	375
0.4/0.8/T 0.5/1.05	0.2/T/-	40/40
15/T 13/T	—	704/704
—	—	1422
Unflavored	Unflavored	Unflavored
Powder	Powder	Liquid
Protein supplement	Carbohydrate supplement	Tube feeding for diabetics, Contains 14 g fiber L
Navaco	Mead-Johnson	Ross

FORMULAS AND SUPPLEMENTS—cont'd

PARTIALLY PRE-DIGESTED		
ISOTEN HN	**PEPTAMEN**	**VITAL HN**
1.2	1	1
Maltodextrin, fructose	Maltodextrin, starch	Hydrolyzed corn starch, sucrose
Delactosed lactalbumin	Hydrolyzed whey protein	Partially hydrolyzed whey & meat & soy, free amino acids
Partially hydrogenated soy oil, MCT	Sunflower oil, MCT, lecithin	Safflower oil, MCT, mono and diglycerides
68 (23%)	40 (16%)	42 (17%)
34 (25%)	39 (33%)	11 (9%)
156 (52%)	127 (51%)	185 (74%)
86:1	130:1	125:1
300	260	500
27/27	22/32	20/34
571/571	600/500	667/667
1770	2000	1500
Vanilla	Unflavored	Vanilla
Powder	Liquid	Powder
Tube feeding, high protein isotonic	Isotonic predigested formula with MCT oil	Tube feeding, elemental, low fat
Sandoz	Clintec	Ross

SPECIAL FORMULATIONS		
HEPATIC-AID II	**PULMOCARE**	**TRAVASORB RENAL**
1.1	1.5	1.35
Maltodextrin sucrose	Hydrolyzed corn starch, sucrose	Glucose oligosaccharides sucrose
Amino acids	Sodium and calcium caseinates	Essential and nonessential crystaline amino acids
Soybean oil, mono and diglycerides	Corn oil	MCT, sunflower oil
44 (15%)	63 (17%)	23 (7%)
36 (26%)	92 (55%)	18 (12%)
169 (57%)	106 (28%)	271 (81%)
340:1	125:1	362:1
560	490	590
<16/<6	57/48	negligible
—	1040/1040	negligible
—	947	2100
Chocolate, Eggnog	Vanilla	Apricot, Strawberry
Powder	Liquid	Powder
Liver formula	Used for COPD patients tube feeding, high fat	Renal formular oral supplement tube feeding
Oral supplement tube feeding 46% BCAA		
McGaw	Ross	Travenol

ENTERAL AND PARENTERAL NUTRITION*

Administration of Enteral Feedings

To determine the appropriate concentration of formula to initiate, a general rule is to start the product at a concentration of 300 mOsm/kg water to avoid hyperosmolar diarrhea.

The following are general rules for the administration of an enteral feeding (unless otherwise indicated):

1. Challenge the gastrointestinal tract with a normal saline solution at a rate of 50 ml/hr. Check residuals and gastric emptying hourly for 6 hours.
2. Initiate the formula at half strength at a rate of 50 ml/hr. The concentration of the formula should not exceed 300 mOsm to avoid hyperosmolar diarrhea.
3. Increase the rate by 25 ml an hour or every 12 hours until the desired rate is achieved.
4. Increase the strength every 12 hours *only after* the desired rate is achieved in gradations of one half to three fourths to full strength *as tolerated.*
5. Flush the feeding tube with 100 ml water every 4 hours if on continuous drip or after each feeding and delivery of oral medications.

TABLE 18-12.—MAINTENANCE FLUID ALLOWANCES

PATIENT AND AGE	FLUID (ml/kg)
Infant, under 1 year	100-120
Child, 1-10 years	60-80
Adolescent, 11-18 years	41-55
Adult, 19+ years	20-30

Modified from Segar (1972).
NOTE: For fever add 360 ml/degree centigrade/day.

TABLE 18-13.—T<small>UBE</small> F<small>EEDINGS</small>

Tube Feedings
Tube feedings should be used if possible before instituting parenteral hyperalimentation. Orders should include the following:
  Strength: Should approximate isotonic, if possible (300 mOsm).
  ml hr: Bolus = 300-400 ml every 4-6 hours, or give via pump as constant infusion
  Total volume and calories/24-hours:
    Calories should be 1800-3000/day (most formulas = 1 cal/ml)
    Most commercial products are vitamin enriched
    Water should be added for a total volume of at least 1 ml/kcal. A minimum of 2000-2500 ml/day should be provided

Recommended Parameters to Monitor
Weight: Weigh daily for 1 week, then once a week
Intake/output daily
Labs (initially, then every week):
  CBC
  Total protein
  Albumin
  BUN
  Sodium
  Potassium
  Glucose
  Urine for glucose and ketones (3 times a week)

TABLE 18-14.—COMPLICATIONS AND SUGGESTED TREATMENTS FOR FEEDING

COMPLICATION	POSSIBLE REASON	SUGGESTED TREATMENT
Electrolyte imbalance	Composition of formula. *Other causes such as diarrhea, renal failure, or fluid status*	Increase or decrease affected electrolytes
Dehydration	Administration of concentrated formulas. *Other causes such as diarrhea*	Correct any abnormal losses; provide increased free water; or adjust the formula to decrease renal solute load
Glucosuria	Increased carbohydrate load. *Other causes such as diabetes*	Decrease carbohydrate content of formula
Azotemia	High-protein formula Insufficient water to excrete waste products. *Other causes such as renal impairment, or GI bleeding*	Reduce amount of protein in formula. Increase free water for excretion
Diarrhea and/or cramping	Medications	Medications that can cause diarrhea are antibiotics, Maalox, KCL, and quinidine. Change to another agent if possible
	Tube placement too low in stomach, causing gastric distention with increased gastric emptying	Check tube placement by x-ray film and adjust as needed
	Liquid stools around impaction	Check for impaction. An enema may be indicated. Adequate water intake or a bulking agent should be used to prevent impaction
	Volume overload	Reduce flow rate. Add high-fiber formula (Enrich)
	Osmotic overload (especially with transpyloric feeding)	Dilute formula with water or reduce rate of administration or change to isotonic formula
	Decreased bulk	Switch to formula that provides more fiber. Add high-fiber formula (Enrich)
	Inadequate intestinal flora caused by antibiotic therapy	Administer 50:50 ratio of plain yogurt and sweet acidophilus milk at 50 ml/hr for 24 hours or lactobacillus crystals tid
	Lactose intolerance	Use lactose-free formula
	Fat malabsorption	Decrease fat content of feeding and/or use medium chain triglyceride oil
	Insufficient osmotic pressure for absorption as indicated by low serum albumin	Reduce enteral feeding and supplement with peripheral albumin or administer TPN until albumin is at least 2.5

From *Handbook of clinical dietetics*, New Haven, 1981, Yale University Press, p. A25.

COMPLICATION	POSSIBLE REASON	SUGGESTED TREATMENT
	Bacterial contamination	Change feeding container and administration tubing every 24 hours. Use clean technique when transferring formula. Hang time not > 4 hours
Constipation	Impaction	Check with rectal examination. Give patient a laxative or an enema
	Decreased bulk	Switch to formula that provides more fiber
	Insufficient free fluid	Increase free fluid administered with formula
	Medications that decrease intestinal motility	Change medications if possible or give stool softener, additional fluid, or laxative
	Decreased intestinal motility resulting from inactivity	Increase patient's activity or treat symptomatically
	Complete absorption of elemental formula, resulting in minimal waste products	Patient education and reassurance

TABLE 18-15.—Protocol for Initiating Central Parenteral Nutrition

I. Run basic parenteral nutrition solution without electrolytes as listed:
　500 ml of 50% dextrose with 500 ml of crystalline, amino acids 8.5%
II. Suggested additions to fluids (should be modified in accordance with lab data):

Na	40-50 mEq/L (as acetate or chloride)*
K	30-40 mEq/L (as acetate or chloride)*
$MgSO_4$	4-8 mEq/L
Ca	4-5 mEq/L (as gluconate)
PO_4	10-15 mEq/L (as sodium or potassium)
MVI_{12}	1 ampule/day
Zn	4 mg/day
Cu	2 mg/day (liver function should be monitored)

III. IV rate
　40 ml/hr for the first 24 hours
　80 mg/hr for the next 24 hours
　120 ml/hr thereafter
　May be increased as tolerated up to 250 ml/hr, on physician's order.
　Do not increase IV rate if you get behind
IV. IM medications
　10 mg vitamin K weekly or as indicated by prothrombin time
V. Parameters to watch
　Accurate input/output
　Finger-stick glucose 3-4 times a day
　Urine for sugar and acetone every 6 hours; call if greater than 2+
　Orders for sliding scale insulin
　Urine for specific gravity
　Weigh daily

Modified from the Department of Dietetics, Miami Valley Hospital: *Miami Valley Hospital handbook of nutrition,* Dayton, Ohio, 1983, pp. 38-40.
*Exclusive use of chloride may result in hyperchloremic metabolic acidosis.

Continued.

TABLE 18-15.—PROTOCOL FOR INITIATING CENTRAL PARENTERAL NUTRITION—cont'd

VI. Lab studies

	During First 7 Days or When Patient is Ill or Unstable	After First 7 Days and When Patient is Stable
Electrolytes	Daily	3 times weekly
Plasma osmolarity	Daily	3 times weekly
Glucose	Daily	3 times weekly
Prothrombin time	Initially	Weekly
Chemistry profile (BUN, proteins, calcium phosphorus, uric acid, SGOT)	3 times weekly	Weekly
Mg^{2+}	3 times weekly	Weekly
Ammonia	2 times weekly	Weekly
Blood pH	2 times weekly	Weekly
CBC	Weekly	Weekly
Transferrin	Weekly	Weekly
Ferritin	Weekly	Weekly
Zinc	Weekly	Weekly

VII. Insulin

Human regular insulin given either subcutaneously or in the intravenous solution is indicated in the following cases:

Known diabetes mellitus

Elderly patients (5-25 U)

Pancreatic disorders

Posttraumatic period when insulin response is depressed

Critically ill, nutritionally depleted patients in whom positive caloric balance is deemed urgent for survival

VIII. Catheter care (central line)

Change IV tubing daily

Change dressing Monday, Wednesday, and Friday:

Use antiseptic ointment

Dressing must be occlusive

Do not give medications, draw blood, or measure CVP through central catheter unless double lumen catheter is utilized

IX. Intravenous fat emulsion 10% or 20%

Occasional infusions may be necessary to prevent essential fatty acid deficiency

When used as a caloric supplement, 500 ml may be infused daily

Cautious administration is recommended if hepatic dysfunction, blood dyscrasia, or a respiratory disorder exists

X. Discontinuing hyperalimentation

It is recommended that hyperalimentation be tapered over 24-48 hours before cessation

If central hyperalimentation is suddenly discontinued, a peripheral IV of D_5W should be started and the patient observed for signs of hypoglycemia

TABLE 18-16.—METABOLIC PROBLEMS ASSOCIATED WITH TOTAL PARENTERAL NUTRITION

PROBLEM	DIAGNOSIS	POSSIBLE CAUSES	TREATMENT
Glucose metabolism			
Hyperglycemia	Increased blood sugar Glycosuria	Excessive rate of infusion Inadequate insulin	Adjust rate of infusion Administer regular insulin
Hyperosmolar nonketotic coma	Increased blood sugar Increased serum and urine osmolality Glycosuria Coma	Excessive total glucose load or rate of infusion: inadequate insulin, glucocorticoids, latent diabetes, sepsis, pancreatic disease, acute or chronic renal failure	Appropriate fluids and insulin therapy
Ketoacidosis in the diabetic patient	Increased blood sugar Acidosis Ketones	Inadequate endogenous insulin response; inadequate exogenous insulin therapy	Appropriate fluids and insulin
Postinfusion hypoglycemia	Confusion Coma Decreased blood sugar	Unusual in nondiabetic patient; seen in patients with liver depleted of glycogen who have been in severe negative nitrogen balance Persistence of endogenous insulin production by stimulated islet cells	Gradually taper glucose infusion before termination

Modified from Cannon J, Welsh J, Whang R: Gastrointestinal system and nutrition. In Papper S, ed: *Manual of medical care of the surgical patient,* Boston, 1981, Little, Brown, pp. 74-76.

Continued.

TABLE 18-16.—METABOLIC PROBLEMS ASSOCIATED WITH TOTAL PARENTERAL NUTRITION—cont'd

PROBLEM	DIAGNOSIS	POSSIBLE CAUSES	TREATMENT
Amino acid metabolism	Hyperchloremic metabolic acidosis Increased serum chloride Acidosis	Excessive chloride and monohydrochloride content of certain crystalline amino acid solutions	Provide a portion of sodium and potassium as acetate salts rather than chlorides
	Hyperammonemia Increased blood ammonia Lethargy	Pediatric age group and patients with cirrhosis are at high risk. May be caused by relative arginine deficiency, which decreases effectiveness of urea cycle: ornithine, aspartic, and/or glutamic acid deficiencies have been implicated	Add 2 mM/kg/day of arginine glutamate or 3 mM/kg/day of arginine hydrochloride
	Prerenal azotemia Increased BUN	Excessive protein hydrolysate or amino acid infusion	Adjust rate of administration
Essential fatty acid deficiency	Dermatitis, hair loss, thrombocytopenia, poor wound healing Abnormal plasma lipid patterns, serum deficiency of phospholipid linoleic and/or arachidonic acids	Inadequate essential fatty acid administration; inadequate vitamin E administration	Infusion of IV fat emulsion Vitamin E administration
Calcium phosphorus metabolism	Hypophosphatemia 1. Decreased erythrocyte 2,3-DPG 2. Increased affinity of hemoglobin for oxygen 3. Aberrations of erythrocyte metabolism Decreased serum phosphorus	Inadequate phosphorus administration, redistribution of serum phosphorus into cells and bone	Add phosphorus to TPN regimen
	Hypocalcemia Decreased serum calcium Tetany, muscle spasm	Inadequate calcium administration	Add adequate calcuim to TPN regimen

Hypercalcemia	Increased serum calcium	Profound in patients who have phosphorus replacement without calcium replacement; Hypoalbuminemia; Excessive calcium administration with or without high doses of albumin; excessive vitamin D administration	Adjust calcium in TPN regimen; Adjust vitamin D dosage
Potassium imbalance			
Hypokalemia	Decreased serum potassium	Inadequate potassium intake relative to increased requirements or protein anabolism; diuresis	Potassium replacement
Hyperkalemia	Increased serum potassium	Excessive potassium administration particularly in metabolic acidosis and renal decompensation	Decreased potassium in the total parenteral nutrition regimen
Trace metal deficiencies			
Hypomagnesemia	Neuromuscular irritability; disorientation, tremor, and seizure; Low urinary excretion of magnesium	Inadequate magnesium administration relative to increased requirements for protein anabolism and glucose metabolism	10-20 mEq magnesium per day added to the TPN regimen
Zinc	Skin lesions, loss of hair, poor wound healing, diarrhea	Inadequate zinc administration	Zinc acetate
Copper	Anemia, leukopenia, hypoproteinemia	Inadequate copper replacement	Add copper to total parenteral nutrition
Vitamin deficiencies			
Folic acid deficiency	Anemia	Inadequate replacement	5 mg/week IV
Vitamin B_{12} deficiency			1000 µg/month IM
Vitamin K	Bleeding	Inadequate administration	10 mg/week IM or SQ

TREATMENT OF HYPERCHOLESTEROLEMIA

TABLE 18-17.—Mean Serum Total Cholesterol, Lipoprotein Cholesterol, and Triglyceride Levels, U.S. Population 1988 Through 1991, Aged 20 Years and Older

POPULATION GROUP	SERUM CHOLESTEROL, mg/dl (mmol/L)[a]				SERUM TRIGLYCERIDES[b] mg/dl (mmol/L)
	TOTAL	LDL	HDL	VLDL	
Age, Years					
≥20[c]	206 (5.33)	128 (3.31)	51 (1.32)	25 (0.65)	135 (1.52)
20-74[c]	205 (5.30)	128 (3.31)	51 (1.32)	25 (0.65)	134 (1.51)
Race/Ethnicity					
Mexican American	201 (5.20)	123 (3.18)	50 (1.29)	28 (0.72)	149 (1.68)
Men	202 (5.22)	124 (3.21)	47 (1.22)	28 (0.72)	155 (1.75)
Women	200 (5.17)	122 (3.15)	53 (1.37)	27 (0.70)	143 (1.61)
Non-Hispanic Black[d]	201 (5.20)	126 (3.26)	56 (1.45)	19 (0.49)	99 (1.12)
Men	199 (5.15)	126 (3.26)	53 (1.37)	20 (0.52)	105 (1.19)
Women	203 (5.25)	126 (3.26)	58 (1.50)	19 (0.49)	95 (1.07)
Non-Hispanic White[d]	207 (5.35)	129 (3.34)	51 (1.32)	25 (0.65)	138 (1.56)
Men	206 (5.33)	132 (3.41)	46 (1.19)	27 (0.70)	149 (1.68)
Women	208 (5.38)	126 (3.26)	56 (1.45)	24 (0.62)	127 (1.43)
Race/Sex[e]					
Black men	199 (5.15)	126 (3.26)	53 (1.37)	20 (0.52)	105 (1.19)
Black women	203 (5.25)	126 (3.26)	58 (1.50)	19 (0.49)	95 (1.07)
White men	206 (5.33)	132 (3.41)	46 (1.19)	27 (0.70)	149 (1.68)
White women	208 (5.38)	126 (3.26)	55 (1.42)	24 (0.62)	129 (1.46)

Sex/Age, Years[c]

Sex/Age, Years[c]					
Men					
≥20	205 (5.30)	131 (3.39)	47 (1.22)	26 (0.67)	143 (1.61)
20-34	189 (4.89)	120 (3.10)	47 (1.22)	22 (0.57)	112 (1.26)
35-44	207 (5.35)	134 (3.47)	46 (1.19)	26 (0.67)	141 (1.59)
45-54	218 (5.64)	138 (3.57)	47 (1.22)	29 (0.75)	199 (2.25)
55-64	221 (5.72)	142 (3.67)	46 (1.19)	30 (0.78)	164 (1.85)
65-74	218 (5.64)	141 (3.65)	45 (1.16)	31 (0.80)	159 (1.80)
≥75	205 (5.30)	132 (3.41)	47 (1.22)	26 (0.67)	134 (1.51)
Women					
≥20	207 (5.35)	126 (3.26)	56 (1.45)	24 (0.62)	126 (1.42)
20-34	185 (4.78)	110 (2.84)	56 (1.45)	19 (0.49)	101 (1.14)
35-44	195 (5.04)	117 (3.03)	54 (1.40)	21 (0.54)	113 (1.28)
45-54	217 (5.61)	132 (3.41)	57 (1.47)	24 (0.62)	126 (1.42)
55-64	237 (6.13)	145 (3.75)	56 (1.45)	30 (0.78)	168 (1.90)
65-74	234 (6.05)	147 (3.80)	56 (1.45)	29 (0.75)	155 (1.75)
≥75	230 (5.95)	147 (3.80)	57 (1.47)	28 (0.72)	157 (1.77)

From the third National Health and Nutrition Examination Survey, 1988 through 1991.

[a] *LDL*, Low-density lipoprotein cholesterol; *HDL*, high-density lipoprotein cholesterol; *VLDL*, very low-density lipoprotein cholesterol. LDL was estimated from the equation: LDL Cholesterol = (Total Cholesterol − HDL) − (Triglycerides/5); VLDL was calculated as (Triglycerides/5). LDL and VLDL were calculated for persons in the morning fasting subsample who fasted 9 hours or more and whose triglyceride levels were ≤400 mg/dl (4.52 mmol/L). The sum of LDL, HDL, and VLDL may not equal the value for total cholesterol because of the approximation of LDL and VLDL using the above equation.

[b] Persons in the morning fasting sample who fasted 9 hours or more.

[c] Includes race/ethnic groups not shown separately.

[d] All Hispanic persons were excluded.

[e] Includes Hispanic persons.

TABLE 18-18,A.—Cholesterol-Lowering Drugs

	CHOLESTYRAMINE (Questran)	NIACIN	GEMFIBROZIL (Lopid)	PROBUCOL (Lorelco)
Actions	↑ Removal of LDL	Lowers all forms; ↑ HDL	↓ VLDL and ↑ HDL	↓ LDL and total cholesterol
Dose	4 g bid	100 mg tid, up to 3 g tid	300 mg bid initially, then 600 mg bid	250 mg bid initially, then 500 mg bid
Adverse effect	Constipation and bloating	Flushing, pruritus, GI distress	Mild GI distress, increase oral anticoag. eff.	Diarrhea; prolonged QT interval

Modified from Choice of cholesterol-lowering drugs, *Med Lett* 35(891):19, 1994.

TABLE 18-18,B.—HMG-Co Cholesterol-Lowering Drugs*

	LOVASTATIN (Mevacor)	FLUVASTATIN (Lescol)	SIMVASTATIN (Zocor)	PRAVASTATIN (Pravachol)
Dose	20-80 mg	20-40 mg	5-40 mg	10-40 mg
Adverse effects	Severe myopathy (rare), rash, headache	Dyspepsia, headaches	Headaches, GI distress	GI distress, headaches

*Action: Lowering LDL and total cholesterol.

TABLE 18-19.—Components of Diets Recommended for Cholesterol Reduction

	STEP 1 DIET*	STEP 2 DIET†
Total fat	<30% total calories	<30% total calories
Saturated fat	<10% total calories	<7% total calories
Polyunsaturated fat	<10% total calories	<10% total calories
Monounsaturated fat	10%-15% total calories	10%-15% total calories
Carbohydrates	50%-60% total calories	50%-60% total calories
Protein	10%-20% total calories	10%-20% total calories
Cholesterol	<300 mg/day	<200 mg/day
Total calories	As necessary to achieve and maintain desirable weight	

From Griffin GC, Castelli WP: *Postgrad Med* 84(3):56, 1988, as modified from National Cholesterol Education Program: *Arch Intern Med* 148:36, 1988.
*Step 1 diet recommended for patients with cholesterol >240 mg/dl or >200 mg/dl if high risk for CAD.
†Step 2 diet recommended if step 1 ineffective or is used by high-risk patients with total cholesterol >240 mg/dl.

TABLE 18-20.—Risk Status Based on Presence of CHD Risk Factors Other than Low-Density Lipoprotein Cholesterol*

Positive Risk Factors

Age, years

  Male ≥45

  Female ≥55 or premature menopause without estrogen replacement therapy

Family history of premature CHD (definite myocardial infarction or sudden death before 55 years of age in father or other male first-degree relative, or before 65 years of age in mother or other female first-degree relative)

Current cigarette smoking

Hypertension (blood pressure ≥140/90 mm Hg,† or taking antihypertensive medication)

Low HDL cholesterol (<35 mg/dl† [0.9 mmol/L])

Diabetes mellitus

Negative Risk Factor‡

High HDL cholesterol (≥60 mg/dl [1.6 mmol/L])

From Griffin GC, Castelli WP: *Good fat bad fat: how to lower your cholesterol and beat the odds of a heart attack,* 1988, Fisher Books.

*High risk, defined as a net of two or more coronary heart disease (CHD) risk factors, leads to more vigorous intervention. Age (defined differently for men and women) is treated as a risk factor because rates of CHD are higher in the elderly than in the young, and in men than in women of the same age. Obesity is not listed as a risk factor because it operates through other risk factors that are included (hypertension, hyperlipidemia, decreased high-density lipoprotein [HDL] cholesterol, and diabetes mellitus), but it should be considered a target for intervention. Physical inactivity is similarly not listed as a risk factor, but it too should be considered a target for intervention, and physical activity is recommended as desirable for everyone.

†Confirmed by measurements on several occasions.

‡If the HDL cholesterol level is ≥60 mg/dl (1.6 mmol/L), subtract one risk factor (because high HDL cholesterol levels decrease CHD risk).

TABLE 18-21.—Initial Classification Based on Total Cholesterol and HDL Cholesterol Levels*

CHOLESTEROL LEVEL	INITIAL CLASSIFICATION
Total Cholesterol	
<200 mg/dl (5.2 mmol/L)	Desirable blood cholesterol
200-239 mg/dl (5.2-6.2 mmol/L)	Borderline-high blood cholesterol
≥240 mg/dl (6.2 mmol/L)	High blood cholesterol
HDL Cholesterol	
<35 mg/dl (0.9 mmol/L)	Low HDL cholesterol

From Summary of the NCEP adult treatment panel II report *JAMA* 269(23):3017, 1993.
*HDL, High-density lipoprotein.

TABLE 18-22.—Treatment Decisions Based on LDL Cholesterol Level

PATIENT CATEGORY	INITIATION LEVEL	LDL GOAL
Dietary Therapy		
Without CHD and with fewer than two risk factors	≥160 mg/dl (4.1 mmol/L)	<160 mg/dl (4.1 mmol/L)
Without CHD and with two or more risk factors	≥130 mg/dl (3.4 mmol/L)	<130 mg/dl (3.4 mmol/L)
With CHD	>100 mg/dl (2.6 mmol/L)	≤100 mg/dl (2.6 mmol/L)
Drug Treatment		
Without CHD and with fewer than two risk factors	≥190 mg/dl (4.9 mmol/L)	<160 mg/dl (4.1 mmol/L)
Without CHD and with two or more risk factors	≥160 mg/dl (4.1 mmol/L)	<130 mg/dl (3.4 mmol/L)
With CHD	≥130 mg/dl (3.4 mmol/L)	≤100 mg/dl (2.6 mmol/L)

From Summary of the NCEP adult treatment panel II report, *JAMA,* 269(23):3020, 1993.
LDL, Low-density lipoprotein; *CHD,* coronary heart disease.

TABLE 18-23.—SATURATED FAT AND CHOLESTEROL IN COMMON FOODS

FOOD	SATURATED FAT (g)	CHOLESTEROL (mg)
Bread (most varieties, per slice)	0.2	0
Bun or roll	0.5	0
Butter (1 T)	7	30
Margarine (1 T)	2	0
Soft diet margarine (1 T)	1	0
Angelfood cake	0	0
White cake with frosting	3	20
Cream cheese (1 oz)	5	30
Cheese (1 oz)	6	30
Weight Watchers Cheese Product (1 oz)	<1	2
Donut	5	20
Oatmeal (without milk) (1 c)	0.4	0
Egg custard (1 c)	7	275
Instant pudding (with skim milk) (1 c)	0.3	0
Egg	1.7	275
Egg yolk	1.7	275
Egg white	0	0
Egg Beaters egg substitute	0	0
Spaghetti (plain)	Trace	0
Potato (baked, plain)	0	0
French fries (1 order)	7	15
Homogenized milk (1 c)	5	30
Nonfat skim milk (1 c)	0.3	Trace
Creamy yogurt (1 c)	5	30
Nonfat yogurt (1 c)	0.3	Trace
Olive oil (1 T)	2	0
Canola oil (1 T)	1	0
Peanut oil (1 T)	2.3	0
Salad dressing (1 T)	1.5	Trace
Poultry (3 oz light meat, skinless)	1	70
Fried chicken nuggets (9 pieces)	14	125
Ice cream (1 c)	9	60
Blended fruit ice	0	0
Nonfat frozen yogurt (1 c)	0.3	Trace
Salmon (coho) (3 oz)	1	35
Ground beef (3 oz, 27% fat)	7	80
Extra-lean beef (3 oz)	4	50
Cream soups (1 c)	5	20
Vegetable soup (1 c)	0.3	0
Vegetables	0	0
Fruits	0	0
Beans, rice, legumes (1 c)	Trace	0

From Griffin GC, Castelli WP: *Good fat bad fat: how to lower your cholesterol and beat the odds of a heart attack,* Tucson, Ariz, 1988, Fisher Books.

T, Tablespoon; *c,* cup.

EATING DISORDERS

TABLE 18-24.—Signs or Behaviors Suggestive of an Eating Disorder

- Commenting repeatedly about being or feeling fat, and asking questions such as "Do you think I'm fat?" when weight is below average
- Reaching a weight that is below the ideal competitive weight set for that athlete and continuing to lose weight even during the off-season
- Eating secretively, a behavior that may be noted by finding food wrappers in the locker room or locker, or observing an athlete sneaking food from the training table
- Repeatedly disappearing immediately after eating, especially if a large amount of food was eaten
- Appearing nervous or agitated if something prevents him or her from being alone shortly after eating
- Losing and/or gaining extreme amounts of weight
- Complaining frequently of constipation
- Exhibiting excessive flatulence and/or dyspepsia

From Reimers KJ, Grandjean AC, Vanderhoof JA: The Center for Human Nutrition, Omaha, Nebraska.

19 *Endocrine Disorders*

Charles W. Smith, Jr.

DIABETES MELLITUS

TABLE 19-1.—THE DIAGNOSIS OF DIABETES MELLITUS

CONDITION	FASTING SERUM GLUCOSE	2-HOUR POSTPRANDIAL SERUM GLUCOSE
Normal	<115 mg/dl	<140 mg/dl
Impaired glucose tolerance	115-139 mg/dl	140-200 mg/dl and 30, 60, or 90 min sample was >200 mg/dl
Diabetes mellitus	>140 mg/dl on two or more occasions	>200 mg/dl
Gestational diabetes	>105 mg/dl	at 1 hour, >190 mg/dl at 2 hours, >165 mg/dl at 3 hours, >145 mg/dl

Modified from Stein JH, ed: *Internal Medicine*, 1994, Mosby.

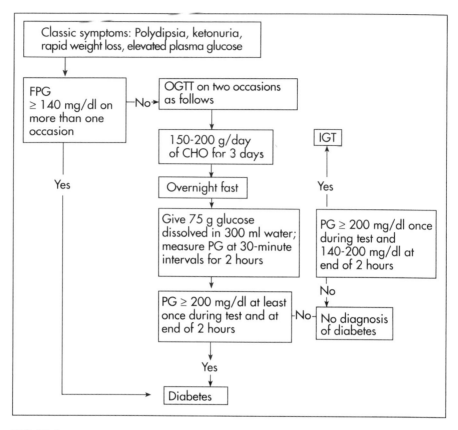

FIG 19-1.

Diagnosis of diabetes. *FPG,* Fasting plasma glucose; *OGTT,* oral glucose tolerance test; *CHO,* carbohydrates; *PG,* plasma glucose; *IGT,* impaired glucose tolerance. (From Bartels DW: Diabetes Mellitus. In Pharmacotherapy self-assessment program, *Module 5: nephrology, endocrinology, immunology,* 1993, p. 149.)

TABLE 19-2.—INSULIN PREPARATIONS

DRUG	DOSAGE			ADVERSE REACTIONS / COMMENTS
	Onset (hr)	Peak (hr)	Duration (hr)	
Insulin				
Rapid				
Regular insulin	0.5-1	2-4	5-7	Only regular insulin can be given IV
Insulin zinc, prompt (Semilente, Semitard)	1-2	4-6	12-16	Human insulin is least antigenic and is the agent of choice for patients with insulin allergy, insulin resistance, all pregnant patients, or intermittent therapy
Intermediate				
Isophane (NPH)	1-1.5	6-14	24+	Pure pork is less antigenic than beef; most insulins available in beef plus pork, purified pork, or purified beef or human form
Insulin zinc (Lente, Lentard)	1-2.5	6-14	24+	Patient should not change order of mixing or change brands without careful monitoring
Long-Acting				
Protamine zinc (PZI)	4-8	14-24	36+	When mixing insulin, regular insulin should be drawn up first; once mixed, these are stable for 30 days (90 days if refrigerated)
Ultralente	4-8	18-24	36+	Complete mixing of regular and NPH insulin takes 15 minutes and regular with Lente takes 15 minutes to 24 hours

TABLE 19-3. —Initiation of Insulin Treatment

Education
Must include injection techniques, characteristics of insulin, monitoring urine
and/or blood sugar, diet, and importance of weight control and exercise

Hospitalization
Indicated for ketoacidosis, severe hyperglycemia (>300-350), infection, or pregnancy

Insulin Dose and Frequency (see Table 19-2)
1. NIDD (type II): Give insulin only to control symptoms. Patients usually do
   well with a single AM dose of NPH.
2. IDD (type I): Usually requires split dose; two thirds of total dose is given in
   the AM, one third in the PM; tight control may require additional regular insulin.
3. Adjustments should be made every 3-7 days. Look for patterns of urine or
   blood sugar responses, not single daily fluctuations. Limit dose increments to
   5 U initially, decreasing to 2- to 3-U increments as better control is attained.

TABLE 19-4.—Approach to Control Problems in Diabetes Mellitus

PROBLEM	TREATMENT
Fasting hyperglycemia	Give evening dose of NPH (5-10 U) and reduce AM dose
Late morning hyperglycemia	Add regular (~5 U) to AM dose
Late evening hyperglycemia	Add regular (~5 U) before dinner (give bed-time snack)
Hypoglycemia (if unexplained by exercise or meal delay)	Reduce insulin in 2- to 5-U decrements

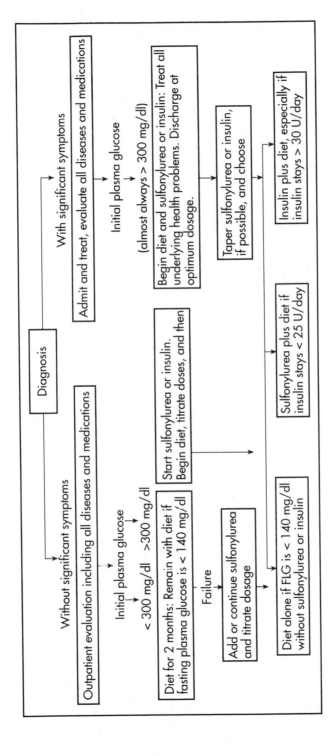

FIG 19-2.
Management of type II diabetes. (From Bartels DW: Diabetes Mellitus. In Pharmacotherapy self-assessment program, *Module 5: nephrology, endocrinology, immunology* 1993, p. 152.)

TABLE 19-5.—INSULIN RESISTANCE

Definition

Requirement of >200 U/day for 2 days without ketoacidosis

Possible Causes

Obesity, infection, steroid treatment (or Cushing's syndrome), or insulin-binding antibodies (most common)

Treatment Approaches

1. Change to Humulin.
2. Use multiple doses of regular, not intermediate or long-acting insulin.
3. Prescribe prednisone, 60 mg/day PO; taper as insulin requirements decrease.
4. Use sulfated insulin (modified for less antigenicity).

TABLE 19-6.—COMPARISON OF ORAL SULFONYLUREA DRUGS

DRUG	DURATION OF ACTION (hours)	TYPICAL DAILY DOSAGE RANGE (mg)	DOSES PER DAY	EQUIVALENT THERAPEUTIC DOSE (mg)	COST*	GENERIC COST*	HEPATIC METABOLITES	EXCRETION	SIDE EFFECTS (%)	HYPOGLYCEMIC REACTIONS (%)
First-Generation										
Tolbutamide (Orinase)	6-12	500-2,000	2-3	1000	$14.40	$2.70	Inactive	Urine	3	<1
Acetohexamide (Dymelor)	12-24	250-1,500	1-2	500	$12.40	$11.90	Very active	Urine	4	1
Tolazamide (Tolinase)	12-24	100-1,000	1	250	$15.00	$6.45	Inactive and weakly active	Urine	4	1
Chlorpropamide (Diabinese)	24-72	100-500	1	250	$19.20	$1.85	Inactive and weakly active	Urine	8	4-6
Second-Generation										
Glipizide (Glucotrol)	12-24	2.5-40	1-2	10	$16.70	—	Inactive	Urine (88%) Feces (12%)	5	2-4
Glyburide (DiaBeta, Glynase Prestab, Micronase)	16-24	1.25-20	1-2	5	$14.70	—	Inactive and moderately active	Urine (50%) Feces (50%)	7	4-6

Modified from Alexander TAL: Oral hypoglycemic agents in the treatment of type II diabetes, *Am Fam Physician* 48(6):1090, 1993.
*Average wholesale price per month for equivalent therapeutic doses based on average prices from Physicians' Generix, Smithtown, N.Y., Data Pharmaceutica Inc., 1992.
Modified from Jackson JE, and Bressler R, Gerich JE: *Physician's guide to noninsulin (type II) diabetes: diagnosis and treatment*, ed 2, Alexandria, VA, 1988, American Diabetes Association.

TABLE 19-7.—Treatment of Diabetic Ketoacidosis

Fluids
1 L/hr of normal saline. Decrease rate according to patient response (begin 5% dextrose when glucose is 250-300 mg/dl)

IV Insulin
0.33 U/kg as IV bolus, then 10 U/hr, prepared as follows:
    100 U regular insulin, diluted with 500 ml of 0.45% NaCl
    Run 100 ml through IV line to allow insulin adsorption to tubing
This makes a solution of 0.2 U/ml. A rate of 50 ml/hr = 10 U/hr

IM Insulin
Can be used as an acceptable alternative to constant infusion, as follows:
    Give 20 U of regular insulin as IV bolus, plus 10-15 units IM
    Give 5-10 U IM every hour
    Blood sugar level (with either method) should fall by 60-120 mg/100 ml/hr

Electrolytes
Na^+: As 0.9% NaCl (1 L/hr)
K^+: Hold if urine output <30 ml/hr; give 40 mEq/L KCl to a total of 100-300 mEq in the first 24 hours
PO_4^-: Follow phosphate levels as glucose falls; if necessary, give 40-60 mEq/L as potassium phosphate instead of KCl if phosphorus is less than 3 mg/dl
HCO_3^-: Give 80-100 mEq in 100 ml of 0.45% NaCl over 1 hour if arterial pH is 7.1 or less

Measurements (use flow sheet)
Vital signs, mental status, fluid intake and output every 30 minutes initially, then every 1-2 hours as indicated
Glucose, sodium, potassium, bicarbonate, and anion gap hourly initially then every 2-4 hours as indicated
Serum ketones (with Acetest Tabs) every 2-3 hours
Creatinine, BUN, Ca^{2+}, arterial blood gas, phosphorus, osmolality, ECG, chest x-ray examination, urinalysis and culture, and blood cultures should be obtained initially and repeated only if indicated

Tubes
Endotracheal if patient is comatose
Foley only if unable to void or otherwise unable to determine output
Nasogastric tube if distention, nausea, or vomiting occurs
CVP should be placed if patient is elderly or debilitated

TABLE 19-8.—Diabetic Management of Surgical Patients

Sliding scales based on urines should *not* be used

If NIDD (type II) and diet is controlled, follow preoperative and postoperative blood sugar and treat only if values are above 300 mg/dl

If NIDD (type II) and patient is taking an oral agent, discharge on day of surgery and if:

   Minor surgery: Treat only if BS > 300 mg/dl

   Major surgery: Give 15-20 U of NPH on day of surgery plus 5% dextrose at 100-125 ml/hr. Give additional insulin as required

If on insulin, begin 5% dextrose preoperatively, and give one half usual daily dose as subcutaneous NPH. Run IV at 125-150 ml/hr, and give additional regular insulin as indicated by frequent (~every 2-3 hours) evaluation of blood sugar levels

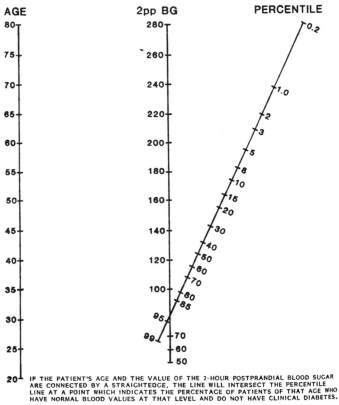

IF THE PATIENT'S AGE AND THE VALUE OF THE 2-HOUR POSTPRANDIAL BLOOD SUGAR ARE CONNECTED BY A STRAIGHTEDGE, THE LINE WILL INTERSECT THE PERCENTILE LINE AT A POINT WHICH INDICATES THE PERCENTAGE OF PATIENTS OF THAT AGE WHO HAVE NORMAL BLOOD VALUES AT THAT LEVEL AND DO NOT HAVE CLINICAL DIABETES.

FIG 19-3.

Nomogram for interpreting 2-hour postprandial blood sugar in relation to patient age. (Modified from *Patient Care,* Darien, Conn, June 15, 1974, Patient Care Communications.)

The Family Practice Desk Reference

TABLE 19-9.— Factors Influencing Urinary Albumin Excretion

Increases Excretion
Exercise
Upright posture
Poor glycemic control
Inflammatory conditions
Hypertension
Decreases Excretion
Steroids
Good glycemic control
Smoking cessation
Antihypertensive therapy
Angiotensin converting enzyme inhibitors

From Konen JC, Shihabi ZK: Microalbuminuria and diabetes mellitus, *Am Fam Physician* 48(8):1423, 1993.

TABLE 19-10.—Conditions in which Microalbuminuria Commonly Occurs

Renal Disorders
Diabetes
Preeclampsia
Immune-related disorders: Systemic lupus erythematosus, IgA nephropathy, Wegener's granulomatosis, rheumatoid arthritis
Acute and chronic renal failure
Reactions to nephrotoxic drugs
Bence Jones proteinuria
Myoglobinuria/hemoglobinuria
Renal transplant

Nonrenal Disorders
Surgery
Anesthesia
Sickle cell disease
Hypertension
Atherosclerosis and infarction

From Konen JC, Shihabi ZK: Microalbuminuria and diabetes mellitus, *Am Fam Physician* 48(8):1422, 1993.

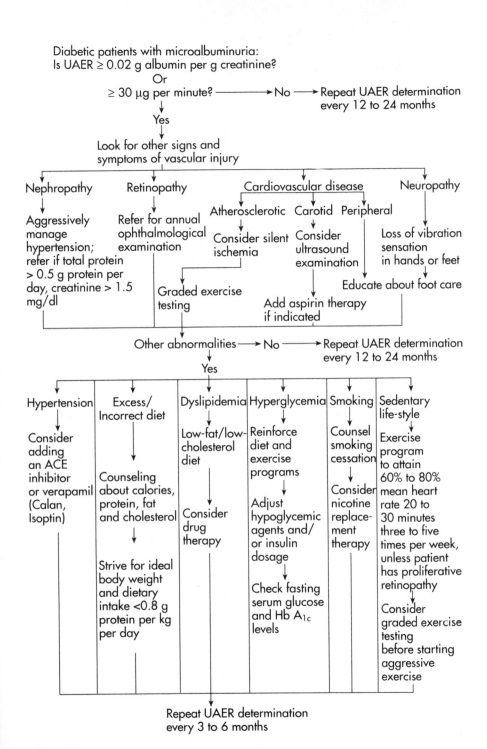

FIG 19-4.

Management of microalbuminuria in diabetic patients. *UAER*, Urinary albumin excretion rate or ratio; *ACE*, angiotensin converting enzyme. (From *Am Fam Physician*, 48(8):426.)

COMPLICATIONS OF DIABETES

TABLE 19-11.—PREVALENCE OF COMPLICATIONS IN PATIENTS WITH IDD

COMPLICATION	CUMULATIVE PREVALENCE (%)
Visual impairment	14
Blindness	16
Renal failure	22
Stroke	10
Amputation	12
Myocardial infarction	21
Median survival after diagnosis of IDD (yr)	36
Median age at death (yr)	49

Data are from Deckert T, Poulsen JE, Larsen M: and are based on 307 patients with IDD followed for at least 40 years (approximately 1933 to 1973).
From Nathan DM: Medical Progress, *N Engl J Med* 328(23):1677, 1993.

TABLE 19-12.—RISK OF MORBIDITY ASSOCIATED WITH ALL TYPES OF DIABETES IN THE UNITED STATES

VARIABLE	RELATIVE RISK*
Blindness	20
End-stage renal disease	25
Amputation	40
Myocardial infarction	2-5
Stroke	2-3

*Data are derived from Kannel WB, McGee DL: . . . National Diabetes Data Group.
Values shown are the relative risks for people with diabetes as compared with people without diabetes.
From Nathan DM: Medical Progress, *N Engl J Med* 328(23):1677, 1993.

TABLE 19-13.—TYPES, CLINICAL MANIFESTATIONS, AND TREATMENT OF DIABETIC NEUROPATHY

TYPE	SYMPTOMS	SIGNS	TREATMENT
Sensorimotor	Paresthesia (numbness and tingling in stocking and, less commonly, glove distribution); progresses to hypoesthesia	Decreased or absent reflexes, and decreased sensation to vibration and light touch; wasting of interosseous muscles with flexion (claw toe) deformity	None, other than foot care to prevent trauma and ulcers
	Painful neuropathy (rare); dysesthesia with lancinating or burning pain; may be accompanied by anorexia and depression	Same as above	Tricyclic antidepressant drugs, phenytoin, carbamazepine, or topical capsaicin; avoid narcotics (high potential for addiction)
Focal motor and compression	Weakness or loss of sensation in distribution of nerve	Cranial (III, IV, V, VI) or peripheral-nerve palsy; carpal tunnel syndrome, footdrop	Improves spontaneously in 2-12 months; surgical decompression for compression lesions

From Nathan DM: Medical progress, *N Engl J Med* 328(23):1679, 1993.

Continued.

TABLE 19-13.—Types, Clinical Manifestations, and Treatment of Diabetic Neuropathy—cont'd

TYPE	SYMPTOMS	SIGNS	TREATMENT
Autonomic gastrointestinal	Gastroparesis (early satiety, nausea, vomiting)		Metoclopramide, erythromycin
	Diabetic diarrhea (nocturnal, with incontinence)		Clonidine
Genitourinary	Impotence, retrograde ejaculation		Penile injections with papaverine, phentolamine, or prostaglandin (or a combination); vacuum or implantable devices
	Overflow incontinence		Bethanechol
Cardiac	Dizziness	Postural hypotension, resting tachycardia	Fludrocortisone, salt

TABLE 19-14.—Diagnosis of Diabetic Complications

COMPLICATION AND DIAGNOSTIC METHOD	COMMENTS
Retinopathy	
Ophthalmoscopy	
Direct	Best results when eyes are dilated; even
Indirect	when eyes are examined by retinal specialists, sensitivity for important lesions may be low
Fundus photography	
Seven-field stereoscopic	Most accurate and sensitive
Nonmydriatic 45-degree	Is as good as ophthalmologist's examination; may be more accurate if eyes dilated
Fluorescein angiography	More sensitive for rare isolated microaneurysms (usually clinically unimportant) than 7-field photography
Nephropathy	
Urinalysis	
Spot test (dipstick or radioimmunoassay)	Semiquantitative for overt proteinuria (>0.5 g/L; approximately 300 mg of albumin/L); new reagent strips detect microalbuminuria and may be useful for screening; urinary microalbumin measurement (by radioimmunoassay) corrected for urinary creatinine excretion may be used for screening
24-Hour urine sample	Necessary to quantitate microalbuminuria, overt proteinuria, and glomerular filtration rate
Serum creatinine level	Crude index of glomerular filtration rate
Glomerular filtration rate	
Creatinine clearance	Less reliable at low glomerular filtration rate
Iothalamate I-125, other tracer methods	More accurate than creatinine clearance but generally not used in clinical setting
Neuropathy	
History, physical examination	Loss of Achilles tendon reflexes and vibratory sensation suggests a patient at risk for foot ulcer; foot-care instructions and special footwear may be required
Semiquantitative examination of sensory function	Electronic tuning fork, multimodal testing of sensory function not necessary other than in research setting
Electrophysiological studies	More sensitive for detection of peripheral neuropathy than physical examination, but clinical relevance not clear; may be useful in diagnosis of focal or compression neuropathy

*Measure serum prolactin and testosterone to rule out hormonal causes. Angiography to identify indicated.
From Nathan DM: Medical progress, *N Engl J Med* 328(23)1681, 1993.

Continued.

TABLE 19-14.—Diagnosis of Diabetic Complications—cont'd

COMPLICATION AND DIAGNOSTIC METHOD	COMMENTS
Autonomic testing	
Gastrointestinal (barium swallow or scan after ^{99}Tc-labeled meal)	May help diagnose delayed gastric emptying characteristic of gastroparesis
Impotence (tests for penile tumescence—e.g., penile plethysmography)*	May help separate organic from psychological causes
Cardiovascular (electrocardiography to examine variation in heart rate with respiration, Valsalva's maneuver, or other maneuvers)	Quantitative tests available, but clinical usefulness questionable

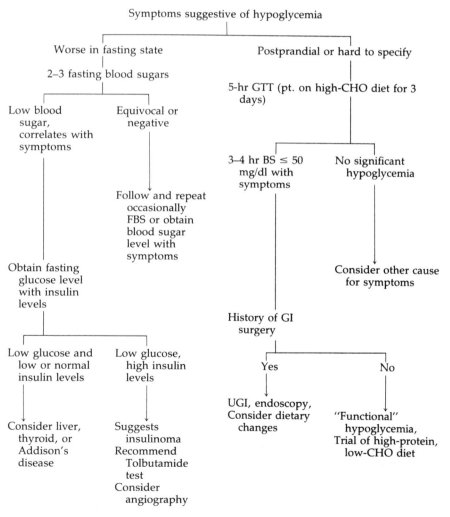

FIG 19-5.
Evaluation of hypoglycemia.

THYROID

TABLE 19-15.—COMMON TESTS OF THYROID FUNCTION

TEST	SUBSTANCE MEASURED	NORMAL VALUES	INDICATION	COMMENT
Serum T_4	Total thyroid hormone (99.97% bound)	5-12 ng/dl	Screening for thyroid disease	False-positive usually caused by increased TBG (see Table 19-16)
Free T_4	Unbound thyroid hormone	2 ng/dl	Confirmation of questionable case	Cumbersome assay, not very precise
T_3 Uptake	Relative saturation of thyroid-binding proteins	25%-35%	Combined with T_4 to give thyroid index	Useful as indirect measure of TBG
Free T_4 index (FT_4I)	Calculated product of T_4 and T_3 uptake	1-4 ng/dl	Screening for thyroid disease	Most useful single indicator of thyroid status
Serum T_3	Triiodothyronine concentration (bound and unbound)	115-190 ng/dl	Evaluation for "hyperthyroid" state, if thyroid index is normal	Often confused with T_3 uptake test; if positive diagnosis is "T_3 toxicosis"
Serum TSH	Total thyroid-stimulating hormone	2-11 µU/ml	Most useful screen for primary hypothyroidism	Use new high-sensitivity test
TRH	Capacity of pituitary to respond to thyrotropin releasing hormone	Raises TSH	Good test to resolve borderline cases	If no rise in TSH, hyperthyroid state exists

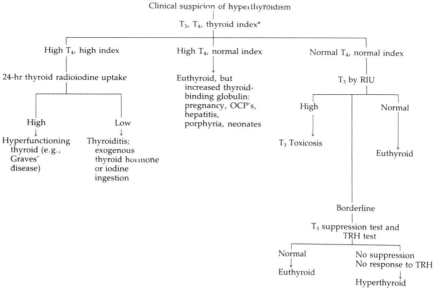

*Calculated as $T_4 \times \dfrac{T_3}{\text{Mean normal } T_3}$

Example: $T_4 = 8$
$T_3 = 36\%$ Thyroid index $= 8 \times \dfrac{36}{32} = 9$
$N1.\ T_3 = 32\%$

FIG 19-6.
Evaluation of hyperthyroidism.

TABLE 19-16.—THYROID-BINDING GLOBULINS

	INCREASED TBG	DECREASED TBG
Causes	Estrogens	Androgens
	Acute hepatitis	Chronic liver disease
	Genetic	Protein loss
	Porphyria	Genetic
	Neonates	
Effect on T_4	Increased	Decreased
Effect on T_3 uptake	Decreased	Increased
Effect on TSH	None	None

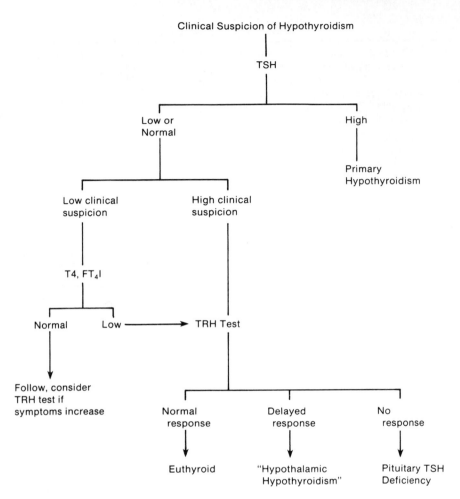

FIG 19-7.
Evaluation of hypothyroidism.

TABLE 19-17.—TRH TEST

The TRH test evaluates the pituitary-thyroid axis. It is a helpful test to resolve previously difficult clinical problems, such as the following:
 Borderline hypothyroidism with minimal elevation of TSH
 Clinical hypothyroidism with normal TSH
 Suspected "hypothalamic hypothyroidism"
 Borderline hyperthyroidism

Procedure
Draw baseline TSH.
Give 500 μg of TRH as IV bolus.
Draw TSH at 15-, 30-, 45-, and 60-minute intervals.
Interpretation: Baseline should double, peaking at 30 minutes
 Primary hypothyroid = High baseline and exaggerated response
 "Hypothalamic hypothyroid" = Delayed peak
 Pituitary failure = No response
 Hyperthyroid = No rise in TSH

Modified from Watts NB, Keffer JH: The thyroid gland. In *Practical endocrine diagnosis,* Philadelphia, 1978, Lea & Febiger.

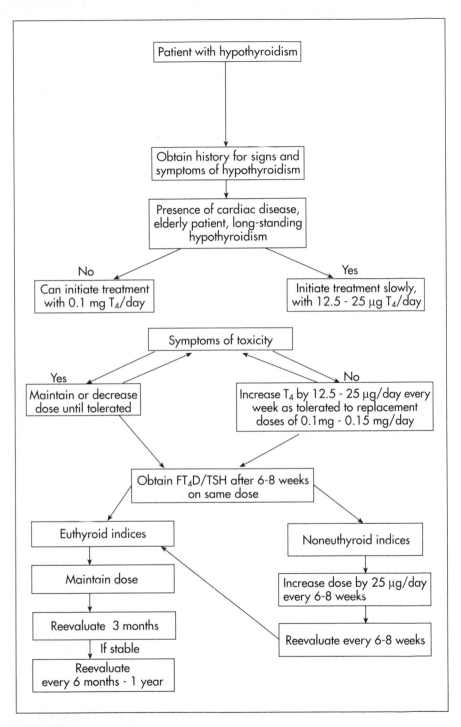

FIG 19-8.
Algorithm for management of hypothyroidism. (From Dong BJ: Thyroid and parathyroid disorders. In Herfindal ET, Gourley DR, Hart LL, eds. *Clinical pharmacy and therapeutics,* ed. 5, Baltimore, 1992, Williams & Wilkins, pp 267-306.)

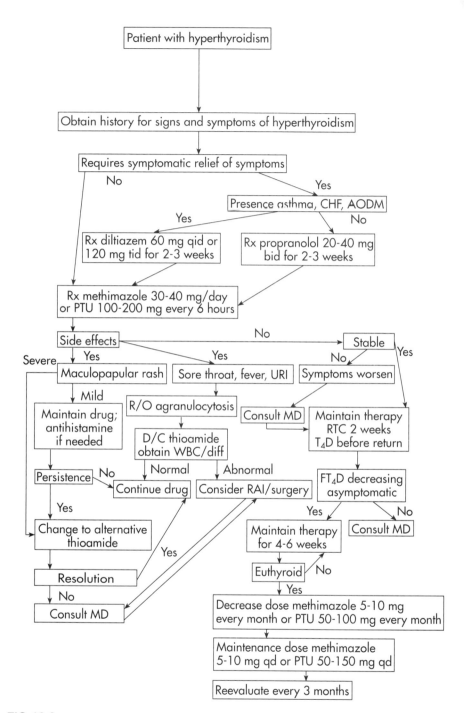

FIG 19-9.
Algorithm for management of hyperthyroidism. From Herfindal ET, Gourley DR, Hart LL, eds. *Clinical pharmacy and therapeutics*, ed. 5, Baltimore, 1992, Williams & Wilkins, pp. 267-306. *COPD,* Chronic obstructive pulmonary disease; *CHF,* congestive heart failure; *AODM,* adult-onset diabetes mellitus; *PTU,* propylthiouracil; *URI,* upper respiratory tract infection; *FT₄D,* free thyroxine by dialysis; *RTC,* return to clinic; *RAI,* radioactive iodine; *WBC/diff,* white blood cell count with differential; *R/O,* rule out; *D/C,* discontinue. (From Dong BJ: Thyroid Disorders. In Pharmacotherapy self-assessment program, *Module 5: nephrology, endocrinology, immunology,* 1993, p. 175.)

TABLE 19-18.—MANAGEMENT OF HYPERTHYROIDISM

METHOD	DRUG	DOSAGE	MECHANISM OF ACTION	TOXICITY	COMMENTS
Thioamides	Propylthiouracil (PTU) 50-mg tablets	100-200 mg every 6 hours initially, maintenance of 50-150 mg/day. Can be formulated for rectal administration	Blocks organification of hormone synthesis, also inhibits peripheral conversion of T_4 to T_3. Immunosuppressive?	Skin rashes, agranulocytosis, gastrointestinal symptoms, hepatitis	Poor remission rate of 20%-30%. Onset of 2-4 weeks. DOC in thyroid storm, pregnancy, and during lactation
	Methimazole (Tapazole 5- and 10-mg tablets	30-40 mg qd initially, maintenance of 5-10 mg/day. Can be formulated for rectal administration	Blocks organification of hormone synthesis. Immunosuppressive?	Same as PTU. Secreted in breast milk, teratogenic: scalp defects	Appears to have no cross-sensitivity to PTU with regard to rashes. Longer duration of action than PTU.
Iodides	Lugol's solution 8 mg iodide/drop Saturated solution of potassium iodide (SSKI) 50 mg/drop	6 mg iodide/day, although larger doses are given	Blocks release of hormone from gland; decreases vascularity of gland and increases the firmness, which facilitates easier removal of gland during surgery	Hypersensitivity reactions-rashes, rhinorrhea, parotid and submaxillary swelling	Can be used for symptomatic control of hyperthyroidism in patients taking thioamides, in thyroid storm, and as a preoperative adjunct. *Do not use prior to RAI.*

From Dong BJ: *Thyroid disorders.* In Carter BL et al, eds: *Pharmacotherapy self-assessment program,* Kansas City, 1993.

Continued.

TABLE 19-18.—Management of Hyperthyroidism—cont'd

METHOD	DRUG	DOSAGE	MECHANISM OF ACTION	TOXICITY	COMMENTS
Adrenergic antagonist (avoid those with ISA activity)	Propranolol (Inderal) 10-, 20-, 40-, 60-, 80-, 60-90-mg tablets, 1 mg/ml IV	20-40 mg PO every 6 hours	Blocks peripheral action of thyroid hormone; no effect on underlying disease state. Blocks T_4 to T_3 conversion peripherally	Bradycardia, congestive heart failure, asthma, inhibits hyperglycemic response to hypoglycemia	Immediate onset provides symptomatic relief while awaiting onset of action of thioamides RAI, or surgery.
	Diltiazem (Cardizem) 30-, 60-, 90-, 120-mg tablets, 60-, 90-, 120-mg SR tablets	60 mg PO qid or 120 mg tid		Hypotension, bradycardia, pedal edema	Alternative in patients unable to use β-blockers; i.e., asthma, diabetes.
Radioactive iodine	^{131}I	80 to 100 µCi/g thyroid tissue	Destruction of gland	Hypothyroidism, fear of malignancy, leukemia, and genetic damage	Slow onset of action approximately 2-4 weeks, full effects seen within 3-6 months
Surgery	Iodides, thioamides, or propranolol preoperative to induce relief of symptoms	5-10 drops/day of iodides for 10-14 days before surgery. See dosages for propranolol and thioamides	Total removal of gland surgical procedure of choice	Hypothyroidism, hypoparathyroidism, complications of surgery and anesthesia	Frequency of hypothyroidism indirectly proportional to gland remnant left
Iodinated contrast media	Ipodate, lopanoic acid	500 mg-1 g/day or 3 g every third day	Blocks T_4 to T_3 conversion; release of iodides. See iodides	Similar to iodides	Rapid onset of action; not for long-term use; effects not sustained

ADRENAL GLAND

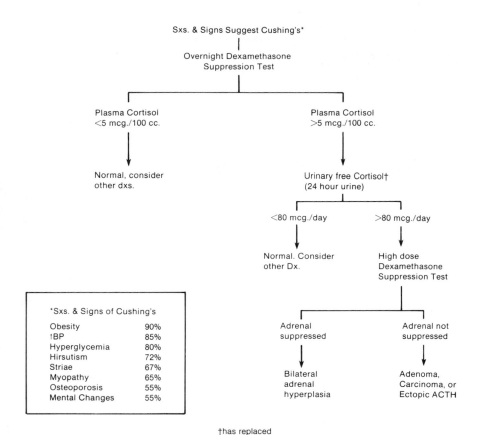

Sxs. & Signs Suggest Cushing's*

Overnight Dexamethasone
Suppression Test

Plasma Cortisol
<5 mcg./100 cc.

Plasma Cortisol
>5 mcg./100 cc.

Normal, consider
other dxs.

Urinary free Cortisol†
(24 hour urine)

<80 mcg./day   >80 mcg./day

Normal. Consider
other Dx.

High dose
Dexamethasone
Suppression Test

Adrenal
suppressed

Adrenal not
suppressed

Bilateral
adrenal
hyperplasia

Adenoma,
Carcinoma, or
Ectopic ACTH

*Sxs. & Signs of Cushing's	
Obesity	90%
↑BP	85%
Hyperglycemia	80%
Hirsutism	72%
Striae	67%
Myopathy	65%
Osteoporosis	55%
Mental Changes	55%

†has replaced
17-Keto & Hydroxysteroid
measurements

FIG 19-10.
Evaluation of Cushing's syndrome.

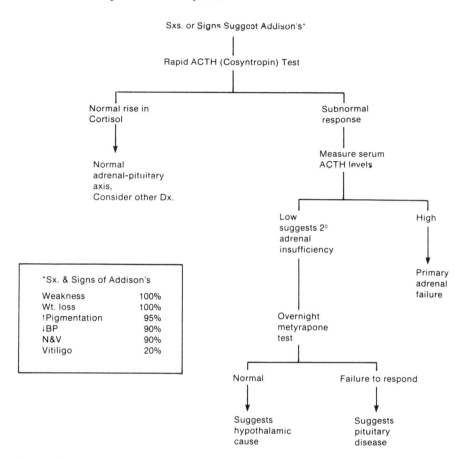

FIG 19-11.
Evaluation of Addison's disease.

TABLE 19-19.—Evaluation of Adrenal Function

Dexamethasone Suppression Test
Give dexamethasone 1 mg and a sedative at bedtime.
Draw fasting cortisol next AM.
Make sure sleep hasn't been disturbed.
Failure to suppress cortisol to <5 μg/100 ml suggests Cushing's syndrome.

High-Dose Dexamethasone Suppression Test
Collect daily 24-hour urine specimin for 4 days for free cortisol and creatinine (first 2 days are baseline measurements).
Measure plasma cortisol at 8 AM and 8 PM for diurnal variation (optional).
At 8 AM on day 3, start dexamethasone, 2 mg PO every 6 hours for 48 hours.
Measure plasma cortisol at 8 AM on day 5 (concludes test).
Plasma and urinary cortisol levels are suppressed in presence of bilateral hyperplasia but not in other conditions.

Rapid ACTH (Cosyntropin) Test
Measure baseline plasma cortisol.
Give 250 μg of cosyntropin (synthetic ACTH) after getting baseline cortisol value.
Obtain cortisol levels at 30 and 60 minutes after injection.
Normal = Rise in cortisol >70 μg/100 ml with a peak response of >18 μg/100 ml.

Overnight Metyrapone Test
Give 3 g of metyrapone as a single oral dose at bedtime with food (to delay absorption).
Measure plasma 11-deoxycortisol at 7 AM the next day.
Normal = >7 μg/100 ml rise in 11-deoxycortisol.

Furosemide Stimulation Test
Give Lasix, 60 mg PO in AM.
Maintain patient in upright posture for 5 hours.
Draw blood into iced tube for plasma renin.
Renovascular hypertensives = 5 times normal values. Normal value on "normal" sodium diet in supine position = 1.6 ng/ml/hr. (Suppressed values = half normal.)

TABLE 19-20.—Perioperative Steroid Replacement

DAYS	INTRAVENOUS HYDROCORTISONE	INTRAMUSCULAR HYDROCORTISONE	ORAL HYDROCORTISONE
Operation day	300 mg *plus*	50 mg preoperative 50 mg postoperative	—
Postoperative day			
1	200 mg *plus*	50 mg every 12 hours	—
2	150 mg *plus*	50 mg every 12 hours	—
3	100 mg *plus*	50 mg every 12 hours	—
4	—	50 mg every 12 hours *plus*	25 mg every 6 hours
5	—	25 mg every 12 hours *plus*	25 mg every 6 hours*
6	—	25 mg daily	
7	—	—	25 mg every 6 hours
8-10	—	—	25 mg every 8 hours
11-20	—	—	25 mg every 12 hours
21 or more	—	—	20 mg 8 AM 10 mg 4 PM

Modified from Tuck M: Adrenal disease. In Hershman JM, ed: *Management of endocrine disorders,* Philadelphia, 1980, Lea & Febiger.
*Add fludrocortisone, 0.05-0.2 mg orally daily. Adjust dose depending on blood pressure, body weight, and serum electrolytes.

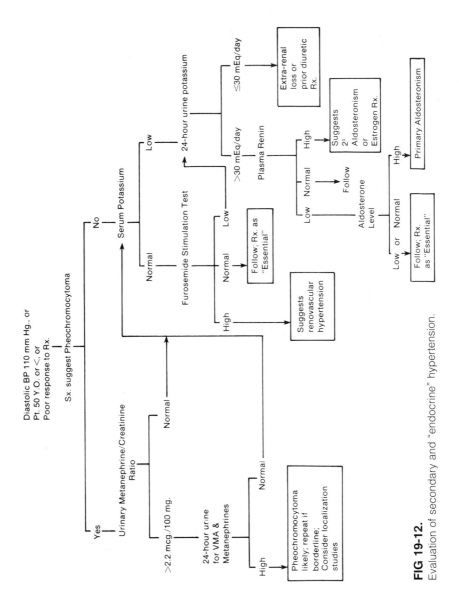

FIG 19-12.
Evaluation of secondary and "endocrine" hypertension.

GYNECOMASTIA

TABLE 19-21.—Conditions Associated with Gynecomastia

Physiological
Neonatal
Pubertal
Involutional

Pathological
Neoplasms
 Testicular (germ cell, Leydig's cell, or Sertoli's cell)
 Adrenal (adenoma or carcinoma)
 Ectopic production of human chorionic gonadotropin (especially lung, liver, and kidney cancer)
Primary gonadal failure
Secondary hypogonadism
Enzymatic defects of testosterone production*
Androgen-insensitivity syndromes*
True hermaphroditism*
Liver disease
Starvation, especially during the recovery phase
Renal disease and dialysis
Hyperthyroidism
Excessive extraglandular aromatase activity
Drugs
Idiopathic gynecomastia

From Braunstein GD: Current concepts, *N Engl J Med* 328(7):491, 1993.
*These conditions are usually associated with ambiguity of genitalia or deficient virilization.

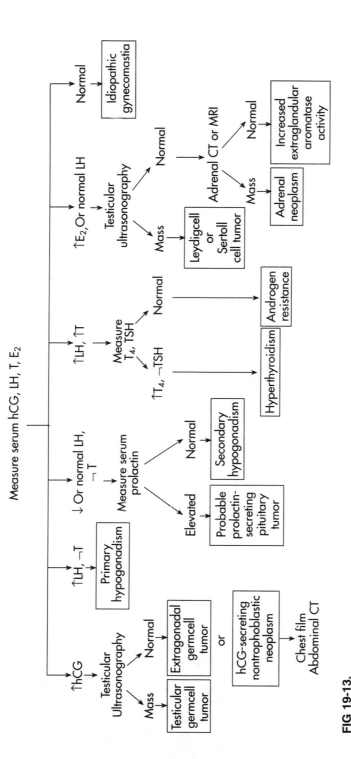

FIG 19-13.

Interpretation of serum hormone levels and recommendations for further evaluation of patients with gynecomastia. Diagnoses are shown in boxes. *LH,* luteinizing hormone; *hCG,* human chorionic gonadotropin; *T,* testosterone, *E₂,* estradiol; *T₄,* thyroxine; *TSH,* thyroid-stimulating hormone; *CT,* computed tomography; *MRI,* magnetic resonance imaging; ↑, increased; ↓, decreased. (From Braunstein: Current concepts, *N Engl J Med* 328(7):494, 1993.)

Normal Values, Calculations, and Equations

Barry L. Carter

TABLE A-1.—Temperature Conversion, Fahrenheit/Centigrade*

°F	°C	°F	°C
97.0	36.1	102.0	38.9
97.5	36.4	102.2	39.0
98.0	36.7	102.4	39.1
98.2	36.8	102.6	39.2
98.4	36.9	102.8	39.3
98.6	37.0	103.0	39.4
98.8	37.1	103.2	39.6
99.0	37.2	103.4	39.7
99.2	37.3	103.6	39.8
99.4	37.4	103.8	39.9
99.6	37.6	104.0	40.0
99.8	37.7	104.2	40.1
100.0	37.8	104.4	40.2
100.2	37.9	104.6	40.3
100.4	38.0	104.8	40.4
100.6	38.1	105.0	40.6
100.8	38.2		
101.0	38.3		
101.2	38.4		
101.4	38.6		
101.6	38.7		
101.8	38.8		

*Fahrenheit to Centigrade: $5(°F - 32)/9 = °C$. Centigrade to Fahrenheit: $(°C \times 9)/5 + 32 = °F$.

TABLE A-2.—Conversion Factors for Length and Weight

Length: Inches to centimeters—inches $\times$ 2.54.
Weight: Calculation of lean body weight (LBW) in lb
        Females: LBW = 100 lb + 5 lb for each inch over 5 feet.
        Males: LBW = 110 lb + 6 lb for each inch over 5 feet.

TABLE A-3.—Equivalent Fat Content as a Percentage of Body Weight for the Sum of Four Skin Folds (Biceps, Triceps, Subscapular, Suprailiac)

SUM OF SKIN FOLDS (mm)	MALES (AGE, YR)				FEMALES (AGE, YR)			
	17-29	30-39	40-49	50+	16-29	30-39	40-49	50+
15	4.8	. . .	. . .	. . .	10.5	. . .	. . .	. . .
20	8.1	12.2	12.2	12.6	14.1	17.0	19.8	21.4
25	10.5	14.2	15.0	15.6	16.8	19.4	22.2	24.0
30	12.9	16.2	17.7	18.6	19.5	21.8	24.5	26.6
35	14.7	17.7	19.6	20.8	21.5	23.7	26.4	28.5
40	16.4	19.2	21.4	22.9	23.4	25.5	28.2	30.3
45	17.7	20.4	23.0	24.7	25.0	26.9	29.6	31.9
50	19.0	21.5	24.6	26.5	26.5	28.2	31.0	33.4
55	20.1	22.5	25.9	27.9	27.8	29.4	32.1	34.6
60	21.2	23.5	27.1	29.2	29.1	30.6	33.2	35.7
65	22.2	24.3	28.2	30.4	30.2	31.6	34.1	36.7
70	23.1	25.1	29.3	31.6	31.2	32.5	35.0	37.7
75	24.0	25.9	30.3	32.7	32.2	33.4	35.9	38.7
80	24.8	26.6	31.2	33.8	33.1	34.3	36.7	39.6
85	25.5	27.2	32.1	34.8	34.0	35.1	37.5	40.4
90	26.2	27.8	33.0	35.8	34.8	35.8	38.3	41.2
95	26.9	28.4	33.7	36.6	35.6	36.5	39.0	41.9
100	27.6	29.0	34.4	37.4	36.4	37.2	39.7	42.6
105	28.2	29.6	35.1	38.2	37.1	37.9	40.4	43.3
110	28.8	30.1	35.8	39.0	37.8	38.6	41.0	43.9
115	29.4	30.6	36.4	39.7	38.4	39.1	41.5	44.5
120	30.0	31.1	37.0	40.4	39.0	39.6	42.0	45.1
125	30.5	31.5	37.6	41.1	39.6	40.1	42.5	45.7
130	31.0	31.9	38.2	41.8	40.2	40.6	43.0	46.2
135	31.5	32.3	38.7	42.4	40.8	41.1	43.5	46.7
140	32.0	32.7	39.2	43.0	41.3	41.6	44.0	47.2
145	32.5	33.1	39.7	43.6	41.8	42.1	44.5	47.7
150	32.9	33.5	40.2	44.1	42.3	42.6	45.0	48.2
155	33.3	33.9	40.7	44.6	42.8	43.1	45.4	48.7
160	33.7	34.3	41.2	45.1	43.3	43.6	45.8	49.2
165	34.1	34.6	41.6	45.6	43.7	44.0	46.2	49.6
170	34.5	34.8	42.0	46.1	44.1	44.4	46.6	50.0
175	34.9	. . .	. . .	. . .	. . .	44.8	47.0	50.4
180	35.3	. . .	. . .	. . .	. . .	45.2	47.4	50.8
185	35.6	. . .	. . .	. . .	. . .	45.6	47.8	51.2
190	35.9	. . .	. . .	. . .	. . .	45.9	48.2	51.6
195	. . .	. . .	. . .	. . .	. . .	46.2	48.5	52.0
200	. . .	. . .	. . .	. . .	. . .	46.5	48.8	52.4
205	. . .	. . .	. . .	. . .	. . .	. . .	49.1	52.7
210	. . .	. . .	. . .	. . .	. . .	. . .	49.4	53.0

Modified from Durnin JVGA, Womersley J: *Br J Nutr* 32:77, 1974.

Men 25-59 Years

Height (feet/ inches)	Small Frame (pounds)*	Medium Frame (pounds)*	Large Frame (pounds)*
5' 2''	128-134	131-141	138-150
5' 3''	130-136	133-143	140-153
5' 4''	132-138	135-145	142-156
5' 5''	134-140	137-148	144-160
5' 6''	136-142	139-151	146-164
5' 7''	138-145	142-154	149-168
5' 8''	140-148	145-157	152-172
5' 9''	142-151	148-160	155-176
5'10''	144-154	151-163	158-180
5'11''	146-157	154-166	161-184
6' 0''	149-160	157-170	164-188
6' 1''	152-164	160-174	168-192
6' 2''	155-168	164-178	172-197
6' 3''	158-172	167-182	176-202
6' 4''	162-176	171-187	181-207

*in indoor clothing weighing 5 lbs, shoes with 1'' heels

Women 25-59 Years

Height (feet/ inches)	Small Frame (pounds)*	Medium Frame (pounds)*	Large Frame (pounds)*
4'10''	102-111	109-121	118-131
4'11''	103-113	111-123	120-134
5' 0''	104-115	113-126	122-137
5' 1''	106-118	115-129	125-140
5' 2''	108-121	118-132	128-143
5' 3''	111-124	121-135	131-147
5' 4''	114-127	124-138	134-151
5' 5''	117-130	127-141	137-155
5' 6''	120-133	130-144	140-159
5' 7''	123-136	133-147	143-163
5' 8''	126-139	136-150	146-167
5' 9''	129-142	139-153	149-170
5'10''	132-145	142-156	152-173
5'11''	135-148	145-159	155-176
6' 0''	138-151	148-162	158-179

*in indoor clothing weighing 3 lbs, shoes with 1'' heels

FIG A-1.
Height-weight correlations for adults.

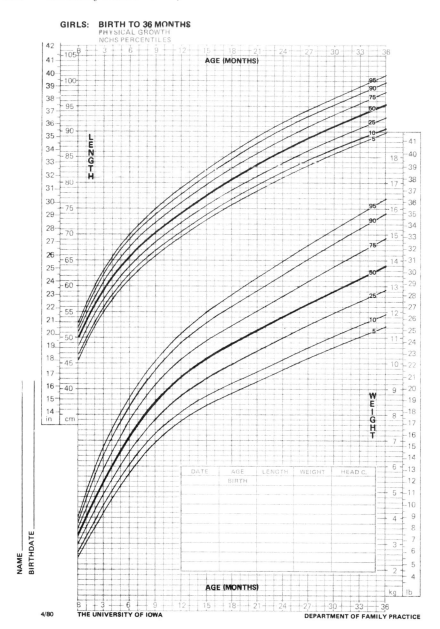

FIG A-2.

Length, weight, and age correlations for girls birth to 36 months of age.

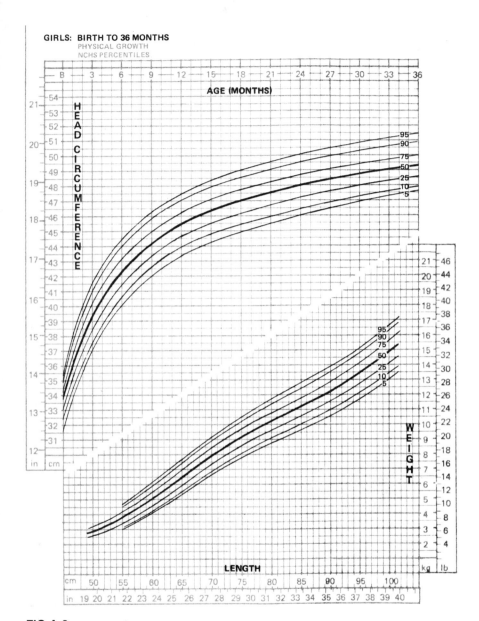

FIG A-3.
Length, weight, age, and head circumference correlations for girls birth to 36 months of age.

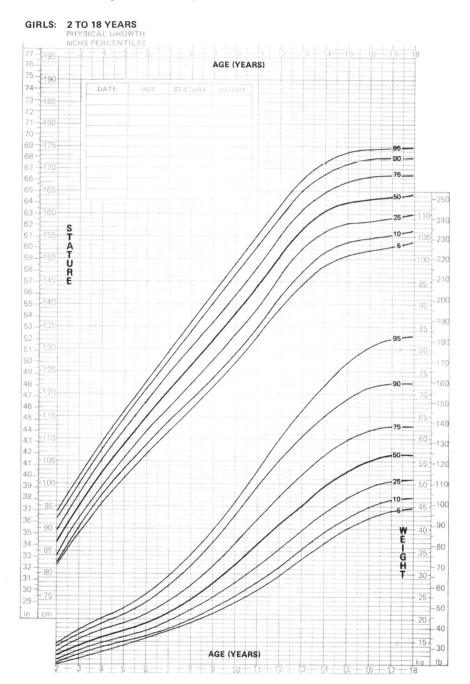

FIG A-4.
Growth profile for girls aged 2-18 years.

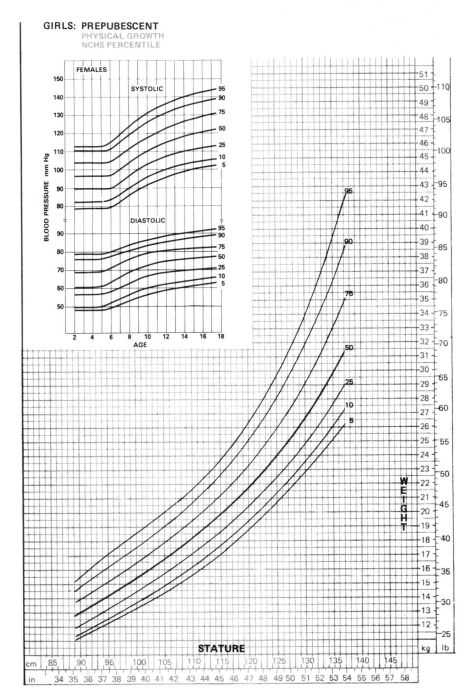

FIG A-5.
Prepubescent growth profiles for girls.

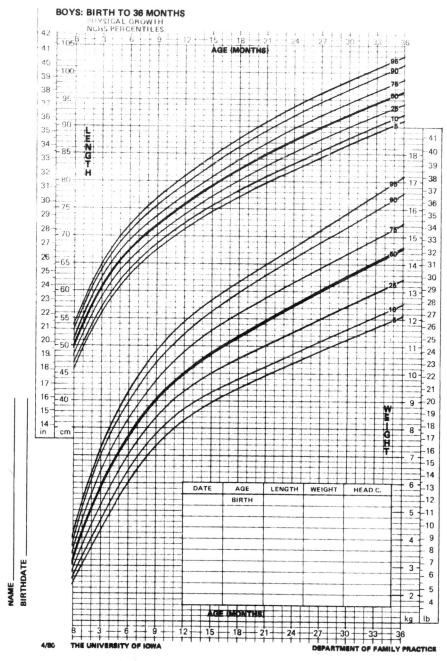

FIG A-6.
Length, weight, and age correlations for boys birth to 36 months of age.

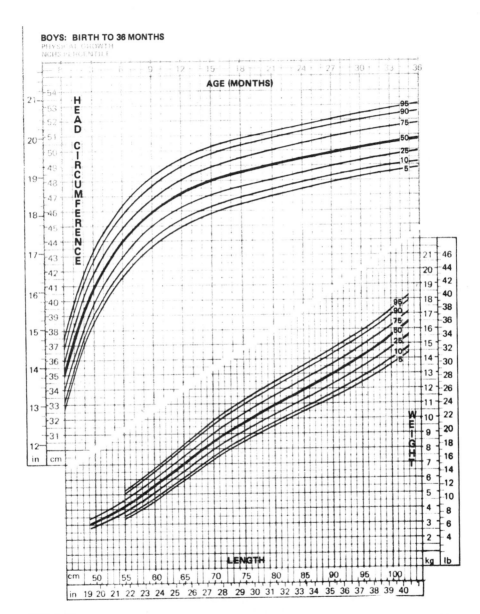

FIG A-7.

Length, weight, age, and head circumference correlations for boys birth to 36 months of age.

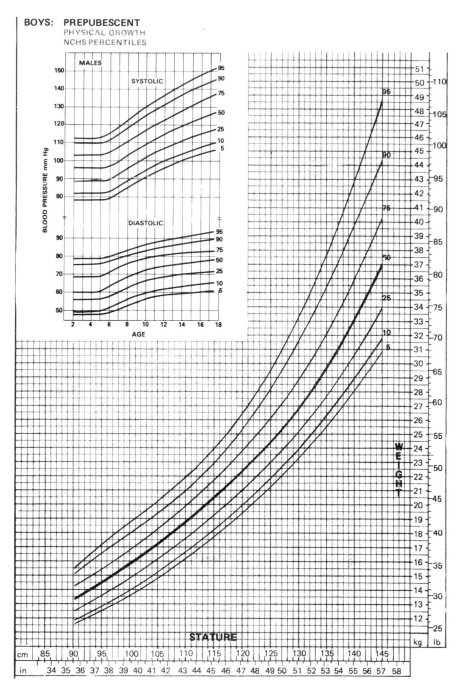

FIG A-8.
Prepubescent growth profiles for boys.

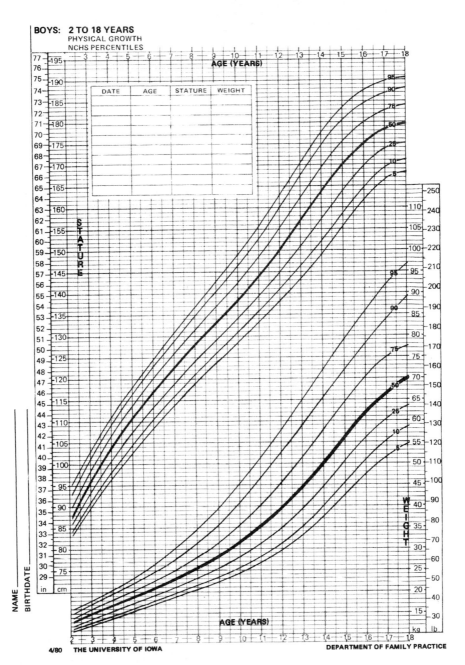

FIG A-9.
Growth profiles for boys aged 2-18 years.

TABLE A-4.—FLUID AND ELECTROLYTE MAINTENANCE THERAPY*

| | LOSSES | | | | REQUIREMENTS | |
	URINE (ml)	STOOL (ml)	INSENSIBLE (ml)	TOTAL (ml)	ML/PERSON	ML/KG
Infant (2-10 kg)	200-500	25-40	75-300 (1.3 ml/kg/hr)	300-840	330-1000	100-165
Child (10-40 kg)	500-800	40-100	300-600	840-1500	1000-1800	45-100
Adolescent or adult (60 kg)	800-1000	100	600-1000 (0.5 ml/kg/hr)	1500-2100	1800-2500	30-45

Modified from Trunkey D: Fluid and electrolyte therapy. In Schrock TR, ed: *Handbook of surgery*, ed. 15, Greenbrae, Calif., 1982, Jones Medical Publication, p. 92.

*Values are for a patient in a normal state of hydration. Daily water losses and water requirements are those for healthy persons not working or sweating.

TABLE A-5.—VOLUME AND COMPOSITION OF GASTROINTESTINAL SECRETIONS AND SWEAT

FLUID	AVG. VOLUME (ml/24 hr)	ELECTROLYTE CONCENTRATIONS (mEq/L)			
		Na^+	K^+	Cl^-	HCO_3^-
Blood plasma		135-150	3.6-5.5	100-105	24.6-28.8
Gastric juice	2500	31-90	4.3-12	52-124	0
Bile	700-1000	134-156	3.9-6.3	83-110	38
Pancreatic juice	>1000	113-153	2.6-7.4	54-95	110
Small bowel (Miller-Abbott suction)	3000	72-120	3.5-6.8	69-127	30
Ileostomy: Recent	100-4000	112-142	4.5-14	93-122	30
adapted	100-500	50	3	20	15-30
Cecostomy	100-3000	48-116	11.1-28.3	35-70	15
Feces	100	<10	<10	<15	<15
Sweat	500-4000	30-70	0-5	30-70	0

Modified from Trunkey D: Fluid and electrolyte therapy. In Schrock TR, ed: *Handbook of surgery,* ed. 15. Greenbrae, Calif, 1982, Jones Medical Publisher, p. 94.

TABLE A-6.—ACID-BASE BALANCE

Normal values:
CO_2	24-30 mM/L
Arterial pH	7.36-7.44
Arterial P_{CO_2}	35-45 mm Hg
Serum chloride	96-106 mEq/L
Arterial P_{O_2}	90-100 mm Hg

Anion gap = (serum Na^+ + serum K^+) − (serum Cl^- + serum HCO_3^-)
  Normal anion gap = 13-17 mEq/L
Bicarbonate deficit − Bicarbonate dose (mEq) = 0.5 × Weight (kg) × Desired increase in serum HCO_3^- (mEq/L) *Or*
  (25 − Observed bicarbonate) × 0.5 (Weight in kg) = Total deficit

TABLE A-7.—COMMON CAUSES OF HYPERCHLOREMIC METABOLIC ACIDOSIS*

Excess Acid Load
Hyperalimentation
Acidifying agents (ammonium chloride, arginine HCl, lysine HCl)
Chloride exchange resin-cholestyramine

Losses of Alkaline Fluids
Diarrhea
Ileostomy
Colostomy
Pancreatic fistula

Decreased Renal Acid Excretion
Renal tubular acidosis
Acetazolamide (Diamox)
Uremia
Hypoaldosteronism

*Associated with a normal anion gap.

TABLE A-8.—COMMON CAUSES OF ACID-BASE DISORDERS

ACIDOSIS	ALKALOSIS
Metabolic	
Renal failure	Nasogastric suction
Renal tubular acidosis	Vomiting
Diabetic ketoacidosis	Diarrhea
Alcoholic ketoacidosis	Diuretics
Starvation ketosis	Glucocorticosteroids
Lactic acidosis	Cushing's disease
Uremic acidosis	Chloride restriction
Drugs (salicylates, ethylene glycol, methanol, par-	Alkali therapy
aldehyde)	Antacid use
Respiratory	
CNS depression	Hyperventilation
Obstructive lung disease	Sepsis
Mechanical hypoventilation	Salicylate intoxication
Status asthmaticus	Mechanical overventilation
Pneumothorax	Pneumonia
Abdominal distention	High altitude

TABLE A-9.—Sodium and Calorie Content of Foods*

FOOD	QUANTITY	mg	mEq	kcal
Snacks				
Salted peanuts	1 tbsp	69	3	95
Unsalted peanuts	1 tbsp	trace	. . .	95
Green olives	2 olives	312	13.6	15
Black olives	2 olives	150	6.5	35
Potato chips	5 chips	34	1.5	60
Pretzels (ring)	1	87	3.8	25
Dairy Products				
Butter, salted	1 pat	99	4.3	45
Butter, unsalted	1 pat	1	. . .	45
American cheese	1 oz	318	13.8	110
Cottage cheese	3 oz	229	10.0	90
Egg	1 large	66	2.9	80
Milk (whole)	8 oz	122	5.3	160
Margarine (salted)	1 pat	99	4.3	45
Vegetables				
Green beans	1 cup			
Fresh		5	0.2	40
Canned		295	12.8	40
Beets	½ cup			
Fresh		36	1.6	55
Canned		197	8.6	55
Broccoli, fresh	⅔ cup	10	0.4	25
Cabbage, raw	1 cup	20	0.9	17
Carrots				
Raw	1 large	47	2.0	40
Canned	⅔ cup	236	10.3	30
Celery	1 outer stalk	63	2.7	7
Corn				
Fresh	1 ear	trace	. . .	70
Canned	½ cup	196	8.5	70
Peas				
Fresh	⅔ cup	1	. . .	75
Canned	¾ cup	236	10.3	90
Frozen	3½ oz	115	5.0	. . .
Potatoes, boiled	1 medium	3	. . .	65
Sauerkraut	⅔ cup	747	32.5	20
Tomatoes				
Raw	1 medium	4	. . .	27
Canned	½ cup	130	5.7	25

*Sodium restrictions: 2 g salt (NaCl) = 800 mg sodium = 34 mEq Na^+.

Continued.

TABLE A-9.—Sodium and Calorie Content of Foods—cont'd

FOOD	QUANTITY	mg	mEq	kcal
Meats				
Bacon	1 strip	71	3.1	45
Hamburger	¼ lb	41	1.8	325
Chicken (broiler)	3½ oz	78	3.4	180
Frankfurter (beef)	⅛ lb	550	23.9	130
Ham, cured	¼ lb	518	22.5	325
Pork chop	6 oz	52	2.3	600
Sausage	3½ oz	740	32.2	325
Salmon canned (water)	3½ oz	387	16.8	130
Sardines canned (oil)	3½ oz	510	22.2	200
Tuna canned (oil)	3½ oz	800	34.8	180
Tuna canned (water)	3½ oz	41	1.8	90
Other				
Bread, white	1 slice	117	5.1	60
Corn flakes	1 cup	165	7.2	110
Noodles, rice		3	. . .	. . .
Fruit juices	6-8 oz	2-4	. . .	. . .
Fresh fruits	3½ oz	1-5	. . .	. . .

TABLE A-10.—Potassium Content of Foods

FOOD	QUANTITY	mg	mEq	kcal
Meats				
Hamburger	3 oz	290	7.4	245
Beef round	3 oz	340	8.7	245
Chicken (fryer)	4 oz	710	18.2	180
Turkey	4 oz	350	9.0	180
Fruits, vegetables				
Banana	1 medium	628	16.1	100
Brussel sprouts	1 cup	300	7.7	56
Cauliflower raw	1¼ cup	500	12.8	30
Dates	1 cup	1,390	35.6	
Fruit cocktail, canned (syrup)	8 oz	410	10.5	170
Grapefruit	1 cup	380	9.7	40
Peach	1 medium	180	4.6	40
Raisins	2 tbsp	144	3.7	60
Spinach	1 cup	600	15.4	40
Sweet corn	1 cup	230	5.9	150
Tomato	1 medium	340	8.7	27
Watermelon	½ slice of ¾ in × 10 in	380	9.7	100
Wheat germ	100 g	737	18.9	
Beverages (8 oz)				
Apricot juice		250	9.5	
Coffee, instant	2 g	238	6.1	. . .
Grapefruit juice, canned		405	10.4	78
Milk, whole (high sodium)		356	9.1	160
Milk, nonfat (high sodium)		278	7.1	90
Orange juice, fresh		496	12.1	120
Prune juice, canned		563	14.4	184
Tea		66	1.7	. . .
Tomato juice, canned (high sodium)		544	14.0	48

TABLE A-11.—Normal Hematology SI Units Values

	NORMAL RANGE	NORMAL RANGE	FACTOR FOR CONVERSION TO SI UNITS
Hematology (Adults)			
Carboxyhemoglobin	<5% of total	0.05 of total	0.01
Erythrocytes			
Men	$4.6\text{-}6.2 \times 10^6/mm^3$	$4.6\text{-}6.2 \times 10^{12}/L$	1
Women	$4.2\text{-}5.4 \times 10^6/mm^3$	$4.2\text{-}5.4 \times 10^{12}/L$	1
Children (depends on age)	$4.5\text{-}5.1 \times 10^6/mm^3$	$4.5\text{-}5.1 \times 10^{12}/L$	1
Leukocytes, total	$4.3\text{-}11.0 \times 10^3/mm^3$	$4.3\text{-}11.0 \times 10^9/L$	1
Band neutrophils	0	0.0-0.05	0.01
Segmented neutrophils	54%-62%	0.54-0.62	
Lymphocytes	25%-33%	0.25-0.33	
Monocytes	3%-7%	0.03-0.07	
Eosinophils	1%-3%	$50\text{-}250/mm^3$	0.01-0.03
Basophils	<1%	0.0-0.01	
Platelets	$150\text{-}350 \times 10^3/mm^3$	$150\text{-}350 \times 10^9/L$	1
Reticulocytes	0.5%-2.5% of erythrocytes	0.005-0.025	0.01
MCH	27-31 pg	27-31 pg	
MCV	$80\text{-}96 \ mm^3$	80-96 fl	
MCHC	32-36 g/dl	320-360 g/L	10
Hematocrit			
Males	40%-54%	0.4-0.54	0.01
Females	37%-47%	0.37-0.47	0.01
Hemoglobin			
Males	14-18 g/dl	8.6-11.2 mmol/L	0.6206
Females	12-16 g/dl	7.4-9.9 mmol/L	0.6206
Hemoglobin, A_{1C}	3.5%-6.0%	0.035-0.06	0.01

Modified from Jordan CD, Flood JG, LaPosata M, Lewandrowsk: KB: Normal reference values, *N Engl J Med* 327:718, 1992.

TABLE A-11.—Normal Hematology SI Units Values—cont'd

	NORMAL RANGE	NORMAL RANGE	FACTOR FOR CONVERSION TO SI UNITS
Sedimentation Rate (Wintrobe)			
Males	0-5 mm/hr		
Females	0-15 mm/hr		
Sedimentation Rate (Westergren)			
Males	0-15 mm/hr		
Females	0-20 mm/hr		
Bone Marrow Differential			
Myeloblasts	0.3%-5.0%		
Promyelocytes	1.0%-8.0%		
Myelocytes			
Neutrophilic	5.0%-19.0%		
Eosinophilic	0.5%-3.0%		
Basophilic	0-0.5%		
Metamyelocytes	13.0%-32.0%		
Polymorphonuclear neutrophils	7.0%-30.0%		
Polymorphonuclear eosinophils	0.5%-4.0%		
Polymorphonuclear basophils	0-0.7%		
Lymphocytes	3.0%-17.0%		
Plasma cells	0.0%-2.0%		
Monocytes	0.5%-5.0%		
Reticulum cells	0.1%-2.0%		
Megakaryocytes	0.3%-3.0%		
Pronormoblasts	1.0%-8.0%		
Normoblasts	7.0%-32.0%		

TABLE A-12.—NORMAL HEMATOLOGY VALUES FOR CHILDREN

AGE	HEMOGLOBIN (g/dl)			RBC COUNT (10⁶/mm³)	HEMATOCRIT (PACKED RBC volume/dl) (%)	MEAN CORPUSCULAR VOLUME (MCV) (μm^3)	MEAN CORPUSCULAR HEMOGLOBIN (MCH) (pg)	MEAN CORPUSCULAR HEMOGLOBIN CONCENTRATION (MCHC) (g/dl)
	TERM BABIES	PREMATURE BABIES (1200-2400 g)	SMALL PREMATURE BABIES (<1200 g)					
Birth (cord values)	13.6-19.6	17.0	15.6	5.4	56.6	106	38	38
1 day	21.2			5.6	56.1	106	38	38
1 week	19.6	15.3	14.8	5.3	52.7	101	37	37
2 weeks	18.0			5.1	49.6	96	35	36
3 weeks	16.6	13.2	12.0	4.9	46.6	93	34	36
4 weeks	15.6	9.6	8.2	4.7	44.6	91	33	35
2 months	13.3			4.5	38.9	85	30	34
3 months	12.5	9.8	8.1	4.5	38.0	84	29	34
4 months	12.4	9.8	9.0	4.5	36.5	79	27	34
6 months	12.3			4.6	36.2	78	27	34
8 months	12.1			4.6	35.8	77	26	34
10 months	11.9			4.6	35.5	77	26	34
1 year	11.6	11.0	11.0	4.6	35.2	77	25	33
2 years	11.7			4.7	35.5	78	25	33
4 years	12.6			4.7	37.1	80	27	34
6 years	12.7			4.7	37.9	80	27	33
8 years	12.9			4.7	38.9	80	27	33
10-12 years	13.0			4.8	39.0	80	27	33
Adult men	16.0			5.4	47.0	87	29	34
Adult women	14.0			4.8	42.0	87	29	34

From Lanzkowsky P, et al, eds: *Primary pediatric care*, St. Louis, 1987, Mosby, p. 860.

TABLE A-13.—Normal Blood and Serum Chemistries

ANALYTE	REFERENCE INTERVAL
Acid phosphatase, serum	0.5-1.9 IU/L* 37° C
Alanine aminotransferase, serum (ALT, SGPT)	5-45 IU/L* 37° C
Albumin, serum	
0-1 yr	29-55 g/L
1-31 yr	35-50 g/L
after 40 yr	declines
Alkaline phosphatase, serum	35-105 IU/L* 37° C
Alpha$_1$antitrypsin, serum neonates have much lower values	0.78-2.0 g/L
Ammonia, plasma	
child 1-5 yr	10-40 umol/L
5-19 yr	11-35 umol/L
adult male	11-35 umol/L
adult female	11-35 umol/L
Amylase, serum	25-115 IU/L* 37° C
Anion gap, serum	5-14 mmol/L
Anticonvulsant drugs, serum	
Carbamazepine, serum	4-12 mcg/mL
Ethosuximide, serum	40-100 mcg/mL
Phenobarbital, serum	15-40 mcg/mL
Phenytoin, serum	10-20 mcg/mL
Primidone, serum	5-12 mcg/mL
Valproic acid, serum	50-120 mcg/mL
Aspartate aminotransferase, serum (AST, SGOT)	15-45 IU/L* 37° C
Bilirubin, total, serum	
0-1 month	1-12 mg/dL
1 mo to adult	0-1.2 mg/dL
Bilirubin, conjugated, serum (direct)	0-0.2 mg/dL
Blood gases, whole blood	
arterial pH	7.35-7.45
pCO$_2$	35-45 mm Hg
pO$_2$	80-100 mm Hg
HCO$_3^-$	22-26 mmol/L
total CO$_2$	23-27 mmol/L
O$_2$ saturation	94-100%
venous pH	7.33-7.43
pCO$_2$	38-50 mm Hg
pO$_2$	30-50 mm Hg
HCO$_3^-$	23-27 mmol/L
total CO$_2$	24-28 mmol/L
O$_2$ saturation	60-85%
Calcium, ionized, plasma	1.14-1.29 mmol/L
Calcium, total, serum	
children	2.2-2.7 mmol/L
adults	2.1-2.55 mmol/L

Modified from Tilton et al: *Clinical laboratory medicine,* St. Louis, 1992, Mosby.
*Enzyme values are method dependent.

Continued.

TABLE A-13.—Normal Blood and Serum Chemistries—cont'd

ANALYTE	REFERENCE INTERVAL
Carbon monoxide, whole blood, (carboxyhemo-globin)	
nonsmoker	<2%
smoker	<8%
Carcinoembryonic antigens, serum (CEA)	
nonsmoker	<2.5 mcg/mL
smoker	<5 mcg/mL
Ceruloplasmin, serum	0.15-0.6 g/L
Chloride, serum	101-111 mmol/L
urine	110-150 mmol/L
sweat	<35 mmol/L
Cholesterol, serum	
desirable	<200 mg/dL
borderline	200-239 mg/dL
high	>=240 mg/dL
Cholinesterase (pseudo), serum	1800-4800 mIU/mL
Cortisol, plasma am	50-230 mcg/L
urine free (extracted)	4.9-35.3 mcg/24 hr
urine (unextracted)	46-131 mcg/24 hr
Creatine kinase, serum (CK)	25-250 IU/L* 37° C
Creatine kinase isoenzymes, serum	
CK (MM)	>95%
CK (MB)	<5%
CK (BB)	about 0%
Creatinine, plasma	
infant 0-1 yr	2-10 mg/L
child 1-5 yr	2-10 mg/L
5-19 yr	4-13 mg/L
adult male	5-12 mg/L
adult female	4-10 mg/L
Creatinine, urine	
male	1.0-2.0 gm/24 hr
female	0.8-1.8 gm/24 hr
Epinephrine, plasma	25-50 pg/mL
Epinephrine, free, urine	0.5-25 mcg/24 hr
Estrogen receptor, breast tissue	>10 fmol/mg
Ferritin, serum	20-200 ng/mL
Folate, serum	<3.0 mcg/L
Follicular stimulating hormone, serum (FSH)	
Prepubertal, male & female	<9 mIU/mL
adult, male	<20 mIU/mL
adult, female	
follicular	<17 mIU/mL
mid-cycle	20-30 mIU/mL
post menopausal	30-150 mIU/mL

TABLE A-13.—Normal Blood and Serum Chemistries—cont'd

ANALYTE	REFERENCE INTERVAL
Follicular stimulating hormone, urine (FSH)	
male to age 8 yr	<5 mIU/mL
male greater 8 yr	<22 mIU/mL
female to age 8 yr	<5 mIU/mL
female age 9 to 15 yr	<22 mIU/mL
female greater 15 yr	<30 mIU/mL
FTI Free thyroxine index	1.2-3.2
Gamma glutamyltransferase, serum	15-70 IU/L* 37° C
Gastrin, serum	30-100 pg/mL
Glucose, serum	70-110 mg/dL
Glycohemoglobin, whole blood	6-8%
Growth hormone, plasma, males	0-5 ng/mL
females	0-10 ng/mL
Haptoglobulin, serum	0.4-1.8 g/L
HDL-Cholesterol, serum	
desirable	>65 mg/dL
borderline	35-65 mg/dL
at risk	<35 mg/dL
Human chorionic gonadotropin, serum (beta-hCG) males and nonpregnant	
premenopausal females	<5 IU/L
postmenopausal females	<7 IU/L
pregnant females	>20 IU/L
rising to in first trimester	>100,000 IU/L
IgA, serum	0.7-3.2 g/L
IgD, serum	0.015-0.2 g/L
IgE, serum	6×10^{-4} g/L
IgG, serum	8.0-12 g/L
IgM, serum	0.5-2.8 g/L
Insulin, serum	<1042 pg/mL
Iron, serum	
males	500-1600 mcg/L
females	400-1500 mcg/L
Iron binding capacity, total serum	2500-4000 mcg/L
Iron saturation, serum	20-55%
Lactic dehydrogenase, serum (P->L)	90-320 IU/L* 37° C
Lactic dehydrogenase isoenzymes	
LD 1	18-33%
LD 2	28-40%
LD 3	18-30%
LD 4	6-16%
LD 5	2-13%
Lead, whole blood	0-200 mcg/L
chronic exposure	200-700 mcg/L
acute exposure	>700 mcg/L

Continued.

TABLE A-13.—NORMAL BLOOD AND SERUM CHEMISTRIES—cont'd

ANALYTE	REFERENCE INTERVAL
LDL-Cholesterol, serum	
desirable	<130 mg/dL
borderline	130-159 mg/dL
high	>=160 mg/dL
Lipase, serum	4-24 U/dL
Luteinizing hormone, serum	
Prepubertal, male & female	<15 mIU/mL
adult, male	<26 mIU/mL
adult, female	
follicular	<33 mIU/mL
mid-cycle	30-200 mIU/mL
post menopausal	30-130 mIU/mL
Luteinizing hormone, urine	
Prepubertial	<7 mIU/mL
Childhood	<40 mIU/mL
Adult	<45 mIU/mL
Magnesium, plasma	0.6-1.1 mmol/L
Norepinephrine, plasma	100-400 pg/mL
Norepinephrine, free, urine	10-70 mcg/24 hr
Osmolality, serum	282-300 mOsm/kg
Osmolality, urine	50-1200 mOsm/kg
Parathyroid hormone, plasma	0-97 pg/mL
Phosphorus, serum	1.45-2.76 meq/L
Porphyrin, blood	500-600 mcg/L
urine	<200 mcg/L
feces	<60 mg/dry gram stool
Potassium, serum	3.6-5.0 mmol/L
Progesterone, serum	
male prepubertal	0.11-0.26 ng/mL
male adult	0-0.4 ng/mL
female prepubertal	0.10-0.34 ng/mL
female adult follicular	0.10-1.5 ng/mL
luteal	2.5-28 ng/mL
pregnant	9-255 ng/mL
postmenopausal	0.03-0.3 ng/mL
ectopic pregnancy	<13-13.5 ng/mL
normal pregnancy	>15-20 ng/mL
Progesterone receptor, breast tissue	>10 fmol/mg
Prolactin, serum, males	6-15 ng/mL
females	8-25 ng/mL
Prostate specific antigen, serum (PSA)	<4 mcg/mL
Protein, total, serum	6.6-6.8 g/dL
urine	40-150 mg/dL
cerebrospinal fluid	15-45 mg/dL

TABLE A-13.—Normal Blood and Serum Chemistries—cont'd

ANALYTE	REFERENCE INTERVAL
Seminal fluid analysis	
volume	2.0 or more
pH	7.2-7.8
sperm concentration	20×10^6 sperm/mL or more
total sperm	40×10^6 spermatozoa
motility	50% with forward progression
morphology	50% with normal morphology
viability	50% or more live
WBC	$<1 \times 10^6$/mL
Zinc	2.4 mcmol or more/ejaculate
Citrate	52 mcmol or more/ejaculate
Fructose	13 mcmol or more/ejaculate
MAR	Fewer than 10% spermatozoa with adherent particles
Immunobead test	Fewer than 10% spermatozoa with adherent beads
Sodium, serum	135-145 mmol/L
urine	40-220 mmol/L
T3-Uptake, serum	25-35%
Testosterone, total, serum	
males	270-1070 ng/dL
females	6-86 ng/dL
urine	
males	25-125 ng/dL
females	5-35 ng/dL
Thyroid stimulating hormone, serum	2 mcU/mL (mean)
Thyroxine, free, serum	2.2 ng/dL (mean)
Thyroxine, total, serum (T4)	8 mcg/dL (mean)
cord blood	6.6-18.1 mcg/dL
2-5 days	8.5-22.0 mcg/dL
3-12 months	7.6-16.0 mcg/dL
1-5 yr	7.3-15.0 mcg/dL
6-10 yr	6.4-13.3 mcg/dL
11-16 yr	5.6-11.7 mcg/dL
>16 yr	4.5-11.5 mcg/dL
Transferrin, serum	2.52-4.29 g/L
Triglycerides, serum	
1-29 yr	<140 mg/dL
30-39 yr	<150 mg/dL
40-49 yr	<160 mg/dL
50-59 yr	<170 mg/dL
>60 yr	<200 mg/dL
Triiodothyronir e, free, serum (T3)	0.4 ng/dL (mean)
Triiodothyronine, reverse, serum (rT3)	25 ng/dL (mean)

Continued.

TABLE A-13.—NORMAL BLOOD AND SERUM CHEMISTRIES—cont'd

ANALYTE	REFERENCE INTERVAL
Triiodothyronine, total, serum (T3)	130 ng/dL (mean)
cord blood	24-77 ng/dL
2-5 days	99-227 ng/dL
3-12 months	96-219 ng/dL
1-5 yr	92-215 ng/dL
6-10 yr	84-194 ng/dL
11-16 yr	75-172 ng/dL
>16 yr	94-168 ng/dL
Urea-nitrogen, serum	
infant, 0-1 yr	60-450 mg/L
child, 1-5 yr	50-170 mg/L
5-19 yr	80-200 mg/L
adult male	100-210 mg/L
adult female	100-210 mg/L
Uric acid, serum	
infant, 0-1 yr	10-76 mg/L
child, 1-5 yr	18-50 mg/L
5-19 yr	30-60 mg/L
adult male	40-90 mg/L
adult female	30-60 mg/L
Urine protein, total	40-150 mg/24 hr
Vanillylmandelic acid, urine (VMA)	2-7 mg/24 hr
Vitamin B_{12}, true-serum	<100 ng/L
Vitamin D, plasma	20-76 ng/L
Zinc, serum	700-1500 mcg/L
urine	0.15-1.0 mg/24 hr
hair	100-280 mcg/g

TABLE A-14.—Amniotic Fluid

Amniotic fluid		
Amniotic fluid analysis absorbance at 450 mm bilirubin	28 weeks	0.0-0.048 A
	40 weeks	0.0-0.020 A
	28 weeks	0.0-0.075 mg/dl
	40 weeks	0.0-0.025 mg/dl
Creatinine		>2.0 mg/dl generally indicates fetal maturity when maternal serum creatinine is normal
Lecithin/spingomyelin (L/S) ratio		2.0-5.0 indicates probable fetal lung maturity
Lecithin phosphorus		>0.10 mg/dl indicates probable adequate fetal lung maturity
Osmolality	28 weeks	255-275 mOsm/kg
	40 weeks	241-264 mOsm/kg
pH		6.96-7.20
Sodium	28 weeks	124-148 mmol/L
	40 weeks	115-139 mmol/L
Volume	10 weeks	Approximately 25 ml
	40 weeks	300-1700

Lumbar CSF
  Albumin/globulin ratio   16.2-2.2
  Albumin, quantitative   10-30 mg/dl
  Calcium   4.2-5.4 mg/dl
  Cell count   WBCs/mm^3

	POLYMORPHONUCLEAR	MONONUCLEAR	RBCs/mm^3
Premature	0-100*	0-25*	0-1000
Newborn	0-70*	0-20*	0-800*
Neonate, early	0-25	0-5	0-50
Neonate, late	0-5	0-5	0-10
Thereafter	0	0-5	0-5

Chloride	Newborn	108-122 mmol/L
	Thereafter	118-132 mmol/L
Cholinesterase		13-21 mU/ml
Glucose (40%-60% of	Newborn	30-80 mg/dl
blood or serum glucose	Infant/child	60-80 mg/dl
level)		
	Thereafter	40-70 mg/dl
Immunoglobulins		IgG: 0.8-6.4 mg/dl
		IgA: 0.4-0.6 mg/dl
		IgM: Negative
Lactate		0.1-1.0 mmol/L
Lactate dehydrogenase (LDH)	Newborn	2.3-8.4 U/L
(1 → p; 30° C)	Child	0.0-20.0 U/L
	Adult	6.3-30.0 U/L
Magnesium		2.2-3.0 mmol/L
Pándy's test		Negative
pH (37° C)		7.33-7.42
Potassium		2.8-4.1 mmol/L
Protein, total	Premature	40-300† mg/dl
	Newborn	45-100
	Child	10-20
	Adolescent	15-30
	Thereafter	15-45 (turbidimetric method)
		8-32 (column method)
Protein electrophoresis		Prealbumin, 2.9%-5.3%
		Albumin, 56.8%-68.0%
		α_1-globulin, 4.1%-6.4%
		α_2-globulin, 6.2%-10.2%
		β-globulin, 10.8%-14.8%
		γ-globulin, 6.1%-8.3%
Sodium		138-150 mmol/L
Specific gravity		1.007-1.009
Transaminases:		
Aspartate aminotransferase		2-10 U/L
(SGOT, AST; 30° C)		
Alanine aminotransferase		None detected
(SGPT, ALT; 30° C)		
Xanthochromia*		Absent

*Number of cells greater than observed in older infants' CSF occurs in many newly born infants who grow and develop normally.

†Values greater than 100 mg/dl are seen in many prematurely born infants who grow and develop normally.

TABLE A-16.—URINE NORMAL VALUES

Acidity, titratable	20-40 mEq/24 hr
Ammonia	30-50 mEq/24 hr
Amylase	35-260 Somogyi units/hr
Bence Jones protein	None detected
Bilirubin	None detected
Calcium	
Unrestricted diet	<300 mg/24 hr (men)
	<250 mg/24 hr (women)
Low-calcium diet	<150 mg/24 hr
(200 mg/day for 3 days)	
Chloride	120-240 mEq/24 hr (varies with dietary intake)
Copper	0-32 μg/24 hr
Creatine	
Male	0-40 mg/24 hr
Female	0-100 mg/24 hr
Creatinine	1.0-1.6 g/24 hr or 15-25 mg/kg body weight/24 hr
Cysteine, qualitative	Negative
Glucose	
Qualitative	None detected
Quantitative	16-300 mg/24 hr
Hemoglobin	None detected
Iron	40-140 μg/24 hr
Lead	0-120 μg/24 hr
Osmolality	50-1200 mOsm/L
pH	4.6-8.0
Phosphorus	0.8-2.0 g/24 hr
Porphobilinogen	
Qualitative	None detected
Quantitative	0-2.4 mg/24 hr
Porphyrins	
Coproporphyrin	50-250 μg/24 hr
Uroporphyrin	10-30 μg/24 hr
Potassium	25-100 mEq/24 hr
Protein	
Qualitative	None detected
Quantitative	10-150 mg/24 hr
Sodium	130-260 mEq/24 hr (varies with dietary sodium intake)
Specific gravity	1.003-1.030
Uric acid	80-976 mg/24 hr
Urobilinogen	0.05-3.5 mg/24 hr <1.0 Ehrlich units/2 hr

Modified from: Stein JH, ed: *Internal medicine,* ed 4, 1994, Mosby.

Index